Second Edition

Focus on
PHARMACOLOGY

ESSENTIALS FOR HEALTH PROFESSIONALS

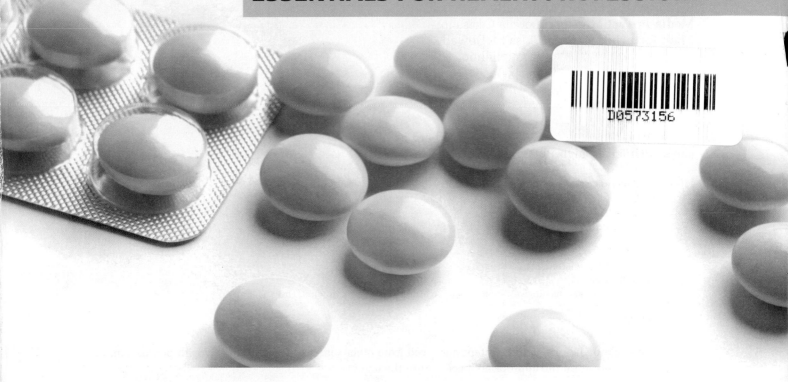

D0573156

Jahangir **Moini**, MD, MPH

Professor, Everest University, Melbourne, Florida

PEARSON

Boston   Columbus   Indianapolis   New York   San Francisco   Upper Saddle River
Amsterdam   Cape Town   Dubai   London   Madrid   Milan   Munich   Paris   Montréal   Toronto
Delhi   Mexico City   São Paulo   Sydney   Hong Kong   Seoul   Singapore   Taipei   Tokyo

Publisher: Julie Levin Alexander
Publisher's Assistant: Regina Bruno
Editor-in-Chief: Mark Cohen
Executive Editor: Joan Gill
Associate Editor: Melissa Kerian
Developmental Editor: Alexis Breen Ferraro, iD8-TripleSSS Media Development, LLC
Editorial Assistant: Mary Ellen Ruitenberg
Director of Marketing: David Gesell
Marketing Manager: Katrin Beacom
Marketing Specialist: Michael Sirinides
Managing Production Editor: Patrick Walsh
Production Liaison: Julie Boddorf
Senior Media Editor: Amy Peltier
Media Project Manager: Lorena Cerisano
Manufacturing Manager: Lisa McDowell
Senior Art Director: Maria Guglielmo
Interior Designer: Wanda España
Cover Designer: Wanda España
Cover Photo: Shutterstock
Composition: PreMediaGlobal
Printing and Binding: R.R. Donnelley/Willard
Cover Printer: Lehigh-Phoenix Color/Hagerstown

Library of Congress Cataloging-in-Publication Data

Moini, Jahangir, (Date)
  Focus on pharmacology: essentials for health professionals / Jahangir Moini.—2nd ed.
    p.; cm.
  Includes index.
  ISBN-13: 978-0-13-249966-8
  ISBN-10: 0-13-249966-5
  I. Title. [DNLM: 1. Pharmacological Phenomena. 2. Allied Health Personnel. 3. Drug Therapy.
  4. Pharmacokinetics.   QV 4]
  615'.1—dc23   2011041618

Credits and acknowledgments for content borrowed from other sources and reproduced, with permission, in this textbook appear on the appropriate page within the text.

10 9 8 7 6 5 4 3 2

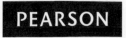

ISBN 13: 978-0-13-249966-8
ISBN 10:   0-13-249966-5

Dedication

This book is dedicated to my granddaughter, Laila Jade Mabry.

Brief Contents

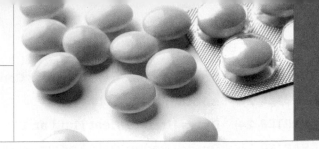

Preface

This second edition of *Focus on Pharmacology: Essentials for Health Professionals* has been updated with the latest drug information available. It is accompanied by a new student workbook, which contains many different types of review questions, including multiple-choice, fill-in-the-blank, true/false, and critical thinking questions.

Pharmacology is often a challenging subject for allied health students. To the rescue comes this text, which is uniquely designed to use a *focused* approach to learning pharmacology. Introductory chapters lay the groundwork for learning this subject by explaining the history of pharmacology, discussing the legal and ethical principles involved, illustrating drug administration techniques, reviewing math, explaining drug calculations, and discussing medication errors and their prevention. Additionally, substance abuse is focused on in detail. The chapters that follow focus on drugs specific to body systems, pharmacotherapy of certain age groups (pediatrics and geriatrics), pharmacology for pregnant women, and broad drug categories, such as antibiotics.

New to This Edition

The following changes and additions have been made to this second edition of *Focus on Pharmacology: Essentials for Health Professionals*:

* Chapter 2 has been revised and updated to include all federal laws that have been adopted since the first edition.

* Chapter 8 is a new chapter focusing on medication errors and prevention.

* Chapter 9 discusses the nutritional aspects of pharmacology and has been expanded to include information about herbal substances.

* Chapter 11 is a new chapter focusing on substance abuse.

* Chapter 14 has been revised to include information about immune globulins.

* Chapter 33 is a new chapter focusing on drugs used to treat pregnant patients.

* For each chapter, the author has added an additional Practical Scenario so there are now two of these per chapter; all scenarios include Critical Thinking questions with answers.

* The Apply Your Knowledge sections in the chapters now contain Critical Thinking questions with answers.

* A student workbook has been added to this edition, containing a variety of such exercises as multiple-choice, fill-in-the-blank, true/false, and critical thinking questions.

* The PowerPoints, *Instructor's Manual*, Test Bank, and companion website have been revised to contain all the related changes to the chapters.

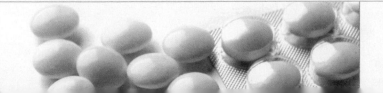

MyHealthProfessionsKit is an online study guide. It provides an array of games and assessment quizzes that have been developed within an automatic grading system. This provides users with instant scoring after users submit their answers. Each student's results can be e-mailed directly to the educator or automatically imported into Grade Tracker.

Go to www.myhealthprofessionskit.com and then select Basic Health Science. Find this book and then register for a username and password.

Structured Presentation of Pharmacologic Principles

Each drug chapter focuses on drugs used to treat a certain body system and its associated disorders. The chapters open with a concise review of anatomy and physiology, providing a foundation for understanding the actions, effects, and uses of each drug. These pharmacologic principles are succinctly explained by using clearly identifiable headings in question format that help focus students' attention on the most important points about a drug class or an individual drug:

* How do they work?
* How are they used?
* What are the adverse effects?
* What are the contraindications and interactions?
* What are the most important points patients should know?

Sometimes, these question headings focus on a class of drugs (for example, beta-adrenergic blockers). Other times, the question headings focus on a *prototype* (representative) drug—that is, the drug that was either the first developed in the class or is the most widely used drug in its class. Whichever approach is taken in the chapter, the five-question headings are used so students can easily focus on the key need-to-know drug information.

Focus On

Aminoglycosides

Aminoglycosides have been very important antibiotics for the treatment of infections caused by gram-negative bacilli. They are **broad-spectrum** antibiotics (effective against a wide range of organisms). The clinically important aminoglycosides are amikacin (Amikin), gentamicin (Garamycin), kanamycin (Kantrex), neomycin (Mycifradin), netilmicin (Netromycin), streptomycin, and tobramycin (Nebcin). Table 12-4 ■ lists various aminoglycosides.

How do they work?

The aminoglycosides combine with bacterial (not human) ribosomes to arrest protein synthesis. This interference prevents cell reproduction, resulting in death of the bacteria.

How are they used?

Large doses of aminoglycosides are given orally before abdominal surgery to reduce the number of intestinal bacteria. The usual route of administration for systemic effects is either IM or IV. Aminoglycosides are also commonly administered via the ophthalmic or otic route in the form of eye or ear drops to treat localized infections.

What are the adverse effects?

The serious adverse effects of aminoglycosides include ototoxicity and nephrotoxicity. Nephrotoxicity may occur, depending on renal function, the age of the patient, and the drug dose. Careful drug dosing is very important with younger and older patients. Prolonged use of aminoglycosides may cause a superinfection.

What are the contraindications and interactions?

Aminoglycosides should not be used during pregnancy because they may cause fetal harm, particularly hearing loss and deafness in newborn babies. When aminoglycosides are used concurrently with penicillins, the desired effects of the aminoglycosides may be greatly decreased. Still, these drugs are often used in combination, especially in the treatment of bacterial endocarditis. These drugs should be given several hours apart. The drug action of warfarin (an oral anticoagulant) can increase if taken simultaneously with aminoglycosides. The risk of ototoxicity increases when ethacrynic acid and aminoglycosides are given.

What are the important points patients should know?

Instruct patients to increase fluid intake while taking aminoglycosides. This measure assists in preventing renal failure from nephrotoxicity. To minimize toxicity problems, short treatment periods (7–10 days) and once-daily administration should be used.

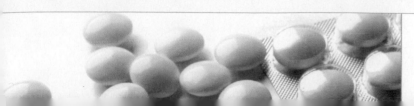

Teach-and-Test Approach

Learning small amounts of information and testing themselves on what they have just learned is a proven way for students to retain new information. This text includes a large number of exercises implemented in three ways: (1) *Practical Scenarios* (two per chapter) with critical thinking questions, (2) within-chapter *Apply Your Knowledge* questions, and (3) end-of-unit *Checkpoint Reviews*. This approach makes learning about pharmacology an engaging, interactive process. The teach-and-test approach truly differentiates this text from others and has been positively received by educators.

PRACTICAL SCENARIOS

Each chapter concludes with two short scenarios involving fictional patients with real-life problems concerning medications. A list of two or three questions follows. These scenarios relate to the knowledge that students have gained from reading each chapter. After completing each chapter, individual students can write short answers to the questions or the class as a whole can discuss the answers.

PRACTICAL SCENARIO 1

A physician orders penicillin for a 15-year-old patient without closely checking the patient's chart. While the medical assistant prepares to explain to the patient and her mother how she should take the medication, he notices that the chart indicates that the patient has an allergy to penicillin.

Critical Thinking Questions

1. What is the first thing the medical assistant should do?
2. How might the medical assistant ensure that the physician sees information about drug allergies in a patient's chart?
3. When taking a patient history, what important question should *always* be asked each time the patient is seen in the office or clinic?

Brian Warling/PH Collage

APPLY YOUR KNOWLEDGE

The second implementation of the teach-and-test approach includes exercises that are strategically placed *within* the chapters (rather than at the end). These exercise sections—called *Apply Your Knowledge*—appear after each component of the chapter content, including anatomy and physiology, and the individual pathophysiology and pharmacology sections.

✹ Apply Your Knowledge 12.1

The following questions test your understanding of the transmission of infection and the types of microorganisms.

CRITICAL THINKING

1. How can infectious disease be controlled?
2. What are "weapons of mass destruction"? Name two examples.
3. What is the chain of transmission of infectious diseases?
4. What are pathogens? Name four classes of these microorganisms.
5. What are subtherapeutic doses?

The exercise sections include a variety of exercises in which students need to recall and apply the content they have just learned. Exercise types include fill in the blank, labeling, matching, and multiple choice as well as more pharmacology-specific exercises, such as dosage calculations and drug name exercises (sound-alike and look-alike and generic-to-brand conversions). The goal of these sections is to provide students with an immediate review of all vital content. All drugs and drug classes mentioned in the content are tested in these exercise sections.

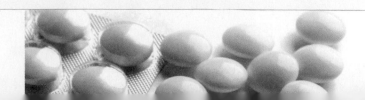

CHECKPOINT REVIEWS

The third component of our teach-and-test approach is unit "tests" called *Checkpoint Reviews*. These review questions reflect the format on most certifying and licensing exams and include multiple-choice and essay questions. Answers to the Checkpoint Reviews and Apply Your Knowledge questions are found at the end of the book in Appendices D and E, respectively.

Checkpoint Review 3

Select the best answer for the following questions.

1. Vitamin requirements are measured by which of the following units?
   a. Milligrams
   b. Centigrams
   c. Micrograms
   d. a and c

2. Vitamin B_1 is also called:
   a. Riboflavin
   b. Cobalamin
   c. Thiamine
   d. Retinol

3. Which of the following is the newest COX-2 inhibitor for the treatment of osteoarthritis?
   a. Celecoxib (Celebrex)
   b. Meloxicam (Mobic)
   c. Oxycodone (Percolone)
   d. Fentanyl (Duragesic)

4. Which of the following vaccines is used for the prevention of viral infections?
   a. Q fever
   b. Pertussis
   c. Yellow fever
   d. Plague

5. Which of the following minerals acts in bone formation, impulse conduction, myocardial contractions, and the blood-clotting process?
   a. Sodium
   b. Phosphorus
   c. Iodine
   d. Calcium

6. Which of the following is the trade name of naloxone?
   a. Demerol
   b. Talwin
   c. Narcan
   d. Stadol

7. Zinc is a very important trace element for which of the following conditions?
   a. During hemoglobin synthesis and energy production
   b. During periods of rapid tissue growth
   c. Gaining too much weight
   d. Kidney failure

8. Which of the following vitamins is an antioxidant?
   a. Tocopherol (vitamin E)
   b. Cholecalciferol (vitamin D)
   c. Phylloquinone (vitamin K)
   d. Cobalamin (vitamin B_{12})

9. Patients should be instructed to drink several full glasses of water when taking which of the following antimicrobial drugs?
   a. Penicillins
   b. Sulfonamides
   c. Fluoroquinolones
   d. Aminoglycosides

10. Acetaminophen should be avoided in which of the following patients?
    a. Those taking antacids
    b. Those drinking milk
    c. Those drinking alcohol
    d. Those taking antibiotics

11. The sulfonamides block the biosynthetic pathway of which of the following?
    a. Folic acid
    b. Bacterial proteins
    c. Bacterial nucleic acid
    d. Bacterial lipids

12. The presence of food in the GI tract reduces is the absorption of many anti-infective agents except:
    a. Penicillin V
    b. Doxycycline
    c. Minocycline
    d. All of the above

13. Which of the following foods contains very high amounts of tyramine, which may interact with MAO inhibitors and cause hypertensive crises?
    a. Bananas
    b. Cottage cheese
    c. Red meat
    d. Red apples

14. Ethanol impairs absorption of which of the following vitamins?
    a. Thiamine (vitamin B_1)
    b. Cobalamin (vitamin B_{12})
    c. Ascorbic acid (vitamin C)
    d. Tocopherol (vitamin E)

Drug Dosing Information

Each drug chapter includes tables of all drugs discussed in the chapter arranged by drug classes and formatted to include generic and trade names, adult dosing, and routes of administration.

Table 12-1 ■ Various Sulfa Drugs

GENERIC NAME	TRADE NAME	AVERAGE DOSAGE IN ADULTS	ROUTE OF ADMINISTRATION
mafenide	Sulfamylon	Apply to burned area 1–2 times/d	Topical
silver sulfadiazine	Silvadene, Thermazene, SSD (cream)	Apply to burned area 1–2 times/d	Topical
sulfadiazine	Sulfadiazine	Loading dose: 2–4 g; maintenance dose: 2–4 g/d in 4–6 divided doses	PO
sulfamethizole	Thiosulfil Forte	0.5–1 g tid–qid	PO
sulfamethoxazole	Gantanol	Initial dose: 2 g; maintenance dose: 1 g bid–tid	PO
sulfasalazine	Azulfidine	Initial dose: 1–4 g/d in divided doses; maintenance dose: 2 g/d in evenly spaced doses of 500 mg qid	PO
sulfisoxazole	Gantrisin	Loading dose: 2–4 g; maintenance dose: 4–8 g/d in 4–6 divided doses	PO
trimethoprim (TMP) and sulfamethoxazole (SMZ)	Bactrim, Septra	160 mg TMP/800 mg SMZ q12h	PO
		8–10 mg/kg/d (based on TMP) in 2–4 divided doses	IV

IV, intravenous; PO, oral; qid, four times a day; tid, three times a day.

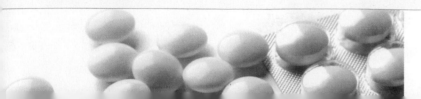

Special Populations and Important Drug-Related Points

✳ **Focus Points:** These features highlight significant or difficult concepts in pharmacology.

✳ **Focus on Pediatrics and Focus on Geriatrics:** Each of these boxes highlights pediatric or geriatric information specific to pharmacology.

✳ **Focus on Natural Products:** This boxed feature highlights drug interactions related to complementary and alternative medicines. Herbs, supplements, and foods are included in these boxes.

✳ **Focus On:** These boxes contain drug profiles that highlight the major information about drugs covered in the chapter.

Focus On

Tetracyclines

The tetracyclines are all very much alike with respect to their antimicrobial spectra and the untoward effects they elicit. They differ mainly in their absorption, duration of action, and suitability for parenteral administration (Table 12-7 ■).

How do they work?

The tetracyclines are broad-spectrum antibiotics and are mainly bacteriostatic. They bind to the bacterial ribosomes and prevent protein synthesis. The tetracyclines have activities against gram-positive and gram-negative bacteria, mycobacteria, rickettsia, and chlamydiae.

How are they used?

The tetracyclines are used in the treatment of infections caused by a wide range of microorganisms. They are effective against *Rickettsia spp.* (Rocky Mountain spotted fever and typhus fever). These drugs are also indicated for therapy of chlamydial infections, cholera, brucellosis, tularemia, and amebiasis. Tetracyclines are prescribed as an alternative to penicillin for the treatment of gonorrhea, syphilis, Lyme disease, anthrax, and *Haemophilus influenzae* respiratory infections. Doxycycline (Vibramycin) is highly effective in the prophylaxis of "traveler's diarrhea."

What are the adverse effects?

The tetracyclines cause a number of untoward effects. GI toxicity is common with oral use; it is probably caused by the combined effect of local irritation and alteration of the intestinal flora. Manifestations are heartburn, nausea, vomiting, and diarrhea. They are also associated with photosensitivity reactions, predisposing patients to severe sunburn.

The broad-spectrum antibacterial activity of the tetracyclines may cause superinfections, as can that of penicillins, cephalosporins, and sulfa drugs. This occurs most commonly in the bowel, but it may also readily occur in the mouth, lungs, and vagina. The most common

superinfection is **candidiasis**, which is an infection or disease caused by *Candida spp.*, especially *Candida albicans*—usually resulti[ng ...] change, prolonged adm[...] barrier breakage. Overgr[...] also occur. Staphylococc[...] frequently fatal.

Various hypersensitiv[...] may occur. Tetracyclines [...] (graying) in developing t[...] 8 years old and may impair bone growth.

What are the contraindications and interactions?

The tetracyclines should [...] persensitivity or liver dise[...] than 8 years old. These dr[...] pregnant and lactating wo[...]

Certain foods (such [...] (such as laxatives, antaci[...] calcium, and iron prepara[...] tion of tetracyclines. Ther[...] tetracyclines be taken on an empty stomach. Phenytoin and barbiturates can decrease the effectiveness of tetracyclines.

What are the important p[...]

Instruct patients that te[...] on an empty stomach (1 [...] meals) to facilitate absor[...] cyclines is strongly influe[...] and other drugs. Advise [...] clines can cause photose[...] avoid the sun during the [...] 2 PM), use a sunblock, an[...] tive clothing. Tetracyclines should be stored away from light and extreme heat because the effects of light and heat cause tetracyclines to decompose and produce toxic breakdown products[...] be disposed of immediate[...]

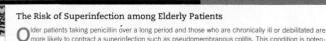

Focus Point

Handwashing Reduces Transmission

Frequent handwashing with soap, friction, and warm running water is one of the most effective ways to reduce pathogenic transmission.

Focus on Pediatrics

Avoid Fluoroquinolones in Children

Fluoroquinolones should be avoided in children because studies in young animals have documented the erosion of cartilage. However, these agents have been used safely in children with cystic fibrosis without harm.

Focus on Geriatrics

The Risk of Superinfection among Elderly Patients

Older patients taking penicillin over a long period and those who are chronically ill or debilitated are more likely to contract a superinfection such as pseudomembranous colitis. This condition is potentially life threatening and produces a toxin that affects the lining of the colon. Signs and symptoms include abdominal cramping and severe diarrhea containing visible blood and mucus. Use of antibiotics should be discontinued, and severe cases may require treatment with intravenous (IV) fluids and electrolytes, oral vancomycin, and protein supplements.

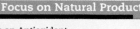

Focus on Natural Products

Green Tea as an Antioxidant

Green tea has a reputation as a healthful drink, with studies suggesting it may reduce the incidence of a variety of cancers, including cancers of the colon, pancreas, and stomach. Green tea contains high levels of polyphenols, which exhibit antioxidant and chemopreventive properties. However, green tea is not a proven cure for cancer. As often happens with natural supplements that are supported primarily by observational trials, results of these studies are inconsistent. Also, green tea should not be given to infants or young children.

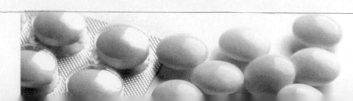

Other Elements

Each chapter includes:

* Chapter Objectives
* Key Terms with pronunciations
* Chapter Capsule: A review of each chapter objective, with bulleted summaries of the key information for each objective

The focused teach-and-test approach of this textbook provides allied health students with the perfect blend of concise content and an enjoyable—even fun—learning process. Pharmacology and fun have never been joined in the same sentence—until now!

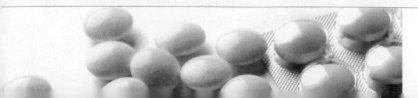

Acknowledgments

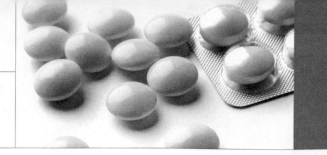

This textbook is the culmination of the efforts of many people, including my students of many years who inspired me to write it. Thank you to Julie Levin Alexander (Publisher), Mark Cohen (Editor-in-Chief), and Joan Gill (Executive Editor)—all of whom believed in this project from the start—and those dedicated professionals on the editorial team who helped produce this book. Melissa Kerian (Managing Editor) has been invaluable in helping me with the media. Alexis Breen Ferraro (Developmental Editor) was vital in coordinating all the steps needed to create this edition from the initial book. The design staff at Pearson Health, especially Wanda España (Designer), created a magnificent text design. Overseeing the production process with finesse were Patrick Walsh (Production Manager) and Julie Boddorf (Production Liaison). Katy Gabel and the staff at PreMediaGlobal provided expert guidance in all aspects of the art and production process.

My special thanks go to Greg Vadimsky, who has been my personal editorial assistant from the first edition through the completion of this second edition. He also assisted me in completing the *Instructor's Manual*, student website, and PowerPoint presentations.

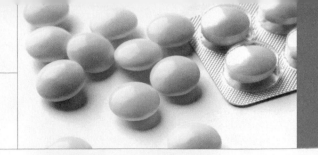

About the Author

Jahangir Moini, MD, MPH, was assistant professor at Tehran University School of Medicine for 9 years, teaching medical and allied health students. The author is a professor and former director (for 15 years) of allied health programs at Everest University. Dr. Moini re-established the medical assisting program in 1990 and the associate degree program for pharmacy technicians in 2000 at Everest's Melbourne campus. He also established several other new allied health programs for Everest University.

Dr. Moini is actively involved in teaching and helping students prepare for service in various health professions, including the roles of pharmacy technicians, medical assistants, and nurses. He has authored 16 allied health books since 1999. In 2011, Dr. Moini became a part of the advisory committee of the National Accrediting Commission of Career Arts & Sciences (NACCAS).

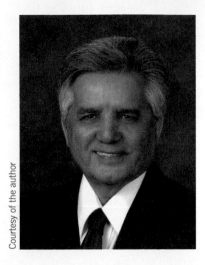

Courtesy of the author

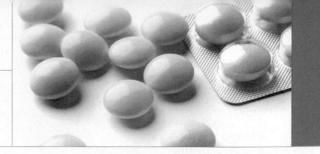

Contributors/Reviewers

CONTRIBUTORS

Karen Bills, PharmD, CPH
HealthFirst, Palm Bay Hospital
Palm Bay, Florida

Jeffrey R. Mabry, DMD
West Palm Beach, Florida

Mahkameh Moini, DMD
West Palm Beach, Florida

Stephanie K. Mullen, RN, MSN, CPNP
Private Practice
Cleveland, Ohio

Norman Tomaka, CRPh, LHCRM
HealthFirst Pharmacist Consultant
Melbourne, Florida

THANK YOU TO OUR REVIEWERS

Reviewers of the Second Edition

Elenora Alvarado
Nashville State Community College
Nashville, Tennessee

Sonya Burns, CMA (AAMA), BBA
Augusta Technical College
Waynesboro, Georgia

Sue Coleman
National College
Lynchburg, Virginia

Chanta Hall
Mountain View College
Dallas, Texas

Barbara Jareo, RN, BSN, CCM, CEN
Davenport University
Saginaw, Michigan

Patricia Sell, RMA(AMT), RN, AAS, BS, MSEd
National College
Princeton, West Virginia

Paula Silver, PharmD
Medical Careers Institute
Newport News, Virginia

Phaedra Spartan, RMA, BS
Vatterott College
Springfield, Missouri

Cindy Thompson
Davenport University
Saginaw, Michigan

Christy Tinnin, RN
Vatterott College
Fairview Heights, Illinois

Cynthia Watkins, RN, BSN
Lorain County Community College
Elyria, Ohio

Stephanie Weller
Carrington College California
Stockton, California

Reviewers of the First Edition

Patricia J. Allee, RN
Blinn College
Brenham, Texas

Kristen Anderson, RN, BSN
Southwest Wisconsin Technical College
Fennimore, Wisconsin

Deborah Bedford, CMA
North Seattle Community College
Seattle, Washington

Susan Boggs, RN, CNOR
Piedmont Technical College
Greenwood, South Carolina

Vince Druash, CMA, BS
Medical Careers Institute
Virginia Beach, Virginia

Judy Ehninger, MA
Lehigh Carbon Community College
Schnecksville, Pennsylvania

Rosemary Fischer, RN, BSN, MS
Alfred State College (retired)
Alfred, New York

Steve Forshier, RT(R), MEd
Pima Medical Institute
Mesa, Arizona

Nancy D. Glass, RN, PhD
Austin Community College
Austin, Texas

Robyn Gohsman, RMA, CMAS, AAS
Medical Careers Institute
Newport News, Virginia

Henry Gomez, MD
ASA Institute
Brooklyn, New York

Jeanette Goodwin, CMA, BSN
Southeast Community College
Lincoln, Nebraska

Corrine C. Harmon, RN, MS, EdD, AOCN
Clemson University
Clemson, South Carolina

Elizabeth Hoffman, MAEd, CMA, CPT, (ASPT)
Baker College of Clinton Township
Clinton Township, Michigan

Robin Kern, RN, BSN
Moultrie Technical College
Moultrie, Georgia

Len Lichtblau, PhD
University of Minnesota School of Nursing
Edina, Minnesota

Douglas Lytle, PhD, MBA
Widener University
Pottstown, Pennsylvania

David Martinez, RHE, BA
International Business College
El Paso, Texas

Nancy Matyunas, PharmD
Jefferson Community & Technical College
Louisville, Kentucky

Gayle Mazzocco, RN, CMA, BSN
Oakland Community College
Waterford, Michigan

Carol McMahon, RN, BSN, MEd
Capital Community College
Simsbury, Connecticut

Michele G. Miller, MEd, CMA, COMT
Lakeland Community College
Kirtland, Ohio

Lisa Nagle, BSed, CMA
Augusta Technical College
Augusta, Georgia

Eva Ruth Oltman, CMA, CPC, EMT, LMR, MA
Kentucky Community & Technical College System
Prospect, Kentucky

Christopher Owens, PharmD, BCPS
Idaho State University
Pocatello, Idaho

Steve Peterson, CPhT, MEd
Apollo College
Scottsdale, Arizona

Diane Premeau, RHIA, CHP, MBA
Chabot College
Fremont, California

Myra Resnick, RN
Southwestern College
Florence, Kentucky

Jackie Smith, RN, CPhT
National College of Business and Technology
Pounding Mill, Virginia

Karen Snipe, CPhT, MAEd
Trident Technical College
Charleston, South Carolina

Pat Stroupe, RN, MSN
Waukesha County Technical College
Pewaukee, Wisconsin

Joe Tinervia, CPhT, MBA
Community Care College
Tulsa, Oklahoma

Robert Tralongo, RRT-NPS, MBA
Molloy College
Rockville Centre, New York

Jana Tucker, CMA, LPRT
Salt Lake Community College
Salt Lake City, Utah

Gail Tuohig, RN, PhD
St. Mark's Hospital
Salt Lake City, Utah

Lori Warren, RN, CPC, CCP, CLNC, MA
Spencerian College
Louisville, Kentucky

Tonia Webster, RN, CMA
Southwest Wisconsin Technical College
Platteville, Wisconsin

Mary Ann Woods, RN, CMA, MS, PhD
Fresno City College
Fresno, California

Judith Wulff, RN, BSN
D.G. Erwin Technical Center
Tampa, Florida

MEDIA REVIEWERS

Reviewers of the Second Edition Media

Sonya Burns, CMA (AAMA), BBA
Augusta Technical College
Waynesboro, Georgia

Barbara Jareo, RN, BSN, CCM, CEN
Davenport University
Saginaw, Michigan

Patricia Sell, RMA(AMT), RN, AAS, BS, MSEd
National College
Princeton, West Virginia

Paula Silver, PharmD.
Medical Careers Institute
Newport News, Virginia

Phaedra Spartan, RMA, BS
Vatterott College
Springfield, Missouri

Cindy Thompson
Davenport University
Saginaw, Michigan

Christy Tinnin, RN
Vatterott College
Fairview Heights, Illinois

Cynthia Watkins, RN, BSN
Lorain County Community College
Elyria, Ohio

Reviewers of the First Edition Media

Joyce B. Benedetti, RN, MS, JD, CMA-AC
Allan Hancock College
Santa Maria, California

Peggy Bush, PhD, RPh
Durham Technical Community College
Durham, North Carolina

Carol Buttz
Dakota County Technical College
Rosemount, Minnesota

Jennifer Chang, BS, MS
College of Marin
Kentfield, California

June A. Griffith, PharmD, CGP
Florida Community College
Jacksonville, Florida

Lynda Harkins, PhD
Texas State University–San Marcos
San Marcos, Texas

Anne P. LaVance, BS, CPhT
Delgado Community College
New Orleans, Louisiana

Vivian C. Lilly, PhD, MBA, RN
North Harris College
Houston, Texas

Patricia McLane, RHIA, MA
Schoolcraft College
Garden City, Michigan

Michele G. Miller, MEd, CMA, COMT
Lakeland Community College
Kirtland, Ohio

Lisa Nagle, BSed, CMA
Augusta Technical College
Augusta, Georgia

Geraldine Twomey, MEd, RRT, RN
North Shore Community College
Danvers, Massachusetts

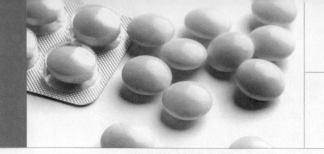

Contents

Unit 1

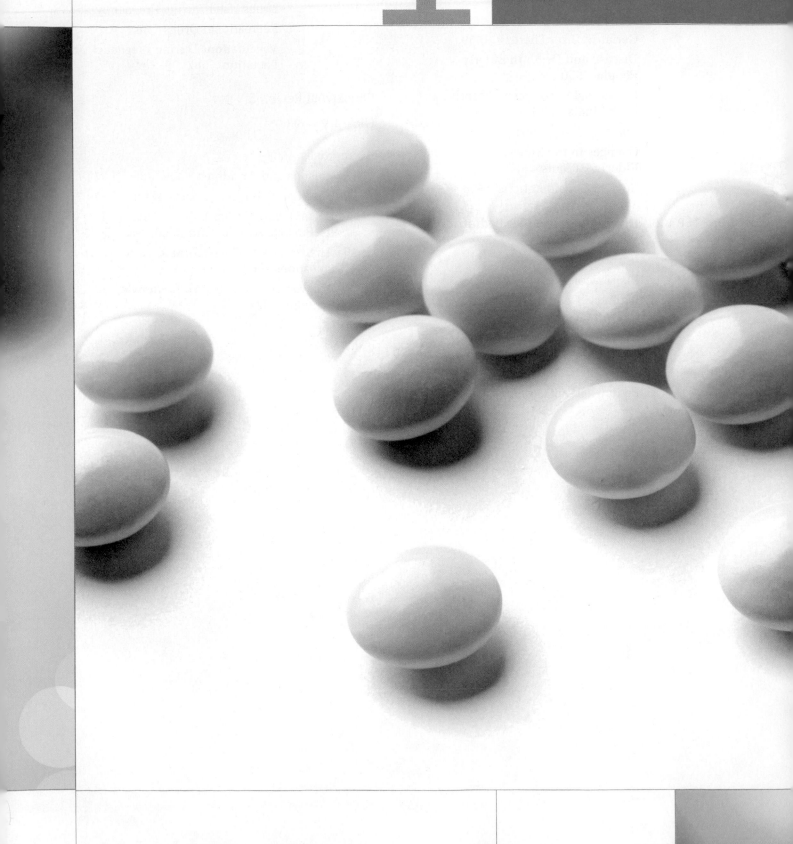

GENERAL PRINCIPLES

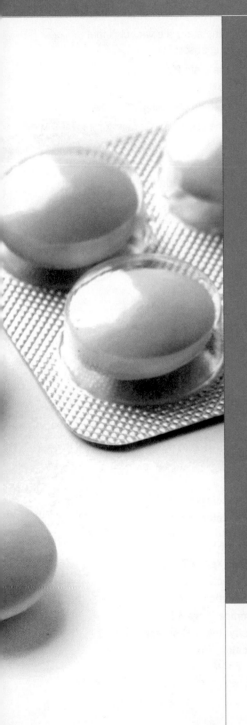

" To administer a drug safely, one must know its usual dose, frequency, route of administration, indications, contraindications, significant adverse reactions, and major drug interactions. "

Chapter 1

Introduction to Pharmacology

Chapter Objectives

After completing this chapter, you should be able to:

1. Define and differentiate the terms *pharmacodynamics* and *pharmacokinetics*.
2. Explain the mechanism of drug action.
3. List various factors that affect drug action.
4. Discuss the main site variables that affect drug absorption.
5. Define the systemic bioavailability of a drug.
6. Describe the metabolism of drugs.
7. Explain the excretion of drugs through the kidneys.
8. Define the term *idiosyncratic reaction*.
9. Explain adverse drug reactions and adverse effects.
10. Define the terms *tolerance, synergism, overdose,* and *potentiation.*

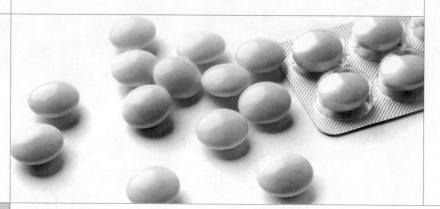

Key Terms

absorption (page 9)
adverse effects (page 6)
affinity (page 7)
agonist (AH-gah-nist) (page 7)
anaphylactic shock
   (an-nuh-fih-LAK-tik SHOK) (page 11)
antagonist (an-TAH-gah-nist) (page 7)
bioavailability (page 9)
biotransformation (page 10)
dissolution (dis-oh-LOO-shun)
   (page 9)
distribution (page 10)

dose-effect relationship (page 6)
excretion (page 11)
first-pass effect (page 9)
half-life ($t\frac{1}{2}$) (page 7)
metabolism (page 5)
overdose (page 11)
pharmacodynamics
   (far-muh-koh-dy-NAM-mix) (page 5)
pharmacognosy (far-muh-KOG-nuh-see)
   (page 6)
pharmacokinetics
   (far-muh-koh-kih-NEH-tix) (page 5)

pharmacology (page 5)
pharmacotherapeutics
   (far-muh-koh-thayr-ruh-PYOO-tix)
   (page 6)
receptor (page 7)
side effects (page 11)
therapeutic (page 6)
tolerance (page 11)
toxicity (tok-SIH-sih-tee) (page 11)
toxicology (tok-sih-KAW-luh-jee)
   (page 6)

Introduction

Pharmacology is the study of drugs, including their action and effects in living body systems. Drugs do not create effects in the body, but they do modify physical processes by mimicking or blocking effects of substances found within the body. The term *drug* is defined as "any substance or product that is used or intended to be used to modify or improve a physiologic or pathologic condition." The terms *medication* and *medicine* refer to drugs mixed in a formulation with other ingredients to improve the stability, taste, or physical form to allow appropriate administration of the active drug.

Pharmacology deals with all the drugs used in society today—those that are legal, illegal, prescription, and over-the-counter (OTC) medications. Healthcare professionals should be well informed about each medication before administering or dispensing it to a patient and should consider what drugs the patient is taking (whether prescribed or self-administered for medical or recreational reasons). To administer a drug safely, one must know its usual dose, frequency, route of administration, indications, contraindications, significant adverse reactions, and major drug interactions. Knowledge of the patient's medication allergies, weight, and liver and kidney functions is also essential.

Pharmacodynamics refers to the biochemical and physiologic effects of drugs and mechanisms of drug action (the effects of a drug on the body or organism). **Pharmacokinetics** is the study of the absorption, distribution, biotransformation (**metabolism**—the sum of chemical and physical changes in the tissues, consisting of anabolism and catabolism), and excretion of drugs (Figure 1-1 ■). Each of these factors is related to the concentration of the drug, its metabolites, and its mechanism of action.

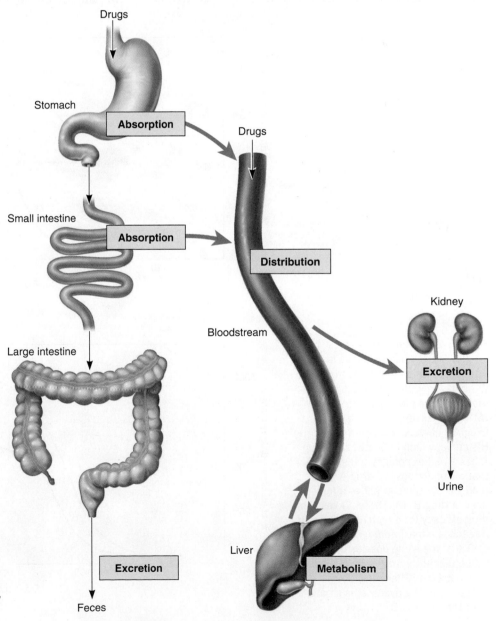

Figure 1-1 ■ The four processes of pharmacokinetics (that is, movement) are absorption, metabolism, distribution, and excretion.

Pharmacognosy is the study of drugs derived from herbal and other natural sources. By studying the compositions of natural substances and how the body reacts to them, one gains better knowledge for developing purified versions. **Pharmacotherapeutics** is the study of how drugs may be best used in the treatment of illnesses and which drug is most or least appropriate to use for a specific disease. **Toxicology** is the study of poisons and poisonings; almost all drugs are capable of being toxic. Toxicology deals with the toxic effects of substances on the living organism. Pharmacodynamics, pharmacokinetics, and toxicology are the principal subjects of pharmacology that are discussed in depth in this chapter.

Pharmacodynamics

The pharmacodynamics process describes all matters concerned with the pharmacologic actions of a drug—whether they are determinants of **therapeutic** effects (effects meant to treat a disease or disorder) or **adverse** effects (harmful effects). A basic understanding of the factors that control drug concentration at the site of action is important for the optimal use of drugs. Blood is the most commonly sampled fluid used to characterize the pharmacologic actions of drugs. The drugs must dissolve before being absorbed. Then, they are able to pass through the small intestine and enter the blood circulation. Some of these drugs are absorbed and metabolized before reaching the site of action. The factors that may influence the onset, duration, and intensity of drug effects include absorption, metabolism, reabsorption, excretion, site of action, and observed response. Usually, there are correlations between pharmacokinetics and pharmacodynamics that demonstrate the relationship between drug dose and blood or other biological fluid concentrations. Pharmacokinetics and pharmacodynamics can determine the **dose-effect relationship** (also called *dose-response relationship*), which is the relationship between the dose of a drug (or other agent) that produces therapeutic effects and the potency of the effects on the person (Figure 1-2 ■).

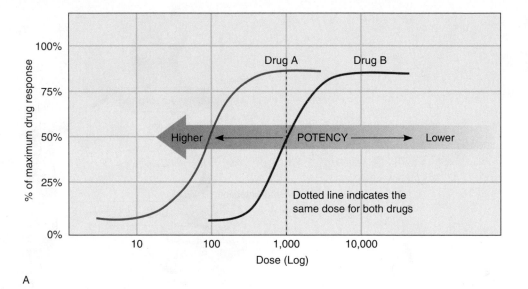

A

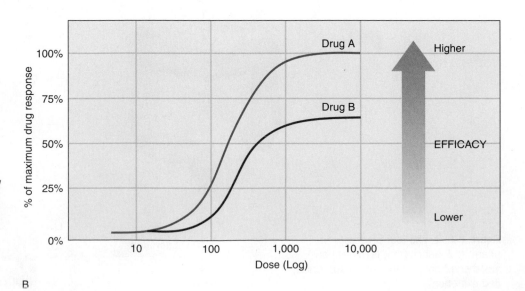

Figure 1-2 ■ The dose-effect relationship. Along the *x*-axis is the drug dose, which increases from left to right. Along the *y*-axis is the maximum response for each drug (%). (**A**) These curves show drug potency. Drug A's curve is to the left of drug B's curve, which indicates that drug A has a higher potency. This means that a smaller dose of drug A will produce the same effect as a larger dose of drug B. (**B**) These curves show drug efficacy (or effectiveness). Drug A reaches a maximum response of 100% at the same dose as drug B, which reaches a maximum response of about 60%. Therefore, drug A's efficacy (or effectiveness) is greater than that of drug B.

B

A graph is used to illustrate the relationship: The response is plotted along the *y*-axis and the dose along the *x*-axis. The resulting plotted relationship is a characteristic curve, as the figure shows. The body's response to a drug (or toxic agent) increases as its overall exposure to the substance increases; for example, in the case of toxic agents, a small dose of carbon monoxide may cause drowsiness, but a large dose can be fatal.

MECHANISM OF DRUG ACTIONS AND RECEPTORS

Drugs produce their effects by altering the function of the cells and tissues of the body or of organisms such as bacteria. Each drug has a specific **affinity** (attractive force) for a target receptor. The cell recipient is known as a **receptor**—usually a specific protein—situated either in cell membranes on cell surfaces or within the cellular cytoplasm. However, some drugs act on intracellular receptors; these include corticosteroids, which act on cytoplasmic steroid receptors. As drugs bind to their specific receptors, one of two actions are produced—an agonist or antagonist action.

Agonists

An **agonist** is a drug that binds to a receptor and produces a stimulatory response that is similar to what an endogenous substance (such as a hormone) would have done if it were bound to the receptor. For example, adrenaline is an agonist at beta (β)-adrenoceptors. When adrenaline binds to β-adrenoceptors in the heart, the heart rate increases.

Antagonists

An **antagonist** is a drug or another agent that blocks or antagonizes the effects of another substance or function. In most cases, antibacterial therapy involves the use of a single drug. Combining two antibiotics may actually decrease each drug's effects. If incorrect combinations are prescribed, the use of multiple antibiotics may also increase the potential to promote resistance.

VARIOUS FACTORS THAT AFFECT DRUG ACTIONS

Drug actions depend on various factors that are important in determining the correct drugs for a patient. These factors include age, gender, body weight, diurnal body rhythms, diseases, and drug half-life.

Drug Half-Life

A drug's **half-life** ($t\frac{1}{2}$) is defined as the time taken for the blood or plasma concentration of the drug to decrease from full to one-half (50%). The half-life is the major determinant of the duration of drug action. The longer the half-life of the drug, the longer the drug remains in the body.

The half-life of each drug may be different; for example, a drug with a short half-life of 2 or 3 hours must be administered more often than one with a longer half-life of 12 hours. Another method of explaining drug action is shown in Figure 1-3 ■, a graphic depiction of the plasma concentration of the drug versus time.

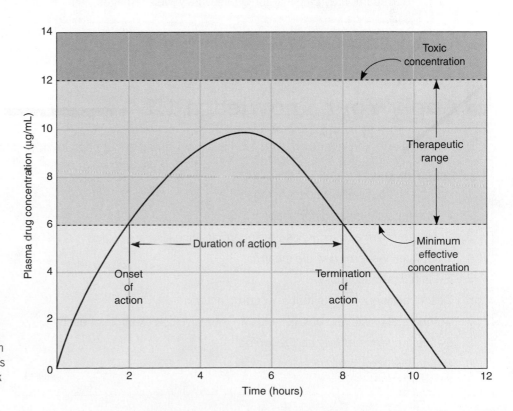

Figure 1-3 ■ Plasma concentration of a drug versus time. The onset of action occurs at 2 hours, the duration of action is 6 hours, peak plasma concentration is 10 mcg/mL, and the time to reach peak drug effect is 5 hours.

Age

Drug effects may vary in patients according to their different metabolic rates. Age often affects metabolic rates. Drug dosages may need to be adjusted in children or elderly patients. The rule of thumb with pediatric and geriatric individuals is "start low and go slow!"

Gender

Male and female patients respond to drugs differently. Drugs administered intramuscularly are absorbed faster by men than by women. Such drugs remain in women's tissues longer than in men's tissues because women have higher body fat content.

Body Weight

Body weight is an important factor for drug action. The same dosage of medication can have varied effects in patients whose weights differ. Some medication doses must be adjusted based on body weight and body surface area, especially in children. The calculation of correct dosage of drugs based on body weight is discussed in Chapter 7.

Diurnal Body Rhythms

Diurnal, or circadian, rhythms can affect the intensity of a person's response to a drug. For example, at night, the circadian clock sets the stage for sleep. By administering sleep-inducing medications at night, the drug actions may be more pronounced. In contrast, administering corticosteroids during the day is meant to mimic the circadian variations in endogenous cortisol.

Diseases

Because the liver is the major site of detoxification and the kidneys are the major sites of elimination of chemical substances, a person with liver or kidney disease may respond differently to medications than does a healthy individual.

Focus on Geriatrics

Drug Elimination in Elderly Patients

Acute or chronic diseases that affect liver architecture or function also markedly affect hepatic metabolism of some drugs. Elderly patients with chronic active hepatitis, cirrhosis of the liver, or drug-induced hepatitis can have markedly affected drug elimination. Consequently, some drugs, such as diazepam, may cause a coma in severely liver-damaged patients when given in ordinary doses.

✳ Apply Your Knowledge 1.1

The following questions focus on what you have just learned about pharmacodynamics.

CRITICAL THINKING

1. What is the dose-effect relationship?
2. Define the term *biotransformation*.
3. Compare pharmacodynamics with pharmacokinetics.
4. What does the term *half-life* mean?
5. Explain pharmacognosy.
6. Describe various factors that affect drug action.
7. Compare agonists and antagonists and then give one example of each.
8. Define the terms *affinity* and *receptor*.
9. Define the terms *tolerance* and *toxicity*.

Pharmacokinetics

As noted earlier in this chapter, pharmacokinetics is the study of the action of drug absorption, drug distribution, drug metabolism, and drug excretion.

DRUG ABSORPTION AND SYSTEMIC AVAILABILITY

The process of drug movement into the systemic circulation is **absorption**. Absorption depends on the drug's ability to cross cell membranes and resist extensive breakdown by the stomach, liver, and intestines. Presystemic metabolism occurs when enzymes in the gastrointestinal (GI) tract begin to break down the drug before it is absorbed. Presystemic metabolism affects the amount of drug that reaches the systemic circulation intact and the speed at which this happens—a concept termed **bioavailability**.

Bioavailability depends on pharmaceutical factors (such as the rate at which a tablet or capsule dissolves or the use of binding products in formulating the medication) and variable factors that affect GI absorption (such as food in the stomach, other drugs taken concurrently, intestinal motility, or certain disease states). The extent of bioavailability depends mostly on absorption and somewhat on presystemic metabolism. Lipid-soluble drugs (for example, diazepam and phenytoin) and weak acids (such as acetylsalicylic acid and penicillin V) may be absorbed directly from the stomach. Weak bases (for example, morphine and atropine) are not normally absorbed from the site. The small intestine is the primary site of absorption because of the very large surface area across which drugs may diffuse. Acids (such as ibuprofen and warfarin) are normally absorbed more extensively in the intestines than in the stomach even though the intestines have a higher pH.

Factors That Affect the Rate of Drug Absorption

In the GI tract, many factors influence the rate of drug absorption, including:

1. **Acidity of the stomach**—Aspirin and other drugs that have an acidic pH are easily absorbed in the stomach's acidic environment. The small intestine, which has an alkaline environment, more readily absorbs alkaline medications. The pH of the stomach tends to be changed by milk products and antacids. Some drugs are not absorbed properly as a result. For this reason, infants who are consuming milk or formula may need to be given certain medications on an empty stomach.

2. **Physiochemical properties**—The rate of a drug's absorption may be greatly affected by the rate at which the drug is made available to the biologic fluid at the administration site. Some of the factors that affect a drug's rate of **dissolution** (the process of dissolving) from a solid form include intrinsic physiochemical properties, such as solubility and thermodynamics (having to do with energy).

3. **Presence of food in the stomach or intestine**—The rate and extent of drug absorption may be greatly influenced by the presence of food. Whereas an empty stomach increases the rate of absorption of some medications, food in the stomach decreases the absorption rate. However, if a medication causes irritation to the stomach, the patient should eat food with the medication; the food serves as a buffer to decrease irritation.

4. **Routes of administration**—Routes that protect drugs from chemical decomposition that may occur in the stomach or liver include sublingual (under the tongue), buccal (in the folds of the cheeks), and rectal (within the rectum). Orally administered drugs are usually absorbed in the upper GI tract. They are immediately exposed to metabolism by liver enzymes before they reach the systemic circulation. This exposure is called the **first-pass effect**. After the drug is in the liver, it is partly metabolized before being sent to the body, where systemic effects occur. As a result, medications that are metabolized too quickly in the liver should not be given orally. Alprenolol (Alfeprol), dopamine (Intropin), and lidocaine (Xylocaine) are some examples of drugs that exhibit first-pass metabolism. To determine the suitability of a drug for each patient, it is crucial that the route of administration be correctly chosen. Depending on the degree of first-pass elimination and the formulation of some drugs, oral administration is feasible for some drugs and not for others.

Drugs that are directly injected into the bloodstream via the veins or arteries bypass the process of absorption and are distributed throughout the body. The time before the drug becomes effective for these injections is typically short compared with other types of injections. Also, drugs may be injected deeply into skeletal muscle. The vascularity of the muscle site and the lipid solubility of the drug determine the rate of absorption. Because the subcutaneous region is less vascular than the muscle tissues, subcutaneous injections (given beneath the skin) are absorbed less rapidly. Transdermal injections (such as those used for tuberculin skin testing), transdermal patches, and otic or ophthalmic administration are other routes. Topical drugs may be absorbed through several layers of skin for a local effect. Transdermal nitroglycerin (Nitrostat, Nitro-Bid) is absorbed rapidly and provides sustained blood levels after application to the skin in the form of either an ointment or a transdermal patch. Some drugs, such as morphine patches (Duramorph), also provide certain systemic effects, such as pain relief. Drugs administered in low concentrations tend to be less rapidly absorbed than those administered in high concentrations.

DRUG DISTRIBUTION

Many drugs are bound to circulating proteins—usually albumin (acid drugs) but also globulins (hormones), lipoproteins (basic drugs), and acid glycoproteins (basic drugs). Only the fraction of drugs that is not bound to protein can bind to cellular receptors, pass across tissue membranes, and gain access to cellular enzymes, thus being distributed to body tissue, metabolized, and excreted (for example, by the kidneys). Changes in protein binding can therefore sometimes cause changes in drug **distribution** (the passage of an agent through blood or lymph to various body sites). The initial rate of distribution of a drug depends heavily on the blood flow to various organs. Lipid-soluble drugs enter the central nervous system (CNS) rapidly. Because of the blood–brain barrier, certain drugs are poorly distributed to the CNS because they pass through the barrier.

DRUG METABOLISM

Most drug metabolism occurs in the liver through the same biochemical pathways and reactions that affect nutrients, vitamins, and minerals. The first-pass effect is an important mechanism that influences drug action and metabolism. Metabolism accomplishes the conversion of molecules as well as biodegration of foreign substances. Substances absorbed across the intestinal wall enter blood vessels. This is known as *hepatic portal circulation*, a process that carries blood directly to the liver (Figure 1-4 ■).

Enzymes act on most drugs in the body and convert drugs to end products called *metabolites* during metabolism. **Biotransformation** is the process of conversion of drugs. Biotransformation may be divided into four main stages:

1. **Oxidation**—combination with oxygen
2. **Reduction**—a reaction with a substance that involves the gaining of electrons
3. **Hydrolysis**—the cleaving of a compound into simpler compounds with the uptake of the hydrogen and hydroxide parts of a water molecule
4. **Conjugation**—the combination of substances with glucuronic or sulfuric acid, terminating biologic activity and making them ready for excretion

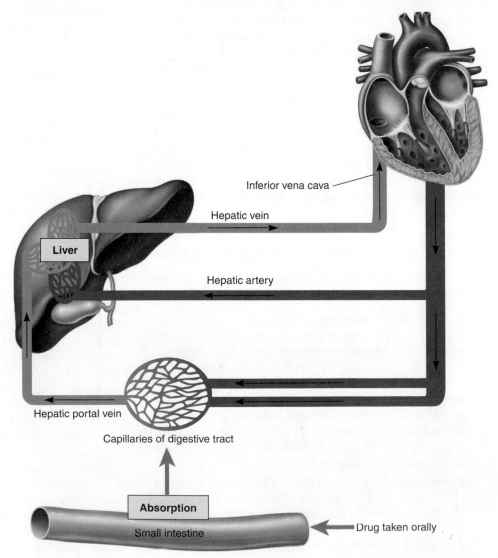

Figure 1-4 ■ First-pass effect. Oral drugs are absorbed through the intestinal wall and enter the hepatic portal circulation. They are taken directly to the liver for metabolism before reaching the heart and circulating throughout the body.

Inferior vena cava

Hepatic vein

Liver

Hepatic artery

Hepatic portal vein

Capillaries of digestive tract

Absorption

Small intestine

Drug taken orally

All these activities occur primarily in the liver via *microsomal enzymes*. One of these enzymes is cytochrome P-450, which has an essential role in drug metabolism. Toxic drug action can be influenced by drug metabolism, interactions, activation, toxicity, and adverse effects (often referred to as **side effects**). Side effects are usually (but not always) undesirable.

DRUG EXCRETION

The main route of drug **excretion**, the last stage of pharmacokinetics that removes drugs from the system, is via the kidneys. The kidneys remove waste and harmful agents in the blood circulation. Because most drugs are excreted by the kidneys, diseases of the kidneys can significantly prolong the duration of drug action. Drugs that affect the kidneys and the processes the kidneys use to remove substances from the body are discussed in Chapter 23.

Other routes of excretion include:

* **Lungs**—important for the excretion of alcohol
* **Breast milk**—important for the excretion of aspirin, barbiturates, and other drugs
* **Sweat, tears, urine, and feces**—excretions that may be alarming if the patient is not expecting the orange-red discoloration caused by phenazopyridine or rifampicin

* **Bile**—leading to the recirculation of compounds, such as chloramphenicol (its inactive metabolites are reactivated by hydrolysis in the gut), morphine, rifampicin, tetracycline, and digitoxin
* **Saliva**—sometimes used in monitoring drug concentrations in body fluids

To aid in the proper excretion of drugs, the patient should follow these guidelines:

* Take medications as ordered.
* Cough and breathe deeply after general anesthesia to help eliminate anesthetics more quickly.
* Chew gum or suck on hard candy to decrease the unpleasant effects of drugs that are eliminated through saliva.
* Increase intake of fluids because this will increase the filtration of urine and increase blood volume, thereby assisting in proper excretion.
* Maintain proper diet and amount of physical activity because both of these speed drug excretion.
* Keep skin clean to help avoid irritation from drugs that are eliminated through the sweat glands.
* Discuss use of all medications, including OTC drugs, with your physician to avoid possible risks to the fetus if you are pregnant.

✳ Apply Your Knowledge 1.2

The following questions focus on what you have just learned about pharmacokinetics.

CRITICAL THINKING

1. List the main route of drug excretion and the factors that may change it.
2. Explain the four main stages of biotransformation.
3. List the factors that affect the rate of drug absorption.
4. What are the four stages of pharmacokinetics?
5. What is meant by the side effects of a drug?
6. Where are the microsomal enzymes found and what are their roles?
7. Define the terms *blood–brain barrier* and *bioavailability*.
8. Why do drugs that are absorbed across the intestinal wall enter the hepatic portal vein?

Other Pharmacologic Principles

Many of the concepts applicable in the study of pharmacology apply equally to unforeseen or inadvertent reactions, including adverse drug reactions, adverse effects, drug allergies, drug interactions, and idiosyncratic reactions.

TOXICITY AND OVERDOSE

Toxicity is the state of being noxious and refers to a drug's ability to poison the body. There may be an antidote for the poison—a drug that has the opposite effect and can reverse the toxic symptoms. Sometimes, through medication errors or poor judgment or as a result of attempted suicide, a patient may receive a drug **overdose**, a toxic dose of the drug that causes harm.

This can be dangerous because any drug can act like a poison if taken in too large a dose.

ADVERSE DRUG REACTIONS AND ADVERSE EFFECTS

An *adverse drug reaction (ADR)* has been defined as any response to a drug that is noxious, unintended, and occurs at doses normally used in humans for the prophylaxis, diagnosis, or therapy of disease (World Health Organization, 1984). Clinical responses to an ADR include discontinuing the drug, modifying the dose, hospitalizing the patient, or providing supportive measures. Examples of an ADR are severe nausea, vomiting, and diarrhea.

ADRs occur in people of all ages. They are a major cause of morbidity and mortality, especially among elderly patients. Little attention has been given to the incidence of ADRs in neonates, infants, children, and adolescents. Before release of a new drug, few (if any) studies are undertaken in children because of issues including ethics, responsibility, cost, and regulations. This often leads prescribers to estimate dosage and hence increases the risk of ADRs in this young population. Today, ADRs are a significant issue in elderly and pediatric patients.

The term *side effect* is frequently used by healthcare professionals and often appears in drug advertisements and consumer information. It refers to effects not necessarily intended, but side effects can be beneficial. Therefore, if one is referring to harmful, unexpected effects, the more accurate term to use is *adverse effect*.

DRUG INTERACTIONS

A *drug interaction* occurs when the effects of one drug are altered by the effects of another drug. The interaction can result in either an increased or a decreased effect of the object drug. For example, amiodarone (Cordarone) inhibits cytochrome P-450 isoenzyme, leading to reduced metabolism of warfarin (Coumadin) and increased anticoagulant effects. The drug carbamazepine (Tegretol) reduces the anticoagulant effect of warfarin by increasing its liver metabolism.

Occasionally, in an interaction, the effects of both drugs are altered, as occurs in the complex interaction of phenytoin (Dilantin) with phenobarbital (Luminal). Although drug interactions usually result in an ADR, in some cases, an interaction is beneficial. One example of this beneficial effect is the pharmacodynamic synergy between diuretics and angiotensin-converting enzyme (ACE) inhibitors in the treatment of hypertension.

Drug reactions can involve prescription drugs as well as OTC drugs. When a drug interacts with another drug, it may cause *duplication, opposition (antagonism),* or *alteration* of the drugs' effects. *Duplication* occurs when two drugs that have the same effect are taken. This may intensify their effects. For example, if a patient takes an OTC cold remedy along with a sleep aid, both of which commonly contain *diphenhydramine*, the effects may be doubled. Other examples of duplication include taking a cold remedy with a pain reliever, which both commonly contain *acetaminophen*. It is important to check drug ingredients carefully to avoid drug duplication and potential toxicity. It is also important to make sure that any doctors who are treating an individual patient are aware of all other prescribed and OTC medications being used. This helps to avoid prescribing a medication containing an ingredient that is already a part of a previously taken medication.

Opposition (antagonism) occurs when two drugs with opposing actions interact, reducing the effectiveness of one or both. For example, nonsteroidal anti-inflammatory drugs (NSAIDs), such as ibuprofen, help to relieve pain while causing the body to retain salt and fluid. Diuretics, such as hydrochlorothiazide, help remove excess salt and fluid. If taken together, the NSAID's effects may reduce the effects of the diuretic. *Alteration* affects how the body absorbs, distributes, metabolizes, or excretes a drug. An example of a drug altering another drug's effects is when a proton pump inhibitor, taken to reduce stomach acid, decreases absorption of the antifungal drug *ketoconazole*.

Drugs may also interact with foods. Examples include *tetracycline*, which should not be taken with milk or other dairy products. This is because calcium reduces the absorption of the drug. Another example is when grapefruit juice is consumed with certain benzodiazepines, estrogen, or statins. It inhibits the enzymes involved in metabolism of these drugs and can intensify their effects.

IDIOSYNCRATIC REACTIONS

When a patient experiences a unique, strange, or unpredicted reaction to a drug, it is termed an *idiosyncratic reaction*. Idiosyncratic reactions may be caused by underlying enzyme deficiencies resulting from genetic or hormonal variation. For example, carisoprodol (Soma) may cause such idiosyncratic reactions as transient quadriplegia, dizziness, or temporary loss of vision.

ANAPHYLACTIC SHOCK

An idiosyncratic, sudden, and severe allergic reaction that may be life threatening is termed **anaphylactic shock**. It can cause a sharp loss of blood pressure, urticaria (lesions known as *hives* or *wheals*), paralysis of the diaphragm, and swelling of the oropharynx; the end result may be cardiac collapse. Anaphylactic shock, a true medical emergency, occurs so swiftly and with such severity that controlled clinical studies of treatment have never been possible. Prevention is, of course, most important. A history of previous allergic reactions to drugs, vaccines, serum, or blood transfusions must be obtained from anyone about to undergo treatment to prevent or at least be prepared for the slightest hazard of this kind. Patients who are predisposed to allergic reactions should wear an alerting bracelet or necklace (for example, Medic Alert®). Epinephrine (adrenaline) is frequently injected to combat anaphylactic shock but must be administered soon after shock begins.

ALLERGIC REACTIONS

Drug allergy is an abnormal response characterized by:

✳ Occurrence in a small number of individuals

✳ Previous exposure to either the same or a chemically related drug

✳ Rapid development of an allergic reaction after re-exposure

✳ Production of clinical manifestations of an allergic reaction

The term *hypersensitivity* is often used synonymously with *allergy*.

The diagnosis of a drug allergy is often difficult to establish because no reliable laboratory tests can identify the relevant drug, and in some cases, the symptoms can imitate infectious disease symptoms. A health-care practitioner must clarify whether the patient is experiencing a true allergic reaction or drug intolerance. For example, administration of penicillin by injection may cause a severe allergic reaction, which may be life threatening. Conversely, when a patient takes penicillin orally, allergy to the substance may cause nausea and vomiting to an intolerable degree. Allergic reactions to drugs generally follow the type I to IV classification as listed in Table 1-1 ■.

Table 1-1 ■ Allergic Drug Reactions

TYPE	EXAMPLES OF DRUGS OR CLASSES OF DRUGS
I. Immediate hypersensitivity	Penicillins, streptomycin, local anesthetics, neuromuscular-blocking drugs, radiologic contrast medicine
I. Antibody dependent, cytotoxic	Quinine, quinidine, rifampicin, metronidazole
III. Complex mediated	Anticonvulsants, antibiotics, hydralazine, diuretics
IV. Cell mediated or delayed hypersensitivity	Local anesthetic creams, antihistamine creams

TOLERANCE

Drug **tolerance** is the development of resistance to the effects of a drug such that the drug's doses must be continually raised to elicit the desired response. Tolerance is often experienced in relation to drugs of abuse. Drugs that commonly produce tolerance are opiates, nitrates, barbiturates, alcohol, and tobacco. Cross-tolerance occurs when a person develops a resistance to chemically similar drugs. *Dependence*, a frequently confused term, refers to a drug's ability to stimulate pleasure centers in the brain, causing the patient to desire more or continued use of the drug.

CUMULATIVE EFFECT

When the body is not able to metabolize and excrete one dose of a drug completely before the next dose is given, a *cumulative effect* occurs. With repeated doses, the drug starts to collect in the blood and body tissues, resulting in cumulative toxicity. Cumulative toxicity may occur rapidly, such as with ethyl alcohol, or slowly over time, such as with lead poisoning.

SYNERGISM

The combined action of two or more agents that produce an effect greater than that which would have been expected from the two agents acting separately is called *synergism*. Some drug interactions exhibit synergism, which, depending on the circumstances, may be beneficial or harmful. For example, the combination of the antibacterial drug trimethoprim with sulfamethoxazole (Bactrim, Septa) is more effective for treating infections than either drug acting alone. However, the combination of aspirin and the anticoagulant warfarin (Coumadin) can act synergistically to reduce blood clotting to the extent of spontaneous hemorrhage if doses are not carefully monitored.

POTENTIATION

An interaction between two drugs that causes an effect greater than that which would have been expected from the additive properties of the drugs involved is called *potentiation*. For example, alcohol potentiates the sedating effects of the tranquilizer diazepam (Valium) when the two drugs are ingested at the same time.

Focus Point

Allergy History

 sk all patients if they have a history of allergies, such as hay fever, rashes, or asthma, or have had unusual reactions to any drugs taken orally or by injection in the past.

✳ Apply Your Knowledge 1.3

The following questions focus on what you have just learned about toxicology.

CRITICAL THINKING

1. Classify various types of allergic drug reactions.
2. Define drug interactions and then give four examples.
3. What is anaphylactic shock? Give four examples.
4. Define *synergism* and *potentiation*, giving one example of each.
5. What are idiosyncratic reactions? Identify their causes.
6. List at least five drugs that produce drug tolerance.

PRACTICAL SCENARIO 1

A 73-year-old man with a 25-year history of alcoholism was prescribed the sedative phenobarbital by his family physician after he reported anxiety and trouble sleeping. The patient was also taking the antico-agulant warfarin (Coumadin) that had been prescribed by his cardiologist. Warfarin is a drug that is metabolized more rapidly when given with phenobarbital. This patient was later brought into the emergency room with a possible hemorrhagic stroke.

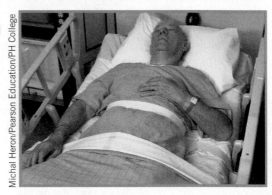

Michal Heron/Pearson Education/PH College

Critical Thinking Questions

1. How might the patient's age be related to the drug toxicity?
2. How could the family physician have helped prevent this emergency?

PRACTICAL SCENARIO 2

Renee, a medical assistant, works in a walk-in clinic. A child is brought in to be treated for strep throat, and the physician orders a penicillin intramuscular (IM) injection. Renee asks the child's mother if the child has any allergies to antibiotics, and the mother says he does not. Renee administers the IM injection. Ten minutes later, the child experiences anaphylactic shock. The pediatrician begins to treat the condition.

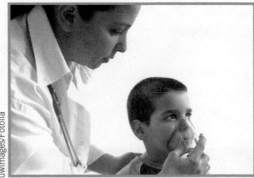

uwimages/Fotolia

Critical Thinking Questions

1. What was the reason that the patient had anaphylactic shock?
2. Explain the signs and symptoms of anaphylactic shock.
3. What did Renee do wrong?

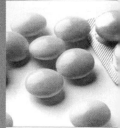

Chapter Capsule

This section repeats the objectives from the beginning of the chapter and then provides a summary of the most important concepts for that objective. Use this section as a quick review and to check your knowledge.

Objective 1: Define and differentiate the terms *pharmacodynamics* and *pharmacokinetics*.

- The study of the biochemical and physiologic effects of drugs and the mechanism of drug action

Objective 2: Explain the mechanism of drug action.

- Alters the normal function of the cells and tissues of the body by mimicking or blocking the effects of normal endogenous substances
- Specific cells (known as receptors) are chosen because the drug has a specific affinity for a particular cell
- Each receptor type attracts a specific group of drugs capable of binding to the receptor, thereby producing a pharmacologic effect

Objective 3: List various factors that affect drug action.

- Age
- Gender
- Body weight
- Diurnal body rhythms
- Diseases
- Drug half-life, absorption, administration route, distribution, metabolism, and excretion

Objective 4: Discuss the main site variables that affect drug absorption.

- Acidity of the stomach—acidic drugs such as aspirin are easily absorbed here; the pH of the stomach tends to be changed by milk products and antacids, thus some drugs are not absorbed properly; certain medications should be given on an empty stomach to ensure proper absorption
- Physiochemical properties—factors that affect the rate of drug dissolution from a solid form, including intrinsic physiochemical properties, such as solubility and rate of dissolution
- Presence of food in the stomach or intestine—an empty stomach increases the rate of absorption of some medications; food in the stomach decreases the absorption rate
- Routes of administration—sublingual (under the tongue), buccal (inner lining of the cheeks), and rectal (within the rectum); orally administered drugs are usually absorbed in the upper GI tract and are immediately exposed to metabolism via liver enzymes before reaching systemic circulation (the first-pass effect)

Objective 5: Define the systemic bioavailability of a drug.

- The amount of administered drug that reaches the systemic circulation intact and the speed at which this happens

Objective 6: Describe the metabolism of drugs.

■ Mostly occurs in the liver but some occurs in the plasma, kidneys, and cells; at synapses; or within nerves

■ First-pass effect—influences drug action and metabolism (the amount of drug that is able to reach the systemic circulation)

■ Substances absorbed across the intestinal wall enter blood vessels (known as the hepatic portal circulation) and are carried with the blood directly to the liver

■ Most drugs are acted on by enzymes (such as cytochrome P-450) and converted to metabolic derivatives (biotransformation)

■ Biotransformation—divided into oxidation, reduction, hydrolysis, and conjugation

Objective 7: Explain the excretion of drugs through the kidneys.

■ The main route of excretion

■ Remove waste and harmful agents in the blood circulation, including the majority of drugs

■ Diseases of the kidneys—significantly prolong the duration of drug action

Objective 8: Define the term *idiosyncratic reaction*.

■ A unique, strange, or unpredicted reaction to a drug

■ May be caused by enzyme deficiencies, resulting from genetic or hormonal variation, allergy, or sensitivities

Objective 9: Explain adverse drug reactions and adverse effects.

■ Adverse drug reactions (ADRs)—any responses to a drug that are noxious and unintended and occur at doses normally used in humans for the prophylaxis, diagnosis, or therapy of disease

■ ADRs—occur in people of all ages; a significant issue concerning children and elderly patients

■ Adverse effects—ADRs that are sometimes called side effects; the term *side effect* implies that the adverse reaction is insignificant, medically trivial, or acceptable

■ Use of the term *side effect* should be avoided if possible; *adverse effect* is the preferred term

Objective 10: Define the terms *tolerance, synergism, overdose,* and *potentiation*.

■ Tolerance: the development of resistance to the effects of a drug

■ Synergism: the combined action of two or more agents that produce an effect greater than that which would have been expected from the two agents acting separately

■ Overdose: a toxic dose of a drug that causes harm

■ Potentiation: an interaction between two drugs that causes an effect greater than that which would have been expected from the additive properties of the drugs involved

Internet Sites of Interest

■ An encyclopedia of medical and pharmacology terms, health news, and information on disorders can be found at Science Daily's website: **www.sciencedaily.com**

- The U.S. Food and Drug Administration's (FDA) website includes new drug approvals, prescription and OTC drug information, drug safety and side effect information, and more: **www.fda.gov/cder/drug**

- The INCHEM website posts a study on the effects of human exposure to various chemicals and toxicity tests. The site is part of the International Programme on Chemical Safety. The report was prepared in conjunction with the World Health Organization: **www.inchem.org**

- Medscape Pharmacists contains a wealth of information about drugs, natural therapies, FDA drug warnings, and even continuing education programs for health professionals at: **www.medscape.com/pharmacists**

- The topic of drug allergies can be found on the National Institutes of Health's MedLink site: **www.nlm.nih.gov/medlineplus**. Search the site for "drug allergies."

- An excellent article on ADRs and treatment options is offered by Riedl and Casillas in *American Family Physician*. 2003; 68:1781–90. It is available at: **www.aafp.org**. Search for this article on the journal's home page.

PEARSON
myhealthprofessionskit™

Go to www.myhealthprofessionskit.com to access the Companion Website created for this textbook. Simply select "Basic Health Science" from the choice of disciplines. Find this book and then log in using your username and password to access interactive learning games, assessment questions, animations, and more.

Chapter 2

Law and Ethics of Medications

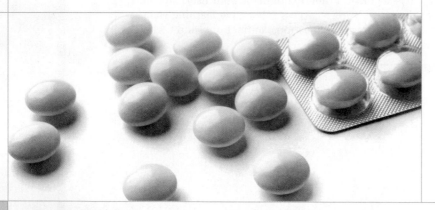

Introduction

All health-care workers who deal with dispensing, preparing, and administering medications must be familiar with the legal and ethical requirements that relate to these procedures. In the United States, the early 1900s marked the beginnings of drug legislation. Today, federal regulations are in place to help protect consumers from the harmful effects of improperly using drugs; however, drug-related adverse effects still occur even with "approved" over-the-counter (OTC) and prescription drugs. The use of dangerous or illicit drugs is prohibited by state and federal governments. The sale and distribution of drugs in the United States is controlled primarily by two major legislative acts: the Federal Food, Drug, and Cosmetic Act (FDCA) and the Federal Controlled Substances Act (CSA). These acts give the Food and Drug Administration (FDA) and other federal and state agencies the power to enforce legislative decisions. The FDCA is predominantly concerned with fixing the rules and regulations by which drugs are imported, manufactured, distributed, and sold in the United States. The CSA is part of the Comprehensive Drug Abuse Prevention and Control Act of 1970, which, as the title suggests, is concerned with the prevention and control of the abuse of certain drugs called **controlled substances**—or drugs whose possession and use are controlled by the act.

The CSA is administered and enforced by the Department of Justice under the attorney general and is a unit of the Federal Bureau of Investigation (FBI) known as the Drug Enforcement Administration (DEA). Although the two agencies have separate missions, they do cooperate in the administration of the federal drug abuse treatment program. The DEA is required to obtain the expert scientific advice of the FDA when seeking to add a substance to the list of controlled substances.

These two acts are supplemented on the federal level by a series of legislative acts designed to address specific problems, including the Poison Prevention Packaging Act of 1970 and the Federal Hazardous Substances Act.

The Need for Drug Control

During the nineteenth century, there was virtually no regulation of the sale of drugs in the United States. Opium was readily and legally available OTC in pharmacies, in grocery and general stores, and from mail order houses. The medications containing opium were advertised extensively in newspapers. Labels often did not reveal the contents. No law required that the contents of a drug be stated.

Case after case of addiction to opiates and fatal delay in seeking medical treatment—caused by reliance on the claims of charlatans or drug-clouded perceptions—occurred (Figure 2-1 ■). To combat this situation, Congress passed the first Pure Food and Drug Act in 1906.

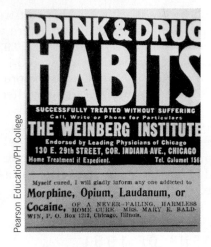

Pearson Education/PH College

Figure 2-1 ■ During the nineteenth century in the United States, over-the-counter opium could be purchased at pharmacies and grocery stores. As a result, addiction became a problem, leading to programs such as the one advertised in this poster. However, in 1906, the Pure Food and Drug Act put an end to the sale of unsafe and untested drugs, such as opium.

Federal Law

Congress found the authority to pass drug legislation within its constitutional right to control **interstate commerce**—that is, the commerce, traffic, transportation, and exchange between states of the United States. The purpose of the Federal Food, Drug, and Cosmetic Act of 1938 was the same then as it still is today: to limit interstate commerce of drugs to those that are safe and effective.

Whereas the act (which is described more completely later in this chapter) requires that drugs comply with the standards of safety and efficacy, the earlier Pure Food and Drug Act of 1906 focused on standards of strength and purity as well as proper labeling that indicated the kind and amount of ingredients present. In 1912, Congress passed the Sherley Amendment, prohibiting the use of fraudulent therapeutic claims.

To fulfill the obligation undertaken in 1912, Congress adopted the Federal Narcotic Drug Act in 1914. This law became popularly known as the Harrison Narcotic Act.

SULFANILAMIDE DISASTER OF 1937

A manufacturer decided to market the antimicrobial *sulfanilamide* in a liquid form for sore throats and mixed the sulfanilamide with diethylene glycol, which is the same ingredient used today as antifreeze in car radiators. Because sulfanilamide was poorly soluble in known solvents, drug marketers rushed to be the first to find a suitable solvent and develop a liquid version of the drug, particularly for use in young children. Diethylene glycol was chosen because of its pleasant color and taste. However, it was a deadly poison, and because no clinical safety or efficacy studies were required before marketing, this fact went overlooked until patients started dying. There were 107 reported deaths from this product. The 1938 Food, Drug, and Cosmetic Act, which followed this disaster, prevented the marketing of new drugs before they had been properly tested for purity, strength, effectiveness, safety, and packaging quality. This act gave the FDA the authority to approve or deny new drug applications. As a result of this law and further legislation, the FDA now approves the investigational use of drugs on humans and ensures that all approved drugs are safe and effective.

THE DURHAM–HUMPHREY AMENDMENT OF 1951

The Durham–Humphrey Amendment of 1951 exempted certain drugs from the requirement that their labeling must contain adequate directions for use. These drugs, which could be taken safely only under medical supervision, were exempted provided they were sold pursuant to the order of a licensed physician or administered under a prescriber's supervision. The Durham–Humphrey Amendment of 1951 prohibits the dispensing of legend drugs without a prescription. Federal law requires **legend drugs**

(prescription drugs) to bear the following statement: "Caution: Federal law prohibits dispensing without prescription." Nonlegend, or OTC, drugs were not restricted for sale and use under a physician's supervision. They were deemed safe for use by the public for self-limited use in minor conditions. Their sale is not restricted, and their use is thought, in most cases, to require neither prescription nor medical supervision.

THALIDOMIDE DISASTER OF 1962

In 1962, thalidomide, used as a sleeping pill and antinausea agent during pregnancy, was being widely used abroad. Before it could be approved for use in the United States, its adverse effects on developing fetuses were discovered. Meanwhile, women in other countries who took thalidomide during their first trimester of pregnancy delivered babies with severe deformities, including malformed or missing limbs.

These events led to the passage of the Kefauver–Harris Amendment in 1962. Currently, thalidomide has limited availability in the United States for the treatment of leprosy, bone marrow transplantation, acquired immunodeficiency syndrome (AIDS), and several other conditions.

Focus on Pediatrics

Drugs and Birth Defects

Thalidomide is not the only drug known to cause birth defects if taken by pregnant women. Studies have proven that drinking alcohol while pregnant can cause fetal alcohol syndrome, characterized by abnormalities of the face and head, growth disturbances, and mental deficiency. Smoking during pregnancy has been linked to smaller birth-weight babies and to abnormal infant reflexes.

✳ Apply Your Knowledge 2.1

The following questions focus on what you have just learned about drug control, federal law, and early legislation that related to drug control.

CRITICAL THINKING

1. What law was passed in Congress to combat the lack of drug regulation in the United States?
2. Which law gave the FDA the authority to approve or deny new drug applications and what happened that caused Congress to pass this law?
3. What was the thalidomide disaster of 1962?
4. Describe legend and nonlegend drugs.
5. Define the DEA and then describe its requirements.

DRUG ABUSE CONTROL AMENDMENT OF 1965

This amendment, the effective precursor of the Drug Abuse Control Act, permitted only certain authorized registrants to manufacture stimulant drugs. This drug abuse control legislation provided the first guidelines for determining the classifications of drugs subject to abuse. By and large, they were incorporated into the 1970 act, which follows.

COMPREHENSIVE DRUG ABUSE PREVENTION AND CONTROL ACT OF 1970

One of the primary functions of this act was to encompass all federal laws dealing with narcotic drugs, stimulants, depressants, and abused **designer drugs** that did not fit the historical classifications. (*Designer drugs* are defined as drugs produced by a minor modification in the chemical structure of an existing drug, resulting in a new substance with similar pharmacologic effects. Scientists also call these drugs *analogues*.) This act also served to consolidate the government's enforcement activities that had previously been handled by various competing agencies. For example, the Bureau of Narcotics and the Bureau of Drug Abuse Control became the Bureau of Narcotics and Dangerous Drugs (BNDD). Finally, in 1973, all agencies involved in drug abuse control and the enforcement of drug abuse laws were combined into one agency: the DEA. The DEA, housed within the Department of Justice, became the nation's sole legal drug enforcement agency.

The Comprehensive Drug Abuse Prevention and Control Act of 1970, also called the CSA, became effective on May 1, 1971. This law was designed to:

✳ Provide increased research into and prevention of drug abuse and drug dependence.

✳ Provide for the treatment and rehabilitation of drug abusers and drug-dependent persons.

✳ Improve the administration and regulation of the manufacture, distribution, and dispensing of controlled substances by legitimate handlers of these drugs to help reduce their widespread dispersion into illicit markets.

Drugs covered by this act have a potential for causing drug dependence, abuse, or both and are classified according to their use and **abuse potential** (possibility of causing abuse or dependence in a user).

Drugs with the potential for abuse are classified into five schedules: I, II, III, IV, and V. Drugs in Schedule I have the highest potential for abuse and addiction, and those in Schedule V have the least potential.

Schedule I: These drugs have a high potential for abuse, and they are not accepted for medical use in the United States. Properly registered individuals may use Schedule I substances for research, analysis, or instruction purposes.

Schedule II: These drugs also have a high potential for abuse, but they are currently accepted for medical use in the United States. The abuse of these drugs may result in severe psychological or physical dependence. The quantity of the substance in a drug product often determines the schedule that will control it. For example, amphetamines (Figure 2-2 ■) and codeine are usually classified in Schedule II; however, specific products containing smaller quantities of Schedule II substances, most often manufactured in combination with a noncontrolled substance, are controlled by Schedules III and IV. An example is Tylenol mixed with codeine, which is considered a Schedule III drug.

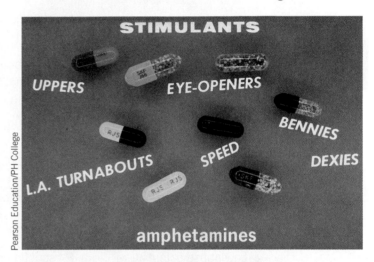

Figure 2-2 ■ Amphetamines, Schedule II drugs, have a high abuse potential and are sold illegally under many street names.

Schedule III: These drugs have less abuse potential than those in Schedules I and II and cause only low to moderate physical dependence if abused. They have accepted medical uses in the United States. Schedule III drugs contain limited quantities of certain narcotic and nonnarcotic agents.

Schedule IV: These drugs have only slight abuse potential and accepted medical uses in the United States. They are still more potent than Schedule V drugs and require a prescription.

Schedule V: These drugs have the lowest abuse potential of all the controlled substances and consist of preparations containing limited quantities of certain narcotic drugs that are generally used for antitussive and antidiarrheal purposes. Schedule V drugs are OTC preparations that may be sold without a prescription to individuals 18 years or older. Diphenoxylate with atropine (Lomotil), which is listed as a Schedule V drug, is an exception: It requires a prescription. Paregoric (a drug that causes emesis, or vomiting) is now restricted to prescription sales only and is included in Schedule III (Table 2-1 ■).

Focus Point

Keeping Medications Safe in the Hospital

In the hospital, all restricted substances must be stored in locked storage facilities to prevent access by unauthorized persons. The nurse in charge of the shift or the pharmacy technician working directly under the supervision of the in-charge pharmacist carries the keys to the locked storage. Likewise, restricted substances kept in other medical settings, such as physicians' offices, must be kept in locked storage facilities.

Table 2-1 ■ Drug Schedules

SCHEDULE	ABUSE POTENTIAL	PRESCRIPTION REQUIREMENTS	EXAMPLES
I	High abuse potential; no accepted medical use	No prescription permitted	Heroin, lysergic acid (LSD), marijuana, mescaline, and peyote
II	High abuse potential; accepted medical use	Prescription required; no refills permitted without a new written prescription	Cocaine, codeine, methamphetamine (Desoxyn), methadone (Methadose), morphine (Astramorph), opium (deodorized), methylphenidate (Ritalin), and secobarbital (Seconal)
III	Low to moderate abuse potential; accepted medical use	Prescription required; five refills permitted in 6 months	Certain drugs compounded with small quantities of narcotics; also other drugs with high potential for abuse (Tylenol with codeine tablets) and certain barbiturates
IV	Low abuse potential; accepted medical use	Prescription required; five refills permitted in 6 months	Barbital, chloral hydrate (Noctec), diazepam (Valium), chlordiazepoxide (Librium), and pentazocine (Talwin)
V	Low abuse potential; accepted medical use	No prescription required for patients 18 years or older	Cough syrups with codeine, diphenoxylate with atropine (Lomotil)*, and kaolin/pectin/opium (Parepectolin)*

*These Schedule V drugs *do* require a prescription.

Focus Point

Ensuring Specificity of Orders

An order or prescription must clearly state the specific circumstances and conditions under which the drug may be given. Health-care providers must not accept conditions that are nonspecific (for example, "if needed," "if indicated," or "as warranted").

ORPHAN DRUG ACT OF 1983

Substantial evidence of both safety and effectiveness is required before a new drug can be marketed in the United States; this requirement causes the drug development process to be extremely expensive, lengthy, and difficult. Therefore, because drug companies are businesses trying to make money, they are more likely to invest the millions of dollars and years of research necessary to secure approval for drugs that would be used to treat millions of people with common diseases and disorders. This means that effective new drugs for rare diseases would likely go undeveloped. Recognizing this as a problem in drug research and development, the government passed the Orphan Drug Act of 1983, which offers federal financial incentives to non-profit and commercial organizations to develop and market drugs to treat rare diseases that affect fewer than 200,000 people in the United States—that is, **orphan drugs**.

This act offers a 7-year patent exclusivity on drug sales and tax breaks to induce drug companies to undertake development and manufacturing of such drugs. Since going into effect, more than 100 orphan drugs have been approved, including those used to treat AIDS, cystic fibrosis, blepharospasm (uncontrolled, rapid blinking), and snake bites.

THE PRESCRIPTION DRUG MARKETING ACT OF 1987

This act prohibits the **reimportation** (importation of a drug into the United States that was originally manufactured here) of a drug by anyone but the manufacturer. It also deals with safety and competition issues raised by secondary drug markets and prohibits the trading or sale of drug samples, the distribution of samples except by mail or common carrier, and the distribution of samples to persons other than those licensed to prescribe them.

SAFE MEDICAL DEVICES ACT OF 1990

This act requires that medical device users report to manufacturers and the FDA occurrences in which a medical device has contributed to or caused the death or illness of or serious injury to a patient. The illness or injury must be life threatening or result in permanent impairment of body function or permanent damage to body structures. Medical devices may include dialyzers, electronic equipment, implants, monitors, restraints, syringes, catheters, in vitro diagnostic test kits and reagents, disposables, components, parts, accessories, related software, thermometers, ventilators, and other types of devices.

ANABOLIC STEROIDS CONTROL ACT OF 1990

Anabolic steroids are hormonal substances related to estrogen, progestins, testosterone, and corticosteroids, which promote muscle growth. Athletes sometimes use these agents to increase their physical performance. This act, which became effective in February 1991, placed anabolic steroids under the CSA's regulatory provisions. It is important because it reflects an essential change of direction for drug abuse control. Anabolic steroids may lead to cardiovascular problems, including heart attack or endocarditis, as well as liver cancer, depression, suicidal thoughts, and a higher risk of viral or bacterial infections. This act was amended in 2004 to modify the definition of the term "anabolic steroids" to include additional related chemicals. Frequently, abusers take both oral and injectable anabolic steroids in doses that are up to 100 times higher than those used for medical conditions.

Focus Point

Ensuring Clarity of Orders

Health-care providers must ensure that orders and prescriptions clearly include in writing the drug's name, dosage, route, and frequency of administration. The order must be signed with clear notation of the prescribing physician's name.

OMNIBUS BUDGET RECONCILIATION ACT (OBRA) OF 1990

This act requires that pharmacists offer to counsel Medicaid and Medicare patients about drug information and potential adverse effects for all new and refilled prescriptions. OBRA '90 reduced state entitlements to reimbursement from the federal government and requires states that seek such reimbursement to adopt programs directly affecting the pharmacy profession. Only costs for drugs approved as "safe and effective" are reimbursed—with just a few exceptions. States must require pharmacists who provide services under this program to give consulting services. These pharmacists may discuss with their patients dosage form, dosage, route of administration, duration of drug therapy, name and description of medication, interactions with other drugs or food, therapeutic contraindications, common adverse effects, proper storage, self-monitoring of medication therapy, special directions for and precautions to be taken, and action in the event of a missed dose.

✳ Apply Your Knowledge 2.2

The following questions focus on what you have just learned about orphan drugs and recent drug legislation.

CRITICAL THINKING

1. Describe orphan drugs and then give two examples.
2. What was the purpose of the Controlled Substances Act?
3. Describe the classifications of scheduled drugs and determine which class has a high potential for abuse but is currently accepted for medical use in the United States.
4. Why is the abuse of anabolic steroids dangerous?
5. What law mandates that pharmacists offer to counsel Medicaid and Medicare patients about drug information and potential adverse effects for all prescriptions?

OCCUPATIONAL SAFETY AND HEALTH ACT OF 1970 (REVISED IN 1992)

This act, originally signed in 1970 by President Richard M. Nixon, is administered by the Occupational Safety and Health Administration (OSHA), which is part of the Department of Labor. In the late 1980s, the medical industry became involved with OSHA-related publicity surrounding the threat of human immunodeficiency virus (HIV) infection as it extended to health-care workers. OSHA's mission is to ensure workplace safety and a healthy workplace environment. The HIV/AIDS crisis provoked improvements in protection of health-care workers who cared for patients with the disease. Before HIV/AIDS, OSHA had focused more directly on viral hepatitis and other pathogens as they affected medical staff members. In July 1992, OSHA's Final Ruling on Bloodborne Pathogens became fully effective. Medical facilities must now comply with the Bloodborne Pathogens Standard and be able to prove their compliance to OSHA inspectors (Figure 2-3 ■). Common OSHA violations include missing or improper labeling of hazardous chemicals, lack of eyewash facilities, inadequate documentation of annual and initial employee training, lack of proof of destruction of hazardous waste, deficient records of the required Written Exposure Control Plan and Emergency Action Plan, missing records of hepatitis B vaccinations on declaration forms, inadequate annual hazard assessment, and neglected posting of OSHA Form 300A during the required time period.

The first specialty area in the pharmacy profession, for which a special regulation at the state level has been established, is the area of **nuclear pharmacy** (a specialty area of pharmacy dealing with radioactive materials for

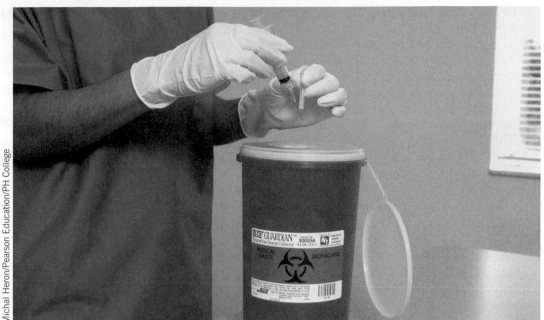

Figure 2-3 ■ In 1992, the Occupational Safety and Health Administration's Final Ruling on Bloodborne Pathogens became law. Safety measures, such as sharps containers for the disposal of needles and syringes, were implemented to stem the spread of HIV/AIDS and other bloodborne diseases.

Michal Heron/Pearson Education/PH College

nuclear studies). In nuclear medicine, exposure to chemotherapy requires safety procedures and special precautions. Most regulations make it unlawful for any persons to provide nuclear pharmaceutical services unless they are under a qualified nuclear pharmacist's supervision.

THE HEALTH INSURANCE PORTABILITY AND ACCOUNTABILITY ACT (HIPAA) OF 1996

This act, known as HIPAA, was signed into law in August 1996 by President Bill Clinton, amending the Internal Revenue Service Code of 1986 (also known as the Kassebaum–Kennedy Act). Each of its four administrative simplification parts has generated various standards and rules, with different compliance deadlines from 2000 to 2005. The four parts are:

1. **Electronic health transaction standards**—Standard code sets must be adopted by health organizations and used in all health transactions. All parties to any transaction must use and accept the same coding systems, which describe diseases, injuries, and other health problems (as well as their symptoms, causes, and actions taken). The goal is to reduce mistakes, duplication, and costs.

2. **Unique identifiers**—HIPAA aims to reduce multiple identification numbers when organizations deal with each other to reduce confusion, errors, and costs.

3. **Security and electronic signature standards**—Physical storage and maintenance, transmission, and individual health information access standards were improved by this section, governing all individual health information that is maintained or transmitted (Figure 2-4 ■). The loophole is that this section applies only to transactions adopted under HIPAA.

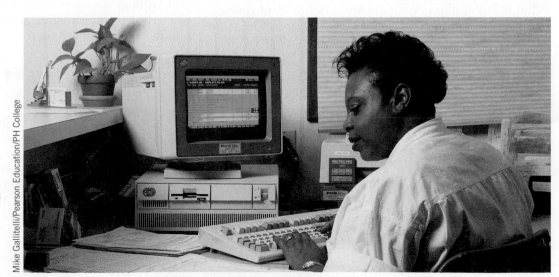

Figure 2-4 ■ The electronic transmission and storage of medical records is protected by the Health Insurance Portability And Accountability Act.

Mike Gallitelli/Pearson Education/PH College

4. **Privacy and confidentiality standards**—This section limits nonconsensual use and release of private health information (now called *protected health information*). It gives patients new rights to access their medical records and to be informed of others who have accessed them. It also restricts most disclosure of health information to the minimum required for the intended purpose. This section also developed new civil and criminal sanctions for the improper use or disclosure of health information and new requirements for access to records by researchers and others.

FDA MODERNIZATION ACT OF 1997

The FDA Modernization Act of 1997 reformed the regulation of cosmetics, food, and medical products by focusing mostly on safe pharmacy compounding, user fees, food safety, and medical devices. Under this act, patients now have increased access to experimental drugs and devices. It also gave manufacturers 6-month extensions on new pediatric drugs, with drug trial test data on file and mandated risk assessment reviews of any foods or drugs containing mercury. This act, also known as the FDAMA, changed the promotion of off-label drugs and required legend drugs to be packaged with the "Rx" symbol included. This act was intended to speed up the drug approval process and address changing technologies and drug marketing.

MEDICARE PRESCRIPTION DRUG, IMPROVEMENT, AND MODERNIZATION ACT OF 2003

The Medicare Prescription Drug, Improvement, and Modernization Act of 2003 is also known as the Medicare Modernization Act (MMA), and it overhauled Medicare more than any other act. It introduced subsidies for prescription drugs as well as tax breaks. It presented new Medicare "Advantage" plans that offered patients better choices about care, providers, coverage, and federal reimbursements. It also established a partially privatized Medicare system, offered pretax medical savings accounts, and raised certain fees for older adults whose net worth is over a certain amount. Overall, this act was designed to help senior citizens by reducing drug costs and to help employers offer drug benefits to their employers.

This act established Medicare Part D, which may be obtained either by joining a prescription drug plan (PDP) or a Medicare Advantage (MA) plan. This is a voluntary program that operates on an annual renewal basis, with varied plans and co-payment amounts. Part D only covers drugs that are approved by the FDA and does not cover people who already have Medicare Part A or B coverage.

COMBAT METHAMPHETAMINE EPIDEMIC ACT OF 2005

The Combat Methamphetamine Epidemic Act of 2005 is focused on the provisions of the Patriot Act extension that dealt with methamphetamine provisions. It was designed to stop illegal use of methamphetamine and regulated trafficking of this drug (and certain others, such as crack cocaine) when these activities are used to finance terrorism. The government can now confiscate the personal property of anyone involved in such activities. Drugs that fall under this act's jurisdiction must be kept behind a counter or in a locked case. It also limits sales of ingredients used to manufacture methamphetamine (ephedrine or pseudoephedrine) to only 9 grams per month per person. To buy these drugs, a customer must provide identification and sign a sales log. Sellers of these drugs must be registered with the U.S. Attorney General's office and receive specialized training.

Federal Regulatory Agencies

The FDA is responsible for cosmetics, medicines, medical devices, radiation-emitting products, food and drugs used for farm animals, domestic and imported food, bottled water, and wine beverages that contain less than 7% alcohol. The DEA oversees controlled substances, including the investigation and prosecution of those who grow or manufacture these substances for illegal distribution. The Centers for Disease Control and Prevention (CDC) oversees foods and foodborne diseases.

FOOD AND DRUG ADMINISTRATION

The FDA is a branch of the U.S. Department of Health and Human Services and controls all drugs for legal use. All drug administration laws are initiated, implemented, and enforced by the FDA.

DRUG ENFORCEMENT ADMINISTRATION

The DEA enforces controlled substance laws and regulations and prosecutes individuals (and organizations) who grow, manufacture, or distribute illegal substances. It also targets people who use violence in the coercion of others to help them in their illegal activities and distributes information about illegal substances to educate the public. The DEA also works with other governments to assist global drug trafficking enforcement.

CENTERS FOR DISEASE CONTROL AND PREVENTION

The CDC provides statistics and information to health professionals about the treatment of common and rare diseases worldwide. Its services include investigating, identifying, preventing, and controlling disease. The CDC's primary function is to issue infection control regulations. Established in 1946 as the Communicable Disease Center, the CDC changed its name to the Centers for Disease Control in 1970, with the words "and Prevention" added in 1992. However, Congress requested that the initials "CDC" remain the same. This agency has been actively involved in the war against AIDS and HIV.

* Apply Your Knowledge 2.3

The following questions focus on what you have just learned about OSHA, HIPAA, and federal regulatory agencies.

CRITICAL THINKING

1. Why must all health professionals obey OSHA guidelines?
2. Describe HIPAA and its four parts.
3. Compare the functions of the FDA, DEA, and CDC.
4. Explain the four parts of Medicare.
5. Describe the Combat Methamphetamine Epidemic Act.

State Law

State governments, not the federal government, are the main regulators of laws that regulate pharmacy practice. Each state is concerned with protecting the health, safety, and welfare of its citizens. Pharmacy laws, although differing from state to state, are based on the same goals, objectives, and principles of pharmaceutical practice.

State law requires minimal qualifications for individuals involved with pharmacy practice—no one may practice pharmacy without a license except those exempted by the state legislation that creates the licensing requirement. Licensed individuals must successfully complete state board of pharmacy requirements. These boards are part of the licensing division of state health departments.

Pharmacy licensure is difficult to gain and not easily revoked. After due process and for just cause as set out in the appropriate legislation, the state can suspend, revoke, or terminate a pharmacist's license. The practice of licensed pharmacists is safeguarded by federal and state constitutions as a property right. Certificates of registration are granted for 1 or 2 years in most states.

Health-care providers must use prescription pads only for writing prescriptions for medications. Prescription pads must be secured at all times. Some states allow medication administration by allied health professionals; other states do not. Therefore, health-care workers must know the laws of the state in which they work. It is also important to understand the rulings that apply to phoning in prescriptions to pharmacists.

Certificates of registration, or pharmacy licenses, can be cancelled or revoked only under special circumstances. Depending on the type of state law violation, a pharmacist's license may be suspended or revoked permanently. An example is the dispensing of a scheduled drug without a prescription or proper documentation. The National Association of Boards of Pharmacy (NABP) developed a Model State Pharmacy Practice Act (MSPPA), which offers flexibility to the states that adopt it but provides a greater degree of uniformity between states.

Ethics in Clinical and Pharmacy Practice

Ethics are standards of behavior and include concepts of right and wrong beyond what legal considerations are in any given situation. Health-care professionals are expected to act in ways that reflect society's ideas of right and wrong even if such behavior is not enforced by law. Allied health professionals must use confidentiality in all areas concerning medications and their administration.

Although drug companies, by law, may provide free supplies of medications to physicians for promoting sales (Figure 2-5 ■), these samples may not be sold.

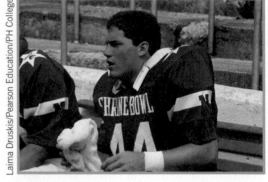

Michal Heron/Pearson Education/PH College

A sample drug is marked "sample," bears a federal legend (Rx), and requires a prescription. Some manufacturers may also provide drug coupons that discount the price of a specific prescribed drug, but these coupons cannot be sold or traded. Samples should be stored immediately where they are not accessible to patients and organized by indication and expiration date. Health-care professionals may not legally supply medicine samples to family, friends, or themselves. Other ethical considerations cover pharmacists' or other health-care providers' professional relationships with their patients and dispensing of medications that may be against their personal beliefs.

Figure 2-5 ■ Pharmaceutical company representatives provide drug samples to physician offices. These samples may not be sold.

PRACTICAL SCENARIO 1

Anabolic steroids are very popular among today's athletes who want to gain a competitive edge over others by building muscle. The evening news often contains stories of professional athletes testing positive for anabolic steroids. One such 20-year-old male athlete illegally obtained anabolic steroids from another athlete at his school and began injecting them regularly to improve his performance in college football. During the season, he collapsed on the field and later died.

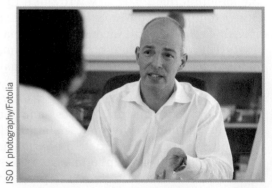

Laima Druskis/Pearson Education/PH College

Critical Thinking Questions

1.   What are the most important side effects of using anabolic steroids?
2.   What types of heart conditions are linked to the use of anabolic steroids?

PRACTICAL SCENARIO 2

Paula, a medical assistant, has worked for a family practitioner for 7 years. In the past, she has been allowed to contact the pharmacy for prescription refills for patients. Her boyfriend has been experiencing back pain after a disc herniation. Paula, wanting to help, writes several prescriptions over a 6-month period for a scheduled drug to relieve his pain. The pharmacist notices the frequency of these prescriptions and calls the family practitioner to ask if he is aware of this patient. The family practitioner says he is not. He confronts Paula, who admits the patient is her boyfriend and that she has been writing the prescriptions herself and stamping them with the family practitioner's signature.

ISO K photography/Fotolia

Critical Thinking Questions

1.   What are the likely consequences of Paula's actions?
2.   What organization or agency oversees scheduled drugs?

Chapter Capsule

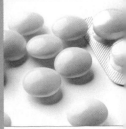

This section repeats the objectives from the beginning of the chapter and then provides a summary of the most important concepts for that objective. Use this section as a quick review and to check your knowledge.

Objective 1: Discuss legal and ethical requirements regarding the use, dispensing, and administration of medications.

- Federal regulations: protect consumers from potential for harm from both legal and illicit drugs
- FDA: controls all drug administration laws

Objective 2: Explain how the need for drug control evolved.

- Absence of laws requiring drug testing or drug labeling in the early nineteenth century
- Pure Food and Drug Act of 1906: developed to require safety and efficacy of drugs

Objective 3: Discuss the poisoning disaster that led to legislation requiring testing for the purity, strength, effectiveness, safety, and packaging quality of drugs.

- Sulfanilamide mixed with diethylene glycol, sold to the public in liquid form for upper respiratory infections: resulted in 107 reported deaths
- Food, Drug, and Cosmetic Act, created in 1938: gave the FDA authority to approve or deny new drug applications
- FDA: approves investigational use of drugs on humans; ensures safety and efficacy of all approved drugs

Objective 4: Explain the major points of the thalidomide disaster of 1962.

- Thalidomide (used in other countries) was tested for marketing in the United States as a sleeping pill or antinausea medication for pregnant women
- Discovery of birth defects (severe deformities) in the children of many women of other countries who took thalidomide during their first trimester of pregnancy
- Kefauver–Harris Amendment passed in 1962: limited thalidomide use to treatment of leprosy, bone marrow transplantation, AIDS, and some other conditions

Objective 5: List the provisions of the Controlled Substances Act.

- Provides increased research into and prevention of drug abuse and drug dependence
- Provides treatment and rehabilitation of drug abusers and drug-dependent persons
- Regulates the manufacture, distribution, and dispensing of controlled substances
- Applies schedules to drugs with potential for causing drug dependence, abuse, or both

Objective 6: Differentiate between each of the five schedules for controlled substances.

- Schedule I—High abuse potential; not accepted for medical use in the United States
- Schedule II—High abuse potential; accepted for medical use in the United States

- Schedule III—Low to moderate abuse potential; accepted for medical use in the United States
- Schedule IV—Slight abuse potential; accepted for medical use in the United States
- Schedule V—Lowest abuse potential of all; includes OTC preparations

Objective 7: Define *orphan drug* and then list some examples.

- Used to treat diseases that affect fewer than 200,000 people in the United States
- Provides a 7-year monopoly on the sale and breaks on taxes given to manufacturers
- 100 orphan drugs approved, including those used to treat AIDS, cystic fibrosis, uncontrolled rapid blinking, and snake bites

Objective 8: Discuss the federal regulatory agencies that deal with food, drugs, and disease control.

- Food and Drug Administration (FDA): controls drugs for legal use
- Drug Enforcement Administration (DEA): enforces controlled substance laws, regulations, and more
- Centers for Disease Control and Prevention (CDC):

  - Provides statistics and information about the treatment of common and rare diseases worldwide
  - Provides facilities and services for investigating, identifying, preventing, and controlling disease
  - Issues infection control regulations

Objective 9: Explain which level of government primarily controls pharmacy licensure.

- States: main regulators of laws governing pharmacy practice
- Licensing required of practicing pharmacies except if exempted by state legislation that creates licensing requirements

Objective 10: Define *ethics* as it relates to pharmacology.

- Expectation of health-care professionals to act in ways that reflect society's ideas of right and wrong even if such behavior is not enforced by law
- Guarantee of confidentiality in all areas that concern medications and their administration
- Security and proper use of prescription pads

 Internet Sites of Interest

- The National Institutes of Health (NIH) website—**www.nlm.nih.gov**—provides information on ethical considerations in research studies. Search for "ethics."
- The abuse of pain medications has led some health-care providers to limit the appropriate use of pain medications in patients who need them. See a discussion among government agents about this issue at: **www.usdoj.gov/dea/pubs/pressrel/pr102301.html**
- Read about laws enforced by the FDA at: **www.fda.gov/opacom/laws**

- Find information about the Orphan Drug Act at: **www.fda.gov/orphan/oda.htm**
- Access an overview of the FDA at:
  www.emedicinehealth.com/fda_overview/article_em.htm

PEARSON
myhealthprofessionskit™

Go to www.myhealthprofessionskit.com to access the Companion Website created for this textbook. Simply select "Basic Health Science" from the choice of disciplines. Find this book and then log in using your username and password to access interactive learning games, assessment questions, animations, and more.

Chapter 3

Terminology, Abbreviations, and Dispensing Prescriptions

Chapter Objectives

After completing this chapter, you should be able to:

1. Explain abbreviations used in pharmacology.
2. Describe how drugs are named.
3. Describe five sources of drug derivation.
4. Explain preparations of oral drugs.
5. Define *solid drug forms*.
6. Describe topical drugs.
7. Explain gaseous drugs.
8. Describe topical drugs and define transdermal patches.
9. List seven component parts of a prescription.
10. Define *standing orders*.

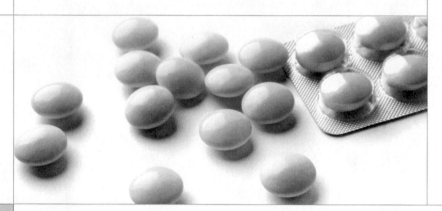

Key Terms

alkaloids (AL-kuh-loyds) (page 37)
approved name (page 36)
chemical name (page 36)

generic name (page 36)
glycoside (GLY-ko-side) (page 37)
parenteral (puh-REN-teh-rul) (page 38)

proprietary name (page 36)
sustained release (page 38)
trade name (page 36)

Introduction

Learning the language of medicine is essential for all fields of the health-care industry. Medical terminology originated primarily from Greek and Latin prefixes, roots, and suffixes, which are known as *word parts.* There are also new terms that are derived from the universal language of English. A majority of terms related to surgery and diagnosis have Greek origins, and most anatomic terms come from Latin origins. To learn medical terminology, it is very helpful to memorize word parts and rules for creating words. By understanding how word parts are combined, it is possible to determine the meanings of medical words.

Health-care professionals who are involved with pharmacology must be familiar with word building, common medical terms, and abbreviations. They must understand general pharmacology terms and concepts.

In this chapter, terminology and abbreviations, drug names, sources of drugs, drug forms, and drug dispensing are reviewed in detail.

Table 3-1 ■ Some Common General Prefixes

PREFIX	MEANING	EXAMPLE
alb-	white	albinism
ante-	before	antepartum
anti-	against	antibiotic
bi-	two, both	bilateral
bio-	life	biology
ecto-	outside	ectoplasm
endo-	into, within	endoscopic
epi-	upon, above	epidermic
multi-	many	multinuclear
myo-	muscle	myocarditis
poly-	many	polyarthritis
semi-	half	semiconscious
ultra-	beyond, excessive	ultrasound

Pharmaceutical Terminology

Allied health-care professionals who must deal with pharmaceutical agents need to be familiar with medical and pharmaceutical terminology. They must understand roots, prefixes, suffixes, and combining vowels.

A *root* is the main part of a word that gives the word its central meaning. It is the basic foundation of a word that can be made more complex through the addition of other word parts. A *prefix* is a structure at the beginning of a word that modifies the meaning of the root; Table 3-1 ■ shows some common general prefixes. A *suffix* is a word ending that modifies the meaning of the root; Table 3-2 ■ gives some common general suffixes.

Medical terms are formed from many different word parts. These parts are often joined by vowels known as *combining vowels.* The most common combining vowel is the letter *o* and, occasionally, the letter *i.* For example, *o* serves as a combining vowel in the term *hyperlipoproteinemia* (hyper / lip / o / protein / emia).

Table 3-2 ■ Some Common General Suffixes

SUFFIX	MEANING	EXAMPLE
-ectomy	excision, removal	hysterectomy
-emesis	vomit	hyperemesis
-gram	record	electrocardiogram
-ism	condition	cryptorchidism
-itis	inflammation	appendicitis
-logy	study of	microbiology
-oma	tumor	carcinoma
-pathy	disease	hemopathy
-phobia	abnormal fear	photophobia
-stomy	surgical creation of a new opening	colostomy
-tomy	incision, cutting	phlebotomy

✳ Apply Your Knowledge 3.1

The following questions focus on what you have just learned about pharmaceutical terminology.

CRITICAL THINKING

1. List the most common combining vowels.

2. Define the terms *prefix, root,* and *suffix.*

3. What are the meanings of the terms *cryptorchidism, hemopathy, photophobia,* and *colostomy?*

4. Describe the meanings of the prefixes *ante-, alb-, semi-, epi-,* and *ecto-.*

Abbreviations Used in Pharmacology

Abbreviations are shortened forms of words representing commonly used medical terms. Many such abbreviations are used in all areas of health-care practice. It is essential for health-care professionals to be familiar with the most common abbreviations used for writing prescriptions (Table 3-3 ■), the abbreviations associated with various measurements (Table 3-4 ■), and general medical abbreviations (Table 3-5 ■).

Table 3-3 ■ Abbreviations Commonly Used in Prescriptions

ABBREVIATION	MEANING	ABBREVIATION	MEANING
āā, aa	of each	per	through or by
Ac	before meals	p.m., PM	afternoon
Ad	to, up to	po, PO	by mouth
ad lib	as desired	PR	through the rectum
a.m., AM	morning	prn, PRN	as needed
amt	amount	PULV	powder
aq	water	q	every
bid, BID	twice a day	q2h	every 2 hours
bin	twice a night	qh	every hour
c̄ (with straight line)	with	qid, QID	four times a day
cap, caps	capsule	QN	every night
comp	compound	qs, qv	as much as you wish (sufficient quantity)
d	day	s̄ (with straight line)	without (sine)
dil	dilute	SIG	write on label
disp	dispense	sol	solution
elix	elixir	sos	if necessary
hr	hour	sp	spirits
IM	intramuscular	stat	immediately
inj, INJ	inject	supp	suppository
IV	intravenous	syr	syrup
liq	liquid	tab	tablet
mixt	mixture	tid	three times a day
noct	at night	top	topically
non rep	do not repeat, no refills	tr., tinct	tincture
NPO	nothing by mouth (*nulla per os*)	vo	verbal order
oint	ointment	X	multiplied by
pc	after meals		

Note: See Internet Sites of Interest at the end of this chapter for the Institute for Safe Medical Practices (ISMP) website, which provides a list of medical abbreviations that are frequently misinterpreted and involved in harmful errors and thus should not be used.

Table 3-4 ■ Abbreviations Commonly Used for Measurements

ABBREVIATION	MEANING	ABBREVIATION	MEANING
°C	Celsius	mEq	milliequivalent
cm	centimeter (2.5 cm = 1 in)	mg	milligram
°F	Fahrenheit	mL	milliliter
fl	fluid	No.	number
g, gm	gram	oz	ounce
gtt	drops	T	temperature
L	liter	Tbs, Tbsp	tablespoon
lb	pound	tsp	teaspoon
kg	kilogram (1 kg = 2.2 lb)	w/v	weight in volume
mcg	microgram		

Table 3-5 ■ General Medical Abbreviations

ABBREVIATION	MEANING	ABBREVIATION	MEANING
AP	anterior–posterior	Dx	diagnosis
BE	barium enema	ECG	electrocardiogram
BP	blood pressure	EEG	electroencephalogram
Bx	biopsy	EENT	eyes, ears, nose, throat
C	carbon	FBS	fasting blood sugar
C&S	culture & sensitivity	Fe	iron
c/o	complains of	FUO	fever of unknown origin
Ca	calcium, cancer	GI	gastrointestinal
CAD	coronary artery disease	GU	genitourinary
cath.	catheter	Gyn	gynecology
CBC	complete blood count	H	hydrogen
CC	chief complaint	H&P	history and physical
CHF	congestive heart failure	HBV	hepatitis B virus
CO	carbon dioxide	HCT	hematocrit
COPD	chronic obstructive pulmonary disease	Hg	mercury
CVA	cerebrovascular accident	Hgb	hemoglobin
CXR	chest x-ray	Hib	*Haemophilus influenzae* type B
D&C	dilatation & curettage	Hx, hx	history
DOB	date of birth	I	iodine
DPT	diphtheria–pertussis–tetanus	IM	intramuscular

(continued)

Table 3-5 ■ General Medical Abbreviations (*continued*)

ABBREVIATION	MEANING	ABBREVIATION	MEANING
IUD	intrauterine device	R/O	rule out
IV	intravenous	RBC	red blood cell
K	potassium	ROM	range of motion
LMP	last menstrual period	SOB	shortness of breath
MI	myocardial infarction	T	temperature
MMR	measles–mumps–rubella	TIA	transient ischemic attack
N	nitrogen	Tx	treatment
Na	sodium	UA	urinalysis
OB	obstetrics	UTI	urinary tract infection
P	pulse	VS, vs	vital signs
PERRLA	pupils equal, round, reactive to light and accommodation	WBC	white blood cell
PO	orally	WNL	within normal limits
Pt	patient	wt	weight
R	respirations, right	y/o, yo	years old
r	take		

✳ Apply Your Knowledge 3.2

The following questions focus on what you have just learned about abbreviations used in pharmacology.

CRITICAL THINKING

1. What terms do the following abbreviations represent: ad, aq, liq, per, QN, supp, and x?
2. What terms correspond to these abbreviations: gtt, fl, mcg, kg, Bx, CVA, Dx, and HBV?
3. What are the abbreviations for potassium, nitrogen, sodium, iodine, and iron?
4. What are the abbreviations for catheter, electrocardiogram, genitourinary, and hemoglobin?
5. What are the abbreviations for intrauterine device, weight, chest x-ray, and microgram?

Drug Names

Each drug may have three different types of names: the **chemical name** (describing the chemical makeup of a drug), the generic name (also called **approved name** or *nonproprietary name*), and the **proprietary name** (also called *brand* or **trade name**). For example, the chemical name of amoxicillin, a commonly prescribed antibacterial antibiotic, is hydroxybenzyl penicillin. Its **generic name** (also known as a drug's *official* or *approved name*) is amoxicillin, a name that is much simpler than its chemical name. All drugs have a generic name, which is not protected by trademark. Amoxicillin is marketed under dozens of proprietary names, including

Alphamox, Amohexal, and Amoxil. This proprietary name is assigned by the manufacturer and is protected by trademark. Because there is only one generic name per drug, the use of a drug's generic name is encouraged over trade names to avoid confusion. Drugs are also classified by their therapeutic use. For example, Tylenol is the brand name of the generic drug acetaminophen, which is classified as an analgesic and an antipyretic agent.

Sources of Drug Derivation

There are basically five sources of drugs: (1) plants, (2) animals (including humans), (3) minerals or mineral products, (4) synthetics (chemical substances), and (5) engineered (investigational) sources. Today, chemicals and even human tissues, such as those used in stem-cell therapy, can be manipulated to create new drug sources.

PLANTS

Plant sources are grouped by their physical and chemical properties. **Alkaloids** are organic nitrogen-containing compounds that are alkaline and usually bitter tasting. They are combined with acids to make a salt. Atropine, nicotine, and morphine are examples of these chemical compounds. An important cardiac **glycoside** (an organic compound that yields sugar and nonsugar substances when hydrolyzed) is digoxin. Digoxin is made from digitalis, a derivative of the foxglove plant.

HUMANS AND OTHER ANIMALS

Animal sources, such as the body fluids and glands of animals, can act as drugs. The drugs obtained from animal sources include such hormones as adrenaline, insulin, and thyroid. Enzymes such as pancreatin and pepsin are also from animal sources.

MINERALS

Minerals from the earth and soil are used to provide inorganic materials unavailable from plants and animals. They are used as they occur in nature. Examples include sodium, iodine, potassium, iron, and gold, which are used to prepare medications. Sodium chloride (table salt) is one of the best-known examples in this group. Gold is prescribed to prevent severe rheumatoid arthritis, and coal tar is used to treat seborrheic dermatitis and psoriasis.

SYNTHETIC SOURCES

Certain drugs may come from living organisms (organic substances) or nonliving materials (inorganic substances). These drugs are known as synthetic or manufactured drugs. They have evolved from the application of chemistry, biology, and computer technology. Because they do not exist in nature, these medications come from artificial substances. Examples of synthetic drugs include oral contraceptives, meperidine (Demerol), and sulfonamides. Certain organic drugs, such as penicillin, are semisynthetic and are made by altering their natural compounds or elements. Some drugs are both organic and inorganic, such as propylthiouracil, which is an antithyroid hormone.

ENGINEERED SOURCES

The newest area of drug origin is gene splicing, or *genetic engineering*. The newer forms of insulin for use in humans have been produced by this technique. A tissue plasminogen activator for heart attack victims is also being developed via this method. Growth hormones (bovine or porcine somatotropin) are being produced from bacteria that have received the appropriate gene (human, cow, or pig). Another new and experimental treatment is gene therapy, which involves replacing a gene that is missing or not functioning correctly with the correct gene. The first successful gene therapy was used in 1990 to treat an immune system defect in children. Genetically engineered products, featuring modified DNA, are being produced to treat malignant brain tumors, cystic fibrosis, and HIV. The public seems to be greatly interested in this new way of developing a wide range of new drugs.

Drug Development

In the United States, the timeline for a drug to be developed and brought to market typically takes between 7 and 15 years. The Food and Drug Administration (FDA) oversees this process. Before a drug can be approved by the FDA, it must go through four phases of drug product development, as follows:

✳ Stage 1: Preclinical investigation
  • Animal pharmacology and toxicology data are obtained over 1 to 3 years.
  • An investigational new drug (IND) application for human testing is submitted to the FDA.

✳ Stage 2: Clinical investigation
  • Clinical phase trials, involving human test participants, are conducted in three different phases, over 2 to 10 years, to determine drug toxicity and tolerance.
  • If the drug is effective without causing serious adverse effects, the approval process may be accelerated or the drug may even be used for treatment in special cases, although close monitoring is required.

✳ Stage 3: Investigational new drug review
  • A final phase of clinical trials and testing may continue for from 2 months to 7 years based on the preclinical results.
  • If the IND is approved, the process continues to stage 4; if it is rejected, the process stops until all concerns are addressed.

✳ Stage 4: Postmarketing studies
  • Testing in humans is continued to check for any new adverse effects in larger, more diverse populations.
  • This is because some adverse effects take longer to appear and are not identified until the drug is used by a larger number of patients.

Removal of a Drug from the Market

In certain situations, the FDA may require that a drug be removed from the market and its use be discontinued. This may be because of a variety of reasons, including improper manufacturing, harmful ingredients, the development of adverse effects not seen in the drug development process, or lack of effectiveness. A drug may be recalled at any time after it has been approved. On an annual basis, the FDA holds public meetings to address comments from health professionals and patients concerning the safety and effectiveness of drugs.

Black Box Warnings

A *black box warning* is the most severe warning from the FDA about a drug. It appears on the prescription label to alert all health-care providers and patients about potentially harmful adverse effects of the drug. The FDA requires a black box warning for each of the following situations:

✳ The medication may cause serious undesirable effects (such as a fatal, life-threatening, or permanently disabling adverse reaction) compared with the potential benefit from the drug.

✳ A serious adverse reaction can be prevented, reduced in frequency, or reduced in severity by proper use of the drug. For example, a medication may be safe for adults but not for children.

Drug Forms

Pharmaceutics is the science of formulating drugs into such different types of preparations as tablets, ointments, injectable solutions, or eye drops. It also includes studying the ways in which various drug forms influence pharmacokinetic and pharmacodynamic activities of the active drug.

Many drugs are available in different formulations. This variety assists the prescriber in choosing a formulation that is best suited for the individual patient and route of administration. Formulations, such as oral pills and tablets, injectable medications, or rectally or vaginally administered drugs, also determine whether a drug acts locally or is absorbed into the systemic circulation. Failure to administer the drug in the correct form results in a medication error. Using an incorrect form can also cause damage to body cells. Therefore, allied health-care professionals need to learn about the various drug preparations and their uses. Drug dosage forms are classified according to their physical state (for example, liquid or solid) and chemical composition. Various forms of drug preparations allow for oral, topical, mucous membrane, or **parenteral** use (introduction of a drug outside of the gastrointestinal [GI] tract; generally in injectable form) and for miscellaneous drug delivery systems.

Some substances can undergo a change of state or phase—from solid to liquid (melting) or from liquid to gas (vaporization). Certain drugs are soluble in water, some are soluble in alcohol, and others are soluble in a mixture of liquids.

PREPARATIONS FOR ORAL USE

An oral drug may appear in solid form (for example, tablets, capsules, or powders) or liquid form (solutions, elixirs, or suspensions). Disintegration of the solid dose form must occur before *dissolution,* a process by which a drug goes into solution and becomes available for absorption. The form of drug dose is important because the more rapid the rate of dissolution, the more readily the compound crosses the cell membrane and is absorbed into the systemic circulation to be circulated to the site where it acts. Oral drugs in liquid form are therefore more rapidly available for GI absorption than those in solid form.

Solid Drugs

The route for administering a medication depends on its form, its properties, and the effect desired. Solid forms of drugs are widely used in drug treatment. The solid forms are also a convenient way to take unpleasant-tasting or irritating drugs. Solid drugs include pills, tablets, capsules, **sustained-release** tablets and capsules (that are specially coated so they dissolve at specific times), enteric-coated tablets and capsules, caplets, gelcaps, powders, granules, and troches or lozenges (Figure 3-1 ■). Some plasters are also considered to be solid drugs, although they are generally semisolids.

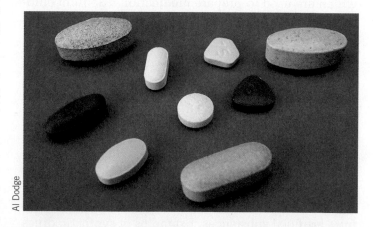

Figure 3-1 ■ Solid drug forms.

PILLS

A single-dose unit of medicine made by mixing the powdered drug with a liquid, such as syrup, and rolling it into a round or oval shape is called a *pill.*

TABLETS

A *tablet* is a pharmaceutical preparation made by compressing the powdered form of a drug and bulk-filling material under high pressure (Figure 3-2 ■). Tablets may appear as simple white disks or may be multilayered or coated with a film to mask an unpleasant taste. Special

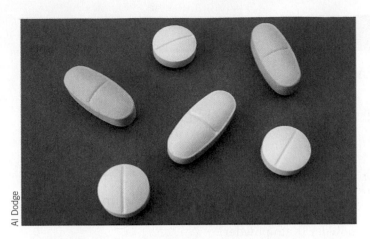

Figure 3-2 ■ Examples of tablets.

forms of tablets include sublingual tablets and enteric-coated tablets. Most tablets are intended to be swallowed whole for dissolution and absorption in the GI tract. Some are intended to be dissolved in the mouth, dissolved in water, or inserted as suppositories. Many times, tablets are mistakenly called pills. Tablets come in various sizes, shapes, colors, and compositions. The various forms of tablets include chewable, sublingual, buccal, enteric-coated, and buffered tablets. Chewable tablets contain a flavored or sugar base and must be chewed. They are commonly used for antacids and antiflatulents and for children who cannot swallow medication. Sublingual tablets must be dissolved under the tongue for rapid absorption; an example is nitroglycerin for angina pectoris. Buccal tablets are placed between the cheek and the gum until they are dissolved and absorbed.

CAPSULES

A *capsule* is a medication dosage form in which the drug is contained in an external shell (Figure 3-3 ■). Capsule shells are usually made of a hard cylindrical gelatin and enclose or encapsulate powder, granules, liquids, or some combinations of these. Liquids may be placed in soft gelatin capsules; examples are vitamin E capsules and cod liver oil capsules. They are used when medications have an unpleasant odor or taste. Capsules can be pulled apart, and the entire contents can be added as powder to food for individuals who have difficulty swallowing. Some forms of capsules come with a controlled-release dosage and are used over a defined period of time (sustained-release [SR] or timed-release capsules). These drugs should *never* be crushed or dissolved because this would negate their timed-release action.

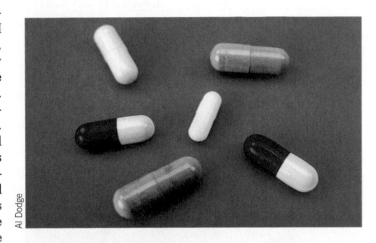

Figure 3-3 ■ Examples of capsules.

Focus on Geriatrics

Coated Aspirin Tablets

Some patients, particularly elderly people who have stomach ulcers, cannot take certain medications, such as aspirin. Therefore, these patients should be given enteric-coated aspirin tablets.

SUSTAINED-RELEASE TABLETS AND CAPSULES

Sustained-release drug forms contain several doses of a drug. The doses have special coatings that dissolve at different rates; therefore, the drug is released into the digestive system gradually. Sustained-release drugs are referred to as *delayed release* and *timed release*. An example is diltiazem (Cardizem SR), a calcium channel blocker used in the treatment of angina pectoris and hypertension.

ENTERIC-COATED TABLETS AND CAPSULES

Some tablets and capsules are covered by a special coating that keeps them from dissolving in the stomach, which contains hydrochloric acid. These drugs do not dissolve until they reach the intestine. Therefore, the strength of these drugs remains undiluted as they pass through the stomach, providing a delayed action that is desirable. An example is Ecotrin, a nonnarcotic analgesic used for pain, an antipyretic used for fever, and a nonsteroidal anti-inflammatory used in the treatment of arthritis. Also important is the fact that enteric coatings may prevent nausea and vomiting that some drugs can induce from dissolving in the stomach. Furthermore, enteric coatings prevent decomposition of chemically sensitive drugs (for example, penicillin G and erythromycin) by gastric secretions. These two drugs are examples of substances that are unstable in the acid pH of the stomach.

Focus Point

Administering Enteric-Coated Tablets

Do not crush or mix enteric-coated tablets or capsules into liquids or foods because it will destroy the enteric coating. This would result in the drug's being released into the stomach instead of the small intestine.

CAPLETS

A caplet is shaped like a capsule but has the form of a tablet. The shape and film-coated covering make swallowing easier.

GELCAPS

A *gelcap* is an oil-based medication that is enclosed in a soft gelatin capsule (Figure 3-4 ■).

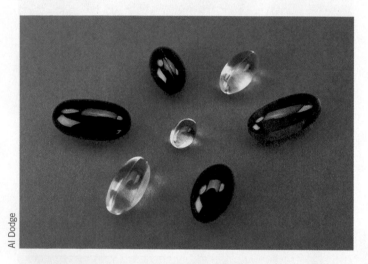

Al Dodge

Figure 3-4 ■ Examples of gelcaps.

POWDERS

A drug that is dried and ground into fine particles is called a *powder*. An example is potassium chloride powder (Kato powder).

GRANULES

A small pill, usually accompanied by many others encased within a gelatin capsule, is called a *granule*. In most cases, granules within capsules are specially coated to gradually release medication over an extended period.

TROCHES OR LOZENGES

A hard or semisolid dosage form containing a medication intended for local application in the mouth or throat is called a *troche* or *lozenge*. These are flattened disks. Typically, a troche is placed on the tongue or between the cheek and gum and left in place until it dissolves. The medications most commonly administered by means of troches include cough suppressants and treatments for sore throat.

Liquid Drugs

Liquid preparations include drugs that have been dissolved or suspended. Examples of liquid drugs are syrups, solutions, elixirs, fluidextracts, mixtures and suspensions, tinctures, emulsions, spirits or essences, liniments, gels or jellies, lotions, most aerosols, and magmas.

Focus on Pediatrics

Liquid Drugs

Infants and young children are not able to take solid drug forms, such as tablets or capsules. Therefore, they should be given liquid drugs.

SYRUPS AND LINCTUSES

Aqueous solutions containing a high concentration of sugars, syrups, and linctuses may or may not have medical substances added (for example, simple syrup and ipecac syrup).

SOLUTIONS

A *solution* is a drug or drugs dissolved in an appropriate solvent. Examples of solutions include elixirs, fluidextracts, spirits, and tinctures, which are highly concentrated forms of drugs.

Elixirs

A drug vehicle that consists of water, alcohol, and sugar is known as an *elixir*. It may or may not be aromatic and may or may not have active medical properties. Their alcohol content makes elixirs convenient liquid dosage forms for many drugs that are only slightly soluble in water. In these cases, the drug is first dissolved in alcohol, and the other elixir components are added. All elixirs contain alcohol (for example, terpin hydrate elixir and phenobarbital elixir). Elixirs differ from tinctures in that they are sweetened. They should be used with caution in patients with diabetes or a history of alcohol abuse. Some pediatric medications retain the name of *elixirs,* although they no longer contain alcohol.

Fluidextracts

A concentrated solution of a drug removed from a plant source by mixing ground parts of the plant with a suitable solvent, usually alcohol, and then separating the plant residue from the solvent is called a *fluidextract.* Typically, 1 mL contains 1 g of the drug. Fluidextracts are not intended to be administered directly to a patient. Instead, they are prescribed to provide a source of drug in the manufacture of final dosage forms. Only vegetable drugs are used (for example, glycyrrhiza fluidextract).

Mixtures and Suspensions

In a *mixture* or a *suspension,* an agent is mixed with a liquid but not dissolved. These preparations must be shaken before being taken by or administered to the patient. Examples include chlorpheniramine/pseudoephedrine (mixture) and betamethasone (suspension).

Tinctures

A *tincture* is an alcoholic preparation of a soluble drug, usually from a plant source. In some cases, the solution may also contain water (for example, digitalis tincture and iodine tincture).

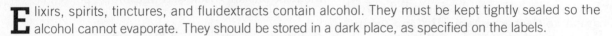

Focus Point

Storing Drugs That Contain Alcohol

Elixirs, spirits, tinctures, and fluidextracts contain alcohol. They must be kept tightly sealed so the alcohol cannot evaporate. They should be stored in a dark place, as specified on the labels.

EMULSIONS

A pharmaceutical preparation in which two agents that cannot ordinarily be combined or mixed is called an *emulsion.* In the typical emulsion, oil is dispersed inside water. Most creams and lotions are emulsions (for example, Petrogalar Plain).

SPIRITS OR ESSENCES

An alcohol-containing liquid that may be used pharmaceutically as a solvent is called a *spirit* or *essence* (for example, essence of peppermint and camphor spirit).

LINIMENTS

Liniments are liquid suspensions for external application to the skin to relieve pain and swelling.

GELS OR JELLIES

A *gel* is a jellylike, semisolid substance in a nonfatty base that may be used for topical application and contains fine particles. An example is the antacid Altern Gel.

LOTIONS

Lotions are suspensions of drugs in a water base for external use. They are patted onto the skin rather than rubbed in. Lotions tend to settle in their containers and thus must be shaken before use. An example is calamine lotion, an antipruritic (anti-itch medication) used to treat exposure to poison ivy.

AEROSOLS

Aerosol medications are frequently delivered by oral inhalers or nebulizers that allow for rapid absorption into the blood circulation. An example is albuterol (Proventil), a bronchodilator used in asthma. Aerosols are generally classified as liquid drugs because they often contain a mist. Those that contain dry powders are considered to be semisolid drugs.

MAGMAS

Magmas contain particles suspended in a liquid and exhibit a more pasty quality in their consistency than other suspensions. The most popular example of a magma is probably milk of magnesia.

INJECTABLE DRUGS

When a rapid response time to medication is desired or if the patient is not able to take the medication orally, parenteral forms of medication can be selected. Injectable drug forms may be available as powders or solutions. A *powder* consists of dry particles of medications. Because the powder itself cannot be injected, it must be reconstituted to a liquid for injection. A diluent, such as sterile water, is added to the powder and then mixed well. A *solution,* as previously explained, is a mixture of one or more substances that are dissolved in another substance. Most solutions are fluids that form a homogeneous mixture. There are a variety of administration routes for parenteral medications, including intra-articular, epidural (into the subarachnoid space), intradermal, subcutaneous, intramuscular (IM), and intravenous (IV).

OTHER FORMS OF MEDICATIONS

There are also other forms of drugs, including topical, ophthalmic, otic, nasal, vaginal, and rectal, as well as drugs that are available in the form of gases.

Topical Drugs

Drugs that are applied to the skin are known as *topical* drugs. They usually provide a local effect. Topical medications include transdermal patches, lotions, ointments, and liniments. Some topical drugs are used to deaden nerves, control itching, or relieve pain and congestion in muscles and joints.

Semisolid Drugs

Semisolid drugs are often used for topical application. These drugs are soft and pliable. Semisolid drugs include creams, ointments, most plasters, and dry-powder aerosols.

CREAMS

A *cream* is a semisolid preparation that is usually white and contains a drug incorporated into both an aqueous base and an oily base. Creams may be applied externally or intravaginally. Examples include benzoyl peroxide (Clearasil, to treat acne topically) and terconazole (Terazol, to treat vulvovaginal candidiasis).

OINTMENTS

An *ointment* is a semisolid preparation in an aqueous or oily base for local protective, soothing, astringent, or transdermal application for systemic effects. Ointments can also be used as anti-inflammatory drugs, topical anesthetics, and antibiotics. Examples are zinc oxide ointment and Bengay ointment.

PLASTERS

A *plaster* is a composition of liquid and powder that hardens when dry. Plasters may be solid but are generally semisolid drugs (for example, salicylic acid plaster used to remove corns).

Transdermal Patches

For a constant, time-released, systemic effect, some medications can be absorbed slowly through the skin. Transdermal patches release a very small amount of a drug at a consistent rate, which is absorbed into the skin and then carried off by the capillary blood supply. Examples of drugs used transdermally include nicotine, estrogen, and nitroglycerin.

Gaseous Drugs (Inhalation Drugs)

Pharmaceutical gases include such anesthetic agents as nitrous oxide and halothane. Compressed gases comprise oxygen or carbon dioxide. Most of the oxygen administered in hospitals for therapy is provided from a central source, where it is stored as a gas or liquid oxygen. Inhalation medications, such as bronchodilators, can be administered through metered-dose inhalers (MDIs) or handheld nebulizers (HHNs). Inhalation medications are discussed in Chapter 28.

Ophthalmic, Otic, and Nasal Drugs

Ophthalmic drugs include drops and ointments that are instilled in the eye for a local effect. They must be sterile and isotonic so they do not cause infections or burning. Ophthalmic medications may be antibiotics, anesthetics, antiviral agents, decongestants, or formulations that provide artificial tears. For the ears, otic medications can control localized infections or inflammation and require very low dosages to be effective. Nasal solutions can treat minor congestion or infection and act locally. They may be in the form of drops or sprays (Figure 3-5A–C ■).

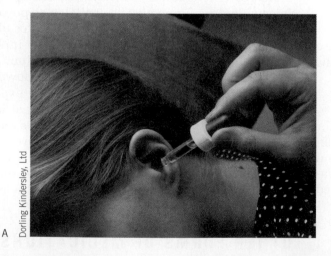
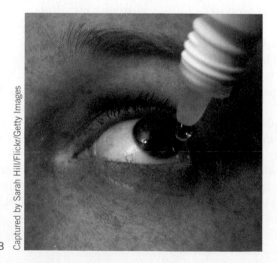

Figure 3-5 ■ Examples of (**A**) otic, (**B**) ophthalmic, and (**C**) nasal drops.

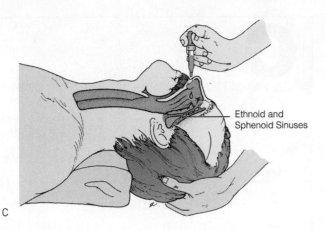

C

Ethnoid and
Sphenoid Sinuses

Figure 3-5 ■ (Continued)

Vaginal Drugs

Vaginal drugs come in a variety of forms, including solutions, creams, tablets, and suppositories. Commonly used vaginal drugs include anti-infectives and contraceptives.

Rectal Drugs

Rectal medications are used for patients with nausea, vomiting, or constipation or for those who may be unconscious and therefore unable to take drugs by mouth. Rectal medications are usually available as cocoa butter or gelatin-based suppositories or as enemas. Most rectal drugs offer systemic effects.

Focus Point

Safe Storage of Drugs

In general, medicines should not be exposed to sunlight, bright light, moisture, or extremes in temperature. Insulin and vaccine preparations should be stored in a refrigerator according to the manufacturer's directions.

✳ Apply Your Knowledge 3.3

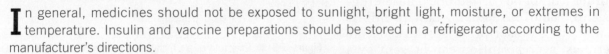

The following questions focus on what you have just learned about drug names, sources of drug derivation, and drug forms.

CRITICAL THINKING
1. List ten examples of solid drugs.
2. Compare caplets, gelcaps, and capsules.
3. Differentiate between syrups and linctuses.
4. Compare emulsions with liniments.
5. Differentiate between creams and ointments.
6. What is the meaning of *sustained release*?
7. What are the differences between tablets and pills?
8. What are enteric-coated tablets and capsules?
9. What is another name for troches? Give an example.
10. What are fluidextracts, tinctures, and magmas?
11. What is the difference between emulsions and lotions?
12. What are the three examples of transdermal patches?

Dispensing Drugs

There are two methods of dispensing drugs: (1) over the counter (OTC) and (2) by prescription. OTC drugs are available to the public for self-medication without a prescription.

An allied health-care professional who is directly involved in patient care should have an understanding of some basic facts regarding OTC drugs. Today, patients are better informed about their personal health care and want to be active participants in health-care decisions. They need facts to make informed choices when using OTC preparations. Most OTC preparations are safe if used as directed on their packages.

Prescription drugs are issued by a licensed prescriber (medical practitioner, dentist, or veterinary surgeon). In some states, nurse practitioners and even pharmacists can write prescriptions with certain restrictions. According to legal terminology, prescription drugs are those that federal law lists as dangerous, powerful, or habit forming and illegal to use except under a prescriber's order. A *prescription* is an order written by an authorized health-care professional for the compounding or dispensing and administration of drugs to a particular patient. A prescription must be signed by a physician or the order cannot be carried out. These drugs have the legend "Caution: Federal Law prohibits dispensing without a prescription" printed on the label. Sometimes, a prescription can be sent by a fax machine, electronically from a physician's computer, or by telephone to the pharmacist. Controlled substances and Schedule I to V drugs are discussed in Chapter 2.

COMPONENTS OF PRESCRIPTIONS

A prescription must be clear, concise, and correct. It has elements that can be correlated with five of the seven nursing rights of medication administration (see Chapter 4 for all seven rights): the patient's name and address (right patient); date written; generic or proprietary drug name (right drug); drug strength and dosage (right dose); route of administration (right route); dosage instruction or frequency of administration (right time); and signature, name, and address of the prescriber (Figure 3-6 ■). Therefore, the component parts of a prescription include:

✳ Name and address of the patient

✳ Address of the prescriber's office

✳ Date

✳ Medication prescribed (*inscription*)

✳ Rx symbol (*superscription*)

✳ Dispensing directions to pharmacist (*subscription*)

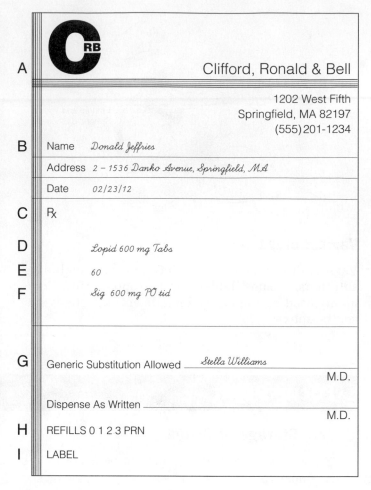

Figure 3-6 ■ Example of a physician's prescription. **(A)** The prescriber's office name, address, and phone number. **(B)** The patient's name, address, and date of prescription. **(C)** The superscription ("Rx" symbol). **(D)** The inscription (names and quantities of ingredients). **(E)** The subscription (tells the pharmacist how many units of medication are needed). **(F)** The signature (Sig), which tells the patient how to take the medication. **(G)** Signature blank(s), where the prescriber signs. **(H)** The repetatur (which tells how many refills are allowed).

✳ Directions for the patient (*signa*)

✳ Refill and special labeling

✳ The prescriber's signature and license or Drug Enforcement Administration (DEA) number

TELEPHONE ORDERS AND STANDING ORDERS

Medications are also sometimes prescribed by physicians who are not present or will not be present when the medication is administered. For example, a physician may telephone a drug prescription (called *telephone orders*) to a pharmacist, who is legally entitled to dispense the prescription, or to a nurse, who is entitled to administer it on oral instructions. In some states, medical assistants are also allowed to do this. The physician must then, as soon as is practicable, write the drug order on a prescription pad, sign it, and post or deliver it to the pharmacy or use the hospital drug chart (see next section of this chapter). A faxed prescription copy can confirm an oral order but is not legally acceptable because the signature has to be original (that is, in the physician's handwriting); the pharmacist must see the original prescription before releasing the drug to the patient. *Standing orders* are written orders sometimes left by physicians as ongoing prescriptions in a hospital, nursing home, or residential-care setting. These orders have no legal validity unless they are properly written, dated, and signed—just as is true for any normal prescription.

HOSPITAL DRUG CHARTS

Prescriptions in hospitals are usually written on a drug chart or physician order sheet and transcribed onto a medication administration record (MAR; Figure 3-7 ■). These can become quite complicated and may run to many pages in a patient's medical record because patients in hospitals are frequently prescribed 10 to 15 drugs during one stay. In the sample chart, note that the users are instructed:

✻ To use approved names for drugs

✻ Not to alter existing orders

✻ To record all instances when drugs are administered or when drugs were not administered, giving reasons

✻ To record IV fluid orders on a separate IV orders chart

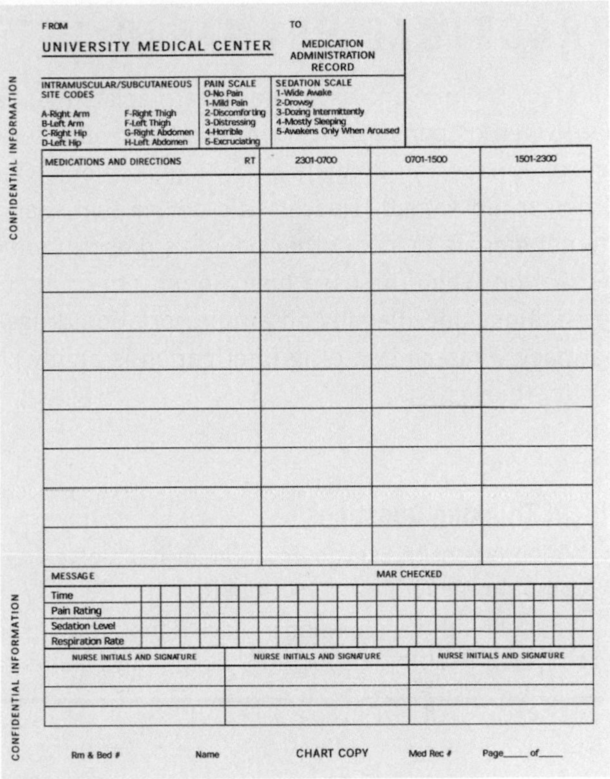
FROM
UNIVERSITY MEDICAL CENTER
TO
MEDICATION ADMINISTRATION RECORD
CONFIDENTIAL INFORMATION

INTRAMUSCULAR/SUBCUTANEOUS SITE CODES		PAIN SCALE	SEDATION SCALE
A-Right Arm	F-Right Thigh	0-No Pain	1-Wide Awake
B-Left Arm	F-Left Thigh	1-Mild Pain	2-Drowsy
C-Right Hip	G-Right Abdomen	2-Discomforting	3-Dozing Intermittently
D-Left Hip	H-Left Abdomen	3-Distressing	4-Mostly Sleeping
		4-Horrible	5-Awakens Only When Aroused
		5-Excruciating	

MEDICATIONS AND DIRECTIONS	RT	2301-0700	0701-1500	1501-2300

MESSAGE
MAR CHECKED
Time
Pain Rating
Sedation Level
Respiration Rate
NURSE INITIALS AND SIGNATURE
NURSE INITIALS AND SIGNATURE
NURSE INITIALS AND SIGNATURE
CONFIDENTIAL INFORMATION
Rm & Bed #
Name
CHART COPY
Med Rec #
Page___ of___

Figure 3-7 ■ Medical administration record as used in many hospitals.

✻ To have nurse-initiated therapy (for example, mild analgesics, laxatives, antacids) countersigned by a physician

Today, the majority of hospitals in the United States (and those in some other countries) use computer charting.

✻ Apply Your Knowledge 3.5

The following questions focus on what you have just learned about dispensing drugs.

1. What are the components of prescriptions?
2. Define the terms *inscription*, *superscription*, and *subscription*.
3. What are standing orders?
4. What are the meanings of the Rx symbol and the term *signa*?
5. What does the abbreviation MAR stand for? Define this.

PRACTICAL SCENARIO 1

Pharmacy technicians as well as pharmacists must always be on guard when dispensing prescriptions for people seeking to defraud their pharmacy and illegally obtain medications. One such individual, a 25-year-old named Brad, used a device that scanned for wireless Internet signals to steal other people's prescription painkiller information. Then, he used his computer to print out altered prescriptions and illegally obtain prescription drugs at his local pharmacy. Prescription drug information is highly prized by today's identity thieves.

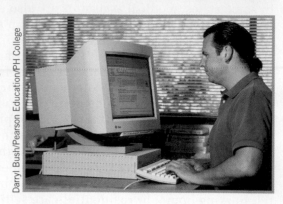

Darryl Bush/Pearson Education/PH College

Critical Thinking Questions

1. Which one of the seven component parts of a prescription could Brad not provide in his computer-generated prescription?
2. What should the pharmacist have done if he or she had any suspicions about the prescription itself or suspected that the physician's signature was a forgery?

PRACTICAL SCENARIO 2

A medical assistant gives some samples of a medication in capsule form to the mother of a 5-year-old patient. Originally, the physician had ordered the powdered form of this medication, which could be dissolved in water or juice. Because the powdered form is unavailable, the medical assistant gives the capsules to the mother and instructs her to simply open and empty them into water or juice for her child.

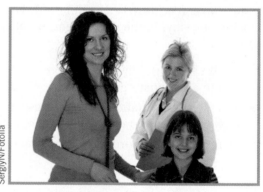

SergiyN/Fotolia

Critical Thinking Questions

1. Do you think that capsules can be opened so their contents can be used in this manner?
2. What was wrong with this medical assistant's actions?

Chapter Capsule

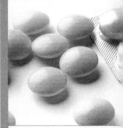

This section repeats the objectives from the beginning of the chapter and then provides a summary of the most important concepts for that objective. Use this section as a quick review and to check your knowledge.

Objective 1: Explain abbreviations used in pharmacology.

■   Abbreviations—shortened forms of words representing commonly used medical terms; terms used for writing prescriptions; and terms associated with various measurements

■   Use of medical abbreviations by health-care professionals—patients' charts, prescriptions, standing orders, preparation of drugs, drug labels, and dosage instructions

Objective 2: Describe how drugs are named.

■   Chemical name—describes the chemical makeup of a drug

■   Generic (official, approved, or nonproprietary) name—simpler than the chemical name; not protected by trademark

■   Proprietary (brand or trade) name—assigned by manufacturer; protected by trademark

Objective 3: Describe five sources of drug derivation.

■   Plants

■   Animals (including humans)

■   Minerals or mineral products

■   Synthetics

■   Engineered (investigational) sources

Objective 4: Explain preparations of oral drugs.

■   Solid forms—tablets, capsules, powders; disintegration of the solid-dose form must occur before dissolution, a process by which a drug goes into a solution and becomes available for absorption

■   Liquid forms—solutions, elixirs, suspensions; more rapidly available for GI absorption than those in solid form

Objective 5: Define *solid drug forms.*

■   Pills—powdered drugs mixed with liquids and rolled into a round or oval shape

■   Tablets—powdered drugs compressed with bulk-filling materials under high pressure

■   Capsules—drugs contained in an external shell

■   Sustained-release tablets and capsules—containing several doses of a drug with special coatings that dissolve at different rates, thereby releasing the drug gradually

■   Enteric-coated tablets and capsules—covered by a special coating that keeps the drugs from dissolving in the stomach; these drugs do not dissolve until they reach the intestines

■   Caplets—drugs shaped like capsules but in the form of tablets, with film coatings

■   Gelcaps—oil-based medications enclosed in soft gelatin capsules

■   Powders—drugs that are dried and ground into fine particles

- Granules—small pills accompanied by many others, encased within gelatin capsules
- Troches or lozenges—flattened disks placed on the tongue or between the cheek and gum and left in place until they dissolve

Objective 6: Describe topical drugs.

- Semisolid—soft and pliable and often used for topical applications
- Creams—semisolid preparations that are usually white and contain a drug incorporated into both an aqueous base and an oily base
- Ointments—semisolid preparations in an aqueous base or a oily base for local protective, soothing, astringent, or transdermal application for systemic effects
- Plasters—compositions of liquid and powder that harden when dry; may be solid or semisolid
- Transdermal patches—used for a constant, time-released systemic effect, as their medications are absorbed slowly through the skin

Objective 7: Explain gaseous drugs.

- Pharmaceutical gases—include such anesthetic gases as nitrous oxide and halothane
- Compressed gases—include therapeutic oxygen or carbon dioxide
- Inhalation medications, such as bronchodilators—can be administered through metered-dose inhalers (MDIs) or handheld nebulizers (HHNs)

Objective 8: Describe topical drugs and define transdermal patches.

- Topical drugs are those that are applied to the skin, usually providing a local effect. Topical medications include transdermal patches, lotions, ointments, and liniments. They may be used to deaden nerves, control itching, or relieve pain and congestion in muscles and joints.
- Transdermal patches allow a time-released systemic effect because they are absorbed slowly through the skin. They release a very small amount of drug at consistent rates into the skin, from where it is carried off by the capillary blood supply. Examples of these drugs include nicotine, estrogen, and nitroglycerin.

Objective 9: List seven component parts of a prescription.

- Patient's name and address
- Date written
- Generic or proprietary drug name
- Drug strength and dosage
- Route of administration
- Dosage instruction or frequency of administration
- Signature, name, and address of the prescriber

Objective 10: Define *standing orders*.

- Orders given by physicians who may not be present at a later time when the medication is needed or ongoing prescriptions for patients in a hospital, nursing home, or residential-care setting; valid only when written, signed, and dated by the physician or other health-care provider with prescribing authority

Internet Sites of Interest

- Information on the parts of a prescription is offered at:
  www.mapharm.com/prescr_parts.htm

- The Institute for Safe Medical Practices provides a list of medical abbreviations, symbols, and dosage designations that are frequently misinterpreted and involved in harmful errors, along with their approved substitutions at:
  www.ismp.org/Tools/errorproneabbreviations.pdf

- Search for any medical abbreviation or term at: **www.medilexicon.com**

- For a list of drugs from "A" to "Z," go to: **www.rxlist.com/drugs/alpha_a.htm**

PEARSON
myhealthprofessionskit™

Go to www.myhealthprofessionskit.com to access the Companion Website created for this textbook. Simply select "Basic Health Science" from the choice of disciplines. Find this book and then log in using your username and password to access interactive learning games, assessment questions, animations, and more.

Chapter 4

Administration of Medications

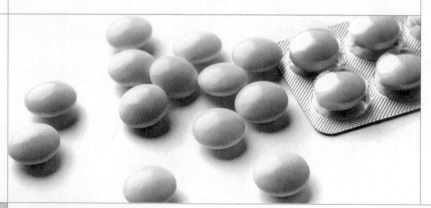

Key Terms

Introduction

It is important to remember that medications have the potential to cause serious harm to the patient. Therefore, the process of dispensing and administering medication orders must always be treated with great care. When you are involved in medication administration, you must be constantly vigilant to prevent errors and deliver quality patient care.

No matter what types of medications are to be administered, the order must come from the physician. If the physician delegates drug administration to the medical assistant, it must be allowable under state laws. Every state has a *medical practice act* that defines whether a medical assistant or other caregiver (besides a nurse) can administer drugs under the supervision of a physician. Some states permit medical assistants to administer only certain types of medications; some prohibit medical assistants from giving injections. To ensure patient safety in drug administration, health-care professionals must perform certain procedures every time a medication is ordered. These procedures are discussed in this chapter.

Principles of Drug Administration

The health-care professionals who may be administering medications should always assess a patient's health status and obtain a medication history before giving any medication. The extent of the assessment depends on the patient's illness or current condition, the intended drug, and the route of administration. For example, if a patient has dyspnea, the nurse or medical assistant must assess respirations carefully before administering any medication that might affect breathing. It is important to determine whether the route of administration is suitable. For example, a patient who is nauseated may not be able to tolerate a drug taken orally. In general, the health-care professional assesses the patient before administering any medication to obtain baseline data for evaluating the effectiveness of the medication.

The medication history includes information about the drugs the patient is taking currently or has taken recently. This includes prescription drugs; such over-the-counter (OTC) drugs as antacids, alcohol, and tobacco; and illegal drugs, such as marijuana. Sometimes, an incompatibility with one or more of these drugs affects the choice of a new medication.

Many patients, especially older adults, often take vitamins, herbs, and food supplements or use folk remedies that they do not list in their medication history. Because many of these have unknown or unpredictable actions and side effects, the health-care professional should always ask about their use and note it in the patient history, with close attention paid to possible incompatibilities with other prescribed medications.

Any problems the patient may have in self-administering a medication must also be identified. For example, a patient with poor eyesight may require special labels for the medication container; elderly patients with unsteady hands may not be able to hold syringes or inject themselves or another person. Obtaining information about how and where the patient stores medications is also important. If the patient has difficultly opening certain containers, he or she may change containers but leave the old labels on, which increases the risk of medication errors.

Socioeconomic factors need to be considered for all patients but especially for elderly people. Two common problems are lack of transportation to obtain medications and inadequate finances to purchase medications. If the health-care professional is aware of these problems, proper resources can be obtained for the patient.

THE SEVEN RIGHTS OF DRUG ADMINISTRATION

Safeguarding the patient during drug administration involves using the seven rights of proper drug administration. (The first five rights were introduced in Chapter 3.) Two more have been added since the original five were created:

1. **The *right* patient.** The easiest way to make sure the drug is being given to the right patient is to ask the patient his or her name or call the patient by name before administering the medication. You cannot assume that the person to whom you are administering a medication is the correct person without verifying his or her name in this manner. Patients can be confused or anxious and may not hear what you say. Therefore, check the patient's chart.

   Always check for allergies before administering medications. Ask the patient directly because recent allergic reactions might not be listed in the record. You should explain the medication's name, dosage, desired action, potential effects, and any precautions that need to be taken.

2. **The *right* drug.** Determining the right drug begins with clarifying the physician's order if needed. Each time a drug is dispensed, the medication label must be checked three times during its preparation to confirm the right drug, right dose, and right strength. Compare the physician's written order with the label. The first check is done when the medication is taken from the storage area. The second is performed just before removing the medication from its container. The third check is performed when the medication is returned to the storage area or just before administration.

   Also check the expiration date to ensure that the medication is still effective. If it has expired, dispose of it appropriately. It is appropriate to flush certain outdated medication into the sewer line. For controlled substances, you must ask someone to witness and document the disposal, referred to as "wasting the medication."

3. **The *right* dose.** If the dose ordered does not match the dose available, perform appropriate dosage calculations to determine the accurate dose (see Chapter 5). Remember to have a colleague check your calculations if you doubt the dose accuracy. Many facilities require health-care workers who set up insulin or heparin doses to check them with a co-worker. After you have calculated the amount to be administered, measure it out carefully. Medication errors are significantly reduced by using unit-dose systems because the medications are already in the correct dose.

4. **The *right* route.** Check the physician's order to clarify the route of administration for the medication—whether it is oral, topical, or parenteral. Many drugs can be given by a variety of routes. Because the route of administration can affect the medication's absorption, it is important that the drug is given by the correct route. If you are not sure what route is intended, confirm it with the physician.

5. **The *right* time.** In the ambulatory care setting, most medications are ordered **stat** (see Chapter 3).

However, it is important to check the physician's order to clarify the appropriate time for medications to be administered. Some medications must be taken on an empty stomach (30 minutes before or 2 hours after a meal), but others should be taken with food.

6. **The *right* technique.** A health-care professional must be familiar with the proper techniques for all routes of administration. If there are any doubts about the ability to administer a particular drug, always ask for help.

7. **The *right* documentation.** Immediately after giving the drug to the patient, document the date and time of administration; the drug's name, strength, dose, and route of administration; any patient reactions to the medication; and details of patient education regarding the drug. If the patient requests a prescription refill, document all pertinent information on the patient chart. The medical record is the legal document recording the order for the medication and its administration. If the medication ordered was not given or the patient refused it, the reason must be included in the record. If the patient refuses to take medication you have prepared, do not return it to its original container. Dispose of it and notify the physician.

Focus Point

Administering Medications

Nurses or medical assistants must be extremely knowledgeable when administering medications in the physician's office. Follow all physician orders exactly as written. If you are unsure about an order, ask for clarification before proceeding. Administer a medication only after the order is written in the patient's chart. This helps eliminate errors and possible omissions in medication therapy. Always implement the *seven rights* and perform three drug order and label checks when dispensing and administering medications.

✳ Apply Your Knowledge 4.1

The following questions focus on what you have just learned about the seven rights of drug administration.

CRITICAL THINKING

1. Describe the principles of drug administration.
2. What are the seven rights of drug administration?
3. What are the problems commonly seen in elderly patients when self-administering a medication?
4. Explain why medication history is important.
5. What are the most important factors to keep in mind concerning drug administration?

SAFETY IN DRUG ADMINISTRATION

Every time a medication is ordered, certain procedures must be performed to ensure patient safety. The physician's order must be completely understood and clearly read; any questions about the medication, dose, route of administration, and its strength must be answered by the physician. When questions arise, the drug should be looked up in a pharmacology reference book (such as a drug handbook) to review its possible side effects, precautions, purpose, and recommended dose. Only after all these steps are taken should the drug be dispensed and administered.

Routes of Drug Administration

Medications may be delivered to the body by different methods. The method of administration depends on the purpose of the medication. Medication may be administered in a variety of ways, but some must be given in specific and limited ways to be effective. Each route has its advantages and disadvantages. Drugs are administered either *enterally* (for absorption through the gastrointestinal [GI] tract) or *parenterally* (by injection) to produce systemic effects. If medications are placed in direct contact with the skin or mucous membranes to be absorbed for a local effect, this is called *percutaneous administration*. When choosing the route and technique of medication administration, the most reliable method of delivery ensures expected results.

ENTERAL ROUTES

The enteral route is the route of drug administration through the GI tract. This method of administration of drugs is safe and convenient for most patients and is relatively economical. Administration of medication through the GI tract may be by the oral, nasogastric or gastrostomy tube, sublingual, or buccal routes.

Oral Route

The oral route is the most common route. It is the easiest and most economical way for a patient to take medication. As long as a patient can swallow and retain the drug in the stomach, this is the route of choice. Medications given by the oral route are absorbed from the stomach and small intestine, traveling first to the liver, where they may be metabolized before they ever reach their target tissues or organs. This process, called *first-pass metabolism*, is discussed in Chapter 1.

Oral medications are contraindicated when a patient is vomiting, has gastric or intestinal suction, or is unconscious and unable to swallow. Generally, oral medications should be taken with enough water to ensure the drug reaches the stomach. Liquid medications are ideal for children. Solid drugs should not be given to children until they are old enough to safely swallow them without the danger of aspiration.

Focus on Geriatrics

Medications May Stain Teeth and Dentures

A dvise elderly patients who have dentures to remove them before taking certain medications. Some oral liquid drugs, such as liquid iron or iodides, may stain the teeth.

Nasogastric and Gastrostomy Routes

For patients who cannot take anything by mouth and have a nasogastric or gastrostomy tube in place, an alternative route for administering medications is through the tube. A **nasogastric (NG) tube** is inserted by way of the nasopharynx (the part of the pharynx that lies above the soft palate and opens into the nasal cavity) and is placed into the patient's stomach for the purpose of feeding the patient or removing gastric secretions. A **gastrostomy tube** is surgically placed directly into the patient's stomach and provides another route for administering medications and nutrition.

Sublingual Route

Medications given via the sublingual route are held under the tongue until completely dissolved (Figure 4-1 ■). This method is used when rapid action is desired because the mucosa of the oral cavity contains a very rich blood supply, offering fast absorption of certain drugs. Absorption via this route bypasses the GI tract, and the medication goes directly from the oral mucosa to the systemic circulation. Medications administered via the sublingual route are not destroyed by digestive enzymes, and they do not undergo first-pass metabolism in the liver. Examples of medications that can be administered by the sublingual

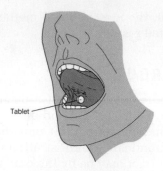

Figure 4-1 ■ Medication given via the sublingual route.

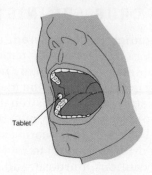

Figure 4-2 ■ Administration of drugs via the buccal route.

route include nitroglycerin (Nitrostat, Nitrobid) for angina pectoris and ergotamine tartrate (Ergostat) for migraines.

Buccal Route

For the administration of drugs via the buccal route (a type of percutaneous route), the medication is placed between the gum and cheek and left there until it dissolves (Figure 4-2 ■). Buccal medications are available in the form of tablets, capsules, lozenges, and troches. These medications should not be swallowed. They are absorbed more slowly from the buccal mucosa than the sublingual area. The buccal route is preferred over the sublingual route for sustained-release delivery because of its greater mucosal surface area.

Focus Point

Buccal and Sublingual Medications

Patients should not drink or eat anything when buccal or sublingual medications are administered until the medication has dissolved completely.

✳ Apply Your Knowledge 4.2

The following questions focus on what you have just learned about enteral routes of drug administration.

CRITICAL THINKING

1. Explain the safest method of medication administration.
2. Compare the nasogastric and gastrostomy routes.
3. What is the buccal route and when should it be used?
4. Name three drugs administered via the sublingual route.
5. What is the enteral route?

PARENTERAL ROUTES

Parenteral administration, as noted in Chapter 3, refers to the injection of a drug into the body with a needle and syringe. Parenteral administration of medications is a common procedure in medical offices, hospitals, ambulatory centers, home care centers, and other facilities by certain medical workers. Parenteral medications may be given via intradermal (ID), subcutaneous (SC), intramuscular (IM), or intravenous (IV) routes. The IV route may be more dangerous than the others because of the possibility of injecting a drug incorrectly into a vein, which may cause serious harm or even death. Because these medications are absorbed more quickly than oral medications and are irretrievable after being injected, the allied health worker must prepare and administer them carefully and accurately. The parenteral route is especially used in emergencies when a drug effect is needed immediately. Administering parenteral drugs requires an **invasive** procedure (one that requires insertion of an instrument or device through the skin or a body orifice), and an **aseptic** technique must be used (hand washing and other techniques to minimize the risk of infection).

Equipment

Syringes, needles, ampules, and vials are used to administer parenteral medications. Ampules and vials contain medications; syringes and needles are used to withdraw the medication and then administer it to the patients.

SYRINGES

Three parts make up a standard syringe: the barrel (the outside part), which has printed scales used to measure medication amounts; the plunger, which fits inside the barrel; and the tip, which connects with the needle (Figure 4-3 ■). The outside of the barrel and the handle of the plunger may be touched, but no unsterile object should ever come into contact with the tip or the inside of the barrel, the plunger's shaft, or the needle's shaft or tip.

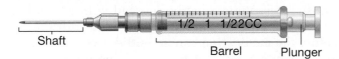

Figure 4-3 ■ The parts of a standard syringe: barrel, plunger, and shaft.

The three most common types of syringes are:

Hypodermic (meaning subcutaneous or under the skin) syringes (available in sizes between 2 mL and 3 mL)—marked in either milliliters or minims

Insulin syringes (available in various sizes)—marked in a specifically designed scale that is used for insulin units; 100-unit syringes are used in North America

Tuberculin syringes (narrow syringes that hold 1 mL or less)—marked in milliliters and minims

Figure 4-4 ■ shows examples of tuberculin, insulin, and 3-mL hypodermic syringes.

Injectable medications are often available in disposable prefilled unit-dose systems:

✳ Prefilled syringes, ready to use

✳ Prefilled sterile cartridges and needles that must be attached to a reusable holder (injection system) before use

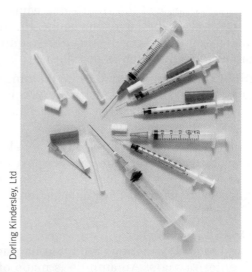

Dorling Kindersley, Ltd

Figure 4-4 ■ (Various types of syringes, including tuberculin, insulin, and hypodermic.

Examples of prefilled unit-dose systems are shown in Figure 4-5 ■.

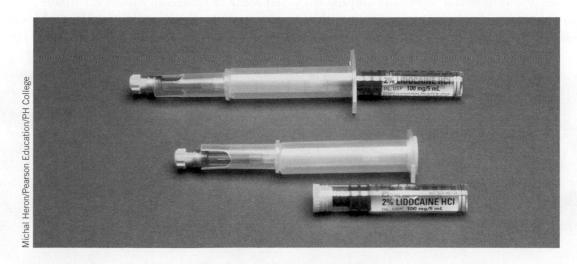

Michal Heron/Pearson Education/PH College

Figure 4-5 ■ Prefilled unit-dose systems.

NEEDLES

Most needles are disposable and are made of stainless steel. Special procedure needles may be reusable and need to be repeatedly sharpened because their points can become dull with use. Dull or damaged needles should never be used.

There are three parts that make up a needle:

* ✻ **Bevel**—the slanted part at the needle's tip

* ✻ **Cannula** or shaft—the actual metal length that makes up the majority of the needle; it is attached to the hub

* ✻ **Hub**—the part of the needle that fits onto the syringe

There are three variable characteristics in needles used for injections:

* ✻ **Gauge** (or diameter of the shaft)—the gauge varies from #18 to #28. The larger the gauge, the smaller the shaft's diameter. Larger gauges are required for thicker medications, such as penicillin.

* ✻ **Length of the shaft**—common lengths range from 1/2 to 2 inches. The correct shaft length is determined by the type of injection, the patient's weight, and the patient's muscle development.

* ✻ **Slant or length of the bevel**—longer bevels cause less discomfort and provide the sharpest needles (these are commonly used for IM and SC injections). Short bevels are used for IV or ID injections.

AMPULES AND VIALS

Sterile parenteral medications are often packaged in either ampules or vials. An ampule is made of clear glass and usually contains a single dose of a drug. It ranges in size from 1 mL to 10 mL or larger. Ampules have a distinctive neck that is tight or constricted; most ampule necks are prescored to be easily opened and are marked with a colored ink at the point at which they are to be opened.

Ampules are broken open at the constricted neck by using a plastic cap over the top of the ampule (to prevent injury from broken glass) and a cutter within the cap that further scores the neck of the ampule when it is rotated. After being broken open, the medication is aspirated into a syringe by using a filter needle, which prevents aspiration of any glass particles. Figure 4-6 ■ shows an example of drawing medication from a vial.

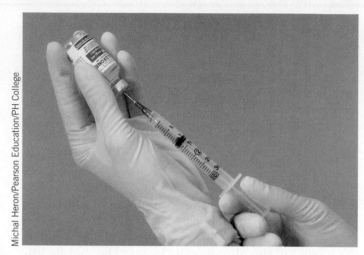

Figure 4-6 ■ Drawing medication from a vial with a syringe.

A *vial* consists of a small glass bottle that is sealed with a rubber cap and may range from single to multidose sizes. Vials must be pierced with a needle to access the medication. Air is injected into the vial before the medication can be withdrawn from it. The air prevents a vacuum from building up within the vial, allowing easier withdrawal of medication.

Drugs that are dispensed as powders in vials (for reconstitution with solvents, such as sterile water or sterile normal saline, or diluents) include penicillin.

Intradermal Injection

ID injections are usually given just below the epidermis into the dermis in the inner forearm or upper back—areas that have little hair growth (Figure 4-7A ■). The ID route is commonly used for tuberculin or allergy skin tests or for the administration of local anesthetics. One method of tuberculin screening is the tine test,

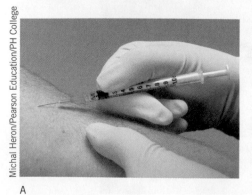

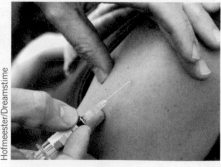

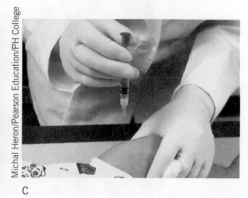

A   B   C

Figure 4-7 ■ **(A)** Intradermal injection. **(B)** Subcutaneous injection. **(C)** Intramuscular injection.

which is administered with individually packaged disposable sterile stamps with four prongs on the end that have been treated with tuberculin solution. However, the tine test is not as accurate as the Mantoux (purified protein derivative [PPD]) ID screening test. Absorption via this route is slow. A 15-degree angle is used when the needle is inserted between the skin's upper layers (Figure 4-8A ■), and the injection of a substance should produce a small **wheal** (a slightly reddened, raised lesion) on the skin's outer surface. With the Mantoux test, a 0.1-mL solution of PPD is injected using a needle gauge of #26 to #27.

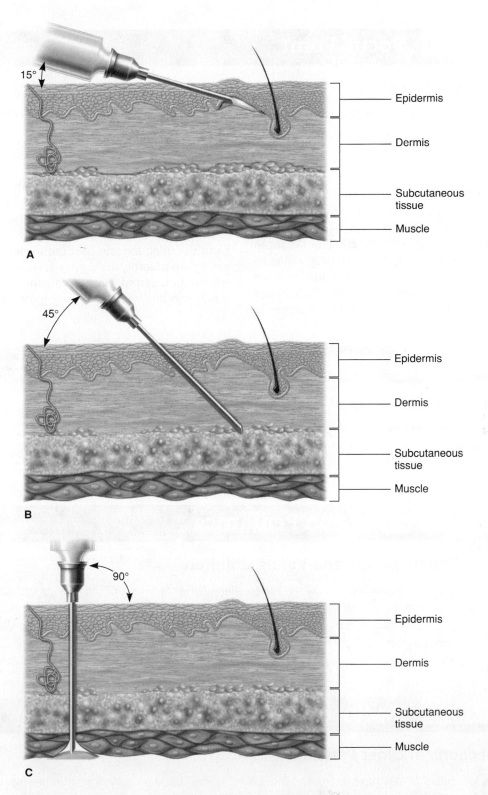

Figure 4-8 ■ Angles and depths of injection for intradermal (**A**), subcutaneous (**B**), and intramuscular (**C**) injections.

Subcutaneous Injection

Subcutaneous injections are usually given into subcutaneous tissue below the dermis in the upper arms, upper back, or upper abdomen (Figure 4-7B ■). The subcutaneous route is commonly used for heparin and insulin injections. Absorption via this route is slower than via IM injections. A 45-degree angle is usually used, although this depends on the patient's body weight, which also influences the length of needle used (Figure 4-8B ■). Small volumes of medication (between 0.5 and 1 mL) are given subcutaneously.

Focus Point

Heparin Injections

For subcutaneous heparin injections, make sure that 0.1 to 0.2 mL of air is in the syringe to prevent heparin leakage into tissue, thus avoiding localized hemorrhaging.

Intramuscular Injection

IM injections are usually given into the deltoid (upper arm), vastus lateralis (thigh), and ventrogluteal or dorsogluteal (hip) muscles (Figure 4-7C ■). The IM route is commonly used for drugs that are irritating to subcutaneous tissue. Absorption via this route is more rapid than other methods because of the rich blood supply found in the muscles. A 90-degree angle is used most commonly (Figure 4-8C ■), although the *Z-track method of IM injection* is also used. To avoid irritation to the skin and subcutaneous tissues, the Z-track injection method prevents any leakage back from the deep muscle into the upper subcutaneous layers by displacing the upper tissue laterally before the needle is inserted. Larger volumes of medication (1 to 3 mL) can be given at one site using IM injections.

Focus Point

Self-Administration of Insulin

Teach diabetic patients who must self-administer insulin at home to rotate insulin administration sites.

Focus on Pediatrics

Injections in Infants and Young Children

Infants and young children usually require smaller, shorter needles (#22 to #25 gauge, 5/8 to 1 inch long) for IM injection. The gluteal muscles are developed by walking. Therefore, do not use the dorsogluteal site in children younger than 3 years unless the child has been walking for at least 1 year. The vastus lateralis site is recommended as the site of choice for IM injections for infants 7 months or younger.

Focus on Geriatrics

Injections in Older Patients

Older patients may have decreased muscle mass, or muscle *atrophy*. A shorter needle may be needed. Assessment of appropriate injection site is critical. Absorption of medication may occur more quickly than expected.

Intravenous Injection

IV injections are given directly into the veins—most commonly those of the arms. The IV route is used for many varieties of drugs and fluids, and distribution via this route is almost immediate. Drugs given via the IV route may be administered slowly, rapidly (IV push), by piggyback infusions (drugs are mixed with compatible fluids and administered over 30 to 90 minutes), into an existing IV line (the IV port), into an intermittent venous access device, such as a heparin lock, or by adding them to an IV solution. IV needles are inserted into veins at short angles (of about 25 degrees) to the skin.

Focus Point

Z-Track Technique of Injection Used for Certain Medications

Some specific medications, such as iron, are irritating or may stain the skin. Therefore, use the Z-track technique of injection for these medications.

✳ Apply Your Knowledge 4.3

The following questions focus on what you have just learned about parenteral routes of drug administration.

CRITICAL THINKING

1. Describe a Z-track injection.
2. Why is the vastus lateralis muscle the preferred injection site for infants?
3. Describe a cartridge syringe and its advantages.
4. Explain a tine test and explain what the abbreviation PPD means.
5. Compare ampules with vials.
6. Describe the parts of a needle.
7. Define the term *hypodermic syringe*.
8. Describe the three parts of a syringe.

OTHER ROUTES OF DRUG ADMINISTRATION

Drugs may be applied to skin and mucous membranes either topically (on the skin's outer layers) or via the eyes (using instillations or irrigations), the ears (using drops of medicated solution), the nose (using drops and sprays), inhalation (drawing breath, vapor, or gas into the lungs), the vagina (using instillations), and the rectum (using suppositories).

Transdermal Applications

Topical skin preparations include creams, ointments, pastes, lotions, powders, sprays, and patches. Transdermal patches allow drugs to be absorbed slowly through the skin to create a constant, time-released systemic effect (Figure 4-9 ■). For example, the nitroglycerin patch is particularly useful for patients with frequent attacks of angina. Other drugs administered via transdermal patches include nicotine (to assist in smoking cessation)

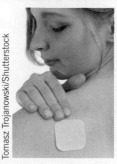

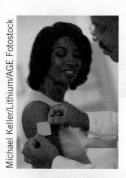

Figure 4-9 ■ Examples of transdermal patches.

Focus Point

Use of Transdermal Patches

Instruct patients to shower with the transdermal patch in place. If the patch is to remain on for 24 hours, a new patch should be applied every day at the same time. Advise patients to rotate sites to prevent skin irritation and to avoid placing the patch on scars and areas with a large amount of body hair.

and estrogen. The rate of delivery of the drug is controlled and varies with each product (12 hours to 1 week).

Ophthalmic Route

Medications are administered to the eye by using instillations or irrigations in the form of liquids or ointments. Eye drops and ointments are used to administer medication by sterile technique. For example, prescribed liquids are usually diluted to less than 1% strength. An eye irrigation is administered to wash out the conjunctival sac to remove secretions or foreign bodies or to remove chemicals that may injure the eye. Figures 4-10 ■ and 4-11 ■ show the instillation of eye ointments and eye drops into the lower conjunctival sac.

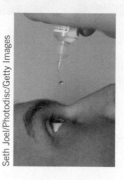

Figure 4-11 ■ Instillation of eye drops.

Otic Route

Localized infection or inflammation of the ear or ears is treated by dropping a small amount of a sterile medicated solution into them. In children younger than 3 years of age, gently pull the earlobe down and back; in adults, gently pull the earlobe up and out (Figure 4-12 ■). The patient must remain lying on his or her opposite side for 5 minutes to allow the medication to run into and coat the surface of the inner ear canal.

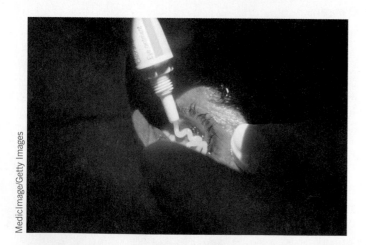

Figure 4-10 ■ Instillation of eye ointment.

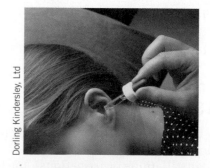

Figure 4-12 ■ Instillation of ear medication. *©Elena Dorfman.*

Focus Point

Otic and Ophthalmic Drops

Otic and ophthalmic drops can be easily confused. Emphasize to patients that otic medications cannot be put in the eyes because they can cause pain and irritation.

Nasal Route

Nose drops and sprays are generally used to shrink swollen mucous membranes or to loosen secretions and facilitate drainage. Sometimes, nasal medications are prescribed to treat infections of the nasal cavity or sinuses. Nasal decongestants are the most common nasal instillations. Many of these medications are OTC drugs.

The medication should be drawn up into a dropper and held over one nostril at a time. Then, the required number of nose drops are administered. Nasal drops are usually used with the patient in the supine position—with the head tilted back (Figure 4-13 ■).

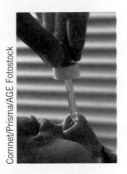

Figure 4-13 ■ Administration of nasal medications.

Focus Point

Self-Administration of Medication by Patients

Correct administration of medications by patients at home requires patient education by the health-care professional. Make sure the patient understands the purpose of the drug; the time, frequency, and amount of the dose; any special storage requirements; and the typical side effects that may occur. Emphasize to the patient the possible serious adverse effects of the medication. Advise the patient to quickly report adverse effects to the physician.

Inhalation Route

Inhalation is the act of drawing breath, vapor, or gas into the lungs. Inhalation therapy may involve the administration of medicines; water vapor; and such gases as oxygen, carbon dioxide, and helium. The medication must be inhaled to achieve local effects within the respiratory tract through aerosols (Figure 4-14A–C ■), nebulizers, Spinhalers, or *metered-dose inhalers* (MDIs). Some inhaled medications are intended to alter the condition of the mucous membranes (albuterol and anti-inflammatory medications), to alter the character of the secretions in the respiratory system (acetylcysteine), or to treat infections of the respiratory tract (antibiotics such as tobramycin).

Oxygen is another medication that is administered by the inhalation route. Because oxygen is a drug, it needs to be prescribed according to the flow rate, concentration, method of delivery, and length of time for administration. Oxygen is prescribed as liters per minute (LPM) and as percentage of oxygen concentration (%). Oxygen toxicity may develop when 100% oxygen is breathed for a prolonged period. A high concentration of inhaled oxygen causes alveolar collapse, intraalveolar hemorrhage, hyaline membrane formation, disturbance of the central nervous system, and retrolental fibroplasias in newborns.

By far, the predominant use of inhaled medications is for the treatment of asthma or other pulmonary disorders. In treating patients with asthma, a common method of administering medications is by nebulizer (see Figure 4-14A ■). A nebulizer is used to deliver a fine spray (fog or mist) of medication or moisture to a client. There are two kinds of nebulization: *atomization* and *aerosolization*. In atomization, a device called an *atomizer* produces rather large

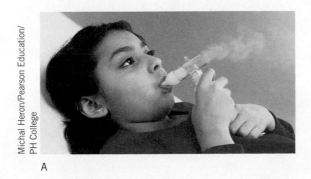

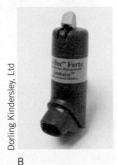

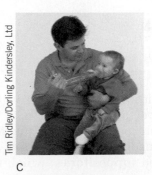

Figure 4-14 ■ (**A**) A girl breathes mist through a nebulizer, with a bite piece in her mouth. (**B**) A breath-actuated inhaler. (**C**) An inhaler with a face mask.

droplets for inhalation. In aerosolization, the droplets are suspended in a gas, such as oxygen. The smaller the droplets, the farther they can be inhaled into the respiratory tract.

The MDI is a handheld nebulizer (Figure 4-15 ■), which is a pressurized container of medication that the patient can use to release the medication through a nosepiece or mouthpiece.

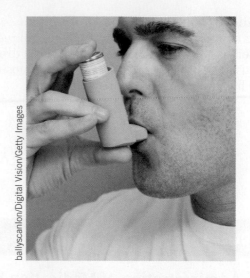

Figure 4-15 ■ Metered-dose inhaler.

Focus Point

Oxygen Precautions

Delivery of oxygen requires specific precautions. Be alert to the flammability of oxygen and make sure no open flames (including lighters, matches, or candles) are being used in the area near the oxygen.

Vaginal Route

Vaginal medications, or instillations, are inserted as creams, jellies, foams, or suppositories to treat infections or to relieve vaginal discomfort, such as pain or itching. Vaginal creams, jellies, and foams are applied by using

a tubular applicator with a plunger. Suppositories are designed to melt at body temperature, so they are usually kept in the refrigerator (Figure 4-16A ■). Vaginal suppositories are gelatin or cocoa butter based and are instilled by using an applicator (Figure 4-16B ■).

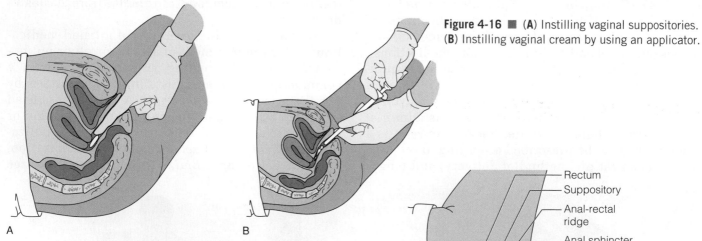

A   B

Figure 4-16 ■ **(A)** Instilling vaginal suppositories. **(B)** Instilling vaginal cream by using an applicator.

Rectal Route

Rectal medications are commonly given in suppository form. The rectal route is useful if the patient is nauseated, vomiting, or unconscious. Manufacturers supply rectal medications in the form of gelatin- or cocoa butter–based suppositories, which melt in the warmth of the rectum and release the medication, or in the form of enemas as a solution. The rectal route of administration is shown in Figure 4-17 ■.

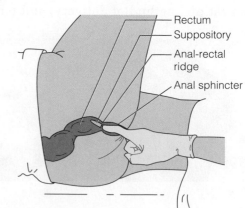

Rectum
Suppository
Anal-rectal ridge
Anal sphincter

Figure 4-17 ■ Inserting a rectal suppository into the anus.

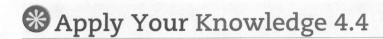

✳ Apply Your Knowledge 4.4

The following questions focus on what you have just learned about other routes of drug administration.

CRITICAL THINKING

1. When may oxygen toxicity occur in patients because of the inhalation route?
2. Compare how the otic route of drug administration is used for infants and adults.
3. Compare the terms *transdermal* and *topical*.
4. What position is the best for administering drugs via the nasal route?
5. What are the most common nasal instillations?
6. What are the indications of the rectal route?

PRACTICAL SCENARIO 1

A 72-year-old woman had a vaginal infection. Her physician prescribed vaginal suppositories for the condition. His medical assistant was busy and did not completely explain how the patient should administer the medication, assuming that she knew. The patient purchased the prescription and administered the suppositories for the 10-day period. After 3 weeks, she returned to her physician and complained that the condition was the same with no relief. Her physician asked her exactly how she was using the suppositories. The patient replied that she had been inserting the suppositories rectally every 12 hours.

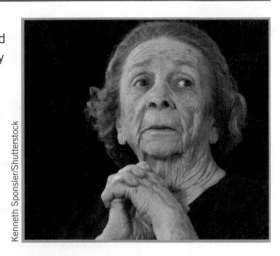

Kenneth Sponsler/Shutterstock

Critical Thinking Questions

1. What mistake did this patient make in administering the suppositories?
2. What should the medical assistant have made sure the patient knew about the proper administration of these suppositories?

PRACTICAL SCENARIO 2

A medical assistant was instructed to give an iron supplement via injection to a pregnant woman who had severe iron-deficiency anemia. She injected the medication subcutaneously. After 3 days, the patient returned with discoloration at the site of injection and complained to the physician.

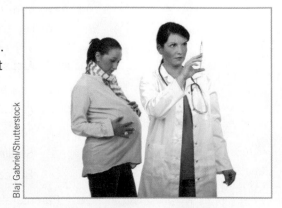

Blaj Gabriel/Shutterstock

Critical Thinking Questions

1. For injectable iron supplementation, what injection technique must be used?
2. What is the result of subcutaneous injection of this medication?

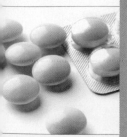

Chapter Capsule

This section repeats the objectives from the beginning of the chapter and then provides a summary of the most important concepts for that objective. Use this section as a quick review and to check your knowledge.

Objective 1: Summarize patient assessment factors that have an impact on medication administration.

- Depends on patient's illness or current condition, intended drug, and route of administration
- Includes other factors, such as breathing problems, nausea, history of or current medication use, and vitamins or food and herbal supplements being taken

Objective 2: Identify the seven rights of drug administration.

- The *right* patient
- The *right* drug
- The *right* dose
- The *right* route
- The *right* time
- The *right* technique
- The *right* documentation

Objective 3: Define percutaneous administration.

- Percutaneous administration involves medications being placed in direct contact with the skin or mucous membranes to be absorbed for a local effect.

Objective 4: Describe when a a nasogastric tube should be used.

- A nasogastric tube should be used to administer medications for patients who cannot take anything by mouth. The tube is inserted by way of the nasopharynx (the part of the pharynx that lies above the soft palate and opens into the nasal cavity) and is placed into the patient's stomach for the purpose of feeding the patient or removing gastric secretions.

Objective 5: Define the meaning of the term *hypodermic*.

- The term *hypodermic* refers to "subcutaneous" or "under the skin." Hypodermic needles are commonly used for many different types of injections.

Objective 6: List and describe the various routes of medication administration.

- Enteral—through the GI tract
  - ❑ Oral—via the mouth
  - ❑ Nasogastric or gastrostomy tube—through the nasopharynx or stomach
  - ❑ Sublingual (percutaneous)—under the tongue
  - ❑ Buccal (percutaneous)—between the gum and cheek
- Parenteral—injected
- Topical (percutaneous)—through the skin

- Skin application
- Ophthalmic route—eye
- Otic route—ear
- Nasal route—nose
- Inhalation—through the airways
- Vaginal—vagina
- Rectal—rectum

Objective 7: Identify equipment and supplies required for parenteral administration of medications.

- Syringes, needles, ampules, and vials

Objective 8: Define terms related to needles used in the parenteral administration of medications.

- Bevel—the slanted part at the needle's tip
- Cannula—the metal needle shaft
- Gauge—the needle shaft's diameter
- Hub—the part of the needle that fits onto the syringe

Objective 9: Identify sites used for intradermal, subcutaneous, and intramuscular injections.

- Intradermal—given within the skin layers of the inner forearm or upper back
- Subcutaneous—given into the upper arms, upper back, or upper abdomen
- Intramuscular—given into the upper arm or the thigh or hip

Objective 10: Explain how to administer an intradermal, subcutaneous, or intramuscular injection.

- Intradermal—a 15-degree angle is used; volumes less than 0.1 mL
- Subcutaneous—a 45-degree angle is used; only small volumes of medication
- Intramuscular—a 90-degree angle, or the Z-track method, is used; larger volumes of medication

Internet Sites of Interest

- The Institute for Safe Medication Practices provides a list of look-alike or sound-alike drugs that are commonly confused at **www.ismp.org/Tools/confuseddrugnames.pdf**.
- An article about strategies to reduce medication errors is offered by the U.S. Food and Drug Administration at **www.fda.gov/fdac**. Search for "medical errors."
- About Senior Health offers much health and medical information for older adults at **www.seniorhealth.about.com**. Search for "taking medications."
- Good teaching information is provided for parents of pediatric patients at **http://www.fda.gov/fdac**. Search "how to give medicine to children."
- Prentice Hall's website for drug guides **www.pearsonhighered.com/drugguides** provides drug updates, administration techniques, a list of common herbal remedies and their interactions, and much more.

- The website Prescription Drug Info allows you to search for most drugs by trade name and provides an overview of each drug, its common dosages, the forms in which it is available, its active chemicals, the pharmaceutical company that manufactures it, and the date that it was approved by the FDA: **www.prescriptiondrug-info.com**.

- The Joint Commission provides an index of articles, such as *Using Medication Reconciliation to Prevent Errors, Medication Errors Related to Potentially Dangerous Abbreviations, Infusion Pumps: Preventing Future Adverse Events*, and others at **http://www.jointcommission.org/sentinel_event.aspx**.

PEARSON myhealthprofessionskit™

Go to www.myhealthprofessionskit.com to access the Companion Website created for this textbook. Simply select "Basic Health Science" from the choice of disciplines. Find this book and then log in using your username and password to access interactive learning games, assessment questions, animations, and more.

Checkpoint Review 1

Select the best answer for the following questions.

1. The half-life is the major determinant of which of the following?
   a. The adverse effects of a drug after a single dose
   b. The interaction with another single dose
   c. The duration of elimination of a drug after administration of multiple doses
   d. The duration of action of a drug after a single dose

2. *Hypersensitivity* is often used synonymously with which of the following terms?
   a. Immunogen
   b. Allergy
   c. Antigen
   d. Allergen

3. Which of the following agencies oversees controlled substances and prosecutes individuals who illegally distribute them?
   a. HIPAA
   b. FDA
   c. DEA
   d. CDC

4. Which of the following federal laws offers a seven-year monopoly on drug sales and tax breaks to induce drug companies to undertake development and manufacturing of such drugs?
   a. Orphan Drug Act of 1983
   b. The Prescription Drug Marketing Act of 1987
   c. The Durham–Humphrey Amendment of 1951
   d. The Comprehensive Drug Abuse Prevention and Control Act of 1970

5. Which of the following is an example of a semisolid drug?
   a. Granules
   b. Caplets
   c. Gelcaps
   d. Gels

6. The angle of insertion for intradermal injections is which of the following degrees?
   a. 30
   b. 90
   c. 15
   d. 45

7. Which of the following is the route of administration of a drug that is placed between the gums and the cheek?
   a. Buccal
   b. Topical
   c. Sublingual
   d. Transdermal

8. Which of the following is the abbreviation for subcutaneous?
   a. SC
   b. Subcutaneous should not be abbreviated to avoid medication errors.
   c. SQ
   d. Sub q

9. The proprietary drug name is also called the:
   a. Chemical name
   b. Generic name
   c. Trade name
   d. None of the above

10. The study of drugs derived from herbal and other natural sources is called:
    a. Pharmacodynamics
    b. Pharmacotherapy
    c. Pharmacognosy
    d. Pharmacology

11. The enteral route is the route of drug administration through which of the following?
    a. Intravenous
    b. Gastrointestinal tract
    c. Intradermal
    d. Topical

12. Which of the following abbreviations means "twice a day"?
    a. bid
    b. qid
    c. qd
    d. tid

13. Administration of corticosteroids may be more effective if administered during what time of the day?

   a. Early morning
   b. Early evening
   c. At noon
   d. At bedtime

14. Which of the following agents is mixed with a liquid but not dissolved?

   a. Elixir
   b. Suspension
   c. Tincture
   d. Fluid extract

15. Bioavailability of a drug means:

   a. The determination of whether two or more drug products release their contents in equal amounts over the same absorption
   b. The degree to which a drug releases itself from its dosage form to become accessible for its intended effect
   c. The process of drug movement into the systemic circulation
   d. The study of the chemical reactions that occur within a living organism

16. The abbreviation qid, as used in prescriptions, means:

   a. Every hour
   b. Every four hours
   c. Every other day
   d. Four times a day

17. The elixir sulfanilamide disaster of 1937 is an example of medication:

   a. Ordering errors
   b. Dispensing errors
   c. Transcribing errors
   d. Formulation errors

18. Which of the following schedule of drugs has the lowest abuse potential of all the controlled substances?

   a. Schedule IV
   b. Schedule III
   c. Schedule V
   d. Schedule II

19. Orphan drugs are used to treat which of the following diseases or conditions?

   a. Shark bite
   b. AIDS
   c. Asthma
   d. Cancer

20. Coal tar is used to treat which of the following disorders?

   a. Rheumatoid arthritis
   b. Scarlet fever
   c. Psoriasis
   d. AIDS

21. Which of the following is the abbreviation for potassium?

   a. Hg
   b. Na
   c. Fe
   d. K

22. Semisolid drugs are most commonly used for:

   a. Topical application
   b. Inhalation
   c. Parental
   d. Oral

23. Which of the following is the most dangerous route of drug administration?

   a. Intradermal
   b. Intramuscular
   c. Intravenous
   d. Subcutaneous

24. Heparin is commonly given by which of the following routes?

   a. Sublingual
   b. Subcutaneous
   c. Intradermal
   d. Rectal

25. Which of the following parts of a prescription is also known as the subscription?

   a. Medication prescribed
   b. Dispensing directions to the pharmacist
   c. Directions for patient
   d. Refill and special labeling

26. Which of the following agents was extensively and legally advertised in newspapers during the nineteenth century, when there was virtually no regulation on the sale of drugs in the United States?

    a. Penicillin
    b. Atropine
    c. Barbital
    d. Opium

27. Short needles are used for which of the following routes of drug injections?

    a. Intravenous or intradermal
    b. Intramuscular and subcutaneous
    c. Intradermal and subcutaneous
    d. Intravenous and intramuscular

28. Which of the following is an example of a sublingual tablet?

    a. Insulin
    b. Heparin
    c. Nitroglycerin
    d. Ampicillin

29. Aqueous solutions containing high concentrations of sugar are called what?

    a. Syrups
    b. Spirits
    c. Elixirs
    d. Tinctures

30. All drug administration laws are initiated, implemented, and enforced by which of the following laws?

    a. MSPPA
    b. OSHA
    c. FDA
    d. HIPAA

31. All the following are examples of the transdermal patch except:

    a. Estrogen
    b. Testosterone
    c. Nicotine
    d. Nitroglycerin

32. Which of the following part of a word gives the word its central meaning?

    a. Suffix
    b. Prefix
    c. Root
    d. Combining vowel

33. Pancreatin and pepsin come from which of the following sources?

    a. Minerals
    b. Humans and other animals
    c. Synthetic sources
    d. Engineered sources

34. Which of the following medications may stain and irritate the skin and for which you should use the "Z-track technique" of injection?

    a. Penicillin
    b. Protein plasma
    c. Iodine
    d. Iron

35. Which of the following is an abbreviation meaning "immediately"?

    a. Sig
    b. SOS
    c. Syr
    d. Stat

36. Which of the following agents promotes muscle growth?

    a. Alkylating drugs
    b. Anabolic steroids
    c. Acetylcholine
    d. Acetylcysteine

37. The DEA is a branch of which department that became the nation's sole legal drug enforcement agency?

    a. U.S. Department of Health
    b. U.S. Department of Labor
    c. U.S. Department of Health and Human Services
    d. U.S. Department of Justice

38. Pharmacy practice regulation is primarily a function of the:

    a. State
    b. Federal government
    c. Board of Pharmacy
    d. U.S. Department of Health

39. Which of the following abbreviations means "by mouth"?

    a. pc
    b. po
    c. prn
    d. pm

40. Which of the following laws was passed to prevent the marketing of new drugs before they had been properly tested for purity, strength, effectiveness, safety, and packaging quality?

    a. The Durham–Humphrey Amendment
    b. The Food, Drug, and Cosmetic Act
    c. The Safe Medical Devices Act
    d. The Controlled Substances Act

41. The abbreviation *mixt* means:

    a. Solution
    b. Liquid
    c. Ointment
    d. A mixture

42. Which of the following syringes are calibrated in units?

    a. Disposable syringes
    b. Needleless syringes
    c. Insulin syringes
    d. Tuberculin syringes

43. A list of officially recognized drug names is known as the:

    a. U.S. Drug Code
    b. National Formulary
    c. National pharmacopeia
    d. International pharmacopeia

44. A wheal occurs on the skin from which of the following injections?

    a. Z-track
    b. Intradermal
    c. Intramuscular
    d. Subcutaneous

45. Which abbreviation means "nothing by mouth"?

    a. Na
    b. NPO
    c. UA
    d. CVA

For questions 46–50, match the lettered drug schedule to the numbered drug.

DRUG

46. _____ Diphenoloxylate hydrochloride with atropine sulfate (Lomotil)

47. _____ Certain drugs compounded with small quantities of narcotics

48. _____ Marijuana

49. _____ Diazepam (valium)

50. _____ Morphine

DRUG SCHEDULE

    a. Schedule I
    b. Schedule II
    c. Schedule III
    d. Schedule IV
    e. Schedule V

For questions 51–55, match the lettered abbreviation to the numbered meaning.

MEANING

51. _____ As directed
52. _____ As needed
53. _____ Four times a day
54. _____ After meals
55. _____ Three times a day

ABBREVIATION

    a. tid
    b. qid
    c. pc
    d. prn
    e. ud

For questions 56–57, please answer in sentences.

56. A 13-year-old girl is picked up at the medical office by her father. Her parents are divorced, and her mother has legal custody. Her father would like to see the girl's medical records. Can he see the medical records by law? Explain.

_____

_____

_____

_____

_____

57. A physician prescribed marijuana for a 35-year-old man who has advanced AIDS. Before the pharmacy technician dispenses the prescription, a health-care person wants to know in which schedule of drugs the marijuana is. On the Internet, the technician should search under which federal law?

_____

_____

_____

_____

_____

Unit 2

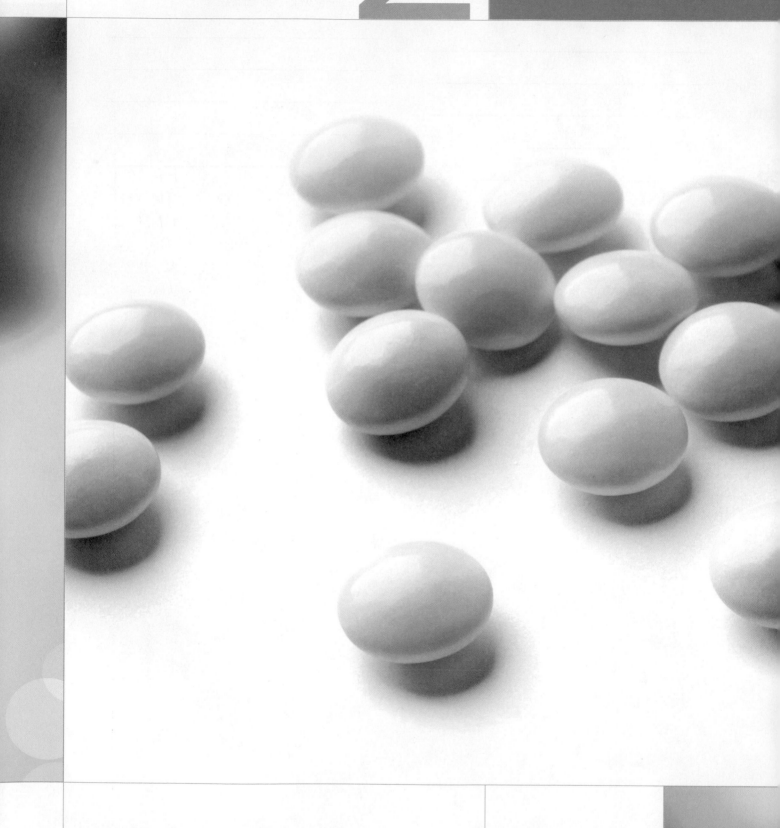

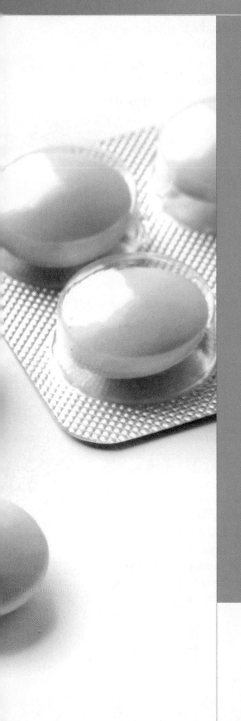

MATHEMATICS AND DOSAGE CALCULATIONS

" It is the health-care professional's responsibility to ensure the patient receives the proper dose of medication and to educate the patient about the proper measurement of doses. "

Chapter 5

Basic Mathematics

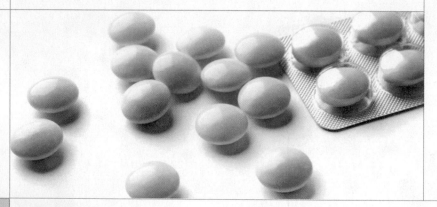

Key Terms

Introduction

The ability to make accurate dosage calculations requires allied health professionals to have skills in adding, subtracting, multiplying, and dividing whole numbers. It is essential that you have a knowledge of basic mathematics, such as Arabic numbers, Roman numerals, fractions, decimals, percents, and ratios, to be able to calculate dosages accurately and quickly.

Arabic System and Roman Numeral System

The **Arabic number** system is commonly used in expressing quantity and value, such as 0, 1, 2, 3, 4, 5, 6, 7, 8, and 9. Any number may be represented by combining these

numbers. Arabic numbers can be written as whole numbers, decimals (for example, 0.6), and fractions (such as 3/4). The **Roman numeral** system consists of letters that represent number values—most commonly of numbers between 1 and 100. When working with numbers that range from 1 to 30, only three Roman numerals (I [1], V [5], and X [10]) are required—used in various combinations.

Example

$$IV = 4$$
$$XXI = 21$$

Roman numerals are commonly used to express units of the apothecary system of weights and measures in writing prescriptions. The most common Roman numerals and their values are shown in Table 5-1 ∎.

Table 5-1 ∎ The Most Common Roman Numerals and Their Arabic Values

ROMAN NUMERAL	ARABIC VALUE	ROMAN NUMERAL	ARABIC VALUE
I	1	XXV	25
II	2	XXX	30
III	3	XL	40
IV	4	L	50
V	5	LX	60
VI	6	LXX	70
VII	7	LXXV	75
VIII	8	LXXX	80
IX	9	XC	90
X	10	C	100
XV	15	D	500
XX	20	M	1,000

READING ROMAN NUMERALS

Roman numerals are read by adding or subtracting the value of the letters. When a letter appears twice in a row, the value of the letter is counted twice, and so on (Example 1). If a lower valued letter follows a larger-valued letter, the letters should be added. The letter representing the largest possible number should be used to represent a value. If a lower-valued letter is placed before a higher-valued letter, the lower letter is subtracted from the higher letter (Example 2).

Example 1

$$VII = 5 + 1 + 1 = 7$$
$$III = 1 + 1 + 1 = 3$$
$$XIV = 10 + 4 = 14$$
$$XXI = 10 + 10 + 1 = 21$$
$$XXXIV = 10 + 10 + 10 + 4 = 34$$

Example 2

$$IV = 5 - 1 = 4$$
$$IX = 10 - 1 = 9$$
$$XL = 50 - 10 = 40$$

✳ Apply Your Knowledge 5.1

The following questions focus on what you have just learned about Arabic numbers and Roman numerals. *See Appendix F for the correct answers.*

DO THE MATH

Convert these Roman numerals to Arabic numbers.

1. VIII = _8_
2. XXV = _25_
3. XV = _15_
4. VI = _6_
5. XXI = _21_

Add or subtract the Roman numerals.

6. VI + VIII = _14_
7. XI + IV = _15_
8. VII + IX = _16_
9. XXI + VI = _27_
10. XIX − XII = _12_
11. XVII − VI = _11_
12. XVIII − XII = _6_
13. XXIV − XIV = _10_

MATCHING

Match the lettered term to the numbered description. Lettered terms may be used more than once.

DESCRIPTION

1. _b_ Commonly used to express units of the apothecary system of weights and measures in prescriptions

2. _b_ Read by adding or subtracting the value of letters

3. _a_ Commonly used in expressing quantity and value

4. _a_ Can be written as whole numbers, decimals, and fractions

5. _b_ Only three of these needed to express numbers from 1 to 30

TERM

a. Arabic numbers

b. Roman numerals

Fractions

Health-care workers who deal with administering medications and dispensing drugs need to understand fractions to interpret and act on practitioners' orders, read prescriptions, and understand patients' records. Fractions are used in apothecary and household measures for dosage calculations. A **fraction** is one or more equal parts of a unit. It is written as a divided number, with one portion considered to be a part of the whole amount, such as 1/2 or 3/4 (one part out of a total of two parts or three parts out of a total of four).

The two parts of a fraction are called the *numerator* and the *denominator*. The **numerator** is the top number of the fraction. The **denominator** is the bottom number and indicates how many equal parts the whole has been divided into. In 3/4, the number 3 is the numerator and the number 4 is the denominator. The numerator shows how many of the parts are used. For example, the fraction 3/4 is read as "three-fourths" and indicates three parts out of the four parts that make up the whole. The fraction bar that separates the numerator and the denominator also means *divided by*. Thus, 3/4 can be read as "three divided by four" or "3 ÷ 4." This definition is important when one changes fractions to decimals.

CLASSIFICATION OF FRACTIONS

Fractions are generally classified into two groups: *common fractions* and *decimal fractions*. A **common fraction** represents equal parts of a whole. A decimal fraction is commonly referred to simply as a *decimal*. Common fractions are subclassified as proper, improper, mixed, and complex.

Proper Fractions

A proper fraction has a numerator that is smaller than the denominator and designates less than one whole unit. For example, 3/4 < 1.

Improper Fractions

An **improper fraction** has a numerator that is greater than or the same as the denominator. The number 5/3 is an improper fraction because the numerator 5 is greater than the denominator: 3.

Example

$$5/3 > 1 \quad \text{or} \quad 5/5 = 1$$

Mixed Fractions

A **mixed fraction** is a whole number and a proper fraction combined. The value of the mixed fraction is always greater than 1.

Example

$$5\text{-}2/3 = 5 + 2/3 > 1$$

A mixed fraction can be converted to an improper fraction by converting the whole number to a fraction and adding (see the section "Adding and Subtracting Fractions with Dissimilar Denominators").

Complex Fractions

A complex fraction has the numerator or the denominator or both as a whole number, proper fraction, or mixed fraction. The value may be less than, greater than, or equal to 1.

Example

$$\frac{\frac{3}{5}}{\frac{1}{2}}, \quad \frac{\frac{1}{3}}{50}, \quad \text{and} \quad \frac{25}{\frac{1}{8}}$$

Adding Fractions

If fractions have the same denominator, simply add the numerators and keep the value of the common denominator the same. Then, reduce the numbers to the lowest terms by dividing the numerator and denominator by the same common divisor (in this case, 2). Remember, by dividing both by 2, you are essentially dividing by 1 because

$$\frac{2}{2} = 1$$

Example 1

$$\frac{1}{10} + \frac{3}{10} = \frac{4}{10} = \frac{2}{5}$$

Example 2

$$\frac{4}{18} + \frac{3}{18} + \frac{6}{18} = \frac{13}{18}$$

Subtracting Fractions

If fractions have the same denominator, subtract the smaller numerator from the larger numerator. Keep the denominator the same and then reduce to the lowest terms to obtain the final answer.

Example

$$\frac{6}{8} - \frac{2}{8} = \frac{4}{8} = \frac{1}{2}$$

Adding and Subtracting Fractions with Dissimilar Denominators

If fractions do not have the same denominator, change the fractions so they have the smallest common denominator, subtract (or add) the numerators, and leave the denominator the same.

Example

$$\frac{10}{24} - \frac{4}{12} = ?$$

Because 12 is a multiple of 24 (24 ÷ 2 = 12), divide 24 by 2 to reach the smallest common denominator of 12:

$$\frac{10}{24} \div \frac{2}{2} = \frac{5}{12}$$

Then, complete the subtraction:

$$\frac{5}{12} - \frac{4}{12} = \frac{1}{12}$$

Sometimes, however, the common denominator is not the smallest number even though both could be divided by 2. In the next example, the numerator 13 cannot be evenly divided by 2. Therefore, multiply the smaller denominator (12) by 2 to get a common denominator of 24. You will also need to multiply the numerator by 2.

Remember, by multiplying the numerator and the denominator by 2, you are essentially multiplying by 1.

Example

$$\frac{13}{24} - \frac{2}{12} = ?$$

$$\frac{2}{12} \times \frac{2}{2} = \frac{4}{24}$$

$$\frac{13}{24} - \frac{4}{24} = \frac{9}{24} = \frac{3}{8}$$

As noted in the section on mixed fractions, you can convert a mixed fraction to an improper fraction by using the following steps:

Example

$$5\text{-}2/3$$

First, convert the whole number to a fraction:

$$5 = \frac{5}{1}$$

Then, find a common denominator:

$$\frac{5}{1} + \frac{2}{3} = \frac{15}{3} + \frac{2}{3}$$

Finally, add the fractions:

$$\frac{15}{3} + \frac{2}{3} = \frac{17}{3}$$

Multiplying Fractions

To multiply fractions, first multiply the numerators; second, multiply the denominators; then, place the product of the numerators over the product of the denominators; and finally, reduce to lowest terms.

Example

$$\frac{3}{5} \times \frac{2}{4} = \frac{6}{20} = \frac{3}{10}$$

Dividing Fractions

To divide fractions, first invert (or turn upside down) the divisor, reduce to lowest terms, and then multiply the numerators and divisors.

Example

$$\frac{4}{8} \div \frac{2}{8} = ?$$

Invert the divisor:

$$\frac{4}{8} \times \frac{8}{2} = ?$$

Reduce to lowest terms and then multiply the numerators and then the denominators:

$$\frac{1}{2} \times \frac{4}{1} = \frac{4}{2} = \frac{2}{1} = 2$$

✳ Apply Your Knowledge 5.2

The following questions focus on what you have just learned about fractions. *See Appendix F for the correct answers.*

FILL IN THE BLANK
Select terms from your reading to fill in the blanks.

1. A proper fraction has a numerator that is _____ than the denominator.
2. The numerator is the _____ of the fraction.
3. A mixed fraction is a whole number and a proper fraction that are _____.
4. If fractions have the same denominator, subtract the _____ numerator from the _____ numerator.
5. To divide fractions, first _____ the divisor and then _____.
6. The numerator in 35/10 is _____.
7. The denominator in 42/100 is _____.
8. The numerator in 88/88 is _____.
9. The denominator in 14/60 is _____.
10. Twelve is the _____ in 12/5.

MULTIPLE CHOICE

Select the correct answer from choices a–d.

1. Determine the proper fraction from the following examples:
   a. 11/11
   b. 32/68
   c. 90/72
   d. 48/38

2. Determine the improper fraction from the following examples:
   a. 14/6
   b. 3/9
   c. 27/45
   d. 17/35

3. Determine the mixed fraction from the following examples:
   a. 2/6
   b. 101/16
   c. 11.238
   d. 6-2/4

DECIMALS

Decimal fractions, or **decimals**, are used with the metric system. Each decimal fraction has a denominator of 10 or a multiple of 10. Instead of writing the denominator, a decimal point is added to the numerator.

Example

$$\frac{3}{4} = \frac{75}{100} = 0.75$$

In writing a decimal fraction, always place a zero to the left of the decimal point so the decimal point can be readily seen.

Example

Fraction	Decimal Fraction
$\frac{2}{10}$	0.2
$\frac{19}{100}$	0.19
$\frac{256}{1,000}$	0.256

Decimals increase in value from right to left (Figure 5-1 ■); they decrease in value from left to right. Decimals increase in value in multiples of 10. Each column

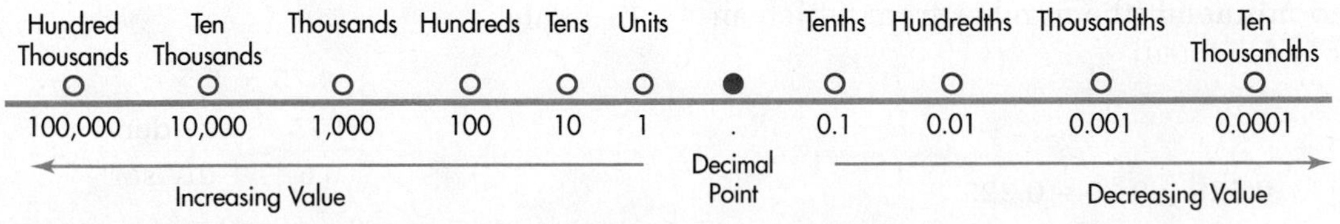

Hundred Thousands	Ten Thousands	Thousands	Hundreds	Tens	Units		Tenths	Hundredths	Thousandths	Ten Thousandths
O	O	O	O	O	O	●	O	O	O	O
100,000	10,000	1,000	100	10	1	.	0.1	0.01	0.001	0.0001

← Increasing Value   Decimal Point   Decreasing Value →

Figure 5-1 ■ Decimal values as they relate to the location of the decimal point.

Focus Point

Zeros in Decimals

When writing decimals, *eliminate* unnecessary zeros ("trailing" zeros) at the end of a decimal figure (for example, write 2.0 as 2) to avoid confusion. For example, if a 1-mg dose of a medication is written as "1.0 mg," the decimal point may not be seen, resulting in a 10-mg dose being administered. This is 10 times the desired dose and may result in a dangerous overdose. However, you should *always* insert a 0 before the decimal point of numbers less than 0 (for example, 0.25 instead of .25). For example, if a 0.5-mg dose of a medication is written as ".5 mg," the decimal point may not be seen, resulting in a 5-mg dose being administered. Again, this is 10 times the desired dose—with the potential to result in a dangerous overdose.

in a decimal has its own value—it depends on where it is situated in relation to the decimal point.

Adding and Subtracting Decimal Fractions

To add decimals, write the decimals in a column, placing the decimal points directly under each other. Then, add as in the addition of whole numbers and place the decimal point in the sum directly under the decimal points in the addends.

Example

$$0.2 + 0.5 + 0.7 = 1.4$$

Align the figures as follows:

$$
\begin{array}{r}
0.2 \\
0.5 \\
+0.7 \\
\hline
1.4
\end{array}
$$

To subtract decimals, write the decimals in columns, keeping the decimal points under each other. Then, subtract as whole numbers (zeros may be added after the decimal without changing the value) and place the decimal point in the remainder—directly under the decimal point in the **subtrahend** (the number that is deducted) and **minuend** (the number from which another number is deducted).

Example

$$0.525 - 0.30 = 0.225$$

Align the figures as follows:

$$
\begin{array}{lr}
0.525 & \text{(minuend)} \\
-0.30 & \\
\hline
0.225 & \text{(subtrahend)}
\end{array}
$$

Multiplying and Dividing Decimal Fractions

To multiply decimal fractions, multiply the two numbers and count off from right to left as many decimal places in the product (answer) as there were in the **multiplier** (the number that multiplies another number) and **multiplicand** (the number that is multiplied by another number).

Example

$$
\begin{array}{lr}
33.86 & \text{(multiplicand)} \\
\times 5.4 & \text{(multiplier)} \\
\hline
182.844 & \text{(product)}
\end{array}
$$

Because the multiplicand has two decimal places and the multiplier has one decimal place, you must count off three places from right to left and then insert the decimal point at this spot in the answer.

To divide by a decimal fraction, first move the decimal point in the divisor (the number that divides another number) enough places to the right to make it a whole number. Then, move the decimal point in the dividend (the number that is being divided) as many places as it was moved in the divisor. Place the decimal point in the answer directly above the one in the dividend.

Example

$$4.75 \div 0.5 = ?$$

$$\frac{4.75}{0.5} = \frac{\text{dividend}}{\text{divisor}}$$

In this example, 4.75 becomes 475 (the decimal point is moved two places). Therefore, 0.5 becomes 50 (the decimal point is moved two places). Now the problem may be divided as follows:

$$475 \div 50 = 9.5$$

✱ Apply Your Knowledge 5.3

The following questions focus on what you just learned about decimals. *See Appendix F for the correct answers.*

DO THE MATH
Calculate these problems.

1. $0.12 + 5.77 + 9.06 + 18 =$ _32.95_
2. $9.75 + 4.6 + 0.21 + 43.4 =$ _57.96_
3. $14.006 - 0.5 =$ _13.06_
4. $7.192 + 0.077 =$ _7.269_
5. $28.4 - 0.188 =$ _28.388_
6. $\$8.12 - \$0.97 =$ _7.15_
7. $\$17.52 - \$1.93 =$ _15.59_
8. $6 + 2.93 + 0.63 + 0.009 =$ _9.569_
9. $5 + 7.2 + 0.07 + 9.33 =$ _21.60_
10. $600 - 275.97 =$ _324.03_

11. $3.002 \times 0.05 =$ _0.150_
12. $16.1 \times 25.04 =$ _403.144_
13. $75.1 \times 1000.01 =$ _____
14. $23.2 \times 15.025 =$ _____
15. $1.14 \times 0.014 =$ _____
16. $45 \div 0.15 =$ _____
17. $73 \div 13.40 =$ _____
18. $25.3 \div 6.76 =$ _____
19. $515 \div 0.125 =$ _____
20. $16 \div 0.04 =$ _____

Ratios

A **ratio** is a mathematical expression that compares the relationship of one number with another number or expresses a part of a whole number. When written, the two quantities are separated by a colon (:). The colon means *division*. The expression 3:4 means there are *three parts to four parts*. Ratios are frequently used to show concentrations of a medication in a solution. They are also used to express measurement equivalents and dosages

of medications per unit (such as tablet or capsule). For example, 1 grain is equal to 15 g, which in a ratio would be expressed as 1 grain:15 g. One tablet containing 500 mg of a medication can be expressed as 1 tablet: 500 mg. When measuring insulin, 100 units are contained in 1 mL, which can be written as 100 units:1 mL.

Example

$\frac{2}{5}$ may be expressed as a ratio: 2:5.

✱ Apply Your Knowledge 5.4

The following questions focus on what you have just learned about ratios. *See Appendix F for the correct answers.*

FILL IN THE BLANK
Select terms from your reading to fill in the blanks.

1. The two quantities are separated by a _____ or _____ (symbol).
2. Ratios are frequently used to show concentrations of medication in a _____
3. A 100-unit insulin syringe contains 100 units in 1 mL, which can be written as a ratio of _____.
4. In administering medications, you can use ratios to express measurement equivalents and dosages of drug per _____.

DO THE MATH
Change the ratios to fractions and then reduce to lowest terms.

1. $0.05:0.15 =$ _____
2. $6:8 =$ _____
3. $3:150 =$ _____
4. $6:10 =$ _____
5. $4:7 =$ _____
6. $9:18 =$ _____

Proportions

A *proportion* is a way of expressing a relationship of equality between two ratios. A proportion may be expressed as:

$$1:4 \;::\; 3:12$$

or

$$1:4 = 3:12$$

or

$$\frac{1}{4} = \frac{3}{12}$$

In the examples above, the relationship of 1 to 4 is the same as the relationship of 3 to 12. In a proportion, these terms have names. The **means** are the two inside terms, and the **extremes** are the two outside terms. This relationship is shown in Figure 5-2 ■.

In a proportion, the product of the means is equal to the product of the extremes, which in turn equals 1. To prove this, convert the proportion into fractions and then cross-multiply the numerators and denominators.

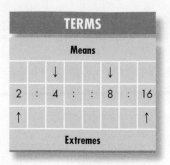

Figure 5-2 ■ The means and extremes of a proportion.

Example

$$1:5 \;::\; 2:10$$

Convert to fractions.

$$\frac{1}{5} = \frac{2}{10}$$

Cross-multiply the numerators and the denominators of the fraction.

$$\frac{1}{5} \times \frac{2}{10} = \frac{10}{10} = 1$$

✳ Apply Your Knowledge 5.5

The following questions focus on what you have just learned about means and extremes. *See Appendix F for the correct answers.*

DO THE MATH
Determine the missing means or extremes values.

1. 10:X :: 5:8 = _____
2. 3:12 :: X:36 = _____
3. 33:39 :: 55:X = _____
4. 10:4 :: 20:X = _____

5. 100:X :: 50:2 = _____
6. 21:27 :: X:45 = _____
7. X:15 :: 100:75 = _____
8. 4:25 :: 16:X = _____

Percents

The term **percent**, or the symbol %, means *hundredths*. Thus, a percentage may also be expressed as a fraction, as a decimal fraction, or as a ratio.

Example

40% means *40 parts per hundred* or 40/100

75% means *75 parts per hundred* or 75/100

Example

Percent		Fraction		Decimal		Ratio
60%	=	60/100	=	0.60	=	60:100

Note: To change a percent to a decimal, move the decimal point two places to the left. In the example, the

decimal point comes before the whole number 60. To change a fraction to a percent, divide the numerator by the denominator and then multiply the results by 100. Then, add a percent symbol (%).

Example 1
To convert 6/10 to a percent:

$$6 \div 10 = 0.6$$
$$0.6 \times 100 = 60\%$$

Example 2
To convert 1/5 to a percent:

$$1 \div 5 = 0.2$$
$$0.2 \times 100 = 20\%$$

✳ Apply Your Knowledge 5.6

The following questions focus on what you have just learned about percents. *See Appendix F for the correct answers.*

FILL IN THE BLANK

Select terms from your readings to fill in the blanks.

1. To convert a percent to a decimal, the decimal point comes before the _____ _____.

2. The symbol % for *percent* means _____.

3. The _____ 25/100 is equivalent to 25%.

4. To change a fraction to a percent, divide the numerator by the _____ and multiply by 100.

5. To change a _____ to a decimal, move the _____ point two places to the left.

DO THE MATH

Convert these percents to decimals.

1. 2% = _____
2. 18% = _____
3. 40% = _____
4. 106% = _____
5. 0.8% = _____
6. 24 1/2% = _____
7. 150.75% = _____
8. 4.5% = _____

Convert these decimals to percents.

9. 0.08 = _____
10. 32 = _____
11. 0.44 = _____
12. 0.5 = _____
13. 0.019 = _____
14. 5.7 = _____
15. 13 = _____
16. 0.99 = _____

PRACTICAL SCENARIO 1

Pharmacy technicians must always be careful when using mathematical equations for compounding. Phil, a pharmacy technician who only recently began working in a pharmacy, is asked by the pharmacist to mix a powdered drug with a solution so the amount of drug is 3%. Phil converts 3% to a decimal (0.03) so he can more easily mix the proper amount. He then mixes 0.03 g of the powdered drug into 100 mL of solution. When the pharmacist checks Phil's calculations, he finds that the mixture is much too weak.

Critical Thinking Questions

1. What miscalculation did Phil make when mixing the solution?
2. What is a good preventive measure when performing calculations for compounding?

PRACTICAL SCENARIO 2

A respiratory care technician was attempting to calculate a 60% solution as a decimal. He calculates this as a 0.06 solution.

Critical Thinking Questions

1. What decimal would have been correct to represent a 60% solution?
2. What would be the ratio of 60% of medication to the solution containing it?

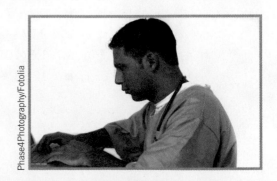
Phase4Photography/Fotolia

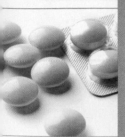

Chapter Capsule

The section repeats the objectives from the beginning of the chapter and then provides a summary of the most important concepts for that objective. Use this section as a quick review and to check your knowledge.

Objective 1: Describe the difference between Arabic numbers and Roman numerals.

- Arabic—use numbers, decimals, and fractions to express values
- Roman—use letters that represent number values

Objective 2: Convert an improper fraction to a mixed fraction.

- 5/3—5 is the numerator and 3 is the denominator
- To convert it to a mixed fraction, divide the numerator by the denominator
- Answers: 1 and 2/3

Objective 3: Add fractions that have the same denominator.

- $1/4 + 2/4 = 3/4$
- $2/5 + 2/5 = 4/5$
- $3/10 + 6/10 = 9/10$

Objective 4: Subtract fractions that have the same denominator.

- $8/12 - 7/12 = 1/12$
- $9/20 - 6/20 = 3/20$
- $27/45 - 19/45 = 8/45$

Objective 5: Multiply fractions and mixed fractions.

- $1/4 \times 1\text{-}3/4 = 1/4 \times 7/4 = 7/16$
- $3/10 \times 2\text{-}7/10 = 3/10 \times 27/10 = 81/100$
- $3/7 \times 1\text{-}2/7 = 3/7 \times 9/7 = 27/49$

Objective 6: Divide fractions and mixed fractions.

- $1\text{-}1/12 \div 9/12 = 13/12 \times 12/9 = 156/108 = 1\text{-}48/108 = 1\text{-}4/9$
- $2\text{-}1/3 \div 2/3 = 7/3 \times 3/2 = 21/6 = 7/2 = 3\text{-}1/2$
- $5\text{-}1/2 \div 1/2 = 11/2 \times 2/1 = 22/2 = 11$

Objective 7: Add, subtract, multiply, and divide decimals.

- $0.2 + 7.13 + 3.067 = 10.397$
- $9.77 - 2.9 - 1.38 = 5.49$
- $1.6 \times 0.77 \times 7.1 = 8.7472$
- $12.33 \div 3.6 \div 1.5 = 2.283333 =$ (rounds to 2.283)

Objective 8: Define *ratios*, *proportions*, and *percents*.

- Ratios—compare one number with another or express a part of a whole number; example: 3:4 means *three parts to four parts*

- Proportions—express a relationship of equality between two ratios; example: 1:4 :: 3:12 means the relationship of 1 to 4 is the same as the relationship of 3 to 12

- Percents—mean *hundredths*; may also be expressed as a fraction, a decimal, or a ratio; example: 40% means *40 parts per hundred*, or 40/100

 ## Internet Sites of Interest

- Get online help with math calculations at S.O.S. Math's site at **www.sosmath.com**.

- On The Math Page, you can click on a chapter in an online textbook to find instructions and plenty of examples for the arithmetic or algebra problem that is confounding you. Find help at **www.themathpage.com**.

- The hot subjects fractions, decimals, and percents are covered by clicking on each topic at **www.math.com**.

PEARSON
myhealthprofessionskit™

Go to www.myhealthprofessionskit.com to access the Companion Website created for this textbook. Simply select "Basic Health Science" from the choice of disciplines. Find this book and then log in using your username and password to access interactive learning games, assessment questions, animations, and more.

Chapter 6

Measurement Systems and Their Equivalents

Chapter Objectives

After completing this chapter, you should be able to:

1. Name the basic units of the metric system for weight, volume, and length.
2. Understand metric abbreviations used in pharmacy and clinical settings.
3. Identify major apothecary and household measurement system units.
4. Discuss milliequivalents and International Units.
5. Convert units of measure to equivalent units of measure within the same system of measurement.
6. Recognize the difference between the Celsius and Fahrenheit temperature scales.

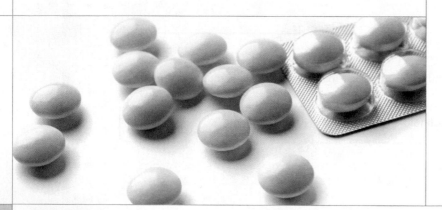

Key Terms

apothecary system (ah-PAW-thuh-keh-ree) (page 89)

drams (page 89)

grain (page 89)

gram (page 87)

household system (page 89)

International Units (page 91)

liter (LEE-ter) (page 87)

meter (MEE-ter) (page 87)

metric system (page 87)

milliequivalents (mil-lee-KWIH-vuh-lentz) (page 90)

minims (MIH-numz) (page 89)

ounces (page 87)

unit (page 87)

Introduction

Health-care professionals who deal with the administration of medications prescribed for patients must ensure the accuracy and correctness of drug dosages. They must have a complete knowledge of the weights and measures used in drug administration for prescribed amounts.

Units of Measure

Three systems of measurement are used in pharmacology and the calculation of drug dosages: (1) metric, (2) apothecary, and (3) household. Today, however, household and apothecary measures, such as teaspoons and **ounces** (equivalent to 480 grains or 31.10349 g), are used less commonly. The most common, most accurate, and safest system of measurement in all countries is the **metric system**—a system based on the decimal system. Medications are administered with three parameters in mind: (1) weight, (2) volume, and (3) length. Weight is the most used parameter and is essential as a dosage **unit** (a unit is defined as a standard of measure, weight, or any other similar quality). Measurement of volume is the next most important parameter and is used for liquids. Length is the least used parameter for dosage calculations.

METRIC SYSTEM

The basic units of weight and volume in the metric system are based on units of "10", as in the decimal system. The metric system uses the basic units of **gram** (g) as the unit of weight (equivalent to 15.432358 grains), **liter** (L) as the unit of volume (equivalent to 1.056688 quarts), and **meter** (m) as the unit of length (equivalent to 39.37007874 inches). In medicine, it is common to use weight for determining medication doses based in kilograms and volume to express liquid amounts. Parts of these basic units are named by adding prefixes that describe multiples or fractions of the standard measures for weight, volume, and length based on units of 10. The prefixes usually relate to Latin and Greek measures. Table 6-1 ■ shows Latin prefixes. Table 6-2 ■ shows Greek prefixes.

Table 6-1 ■ Latin Prefixes

PREFIX*	VALUE	EQUIVALENTS
micro- (mc):	1/1,000,000	= 0.000001
milli- (m):	1/1,000	= 0.001
centi- (c):	1/100	= 0.01
deci- (d):	1/10	= 0.1

*Remember: Latin prefixes denote fractions.

Table 6-2 ■ Greek Prefixes

PREFIX*	VALUE
deca- (da):	10
hecto- (h):	100
kilo- (k):	1,000
mega- (M):	1,000,000

*Remember: Greek prefixes denote multiples.

A system for international standardization of metric units was established throughout the world in 1960 with the introduction of the International System, or SI (from the French *Système International*). Table 6-3 ■ shows SI standardized abbreviation.

Table 6-3 ■ SI Standardized Abbreviations (Metric System)

PARAMETER	UNIT	ABBREVIATION	EQUIVALENTS
Weight	gram (basic unit)	g	1 g = 1,000 mg
	milligram	mg	1 mg – 1,000 mcg = 0.001 g
	microgram	mcg	1 mcg = 0.001 mg = 0.000001 g
	kilogram	kg	1 kg = 1,000 g
Volume	liter (basic unit)	L	1 L = 1,000 mL
	milliliter	mL	1 mL = 1 cc* = 0.001 L
Length	meter (basic unit)	m	1 m = 100 cm = 1,000 mm
	centimeter	cm	1 cm = 0.01 m = 10 mm
	millimeter	mm	1 mm = 0.001 m = 0.1 cm

*This abbreviation should not be used in clinical practice to avoid medication errors.

✺ Apply Your Knowledge 6.1

The following questions focus on what you have just learned about the metric system. *See Appendix F for the correct answers.*

FILL IN THE BLANK

Rewrite the following metric numbers by using numerals and abbreviations.

1. Twenty-five grams _____
2. Eight milliliters _____
3. Fifty-five hundredths of a milligram _____
4. One hundred micrograms _____
5. Seven and two-tenths micrograms _____
6. Sixteen liters _____
7. Two thousand milliliters _____
8. Four meters _____
9. Nineteen millimeters _____
10. Three and one-half centimeters _____

MULTIPLE CHOICE

Select the correct answer from choices a–d.

1. The metric system is based on which of the following?
   a. Units
   b. Fractions
   c. Decimals
   d. Proportions

2. Which of the following is the least used parameter for dosage calculations?
   a. Volume
   b. Length
   c. Unit
   d. Weight

3. In medicine, it is common to use weight for determining medication doses in which of the following increments?
   a. Ounces
   b. Kilograms
   c. Pounds
   d. International Units

4. The abbreviation for the International System is:
   a. INS
   b. IS
   c. SI
   d. SIN

5. The value of the prefix "hecto" is:
   a. 10
   b. 100
   c. 1,000
   d. 1,000,000

APOTHECARY SYSTEM

The **apothecary system** is a very old English system that has slowly been replaced by the metric system. The apothecary system uses **minims** (the basic unit of volume), **drams** (fluidrams—equivalent to 1/8 ounce), ounces (fluidounces), pints, quarts, and gallons to measure volume.

It measures weight by grains, drams, ounces, and pounds. The apothecary system also uses Roman numerals to indicate the amount of drug. The basic unit of weight is the **grain**. Today, the apothecary system is used for only a few drugs, such as acetaminophen, aspirin, and phenobarbital. Table 6-4 ■ shows common apothecary equivalents.

Table 6-4 ■ Apothecary System

PARAMETER	UNIT	ABBREVIATION	EQUIVALENTS
Weight	grain (basic unit)	gr	
	dram	dr or ʒ*	
	ounce	oz or ʒ*	1 oz = 16 dr = 437.5 gr
	pound	lb	1 lb = 16 oz = 7000 (gr)
Volume	minim (basic unit)	M or ♏*	
	fluidram	fl dr	
	fluidounce	ʒ*	pt i = ʒ* 16
	pint	pt	qt i = ʒ* 32
	quart	qt	qt i = pt ii
	gallon	gal	

*These abbreviations should not be used in clinical practice to avoid medication errors.

Note: There are no essential equivalents of weight or length to learn for this system.

✳ Apply Your Knowledge 6.2

The following questions focus on what you have just learned about the apothecary system of measurements. *See Appendix F for the correct answers.*

FILL IN THE BLANK

Select abbreviations or symbols for the apothecary system to fill in the blanks.

1. fluid ounce _____
2. grain _____
3. dram _____
4. quart _____
5. pint _____
6. minim _____

HOUSEHOLD SYSTEM

The **household system** is used in most American homes. This system of measurement is important for a patient at home who has no knowledge of the metric or apothecary systems. However, household measurements, consisting of teaspoons and tablespoons, are not precisely accurate, so they should never be used in the medical setting. The only household units of measurement used to measure drugs are units of volume. These include the drop, teaspoon, tablespoon, ounce (fluid), cup, pint, quart, and gallon. Table 6-5 ■ shows common household units, abbreviations, and equivalents.

Table 6-5 ■ Household Measurements

UNIT	ABBREVIATION	EQUIVALENTS
drop	gtt	15 gtt = 1 mL
teaspoon	t (tsp)	1 tsp = 5 mL
tablespoon	T (tbsp)	1 T = 3 t
ounce (fluid)	oz	2 T = 1 oz
cup	cup	1 cup = 8 oz
pint	pt	1 pt = 2 cups
quart	qt	1 qt = 4 cups = 2 pt
gallon	gal	1 gal = 4 qt

Note: Cups, quarts, and gallons are commonly used to measure medications.

✳ Apply Your Knowledge 6.3

The following exercises focus on what you have just learned about conversions among measurement systems. *See Appendix F for the correct answers.*

FILL IN THE BLANK

Select terms from your reading to fill in the blanks.

1. How many cups equal 2 pints? _____
2. Forty-five teaspoons are equivalent to how many tablespoons? _____
3. How many cups are equivalent to 8 ounces? _____
4. How many teaspoons are equivalent to 1 ounce? _____
5. How many drops are equivalent to 2 tablespoons? _____
6. How many tablespoons are equivalent to 1 ounce? _____
7. How many pints are equivalent to 8 cups? _____
8. How many ounces are equivalent to 4 tablespoons? _____
9. A meter is a metric unit that measures _____.
10. A liter is a metric unit that measures _____.
11. A gram is a metric unit that measures _____.
12. 3 cups = _____ oz
13. 220 drops = _____ tsp

MILLIEQUIVALENT MEASURES AND INTERNATIONAL UNITS

Milliequivalents and units are measurements used to indicate the strength of certain drugs. Pharmacists and chemists define *milliequivalent* measures as an expression of the number of grams of equivalent weight of a drug contained in 1 mL of a normal solution. Electrolytes, such as sodium and potassium, are usually measured in milliequivalents (mEq). Examples of drugs that are ordered by prescribers in milliequivalents include potassium chloride, sodium bicarbonate, and sodium chloride. Because the dosage is individualized, no calculations are involved.

Units mainly measure the potency of heparin, insulin, penicillin, and some vitamins. A unit is the amount of a medication required to produce a specific effect. The size of a unit varies for each drug. Vitamins are measured in standardized units called

International Units. These International Units show the amount of drug required to produce a certain effect, but they are standardized by international agreement. The International Unit does not measure a medication in terms of its physical weight or volume. Units and milliequivalents cannot be directly converted into the metric, apothecary, or household systems.

Conversion Within and Between Systems

Drug doses are usually ordered in metric system amounts, such as grams, milligrams, liters, and milliliters. Sometimes, you need to convert drug dosages between the metric, apothecary, and household systems of measurement. First, you must know how the measure of a quantity in one system compares with its measure in another system. For example, you learned the relationships between gram and kilogram, milliliter and liter, and teaspoon and tablespoon. To convert between systems, you may also need to know the relationship between milliliter and teaspoon. For example, 1 tsp = 5 mL or 1 kg = 1,000 g. Most prescriptions and medication orders are written in the metric system. Medications are usually ordered in a unit of weight measurement, such as grams or grains. You must be able to convert between units of measurement within the same system or convert units of measurement from one system to another. Table 6-6 ■ summarizes equivalent measures for volume in three different systems.

Table 6-6 ■ Approximate Equivalents for Volume and Weight

	METRIC	APOTHECARY	HOUSEHOLD
Volume	5 mL	1 dr	1 tsp
	15 mL	4 dr	1 T
	30 mL	1 fl oz	2 T
	240 mL	8 fl oz	1 cup
	480 mL	16 fl oz	1 pt
	960 mL	32 fl oz	1 qt
Weight	1 mg	gr 1/50 (1/50 grain)	3/100,000 oz
	15 mg	gr 1/4 (1/4 grain)	5/10,000 oz
	30 mg	gr ss 1/2 grain)	1/1,000 oz
	60 mg	gr i (1 grain)	1/500 oz
	0.5 g	gr viii (8 grains)	2/100 oz
	1 g (1,000 mg)	gr xv (15 grains)	2/1,000 lb
	1 kg	15,432 grains	2.2 lbs

✳ Apply Your Knowledge 6.4

The following questions focus on what you have just learned about conversion between different systems for volume and weight. *See Appendix F for the correct answers.*

FILL IN THE BLANK
Convert the following amounts.

1. 5 L = _____ oz
2. 0.25 L = _____ oz
3. 20 oz = _____ L
4. 12 oz = _____ L
5. 4 oz = _____ mL
6. 8-1/2 oz = _____ mL
7. 1/2 oz = _____ mL
8. 60 mL = _____ oz
9. 150 mL = _____ oz
10. 15 mL = _____ oz
11. 5 g = _____ gr

12. 0.5 g = _____ gr
13. 0.1 g = _____ gr
14. 3 gr = _____ g
15. 1-1/2 gr = _____ g
16. 4 gr = _____ mg
17. 1-1/2 gr = _____ mg
18. 7-1/2 gr = _____ mg
19. 150 mg = _____ gr
20. 30 mg = ___1/2___ gr
21. 15 mg = ___1/4___ gr

TEMPERATURE CONVERSION

Two common scales of temperature are used throughout the world: Celsius (Centigrade) and Fahrenheit scales. The Fahrenheit scale is still used in the United States; the Celsius scale is used in most other parts of the world. The abbreviation used in the Fahrenheit scale is an "F," and in the Celsius scale, it is a "C."

Water freezes at 32°F and at 0°C. This difference of 32° is used in converting temperature from one scale to the other. It can also be determined that water boils at 212°F and at 100°C.

There is a 180° difference between the freezing and boiling points on the Fahrenheit scale and a 100° difference between these two points on the Celsius scale. The difference between the boiling point and the freezing point on the Fahrenheit scale and the Celsius scale can be set as a ratio of each Celsius degree being 9/5 times greater than each Fahrenheit degree, as seen in the following formula:

$$180{:}100 \quad \frac{180}{100} = \frac{9}{5}$$

If the fraction 9/5 is expressed as a decimal, it can be stated that each Celsius degree is 1.8 times greater than each Fahrenheit degree. To convert a given temperature from one scale to the other, you may use one of the following formulas:

$$°F = 1.8°C + 32$$
$$°F = 9/5°C + 32$$

Example 1: Convert 100°C to Fahrenheit:

$$°F = 1.8 \times 100°C + 32 \qquad °F = 9/5 \times 100°C + 32$$
$$°F = 180 + 32 \qquad\qquad °F = 180 + 32$$
$$°F = 212 \qquad\qquad\quad\; °F = 212$$

Example 2: Convert 212°F to Celsius:
(Note: Subtract 32 from both sides of the equation.)

$$212°F = 1.8°C + 32$$
$$212°F - 32 = 1.8°C + 32 - 32$$
$$180°F = 1.8°C$$
$$°C = 100$$

or

$$212°F = 9/5°C + 32$$
$$212°F - 32 = 9/5°C + 32 - 32$$
$$180°F = 1.8°C$$
$$°C = 180°F \div 9/5$$
$$°C = 180°F \times 5/9$$
$$°C = 100°F$$

Figure 6-1 ■ indicates that water freezes at 32°F and at 0°C.

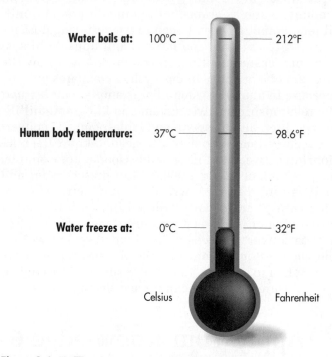

Figure 6-1 ■ Thermometer showing the temperatures at which water freezes (0°C and 32°F) and boils (100°C and 212°F).

✳ Apply Your Knowledge 6.5

The following questions focus on what you have just learned about temperature conversions. *See Appendix F for the correct answers.*

FILL IN THE BLANK

Convert these to the Celsius or Fahrenheit scale.

1. 13°C _____
2. 21°C _____
3. 34°C _____
4. 45°C _____
5. 67°C _____

6. 97°C _____
7. 99.9°C _____
8. 106°C _____
9. 38°F _____
10. 52°F _____

11. 76°F _____
12. 98°F _____
13. 104°F _____
14. –16°F _____

PRACTICAL SCENARIO 1

Tara is a 7-month-old girl who is brought to her doctor's office by her mother. Her body temperature is 103.4°F. Her pediatrician orders acetaminophen 7 mL every 4 hours while her fever is above 101°F. You, the medical assistant, advise Tara's mother about carefully following the physician's order. Tara's mother, who grew up in England and only recently relocated to the United States, asks if you can convert the temperature of 101°F into Celsius degrees, and you agree to do this.

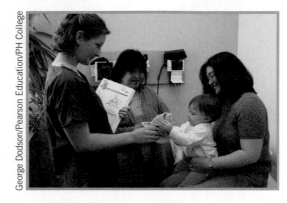

George Dodson/Pearson Education/PH College

Critical Thinking Questions

1. Which formula should you use to convert 101°F into Celsius degrees?
2. What is the answer that you give to Tara's mother?
3. What type of measuring instrument should you instruct Tara's mother to use?

PRACTICAL SCENARIO 2

A physician instructs the mother of a child to give the child 10 milliliters of a medication every 6 hours. The mother of the child asks the medical assistant if she can use a teaspoon to administer the ordered dose.

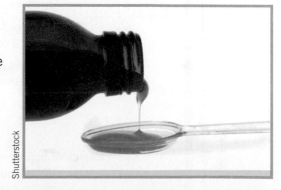

Shutterstock

Critical Thinking Questions

1. How many teaspoons constitute 10 milliliters?
2. How many drops are equal to 10 milliliters?

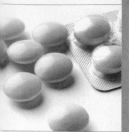

Chapter Capsule

This section repeats the objectives from the beginning of the chapter and then provides a summary of the most important concepts for that objective. Use this section as a quick review and to check your knowledge.

Objective 1: Name the basic units of the metric system for weight, volume, and length.

- ■ Weight—gram (g)
- ■ Volume—liter (L)
- ■ Length—meter (m)

Objective 2: Understand metric abbreviations used in pharmacy and clinical settings.

- ■ Grams (g)
- ■ Milligrams (mg)
- ■ Micrograms (mcg)
- ■ Kilograms (kg)
- ■ Liters (L)
- ■ Milliliters (mL)

Objective 3: Identify major apothecary and household measurement system units.

- ■ Apothecary—minims, drams (fluidrams), ounces (fluidounces), pints, quarts, gallons, grains, drams, pounds
- ■ Household—drops, teaspoons, tablespoons, ounces (fluid), cups, pints, quarts, gallons

Objective 4: Discuss milliequivalents and International Units.

- ■ Milliequivalents and units are measurements used to indicate the strength of certain drugs.
- ■ Milliequivalent measures are defined as expressions of the number of grams of equivalent weight of a drug contained in 1 mL of a normal solution.
- ■ Electrolytes, such as sodium and potassium, are usually measured in milliequivalents.
- ■ Other drugs ordered in milliequivalents include potassium chloride, sodium bicarbonate, and sodium chloride.
- ■ Units mainly measure the potency of heparin, insulin, penicillin, and some vitamins.
- ■ A unit is the amount of a medication required to produce a specific effect, and the size of a unit varies for each drug.
- ■ Vitamins are measured in standardized units (per international agreement) called International Units.
- ■ International Units do not measure a medication in terms of its physical weight or volume.

Objective 5: Convert units of measure to equivalent units of measure within the same system of measurement.

- ■ For example: 1 kg = 1,000 g; 1 g = 1,000 mg; 1 mg = 1,000 mcg
- ■ 1 L = 1,000 mL
- ■ 1 m = 1,000 mm; 1 cm = 10 mm

- 1 lb = 16 oz = 7,000 gr
- 1 pt = 16 fluid ounces
- 2 pt = 1 qt
- 1 T = 3 tsp
- 2 T = 1 oz
- 1 cup = 8 oz

Objective 6: Recognize the difference between the Celsius and Fahrenheit temperature scales.

- Celsius—used in most parts of the world besides the United States; abbreviation for Celsius is C; water freezes at 0°C; water boils at 100°C

- Fahrenheit—used in the United States; abbreviation for Fahrenheit is F; water freezes at 32°F; water boils at 212°F; °F = 1.8°C + 32 or °F = 9/5°C + 32

Internet Sites of Interest

- A conversion calculator for length, weight, pressure, volume, and temperature can be found at **www.worldwidemetric.com/Measurements.html**.

- For a quick check of common weights and measures used by pharmacy technicians and other medical professionals, visit **http://www.rxtrek.net/weights.htm**.

- Click on the appropriate calculator at **www.sciencelab.com/data/conversion.shtml** and then convert between different units of measure for weight and mass, metric weight, temperature, length, distance, volume, speed, pressure, area, force, energy, frequency, power, torque, and astronomical units.

PEARSON myhealthprofessionskit™

Go to www.myhealthprofessionskit.com to access the Companion Website created for this textbook. Simply select "Basic Health Science" from the choice of disciplines. Find this book and then log in using your username and password to access interactive learning games, assessment questions, animations, and more.

Chapter 7

Adult and Pediatric Dosage Calculations

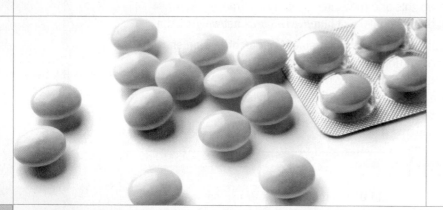

Chapter Objectives

After completing this chapter, you should be able to:

1. Discuss the differences between *dosage ordered, desired dose,* and *dose on hand*.

2. Explain how to use the formula $D/H \times Q = X$ to calculate drug doses.

3. Explain the fraction proportion method and the formula used in this method.

4. Discuss how to calculate parenteral medications and the formula used.

5. Calculate intramuscular doses.

6. Name the most common types of insulin used in the United States.

7. Explain the steps required for the proper injection of insulin.

8. Convert physician orders of heparin to the volume of solution that contains the amount of heparin ordered.

9. Calculate whether the amount of a prescribed pediatric dosage is the safe or appropriate amount for a particular patient.

10. Define the most accurate method of calculating a child's dose and perform correct calculations by using this method.

Key Terms

calibrated (page 97)
capsule (page 99)
conversion (page 97)
desired dose (page 97)
dilutions (dye-LOO-shuns) (page 98)
dose (page 97)
elixir (page 100)

heparin (HEH-puh-rin) (page 98)
injectable (page 103)
insulin (IN-suh-lin) (page 104)
loading dose (page 97)
maintenance dose (page 97)
nomogram (NAW-mo-gram) (page 110)

prophylactic dose (page 97)
scored (page 99)
spirit (page 100)
suspension (page 100)
syrup (page 100)
tablet (page 99)

Introduction

The ability to accurately calculate drug dosages is an essential skill in health care. Serious harm to patients may result from a mathematical error during a calculation and the subsequent administration of a drug dosage. It is the responsibility of those administering drugs to carry out medical orders precisely and efficiently.

General Dosage Calculations

The **dose** of a drug is the amount a patient takes for the intended therapeutic effect, and the *dosage regimen* is the schedule of dosing for a drug. Many factors contribute to determining the dose and dosage regimen, including the potency of the drug and route of administration as well as such patient factors as weight, disease state, and tolerance. A **loading dose** may be required for some drugs to produce an adequate blood level that yields the desired therapeutic effect; this dose would then be followed by smaller **maintenance doses** to maintain an adequate blood level. A **prophylactic dose** of a drug may be given to prevent a disease, but a *therapeutic dose*, which is usually higher than the prophylactic dose, is given to treat an ongoing disease. The dose for most drugs is given in units of weight (for example, 500 mg), but the dose for some drugs, such as biologics, is given based on activity.

The doses for many drugs, such as antihypertensives, are general and usually not patient-specific. However, the doses for some drugs require patient data, such as body surface area (BSA), clinical laboratory values, or pharmacokinetic parameters.

It is the health-care professional's responsibility to ensure that the patient receives the proper dose of medication and to educate the patient about the proper measurement of doses. For solid-dosage forms, the correct dose is easily administered in premeasured tablets or capsules. However, if the drug is a liquid, the dose is usually a volume that must be accurately measured by using a standardized 5-mL teaspoon, **calibrated** dropper (a dropper that is marked with graduated measurements), or syringe. If the pharmacist compounds a specific product for a patient, it is also his or her responsibility to ensure that the correct amount of drug is delivered in each dose.

As a health-care professional, you must also be familiar with the following terms to understand dosage calculations:

✳ Amount to administer—The volume of a medication that contains the desired dose; the number of tablets (or milliliters of a solution) administered once to provide the desired amount of a drug.

✳ **Desired dose**—The amount to be administered at one time. It must be in the same unit of measurement as the dosage unit.

✳ Dosage ordered—The total amount of ordered drug, along with the frequency it is to be administered. Its measurement units may not be the same as the dosage unit.

✳ Dosage strength—The dose on hand per the dosage unit. If the dose on hand is 100 mg per capsule and the dosage unit is 1 capsule, the dosage strength is 100 mg/capsule.

✳ Dosage unit—The volume of medication that contains a quantity of drug as listed on the drug label. If a drug contains 50 mg of drug per capsule, the dosage unit is 1 capsule.

✳ Dose on hand—The amount of drug in a dosage unit. If a drug has 150 mg of drug per capsule, the dose on hand is 150 mg.

Calculating Dosages

The first step in computing medication dosage, regardless of the method used, is to make certain the strength of the drug ordered and the strength of the drug available are in the same unit of measure. If necessary, **conversion** (changing) to a single unit must be carried out. After this is done, the problem can be set up by using this formula:

$$\frac{D}{H} \times Q = X$$

The answer is most commonly signified by the letter X. In this formula, D represents the desired dosage of the drug to be administered. H represents the dosage of the drug available. D and H must always be in the same unit of measure. Q represents the number of tablets, capsules, milliliters, minims, and so forth, that contains the available dosage. X represents the number of tablets, capsules, milliliters, minims, and so on, of the desired dose (the amount to be administered). Q and X must always be in the same unit of measure. Make certain that all the terms in the formula are labeled with the correct units of measure.

Several formulas can be used to calculate drug dosages. One formula uses ratios:

$$\frac{\text{Dose on hand } (H)}{\text{Quantity on hand } (Q)} = \frac{\text{Desired dose } (D)}{\text{Quantity desired } (X)}$$

Example 1

Amoxil 500 mg is ordered. It is supplied in a liquid form containing 250 mg in 5 mL. To calculate the dosage, use this formula:

$$\frac{250 \text{ mg } (H)}{5 \text{ mL } (Q)} = \frac{500 \text{ mg } (D)}{X}$$

Then, cross-multiply:

$$250\,X = 5\text{ mL} \times 500\text{ mg}$$

$$X = \frac{5 \times 500}{250}$$

Therefore, the dose ordered is 10 mL.

You can also use the formula above to calculate dosages:

$$\text{Amount to administer }(X) = \frac{\text{Desired dose }(D)}{\text{Dose on hand }(H)} \times \text{Quantity on hand }(Q)$$

Example 2

Heparin, an anticoagulant, is often distributed in vials in prepared **dilutions** (less concentrated mixtures) of 10,000 units/mL. If the order calls for 2,500 units, you can use the previous formula to calculate:

$$X = \frac{2,500\text{ units}}{10,000\text{ units/mL}} \times 1$$

$$X = 0.25\text{ or }1/4\text{ mL}$$

Focus Point

Double Checking Calculations

Any health-care professional who is unsure about a dosage calculation should have another health-care professional double-check the calculation before the administration of medication.

✳ Apply Your Knowledge 7.1

The following questions focus on what you have just learned about general dosage calculations. *See Appendix F for the correct answers.*

MATCHING

Match the lettered terms to the numbered descriptions. The lettered terms may be used more than once.

DESCRIPTION

1. _____ The amount to be administered at one time
2. _____ The amount of drug in a dosage unit
3. _____ The volume of medication that contains a quantity of drug
4. _____ The volume of a medication that contains the desired dose
5. _____ The total amount of ordered drug, along with the frequency it is to be administered
6. _____ The dose on hand per the dosage unit

TERM

a. Dosage unit
b. Dosage strength
c. Dosage ordered
d. Desired dose
e. Dose on hand
f. Amount to administer

DRUG DOSAGE CALCULATIONS

Calculate the drug dosages.

1. Ordered: cimetidine (Tagamet) 0.2 g PO qid

   On hand: Tagamet 400 mg is available.

   How many tablet(s) would you administer per dose? _____

2. Ordered: methyldopa (Aldomet) 150 mg PO tid

   On hand: Aldomet 250 mg/5 mL is available.

   How many milliliters would you administer per dose? _____

3. Ordered: lorazepam (Ativan) 1 mg PO tid

   On hand: Ativan 0.5 mg is available.

   How many tablet(s) would you administer? _____

4. Ordered: clarithromycin (Biaxin) 100 mg PO qid

   On hand: Biaxin 125 mg/5 mL is available.

   How many milliliters (mL) should the patient receive per dose? _____

Calculating Oral Dosages

Oral medications are divided into solid types (such as tablets and capsules) and liquids. The **tablet** is the most common form of solid oral medication. Certain tablets are specially designed to be administered sublingually (under the tongue) or buccally (between the cheek and gum). Some tablets are chewable; others dissolve in water to make a liquid that the patient can drink. Always check the drug label to find out how a tablet is meant to be administered. **Capsules** are usually oval-shaped gelatin shells that contain medication in powder or granule form. Some tablets and capsules are available in sustained release form. This allows increased duration of drug action and therefore the patient does not have to take as many doses of the drug.

SOLID DOSES

Tablets may be broken into parts only if they are **scored** (notched), and they must be broken only along the line of the scoring. Unscored tablets must *not* be broken into parts.

Before administering medication to a patient, you need to determine how many tablets or capsules will deliver the *desired dose*. If necessary, convert the *dosage ordered* to the *desired dose* by using the same unit of measurement as the dose on hand. Then, you can calculate the *amount to administer* by using the fraction proportion method.

$$\frac{\text{Dose on hand } (H)}{\text{Dosage unit } (Q)} = \frac{\text{Desired dose } (D)}{\text{Amount to administer}}$$

or

$$\text{Desired dose } (D) \times \frac{\text{Dosage unit } (Q)}{\text{Dose on hand } (H)}$$
$$= \text{Amount to administer}$$

Example 1

Ordered: Zocor 40-mg bid

On hand: Zocor 20-mg tablets

The dosage ordered is 40 mg, the dose on hand is 20 mg, and the dosage unit is 1 tablet. The units of the dosage ordered and the dose on hand are the same, so no conversion is needed. The desired dose is 40 mg.

Use the formula:

$$D \times \frac{Q}{H} = X$$

$$40 \text{ mg} \times \frac{1 \text{ tablet}}{20 \text{ mg}} = X$$

$$X = 2 \text{ tablets}$$

Example 2

Ordered: doxazosin mesylate 4 mg PO daily

The label is shown in Figure 7-1 ■. How many tablets will you administer to the patient?

Use this formula:

$$D \times \frac{Q}{H} = X$$

$$4 \text{ mg} \times \frac{1 \text{ tablet}}{4 \text{ mg}} = 1 \text{ tablet}$$

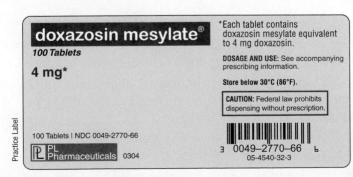

(For educational purposes only)

Figure 7-1 ■ Drug label for doxazosin mesylate.

Example 3

Ordered: amlodipine besylate 5 mg PO daily
The label is shown in Figure 7-2 ■. How many tablets
will you administer to the patient?

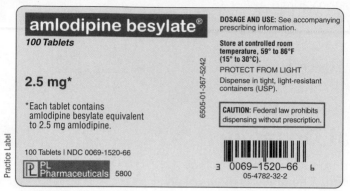

Figure 7-2 ■ Drug label for
amlodipine besylate.

(For educational purposes only)

Use the formula:

$$D \times \frac{Q}{H} = X$$

$$5 \text{ mg} \times \frac{1}{2.5 \text{ mg}} = X$$

$$\frac{5}{2.5} = 2 \text{ tablets}$$

LIQUID DOSES

Liquid medications can be measured in small units of
volume. Therefore, a greater range of doses can be ordered and administered. They are commonly used for
children and elderly patients. Liquid medications can
also be given via feeding tubes. Many medications are
given as liquids, which are supplied initially as powders. Liquid preparations are drugs that have been
dissolved or suspended. Examples of liquid drugs are
syrups, spirits, elixirs, suspensions, and so on. Liquid
drugs can be administered systemically by mouth or by
injection throughout the body.

Three measuring devices used in the administration of oral medications are:

1. The measuring cup—calibrated in fluid ounces, fluidrams, cubic centimeters, milliliters, teaspoons, or
tablespoons
2. The medicine dropper or oral syringe—medicine
droppers are calibrated in milliliters, minims, or
drops, whereas oral syringes are usually calibrated
in cubic centimeters
3. The calibrated spoon—usually calibrated in teaspoons and cubic centimeters

To calculate oral liquid doses, this formula can be
used:

$$D \times \frac{H}{Q} = X$$

Example 1

The physician orders 400 mg of the antibiotic cefdinir
(Omnicef). Figure 7-3 ■ shows the availability of the
drug. Calculate how many milliliters you will administer.

Focus on Pediatrics

Administering Medicine to Young Children

Dosage cups are convenient for children who know how to drink from a cup without spilling, but for
children who cannot drink from a cup, the following options are available:

- *Syringes* are convenient for infants who cannot drink from a cup. A parent can squirt the medicine
into the back of the child's mouth, where it is less likely to spill out, or can measure out a dosage
for a babysitter to use with the child later.

- *Droppers* are safe and easy to use with pediatric patients but must be measured at eye level and
administered quickly to avoid losing any of the medication.

- *Cylindrical dosing spoons* have long handles that can be held easily by small children, with small
cups that fit easily into their mouths.

The label on the bottle indicates that 5 mL contains 125 mg of cefdinir. Therefore,

$$\frac{5 \text{ mL}}{125 \text{ mg}}$$

$$400 \times \frac{5}{125} = \frac{2,000}{125} = 16 \text{ mL}$$

Figure 7-3 ■ Drug label for cefdinir.

Example 2

The pediatrician orders erythromycin 375 mg. Figure 7-4 ■ shows the availability of this drug. Calculate how many milliliters you will administer:

$$375 \times \frac{5 \text{ mL}}{200} = \frac{1,875}{200} = 9.375 \text{ mL} = 9.4 \text{ mL}$$

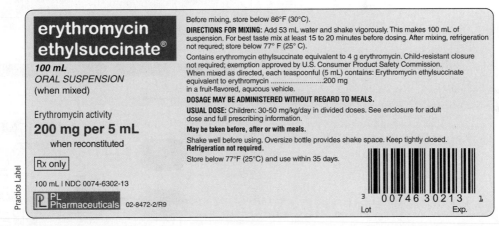

(For educational purposes only)

Figure 7-4 ■ Drug label for erythromycin ethylsuccinate.

Focus on Geriatrics

New Medication-Dispensing Systems Help Elderly Patients

Advances in communication and artificial intelligence are examples of the ways that medication-dispensing systems are improving care for elderly patients. Some systems help to manage home administration of complex, multiple-drug regimens by offering "smart" bottles arranged on a tray that alert the patient when it is time to take a medication. The bottles release the correct amount of medication doses and offer a self-locking feature to prevent accidental overdose. When supplies get low, the system alerts the pharmacist or caregiver. A complete record of all medications dispensed is retained by the system for future reference.

Apply Your Knowledge 7.2

The following questions assess your knowledge about calculating oral drug doses. *See Appendix F for the correct answers.*

LABELING

Calculate the drug dosages by using the labels shown.

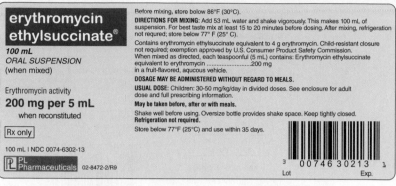

erythromycin ethylsuccinate®

100 mL
ORAL SUSPENSION
(when mixed)

Erythromycin activity
200 mg per 5 mL
when reconstituted

Rx only

100 mL I NDC 0074-6302-13
PL Pharmaceuticals 02-8472-2/R9

Before mixing, store below 86°F (30°C).
DIRECTIONS FOR MIXING: Add 53 mL water and shake vigorously. This makes 100 mL of suspension. For best taste mix at least 15 to 20 minutes before dosing. After mixing, refrigeration not required; store below 77° F (25° C).

Contains erythromycin ethylsuccinate equivalent to 4 g erythromycin. Child-resistant closure not required; exemption approved by U.S. Consumer Product Safety Commission. When mixed as directed, each teaspoonful (5 mL) contains: Erythromycin ethylsuccinate equivalent to erythromycin ....200 mg in a fruit-flavored, aqueous vehicle.

DOSAGE MAY BE ADMINISTERED WITHOUT REGARD TO MEALS.
USUAL DOSE: Children: 30-50 mg/kg/day in divided doses. See enclosure for adult dose and full prescribing information.
May be taken before, after or with meals.
Shake well before using. Oversize bottle provides shake space. Keep tightly closed. **Refrigeration not required.**
Store below 77°F (25°C) and use within 35 days.

3 00746 30213 1
Lot   Exp.

(For educational purposes only)

1. Erythromycin (EryPed 200) 245 mg = _____ mL

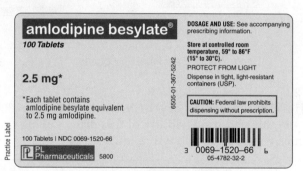

amlodipine besylate®

100 Tablets

2.5 mg*

*Each tablet contains amlodipine besylate equivalent to 2.5 mg amlodipine.

100 Tablets I NDC 0069-1520-66
PL Pharmaceuticals 5800

DOSAGE AND USE: See accompanying prescribing information.

Store at controlled room temperature, 59° to 86°F (15° to 30°C).

PROTECT FROM LIGHT
Dispense in tight, light-resistant containers (USP).

CAUTION: Federal law prohibits dispensing without prescription.

3 0069-1520-66 6
05-4782-32-2

(For educational purposes only)

2. Amlodipine (Norvasc) 2.5 mg = _____ cap

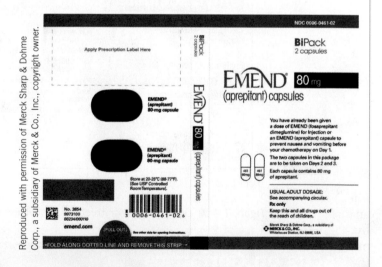

NDC 0006-0461-02

BiPack
2 capsules

EMEND® 80 mg
(aprepitant) capsules

You have already been given a dose of EMEND (fosaprepitant dimeglumine) for Injection or an EMEND (aprepitant) capsule to prevent nausea and vomiting before your chemotherapy on Day 1. The two capsules in this package are to be taken on Days 2 and 3. Each capsule contains 80 mg of aprepitant.

USUAL ADULT DOSAGE:
See accompanying circular.
Rx only
Keep this and all drugs out of the reach of children.

3 0006-0461-02 6

3. Aprepitant (Emend) 240 mg = _____ cap

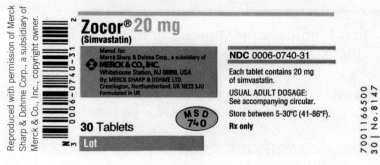

Zocor® 20 mg
(Simvastatin)

Manuf. for:
Merck Sharp & Dohme Corp., a subsidiary of
MERCK & CO., INC.
Whitehouse Station, NJ 08889, USA
By: MERCK SHARP & DOHME LTD.
Cramlington, Northumberland, UK NE23 3JU
Formulated in UK

NDC 0006-0740-31

Each tablet contains 20 mg of simvastatin.

USUAL ADULT DOSAGE:
See accompanying circular.
Store between 5-30°C (41-86°F).
Rx only

30 Tablets
Lot

MSD 740

7001166500
30 I No.8147

4. Simvastatin (Zocor) 80 mg = _____ tab

glipizide®
30 Tablets

2.5 mg

GITS

Rx only

30 Tablets | NDC 0099-1620-30

PL Pharmaceuticals 7220

Each tablet contains 2.5 mg glipizide.
DOSAGE AND USE: See accompanying prescribing information.
Dispense in tight containers (USP).
PROTECT FROM MOISTURE AND HUMIDITY.
Store at controlled room temperature, 59°–86°F (15°–30°C).

N3 0049-1620-30 b
05-5599-32-1

Practice Label

(For educational purposes only)

5. Glipizide (Glucotrol XL) 0.01 g = _____ tab

DRUG DOSAGE CALCULATIONS

Calculate the solid or liquid doses to be administered.

1. Ordered: nifedipine (Procardia) 20 mg PO tid

   On hand: Procardia 10 mg is available.

   How many capsule(s) would you administer? _____

2. Ordered: levothyroxine (Synthroid) 0.3 mg PO daily

   On hand: Synthroid 0.15 mg is available.

   How many tablet(s) would you administer? _____

3. Ordered: Keflex 500 mg PO bid

   On hand: Keflex 250 mg/5 mL

   How many milliliters would you administer per dose? _____

4. Ordered: Augmentin 1 g PO bid

   On hand: Augmentin 400 mg/5 mL is available.

   How many milliliters would you administer per dose? _____

5. Ordered: Singulair 5 mg PO daily

   On hand: Singulair 5 mg is available.

   How many tablet(s) would you administer per dose? _____

Calculating Parenteral Medications

Injections are mixtures that contain the drug dissolved in an appropriate liquid. Medication can be administered by injection intradermally (within the skin), subcutaneously (into fatty tissue under the skin), intramuscularly (IM, into the muscle), and intravenously (IV, into the vein). Such **injectable** medications are prescribed in grams, milligrams, micrograms, grains, or units. The injectable drugs can be prepared in packages as solvents (diluents or solutions) or in powdered form. Drug solutions for injection are commercially premixed and stored in vials and ampules for immediate use.

INTRADERMAL INJECTION

An intradermal injection is usually used for skin testing to diagnose the cause of an allergy or to determine the presence of a microorganism. The common syringe that is used for intradermal testing is the tuberculin syringe with a 25-gauge needle.

The inner portion of the forearm is usually used for diagnostic testing because there is less hair in that area, and the test results are more visible. The upper back may also be used as a testing site. Test results are read 48 to 72 hours after the intradermal injection. A reddened or raised area is a positive reaction.

SUBCUTANEOUS INJECTION

Drugs injected into the subcutaneous tissue are absorbed slowly because there are fewer blood vessels in fatty tissue. The amount of drug solution administered subcutaneously is generally 0.5 to 1 mL at a 45-degree angle.

The two types of syringes used for subcutaneous injections are the tuberculin syringe (1 mL), calibrated in 0.1-mL and 0.01-mL increments, and the 3-mL syringe, calibrated in 0.1-mL increments. To calculate dosages for subcutaneous or IM injections, use the basic formula of $D/H \times V$, or the ratio and proportion method. Heparin is a drug commonly administered subcutaneously.

Medications given by IM injection are absorbed more rapidly than those given by subcutaneous injection. The volume of solution for IM injections is 0.5 to 3.0 mL. For calculating IM doses, the following example can be used:

Example 1

Ordered: gentamicin 60 mg IM
On hand: gentamicin is available 80 mg/2 mL in a vial. To calculate, use this formula:

$$\frac{D}{H} \times V = \frac{60}{80} \times 2 = \frac{120}{80} = 1.5 \text{ mL}$$

Or

$$H{:}V :: D{:}V$$

$$80 \text{ mg}{:}2 \text{ mL} :: 60 \text{ mg}{:}X \text{ mL}$$

$$80 X = 120$$

$$X = \frac{120}{80} = 1.5 \text{ mL}$$

Example 2

Ordered: atropine 0.2 mg subcutaneously Stat
On hand: atropine 400 mcg/mL (0.4 mg/mL)
By using the same formula, you can calculate the amount of atropine to be given.

$$\frac{D}{H} \times V = \frac{0.2 \text{ mg}}{0.4 \text{ mg}} \times 1 \text{ mL} = \frac{0.2}{0.4} \times 1 = 0.5 \text{ mL}$$

INSULIN INJECTION

Insulin is a pancreatic hormone that stimulates glucose metabolism. Patients who have insulin-dependent diabetes often need regular injections of insulin to keep their blood glucose from rising to levels that could be life threatening. These regular injections must be rotated to various sites of the body to prevent scarring of the tissue at a single injection site. Different forms of insulin are available, and insulin may be administered several ways depending on the form. These ways include subcutaneous injections,

IV administration, and continuous administration through an insulin pump.

There are four types of insulin: (1) rapid-acting, (2) short-acting, (3) intermediate-acting, and (4) long-acting types. (See Chapter 22 for complete information on insulins.) Insulin is packaged in two ways: (1) vials containing 10 mL of solution with 100 units of insulin per milliliter and (2) prepackaged syringes that contain smaller amounts of insulin. In the United States, insulin is usually standardized to 100 units/mL. Insulin vials can combine NPH (neutral protamine Hagedorn; Humulin N, Iletin II) and regular insulin (Humulin R, Novolin R) in one solution. The most common is 70/30, but 50/50 is also available (Figure 7-5 ■). It is important to always use *insulin syringes* to administer insulin and not other types of syringes.

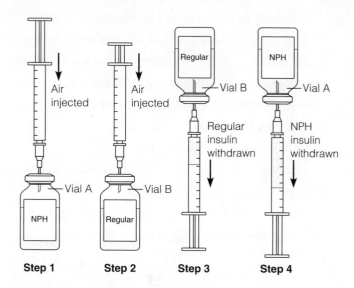

Figure 7-5 ■ Mixing regular and NPH (neutral protamine Hagedorn) insulins in one syringe.

The three types of insulin syringes are:

1. 100-unit syringes
2. 50-unit syringes
3. 30-unit syringes (Figure 7-6 ■)

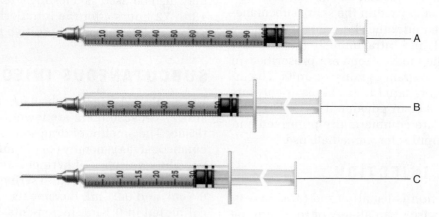

Figure 7-6 ■ Insulin syringes: 100 unit (A), 50 unit (B), and 30 unit (C).

Focus Point

Preparing Insulin Injections

For more accurate measurements, use a 30-unit insulin syringe for insulin doses less than 30 units and a 50-unit insulin syringe for insulin doses less than 50 units if a standard 100-unit syringe is not available. To successfully remove insulin from a vial for injection, first draw up the same quantity of air as the ordered insulin volume before withdrawing the appropriate insulin quantity. If the physician orders two types of insulin to be administered, they may be combined in one syringe to allow for one injection. Draw up the shorter-acting insulin first.

The size of the syringe depends on the size of the dose to be administered. For example, if you needed to give 18 units of regular insulin and 11 units of NPH insulin, you would select a 30-unit syringe. Similarly, if you needed 35 units of regular and 40 units of NPH, you would select a 100-unit syringe to administer these larger unit sizes. The smallest size syringe that will contain the number of units required is best because it is easier to see the unit markings on the syringe.

Example 1

Find how much liquid is in the tuberculin syringe in Figure 7-7 ■.

You can see that the top ring of the plunger is even with one line above 0.60 mL. Each marking line represents 0.01 mL, so the amount of liquid in this syringe is 0.61 mL.

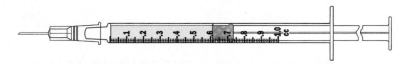

Figure 7-7 ■ Tuberculin syringe.

Example 2

Figure 7-8 ■ shows a 100-unit insulin syringe. In this type of syringe, 100 units is equivalent to 1 mL. Each measurement line on the syringe measures 2 units, or 0.02 mL.

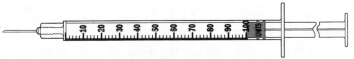

Figure 7-8 ■ 100-unit insulin syringe.

Example 4

Figure 7-10 ■ shows a 30-unit insulin syringe, also known as a Lo-Dose syringe. In this type of syringe, the measurement lines are the same as in the 50-unit insulin syringe, measuring just 1 unit, or 0.01 mL.

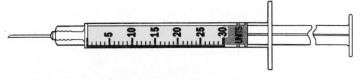

Figure 7-10 ■ 30-unit insulin syringe

Example 3

Figure 7-9 ■ shows a 50-unit insulin syringe. In this type of syringe, each measurement line only measures 1 unit, or 0.01 mL.

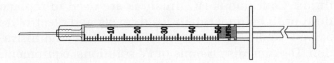

Figure 7-9 ■ 50-unit insulin syringe.

Example 5

Figure 7-11 ■ shows a partially filled 50-unit insulin syringe. You can see that the top ring of the plunger is even with three lines above the number 25. Because each line represents 1 unit, this syringe contains 28 units of liquid.

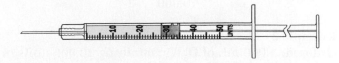

Figure 7-11 ■ A partially filled 50-unit insulin syringe.

Example 6

Figure 7-12 ■ shows a partially filled 100-unit insulin syringe. You can see that the top ring of the plunger is even with one line above 70. Because each line represents 2 units, this syringe contains 72 units of liquid.

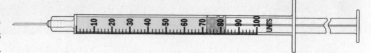

Figure 7-12 ■ A partially filled 100-unit insulin syringe.

Focus Point

Safe Insulin Practices

Avoid keeping insulin on top of medication carts or counters or under pharmacy compounding hoods because it could be confused with heparin (which is also measured in units). Immediately return insulin to a proper storage area after use. If insulin concentration is not 100 units/mL, apply *bold warning labels* to alert the user about the concentration. Always use single standard concentration for all adult IV insulin infusions. Prescribers should order insulin cartridges for outpatients to help ensure correct dispensing.

HEPARIN CALCULATION

The anticoagulant heparin is measured in USP (United States Pharmacopeia) units. It is given to patients to reduce or prevent the blood from clotting. Heparin can be administered to a patient by subcutaneous injection or IV injection.

The abbreviation U should be avoided in practice to prevent medication errors. Vials of heparin are prepared by the manufacturer in a variety of strengths. The vials come in 1,000-unit, 5,000-unit, 20,000-unit, and 40,000-unit sizes. Ampules are supplied in 1,000-unit, 5,000-unit, and 10,000-unit sizes.

Heparin is also available in premixed IV solutions—for example, 12,500 units in 250 mL of 5% dextrose in water (D_5W); or 25,000 units in 500 mL of 0.45% saline solution. With a premixed parenteral solution, you have to convert the physician's order to the volume of solution that contains the amount of heparin ordered.

Example 1

Ordered: heparin 5,000 units subcutaneously q8h
On hand: heparin is available as 10,000 units/mL.
You need to convert units to milliliters.

$$10,000 \text{ units} = 1 \text{ mL} = 5,000 \text{ units}:X \text{ mL}$$
$$10,000\,X = 5,000$$
$$X = \frac{5,000}{10,000} = \frac{1}{2} = 0.5 \text{ mL}$$

Example 2

Ordered: 1,000 mL of D_5W containing 20,000 units of heparin, which is to be infused at 30 mL/h
How much heparin should be given to the patient per hour?

$$20,000 \text{ units}:1,000 \text{ mL} = X \text{ units}:30 \text{ mL}$$
$$1,000\,X = 20,000 \times 30$$
$$\frac{1,000\,X}{1,000} = \frac{60,000}{1,000}$$
$$X = 60 \text{ units/h}$$

INTRAVENOUS CALCULATION

IV fluid therapy is used to administer fluids that contain water, dextrose, vitamins, electrolytes, and drugs. Medications for IV administration are usually available in small-volume vials that are mixed in a large-volume solution by the pharmacist before administration to the patient. The drug added to a parenteral solution is often available in a solution. Therefore, the additive amount is calculated in terms of volume—usually in milliliters.

The amount of drug in a parenteral solution is clearly stated on the label, but the pharmacist must be careful to notice whether the amount is given in terms of concentration (for example, 5 mg/mL) or amount of drug in the vial (for example, 80 mg in a 2-mL vial). The concentration is used to calculate the correct volume to be mixed with a parenteral diluent to produce the prescribed dose.

IV fluids and drugs may be administered by intermittent or continuous IV infusion. Intermittent IV infusion, such as IV piggyback and IV push infusions, are used for IV administration of drugs and supplement fluids. Continuous IV infusions are used to replace fluid or to help maintain fluid levels and electrolyte balance and to serve as vehicles for drug administration. Detailed discussions of IV solutions, equipment, and calculations are not suitable for this pharmacology book. Therefore, for more information, it is advisable to refer to a pharmaceutical calculations textbook.

✳ Apply Your Knowledge 7.3

The following questions assess your knowledge of calculating doses of parenteral medications. *See Appendix F for the correct answers.*

LABELING
Answer the drug labeling questions by using the labels depicted below.

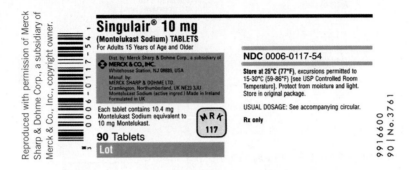

1. How many milligrams are contained in the Singulair bottle? _____

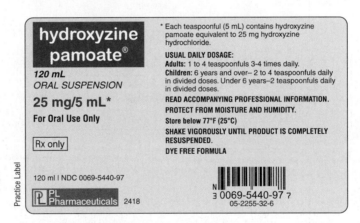

(For educational purposes only)

2. What is the usual daily adult dose of hydroxyzine pamoate? _____

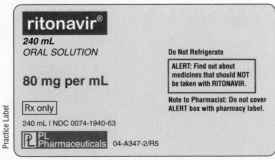

(For educational purposes only)

3. How many milligrams of ritonavir are contained in this package? _____

(*continued*)

Apply Your Knowledge 7.3 (continued)

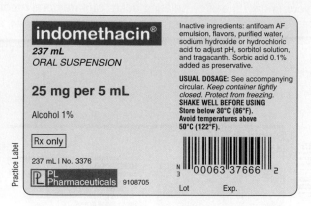

(For educational purposes only)

4. How many milligrams of indomethacin are there in 2.5 mL of solution? _____

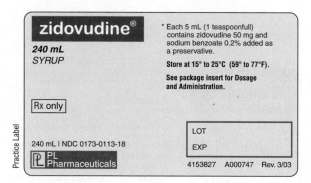

(For educational purposes only)

5. How many milliliters of zidovudine are needed for a 150-mg dose? _____

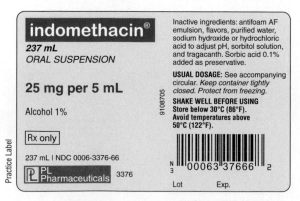

(For educational purposes only)

6. If only half the indomethacin suspension was used, how many milliliters would be left? _____

DRUG DOSAGE CALCULATIONS

Calculate the amount of medications you should administer.

1. Ordered: Humulin R U-500 insulin in 80 units

   Administer: _____

2. Ordered: 150 units Humulin R, IV Stat

   Administer: _____

3. Ordered: Heparin 5,000 units subcutaneously q8h

   On hand: Heparin 10,000 units/mL is available.

   Administer: _____

4. Ordered: Valium 10 mg IM

   On hand: Valium 5 mg/mL is available.

   Administer: _____

5. Ordered: Lidocaine 25 mg subcutaneously

   On hand: Lidocaine 5% solution

   Administer: _____

6. Ordered: Lanoxin 300 mcg IM Stat

   On hand: Lanoxin (digoxin) 500 mcg in 2 mL

   Administer: _____

7. Ordered: Zantac 50 mg IM qid

   On hand: Zantac 25 mg/mL

   Administer: _____

Dosage Calculation in Pediatrics

The pediatrician must determine the proper kind and amount of medication for a child. Dosages for infants and children are usually less than the adult dosages for the same medication. The body mass in children is smaller, and their metabolism is different from that of adults. Therefore, dosage calculations for pediatric patients (infants or children) must be precise.

For many years, pediatric dosage calculations used such pediatric formulas as Clark's rule, Young's rule, or Fried's rule (see pages 110–111). These formulas are based on the weight of the child in pounds or on the age of the child in months, and they aid in determining how much medication should be prescribed for a particular child.

Today, the most accurate methods of determining an appropriate pediatric dose are by weight and body area. You must know whether the amount of a prescribed pediatric dosage is the safe or appropriate amount for a particular patient. If this information is not on the drug label, it can be found on the package insert, in the *Physician's Desk Reference* (*PDR*), on a hospital formulary, in the *United States Pharmacopoeia*, or in pharmacology texts.

Focus Point

Questions to Ask When a Child Is Prescribed Medication

Encourage parents or caregivers of children to ask their physician the following questions:

- What is the drug, and what is it used for?
- Will it cause a problem with other drugs my child is taking?
- How often and for how many days or weeks should I give my child this medicine?
- What if I miss giving my child a dose?
- How soon will the drug start working?
- What side effects does it have, and what should I do if my child has any of these side effects?
- Should I stop giving the medicine when my child gets better?
- Is there a less expensive generic version I can use?

DRUG DOSAGE CALCULATION BY BODY SURFACE AREA

BSA is determined by using a **nomogram** (a numerical relationship chart) and the child's height and weight. This is considered to be the most accurate method of calculating a child's dose. Standard nomograms give a child's BSA according to weight and height (Figure 7-13 ■).

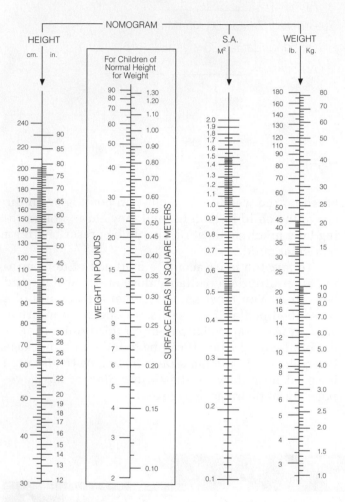

Figure 7-13 ■ Pediatric nomogram used for determining body surface area.

The calculation formula is the ratio of the child's BSA to the surface area of an average adult (1.7 square meters, or 1.7 m²) multiplied by the normal adult dose of the drug:

Example 1

$$\text{Child's dose} = \frac{\text{Surface area of child (m}^2)}{1.7 \text{ m}^2} \times \text{Normal adult dose}$$

A child who weighs 12 kg and is 60 cm tall has a BSA of 0.4 m². Therefore, a child's dose of ampicillin that corresponds to an adult dose of 250 mg would be:

$$\text{Child's dose} = \frac{0.4 \text{ m}^2}{1.7 \text{ m}^2} \times 250 \text{ mg} = 0.23 \times 250$$
$$= 58.32 \text{ mg}$$

Example 2

The pediatrician ordered: digoxin 0.64 mg/m² PO daily The child's BSA is 0.9 m². How many milligrams would you administer to this child as a loading dose?

First, you need to convert BSA to dose in milligrams:

$$0.9 \text{ m}^2 = X \text{ mg}$$

$$0.9 \text{ m}^2 \times \frac{? \text{ mg}}{? \text{ m}^2} = X \text{ mg}$$

Because 0.64 mg = 1 m², the equivalent fraction is:

$$\frac{0.64 \text{ mg}}{1 \text{ m}^2}$$

You then cancel the square meters and obtain the dose in milligrams.

$$0.9 \text{ m}^2 \times \frac{0.64 \text{ mg}}{1 \text{ m}^2} = 0.576 \text{ mg or } 0.58 \text{ mg}$$

Therefore, the child should receive 0.58 mg of digoxin.

DRUG DOSAGE CALCULATION BY BODY WEIGHT

Drug manufacturers sometimes recommend a dosage based on the weight of the child. This method uses a specific number of milligrams, micrograms, or units for each kilogram of body weight (mg/kg, mcg/kg, and units/kg, respectively). Usually, drug data for pediatric dosage (mg/kg) is supplied by manufacturers in a drug information insert.

Example

Ordered: amoxicillin 60 mg PO tid
On hand: 125 mg/5 mL
Child's weight: 12-1/2 lb
To calculate, first change pounds to kilograms.

$$\frac{12.5 \text{ lb}}{2.2 \text{ kg}} = 5.7 \text{ kg}$$

Second: The pediatric dosage for a child who weighs 20 kg is 20–40 mg/kg/day in three equal doses.

$$20 \text{ mg/kg/day} \times 5.7 \text{ kg} = 114 \text{ mg/day}$$
$$40 \text{ mg/kg/day} \times 5.7 \text{ kg} = 228 \text{ mg/day}$$
$$60 \text{ mg} \times 3 = 180 \text{ mg}$$

Because 180 mg falls within the recommended daily dose range for amoxicillin, it is considered a safe dose.

Clark's Rule

Clark's rule is based on the weight of the child, which is much more accurate than Young's or Fried's rules. Clark's rule uses average adult weight (usually considered to be

150 lb or 70 kg) and assumes that the child's dose is proportionately less. To calculate pediatric dose by Clark's rule, use the following formula:

Example

Calculate the dose of cortisone for a 42-lb child (adult dose = 100 mg).

$$\text{Pediatric dose} = \frac{\text{Child's weight in lb}}{150 \text{ lb}} \times \text{Adult dose}$$

$$\frac{42 \text{ lb}}{150 \text{ lb}} \times 100 \text{ mg} = 28 \text{ mg}$$

Young's Rule

Young's rule is used for children older than 1 year of age.

Example

$$\text{Pediatric dose} = \frac{\text{Child's age in years}}{\text{Child's age in years} + 12} \times \text{Adult dose}$$

Calculate the dose of Tylenol for a 5-year-old child (adult dose + 1,000 mg):

$$\frac{5 \text{ years}}{5 \text{ years} + 12} \times 1,000 \text{ mg} = 294 \text{ mg}$$

Fried's Rule

Fried's rule is a method of estimating the dose of medication for infants younger than 1 year of age.

$$\frac{\text{Child's age in months}}{150 \text{ lb}} \times \text{Average adult dose}$$

Example

Calculate the dose of phenobarbital for an 8-month-old infant (adult dose = 400 mg).

$$\frac{8 \text{ mo}}{150 \text{ lb}} \times 400 \text{ mg} = 21 \text{ mg}$$

✳ Apply Your Knowledge 7.4

The following questions focus on what you have just learned about dosage calculations for pediatric patients. *See Appendix F for the correct answers.*

MULTIPLE CHOICE

Choose the correct answer from choices a–d.

1. The most accurate methods of determining an appropriate pediatric dose are:
   a. Clark's rule and Young's rule
   b. Young's rule and Fried's rule
   c. By weight and body area
   d. By weight and Clark's rule

2. Which of the following methods of pediatric dosage calculations is used for children older than one year of age?
   a. Clark's rule
   b. Fried's rule
   c. Freud's rule
   d. Young's rule

3. Body surface area is determined by using the child's height and weight and a:
   a. Nomogram
   b. Sonogram
   c. Child's dose of a similar medication
   d. Loading dose

4. Drug manufacturers sometimes recommend doses based on the:
   a. Height of the child
   b. Weight of the child's parents
   c. Usual daily dosage
   d. Weight of the child

(continued)

Apply Your Knowledge 7.4 (continued)

5. Which of the following dosage calculation methods is the most accurate?

   a. Clark's rule

   b. Young's rule

   c. Fried's rule

   d. The child's height

DO THE MATH

Convert these weights (in pounds) to kilograms.

1. 55 lb   = _____

2. 11 lb   = _____

3. 157 lb = _____

4. 18 lb   = _____

5. 209 lb = _____

6. 27 lb   = _____

7. 93 lb   = _____

8. 135 lb = _____

PRACTICAL SCENARIO 1

A physician orders a medication in the amount of 250 mg per 5 mL for a patient's upper respiratory tract infection. Before dispensing the medication, the medical assistant calculated the amount of medication required as 125 mg/mL. This would have meant the patient might have received 625 mg/5 mL instead of what the physician ordered. A second person in the medical office checked the calculation and found the error before administration. Therefore, it is essential for allied health-care professionals to accurately calculate dose calculations and always consult another coworker or physician to verify accuracy.

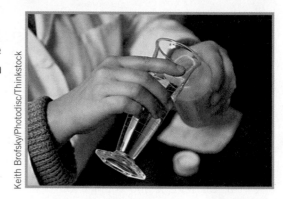

Keith Brofsky/Photodisc/Thinkstock

Critical Thinking Questions

1. What is the formula the medical assistant should have used to calculate the proper dose?

2. Besides checking that the dose calculation was right, what other "rights" does the assistant need to check?

PRACTICAL SCENARIO 2

A physician ordered Keflex 500 mg PO bid. A pharmacy technician has Keflex 250 mg per mL.

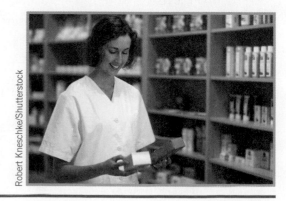

Robert Kneschke/Shutterstock

Critical Thinking Questions

1. If the pharmacy technician wants to dispense this medication, how many milliliters will be needed to contain each required dose?

2. How many milliliters should the patient receive per day?

Chapter Capsule

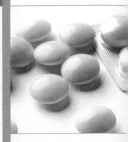

This section repeats the objectives from the beginning of the chapter and then provides a summary of the most important concepts for that objective. Use this section as a quick review and to check your knowledge.

Objective 1: Discuss the differences between *dosage ordered, desired dose*, and *dose on hand*.

- Dosage ordered: total amount ordered and its frequency of administration
- Desired dose: amount to be administered at one time
- Dose on hand: amount of drug in a dosage unit

Objective 2: Explain how to use the formula $D/H \times Q = X$ to calculate drug doses.

- D = desired dose
- H = dose available
- D and H: must always be in the same unit of measure
- Q = number of tablets, milliliters, or other units that contain H
- X = number of capsules, minims, or other units that D will be contained in (also known as the "amount to be administered")

Objective 3: Explain the fraction proportion method and the formula used in this method.

- The fraction proportion method uses the dose on hand (H), dosage unit (Q), desired dose (D), and amount to administer to calculate doses. The formula that is used in this method is:

$$\frac{\text{Dose on hand } (H)}{\text{Dosage unit } (Q)} = \frac{\text{Desired dose } (D)}{\text{Amount to administer}}$$

This can also be expressed in this formula:

$$\text{Desired dose } (D) \times \frac{\text{Dosage unit } (Q)}{\text{Dose on hand } (H)} = \text{Amount to administer}$$

Objective 4: Discuss calculating parenteral medications and the formula that is used.

- For parenteral medications, a drug is dissolved in an appropriate liquid. These medications are commonly prescribed in grams, milligrams, micrograms, grains, or units. To calculate parenteral medications, use this formula.

$$\frac{\text{Desired dose } (D)}{\text{Dose on hand } (H)} \times \text{Volume of parenteral solution } (V)$$

Objective 5: Calculate intramuscular doses.

- $D \times H \times V = X$
- Or: $H{:}V :: D{:}X$

Objective 6: Name the most common types of insulin used in the United States.

- Rapid-acting insulin
- Short-acting insulin
- Intermediate-acting insulin
- Long-acting insulin

Objective 7: Explain the steps required for the proper injection of insulin.

- Step 1: Inject the same quantity of air as the ordered insulin volume into the vial.
- Step 2: Withdraw the appropriate quantity of insulin.
- Step 3: Draw up the shorter-acting insulin first if using two types of insulin.
- Step 4: Inject the insulin per the physician's instructions.

Objective 8: Convert physician orders of heparin to the volume of solution that contains the amount of heparin ordered.

- If required, convert units to milliliters: 10,000 units = 1 mL
- Then, use this formula: X mL = ordered units/available units
- Or: 10,000 units:1 mL :: ordered units:X mL

Objective 9: Calculate whether the amount of a prescribed pediatric dosage is the safe or appropriate amount for a particular patient.

- For the calculation: Use either the child's weight or body area
- To find safe pediatric dosages, check: drug labels, package inserts, the *PDI*, hospital formularies, the *USP*, or pharmacology texts

Objective 10: Define the most accurate method of calculating a child's dose and perform correct calculations by using this method.

- Most accurate method: the body surface area (BSA) method
  - ❏ To find the child's body surface area: Use a nomogram, which compares the child's weight and height
- Use this formula:
  - ❏ Child's dose = m^2 (child's BSA) ÷ 1.7 m^2 × normal adult dose

Internet Sites of Interest

- *Diabetes Health* magazine presents an article at **www.diabeteshealth.com** that discusses errors in calculation of insulin dosage by adolescents and the impact of using an insulin dosage calculator (IDC). Search "insulin dosage calculator adolescents."
- This website offers calculators for math, including equations and formulas: **http://www.rncalc.com**.
- Targeted to medical assistants' needs, the Medical Office Pharmacology Review for Medical Assistant Students and Professionals website at **www.mapharm.com/dosage_calc.htm** provides an overview of dosage calculations.

- This website offers a discussion about the need to correctly split pills in order for safe dosing: **http://www.myfamilywellness.org/MainMenuCategories/ FamilyHealthCenter/Medication/Pill-splitting.html**.

- Prescription Drug Info at **www.prescriptiondrug-info.com/Drugs/Regular_Insulin.asp** offers dosages for regular insulin.

- This website discusses safe pediatric dosage and offers examples: **http://www.alamo.edu/sac/nursing/math/peds5.html**.

PEARSON
myhealthprofessionskit™

Go to www.myhealthprofessionskit.com to access the Companion Website created for this textbook. Simply select "Basic Health Science" from the choice of disciplines. Find this book and then log in using your username and password to access interactive learning games, assessment questions, animations, and more.

Chapter 8

Medical Errors and Prevention

Chapter Objectives

After completing this chapter, you should be able to:

1. Explain why errors can occur in three stages in the medication process.
2. Describe factors that cause medication errors.
3. Explain general recommendations to reduce medication errors.
4. Describe the legal and ethical responsibility of health professionals to report all medication errors.
5. Explain the role of the Food and Drug Administration in medication errors.
6. Define The Joint Commission and its role in preventing medication errors.
7. Explain the steps that may be taken to avoid medication errors and ensure safe administration of medication.
8. Define polypharmacy.

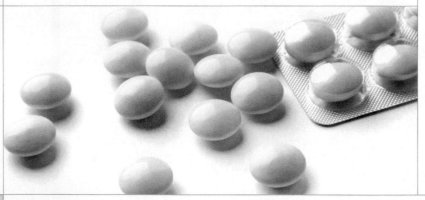

Key Terms

medication error (page 117)

medication reconciliation (page 122)

polypharmacy (pah-lee-FAR-muh-see) (page 122)

risk management department (page 119)

root cause analysis (RCA) (page 120)

sentinel events (page 120)

Introduction

Medication errors occur in small and large communities across the United States. Tens of thousands of Americans die each year from various medical errors while they are receiving care. Errors in quality of care by physicians, nurses, pharmacists, and other allied health professionals routinely harm patients, causing disability, permanent damage, and even death. A system of true quality would greatly help to prevent these occurrences. The current system does not make the best use of its resources. On a daily basis, medical errors, medication errors, lack of access to clinical information, duplication of services, delays, and overusage of medications and natural supplements all combine to increase the risks of patient harm. All health professionals must take their responsibilities seriously in order to help prevent medical and medication errors. Also, patients and their families must be educated about potential errors that can happen at home and take steps to reduce or prevent these errors.

Medication Errors

A **medication error** is the inappropriate or incorrect administration of a drug that should be preventable through effective system controls involving physicians, pharmacists, nurses, risk management personnel, legal counsel, administrators, and patients. Medication errors can occur because of manufacturing mistakes. Thousands of medication errors occur each year in hospitals throughout the United States. These errors often result in pain, injury, and even death. According to the Institute of Medicine (IOM), medical errors have caused up to 98,000 deaths annually in the United States. The IOM suggests that this should be considered a national epidemic. Another study conducted by HealthGrades has shown as many as 195,000 deaths per year in American hospitals because of preventable medical errors.[1]

Medication errors usually occur more frequently than they are reported and are the result of either human error or a flawed system within a health-care facility. Errors can occur in three stages within the medication process:

1. The first stage involves prescribing or ordering medication. During this stage, physicians or other persons prescribing the medication may be distracted or interrupted and as a result provide incomplete orders—greatly increasing the risk of errors. Medication errors are most prevalent when choosing a medication, its dosage, and the schedule.

2. The second stage is when the medication is dispensed to patients or consumers. Dispensing errors can occur as a result of insufficient or inexperienced staffing and a lack of adequate time for patient counseling and can lead to confusion about how to take the medication or how to assist the patient in taking it. It is an extremely important and effective practice for all health-care professionals to double-check medications against the medication administration record (MAR). This practice helps those who are dispensing the medication to catch errors before medications are dispensed.

3. The third stage is when the medication is administered and monitored for side effects. At this stage, medication administration errors are most commonly attributed to nurses or others who are legally allowed to handle administration. Those who administer medications may be accountable for medication errors that can be attributed to poor communication or misread prescriptions, orders, or drug labels. Other factors that contribute to errors include similar labeling and packaging of products and medications with similar names (see Appendix C for a list of medications with similar-sounding names). After administering medication, health-care professionals must also ensure that the patient does not have a reaction to the medication.

The most common error is dosage; errors also often involve antibiotics and analgesics. For example, a community pharmacist misreads a handwritten prescription for 10 mg of Metadate ER and instead dispenses 10 mg of methadone for a 7-year-old boy. Fortunately, the boy's mother reads the information that accompanies the prescription and realizes the error.

A medication error may occur when dealing with outpatients because of the increasing number of prescriptions in the United States and because pharmacists do not adequately counsel patients. In addition, there is a shortage of pharmacists and pharmacy technicians, which contributes to medication errors. Increased usage of over-the-counter (OTC) drugs and herbals and the availability of drugs through the Internet also cause medication errors.

A medication error must be reported as soon as it is noticed, and the patient must be monitored to see if any undesirable effect or injury from the medication develops. Medication errors must be documented in the medical record with the signature of the individual who made the error. If allied health professionals who are involved with prescribing, dispensing, or administering medication follow the seven rights of medication administration and adhere to dispensing guidelines, medication errors should not occur.

WHY MEDICATION ERRORS OCCUR

A number of factors cause medication errors, including:

* Use of incorrect abbreviations: Many abbreviations may be mistaken for different units and different dosages

* Miscommunication: Poor handwriting, similar drug names, dosing unit confusion

[1]Source: www.medicalnewstoday.com

❋ Missing information: Lack of patient information, such as allergies, diseases, drug history, laboratory information, and drug information or warnings

❋ Lack of appropriate labeling: By the manufacturer or the pharmacist

❋ Environmental factors: Noise, lighting, stress, and fatigue affecting health-care providers

❋ Poor management: Unhealthy health-care facility culture

Medication errors may occur in such inpatient settings as hospitals and nursing homes or in such outpatient settings as physicians' offices or clinics. They can also happen during the manufacturing process and include errors in formulation, packaging, labeling, and distribution. They may be the result of undiscovered toxicity. Medication errors are preventable and are the single largest source of all medical errors.

Medication errors may occur as a result of the following:

❋ Wrong patient

❋ Incorrect route

❋ Incorrect drug

❋ Incorrect dose

❋ Incorrect time

❋ Incorrect technique

❋ Incorrect information on the patient chart

Focus Point

Medical Errors During the Prescribing Process

The three most common forms of prescribing errors include dosing errors, prescribing medications to which the patient has had an allergic response, and errors involving the prescribing of inappropriate dosage forms.

Focus Point

Administering Medications

Nurses and medical assistants must be extremely knowledgeable when administering medications in the physician's office. Follow all physician orders exactly as written. If unsure about an order, ask for clarification before proceeding. Administer a medication only after the order is written in the patient's chart. This helps eliminate errors and possible omissions in medication therapy. Always implement the *seven rights* and perform three-drug order and label checks when dispensing and administering medications.

REDUCING MEDICATION ERRORS

Medication errors may relate to professional practice, health-care products, procedures, and systems. The following statements are guidelines for communication, education, and policy to assist in decreasing the rate of medication errors. To reduce medication errors, general recommendations include:

❋ Using an adequate number of allied health staff (nurses, medical assistants, and pharmacy technicians) who are trained to prepare, dispense, and administer medications to patients

❋ Using standardized measurement systems for both inpatients and outpatients

❋ Using prospective error-tracking systems that are run on a consistent basis to target and monitor common patient errors

❋ Clearly defining a system for drug administration, ordering, and dispensing that includes reviews of original drug orders

❋ Compiling medication profiles for inpatients, outpatients, and ambulatory patients with updated allergy histories after each encounter

❋ Providing suitable work environments for safe, effective drug preparation

❋ Electronic medical records and e-prescribing offer automatic surveillance measures that seek out potential medication errors, especially when information is lacking or conflicting with other information.

Focus on Geriatrics

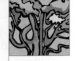

Physiologic Changes Impact Medication Effects

The physiologic changes associated with aging include altered memory, less acute vision, decreased renal function, less complete and slower absorption from the gastrointestinal tract, and decreased liver function. These changes can increase the possibility of cumulative and possibly toxic effects of medications.

✳ Apply Your Knowledge 8.1

The following questions focus on what you have just learned about medication errors.

CRITICAL THINKING
1. What is the definition of *medication errors*?
2. What are the most common medication errors?
3. Why may the Internet cause medication errors?
4. What are risk factors for medication errors?
5. When can medication errors occur?

REDUCING ERRORS IN HEALTH-CARE FACILITIES

In many health-care facilities, medications are stored in locked, automated, computerized cabinets. Each nurse is given a specific code for accessing these cabinets. Automation allows the cabinets to maintain an accurate inventory of medication supplies. In larger facilities, **risk management departments** are used to minimize medication errors and examine risks that may cause them. Risk management specialists track data, investigate incidents, identify problems, and provide recommendations to help improve the accuracy of patient care. Collaboration between nurses and risk management specialists helps to modify the facility's policies and procedures. Errors can be reduced by a variety of methods, including correct storage of medications, avoiding use of expired medications, avoiding transfer of medications between containers, avoiding overstocking, avoiding dangerous abbreviations, and keeping reference materials up to date.

RESULTS OF MEDICATION ERRORS

In hospitals, medication errors are the most common causes of morbidity and preventable death. Medication errors affect not only patients but also their families and responsible health-care professionals. Medication errors may result in extended stays

in the hospital, higher costs, and increased separation from family and normal activities. Each health-care professional involved in medication errors may experience serious emotional trauma because of his or her responsibility for the patient's welfare. High error rates can seriously harm the representations of health-care staff members and entire facilities. Financial penalties may be assessed, and legal cases may result.

The goal of every health-care facility should be to reduce medication errors to the lowest number possible. Each error should be thoroughly investigated and documented. This can greatly help in the prevention of future errors. Investigations should be conducted so they encourage the correct reporting of what occurred and not under threat of penalties. After error patterns have been identified, steps can be taken to eradicate activities that lead to the error occurring.

REPORTING MEDICATION ERRORS

It is the legal and ethical responsibility of staff members to report all occurrences of medication errors. Patients who were harmed seriously enough may have had to undergo lifesaving interventions and may need follow-up supervision and treatments. At the federal level, the Food and Drug Administration (FDA) coordinates the reporting of medication errors by using its MedWatch program. Also known as the FDA Safety Information and Adverse Event Reporting Program, MedWatch provides timely information that is clinically important regarding medical products. This includes information about safety issues for prescription drugs, OTC drugs, biologics, medical devices, radiation-emitting devices, and special nutritional products. Health-care professionals are encouraged to use the MedWatch database to report medication errors and situations that may lead to errors. This reporting may be done anonymously, directly to the FDA, either by the Internet or telephone. MedWatch may be contacted at http://www.fda.gov/Safety/MedWatch/default.htm or by calling 800-332-1088.

The National Coordinating Council for Medication Error Reporting and Prevention (NCC MERP) provides assistance with medication errors. This organization has helped to standardize the medication error reporting system. The NCC MERP coordinates medication error information and provides preventive education. They may be contacted at http://www.nccmerp.org or 800-233-7767.

The Institute for Safe Medication Practices (ISMP) publishes *Safe Medicine*, a consumer newsletter about medication errors. The ISMP accepts consumer and health-care professional reports that relate to medication safety. The ISMP may be contacted at http://www.ismp.org/newsletters/consumer/default.asp. The U.S. Pharmacopeia's MEDMARX medication error reporting program is used by hospitals. Contact https://www.medmarx.com/docs/about.pf.

The Joint Commission has established patient safety standards that address many significant patient safety issues. These include patient safety programs; management practices that focus on safety; and regular analysis of the ordering, preparation, and dispensing of medications. The Joint Commission requires that hospitals inform patients when they have been harmed because of hospital errors. Continually attempting to standardize practices in hospitals nationwide, The Joint Commission has established National Patient Safety Goals (NSPGs). Because of their efforts, the use of bar coding for medication administration is now standard in all hospitals. The Joint Commission's website is http://www.jointcommission.org.

DOCUMENTING MEDICATION ERRORS

Documentation of medication errors should be clear and factual, following the facility's policies and procedures guidelines. Blame and judgment should be put aside with the goal being to determine the causes of the error so they can be eradicated in the future. Documentation of medication errors must include the interventions that were undertaken to counteract the error. The patient's medical record should be updated with complete information about the error. If the patient is hospitalized, the MAR should also be fully updated.

After updating the specific records about a medication error, the person who made the error or the person who observed its occurrence should complete a separate written report (often called an "incident report" or "occurrence report"). A factual, objective recording of the specific details of the error should be assembled. These reports are used by risk management personnel for quality improvement and assurance.

For legal reasons, accurate documentation in a medical record and in an error report is required. These documents help to improve medication administration processes and verify that patient safety was protected. If there is any attempt to delay corrective action or to hide a mistake, the legal ramifications may be much more severe. This is also true if interventions are not documented in the patient's chart.

Quality and improvement programs are used by hospitals and other health-care facilities to monitor medication errors. These may alert practitioners about trends in medication errors and help to create specific solutions. Many facilities use **root cause analysis (RCA)** to prevent future mistakes, asking exactly what happened, why it happened, and what can be done to prevent its recurrence. RCA may also be used to determine whether risk of recurrence has actually been reduced.

Sentinel events are unexpected occurrences involving death or serious physical or psychological injury or risk thereof. They are recognized by The Joint Commission and are always investigated so interventions may be used to ensure zero recurrence. RCA is used to identify causes and the needed type of intervention.

Focus Point

OTC Drugs

Patient use of OTC drugs and herbal substances may cause adverse reactions and medication errors.

✳ Apply Your Knowledge 8.2

The following questions focus on what you have just learned about reporting and documenting medication errors.

CRITICAL THINKING

1. Why must each error be thoroughly investigated and documented?
2. What federal agency coordinates the reporting of medication errors?
3. What is the MedWatch program?
4. Which organization assists in standardizing the medication error reporting system?
5. What are the advantages of documenting medication errors?

STRATEGIES FOR HANDLING MEDICATION ERRORS

The following steps can help in avoiding medication errors and promoting safe administration of medications:

1. Assessment: asking patients about allergies, health condition, use of medications and herbal supplements in correct doses and routes—taken at the right times; educating the patient about all medications he or she needs; and assessing body system functions to determine if pharmacotherapy impairments exist.

2. Planning: avoiding abbreviations that can be misunderstood, questioning orders that are unclear, refusing verbal orders, and following all policies and procedures exactly. Patients should restate dosing directions, including dosage amounts, routes, and times. The patient should be asked to explain the goals of the medication therapy.

3. Implementation: eliminating distractions during medication administration (including noise, talking, and other events); ensuring that the right patient, time, frequency, dose, route, and drug are all exact; and identification verification, correct procedures and techniques, exact dose calculations, correct and timely opening of medications, correct documentation of procedures, confirmation (if an oral medication) that the patient has completely swallowed the dose, and double-checking for long-acting oral dosage forms.

4. Evaluation: assessing the patient for correct outcomes and determining any adverse effects.

There are nine various categories of medication errors, and health-care professionals should be familiar with all of them. These categories are

✳ Category A: circumstances or events that have the capacity to cause errors

✳ Category B: errors that occurred but did not reach the patient

✳ Category C: errors that reached the patient but did not cause any harm

✳ Category D: errors that occurred, reached the patient, and required monitoring to ensure no patient harm or that required intervention to prevent patient harm

✳ Category E: errors that occurred and may have contributed to or resulted in temporary harm to the patient (and required intervention)

✳ Category F: errors that occurred that might have contributed to or resulted in temporary harm to the patient (and required initial or prolonged hospitalization)

✳ Category G: errors that occurred that might have contributed to or resulted in permanent patient harm

✳ Category H: errors that occurred that required intervention necessary to sustain life

✳ Category I: errors that occurred that might have contributed to or resulted in the patient's death

Most types of medication errors involve administration of an improper dose (41%). Nearly half of fatal medication errors occur in patients older than 60 years of age (Figure 8-1 ■). This is likely because older adults often need many different medications, have multiple health-care providers, or experience age-related physiology changes. Children are also more likely to experience medication errors because doses are based on body weight, which increases the likelihood of calculation errors. Up-to-date drug information must be available so health-care practitioners can verify correct data on the medications they are administering.

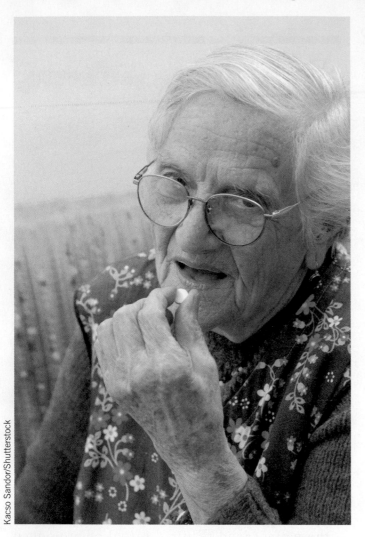

Kacso Sandor/Shutterstock

Figure 8-1 ■ Nearly half of fatal medication errors occur in patients older than 60 years of age.

RECONCILIATION OF MEDICATIONS

In older adults, multiple medications may be taken concurrently. **Polypharmacy** is defined as "receiving multiple medications, sometimes for the same condition, that have conflicting pharmacologic actions." Polypharmacy is most prevalent in the older age groups but may occur in all ages. It is hard to keep track of multiple medications and health-care providers, but this is made even more difficult by poor medication information, documentation, and reporting.

Keeping track of a patient's medications as they change health-care providers is called **medication reconciliation**. This involves accurately listing all medications a patient takes in order to reduce duplications, dosing errors, omissions, and drug interactions. When a patient is hospitalized, nurses document all medications previously being taken at home, including the dose, frequency, and route. This list is maintained and used whenever the patient is admitted to other facilities or transferred to different hospital units and is checked during the hospital discharge procedure. Many potential medication errors have been caught during medication reconciliation procedures. Medications being taken by a patient should be considered to include prescription medications, OTC medications, herbal supplements, and even vitamins.

The Joint Commission has identified many serious medication errors related to medication reconciliation and has developed recommendations for their prevention. The Joint Commission encourages hospitals to completely document all medications used by each patient during the admission process. Prescription medications, OTC medications, vitamins, and herbal supplements must all be documented. These patient medication lists must be communicated to all providers of service—inside and outside the hospital. After a patient is discharged, he or she should receive a complete list of medications to be taken as well as instructions on the use of any newly prescribed medications.

PATIENT EDUCATION

Medication Usage

Regarding their medications, patients should be provided with age-appropriate written information, audiovisual teaching aids when available, and contact information of the professionals to be notified in the case of an adverse reaction. Patients should know the names of all medications they are taking as well as the uses of these medications and dosages and when and how they should be taken. They should understand potential adverse effects that need to be reported immediately. Patients should always use specified medication devices to administer their medications and not household utensils, such as spoons, which may be inaccurate. They should be instructed to carry a list of all their prescription and OTC medications (as well as vitamins and herbal supplements) with them at all times and to use one pharmacy for all their prescriptions. They should be encouraged to ask questions so they can partner in maintaining safe medication principles.

✸ Apply Your Knowledge 8.3

The following questions focus on what you have just learned about strategies for handling and reconciling medications.

CRITICAL THINKING

1. What steps may help in avoiding medication errors?
2. What age group of individuals makes up nearly half of those who experience fatal medication errors?
3. What is the meaning of polypharmacy?
4. What is the meaning of *medication reconciliation*?
5. Why do older adults often need many different medications?

PRACTICAL SCENARIO 1

A physician wrote a prescription for ".5 mg IV morphine for postoperative pain" for a 9-month-old infant. The unit secretary recorded the order in the MAR as "5 mg." An inexperienced nurse followed the directions on the MAR without question and gave the baby 5 mg of IV morphine initially and another 5-mg dose 2 hours later. About 4 hours after the second dose, the baby stopped breathing and experienced cardiac arrest. If the physician had written "0.5 mg," the unit secretary would probably not have had any misunderstanding of the intended amount and the nurse would have administered the correct dose.

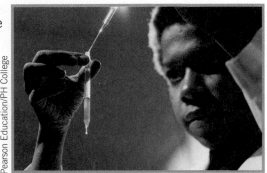

Pearson Education/PH College

Critical Thinking Questions

1. Although the initial error was not the nurse's, what steps should he or she have taken to avoid this medication error?
2. What measures could the facility implement to curtail future medication errors?
3. Explain how using a standardized written measurement system would have prevented this adverse drug event.

PRACTICAL SCENARIO 2

A 75-year-old man was taking several different medications for hypertension, hyperplasia of the prostate, and rheumatoid arthritis. Four of his medications were to be taken before bed, and three were to be taken in the morning. One night, he recalled that he had forgotten to take one of his medications. He got out of bed, went into his kitchen, and avoided turning on the light so as not to disturb his son-in-law, who was sleeping in the adjacent family room. In the darkness, he inadvertently took one of the medications he had already taken earlier. After 2 hours, he woke up to go to the bathroom and felt chest pain and dizziness, which caused him to collapse, awakening his wife.

Monkey Business Images/Shutterstock

Critical Thinking Questions

1. Which of his medications would cause lower blood pressure, chest pain, and dizziness?
2. What are the disadvantages of taking several drugs at the same time?

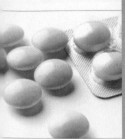

Chapter Capsule

This section repeats the objectives from the beginning of the chapter and then provides a summary of the most important concepts for that objective. Use this section as a quick review and to check your knowledge.

Objective 1: Explain why errors can occur in three stages in the medication process.

- First-stage errors can occur during prescribing or ordering if practitioners are distracted or interrupted.

- Second-stage errors can occur during dispensing because of inexperience, insufficient staff, lack of time for patient counseling, and not double-checking medications against a MAR or other paperwork.

- Third-stage errors can occur during administration and monitoring because of poor communication, misread paperwork, similar labeling and packaging of products, medications with similar names, and not monitoring patients for reactions to medications.

Objective 2: Describe factors that cause medication errors.

- Factors that cause medication errors include use of incorrect abbreviations, miscommunication, missing information, lack of appropriate labeling, environmental factors, and poor management.

Objective 3: Explain general recommendations to reduce medication errors.

- In general, to reduce medication errors, there should be an adequate amount of staff members; standardized measurement systems in place; consistently used error-tracking systems; a clearly defined system for drug administration, ordering, and dispensing with a review of the original drug orders; compilation of medication profiles; and a suitable work environment.

Objective 4: Describe the legal and ethical responsibility of health professionals to report all medication errors.

- The legal and ethical reporting of medication errors by all health professionals is of utmost importance in protecting patients. The FDA and other organizations offer systems for reporting medication errors. Health-care professionals are encouraged to use these systems to report medication errors and situations that may lead to errors.

Objective 5: Explain the role of the Food and Drug Administration in medication errors.

- On a federal level, the FDA coordinates the reporting of medication errors via its MedWatch program. This program provides timely information that is clinically important regarding medical products. Reporting to the FDA may be done anonymously, directly to the FDA, either by the Internet or telephone.

Objective 6: Define The Joint Commission and its role in preventing medication errors.

- The Joint Commission has established patient safety standards that address many significant patient safety issues. They require that hospitals inform patients when they have been harmed because of hospital errors. Continually attempting to standardize practices in hospitals nationwide, The Joint Commission has established National Patient Safety Goals (NSPGs). The use of bar coding for medication administration is now standard in all hospitals.

Objective 7: Explain the steps that may be taken to avoid medication errors and ensure safe administration of medication.

■ Assessment: asking patients about allergies, health condition, use of medications and herbal supplements in correct doses and routes—taken at the right times; educating the patient about all medications needed; and assessing body system functions to determine if pharmacotherapy impairments exist.

■ Planning: avoiding abbreviations that can be misunderstood, questioning orders that are unclear, refusing verbal orders, and following all policies and procedures exactly.

■ Implementation: eliminating distractions during medication administration, ensuring the seven rights, identification verification, correct procedures and techniques, exact dose calculations, correct and timely opening of medications, correct documentation of procedures, confirmation that the patient has completely swallowed an oral dose of medication, and double-checking for long-acting oral dosage forms.

Objective 8: Define polypharmacy.

■ Polypharmacy is defined as receiving multiple medications—sometimes for the same condition—that have conflicting pharmacologic actions.

 Internet Sites of Interest

■ Fatal medication errors: **http://www.suite101.com/content/fatal-medication-errors-occur-more-often-at-home-a62612**.

■ Medication error prevention: **http://cme.medscape.com/viewarticle/550273**.

■ Medication errors: **http://www.fda.gov/Drugs/DrugSafety/MedicationErrors/default.htm**.

■ Polypharmacy: **http://www.modernmedicine.com/modernmedicine/article/articleDetail.jsp?id=172920**.

■ Reducing errors in health care: **http://findarticles.com/p/articles/mi_mOHRO/is_2000_April_1/ai_66706679**.

■ Reducing medication errors: **http://www.nursingceu.com/courses/240/index_nceu.html**.

■ Reporting medication errors: **https://www.ismp.org/orderforms/reporterrortoISMP.asp**.

■ The most common medication errors: **http://www.medicinenet.com/script/main/art.asp?articlekey=55234**.

PEARSON
myhealthprofessionskit™

Go to www.myhealthprofessionskit.com to access the Companion Website created for this textbook. Simply select "Basic Health Science" from the choice of disciplines. Find this book and then log in using your username and password to access interactive learning games, assessment questions, animations, and more.

Checkpoint Review 2

1. Circle the *improper* fraction(s).

$$\frac{3}{4} \qquad 2\text{-}\frac{5}{8} \qquad \frac{4}{4} \qquad \frac{9}{7} \qquad \frac{18}{19} \qquad \frac{1\frac{1}{5}}{2\frac{2}{3}}$$

2. Circle the *complex* fraction(s).

$$\frac{3}{5} \qquad 1\text{-}\frac{3}{4} \qquad \frac{6}{6} \qquad \frac{7}{6} \qquad \frac{8}{9} \qquad \frac{\frac{1}{100}}{\frac{1}{160}}$$

3. Circle the *proper* fraction(s).

$$\frac{1}{3} \qquad \frac{1}{12} \qquad \frac{12}{1} \qquad \frac{16}{16} \qquad \frac{132}{12}$$

4. Circle the *mixed* number(s) *reduced to lowest terms.*

$$\frac{2}{5} \qquad 1\text{-}\frac{1}{6} \qquad \frac{5}{7} \qquad 1\text{-}\frac{2}{9} \qquad \frac{2}{3} \qquad 7\text{-}\frac{7}{9}$$

Change the following proper or improper fractions to fractions, whole numbers, or mixed numbers and reduce to lowest terms.

5. $\frac{12}{16}$ = _____

6. $\frac{4}{4}$ = _____

7. $\frac{30}{9}$ = _____

8. $\frac{44}{16}$ = _____

9. $\frac{100}{75}$ = _____

Change the following mixed numbers to improper fractions.

10. $6\text{-}\frac{1}{2}$ = _____

11. $7\text{-}\frac{5}{6}$ = _____

12. $1\text{-}\frac{1}{5}$ = _____

13. $10\text{-}\frac{2}{3}$ = _____

14. $102\text{-}\frac{3}{4}$ = _____

Circle the correct answer.

15. Which is smaller? $\frac{1}{100}$ or $\frac{1}{1,000}$

16. Which is larger? $\frac{1}{15}$ or $\frac{1}{10}$

17. Which is smaller? $\frac{3}{10}$ or $\frac{5}{10}$

18. Which is larger? $\frac{2}{9}$ or $\frac{5}{9}$

Add and then reduce your answers to lowest terms.

19. $\frac{3}{4} + \frac{2}{3}$ = _____

20. $\frac{3}{4} + \frac{1}{8} + \frac{1}{6}$ = _____

21. $\frac{1}{7} + \frac{2}{3} + \frac{11}{21}$ = _____

22. $\frac{1}{4} + \frac{5}{33}$ = _____

23. $\frac{12}{17} + 5 - \frac{2}{7}$ = _____

24. $7\text{-}\frac{4}{5} + \frac{2}{3}$ = _____

Multiply and then reduce your answers to lowest terms.

25. $\frac{30}{10} \times \frac{1}{12}$ = _____

26. $\frac{1}{100} \times 3$ = _____

27. $\frac{3}{4} \times \frac{2}{3}$ = _____

28. $\frac{5}{8} \times 1\text{-}\frac{1}{6}$ = _____

29. $\frac{3}{4} \times \frac{1}{8}$ = _____

30. $12\text{-}\frac{1}{2} \times 20\text{-}\frac{1}{3}$ = _____

Divide and then reduce your answers to lowest terms.

31. $\dfrac{1}{60} \div \dfrac{1}{2}$ = _____

32. $\dfrac{1}{8} \div \dfrac{7}{12}$ = _____

33. $2\dfrac{1}{2} \div \dfrac{3}{4}$ = _____

34. $\dfrac{1}{150} \div \dfrac{1}{50}$ = _____

Select terms from your reading to fill in the blanks.

35. Liters and milliliters are metric units that measure _____.

36. 1 mg is _____ of a gram.

37. 1 liter = _____ mL.

38. 1,000 mcg = _____ mg.

39. There are _____ mL in a liter.

40. Which is smallest: a kilogram, gram, or milligram? _____

41. Which is largest: a kilogram, gram, or milligram? _____

42. Milligrams are metric units that measure _____.

Circle the correct metric notation.

43. 4 kg   4.0 kg   kg 04   4 kG   4 KG

44. .6 g   0.6 Gm   0.6 g   .6 Gm   0.60 g

45. 2.5 mm   2-1/2 mm   2.5 Mm   2.50 MM   2-1/2 MM

46. mg 20   20 mG   20.0 mg   20 mg   20 MG

Write the term for these abbreviations.

47. g   _____

48. mm   _____

49. cm   _____

50. kg   _____

51. mcg   _____

52. mL   _____

Write the terms for these abbreviations and symbols.

53. qt   _____

54. gr   _____

55. ℥   _____

56. ℨ   _____

Write the terms for these equivalencies.

57. 16 oz = pt   _____

58. qt i = oz   _____

Write the following apothecary quantities using abbreviations and proper notation.

59. ten grains   _____

60. two pints   _____

61. one-half ounce   _____

62. sixteen pints   _____

63. four ounces   _____

64. three grains   _____

Write these measurements using abbreviations.

65. 3 tablespoons   _____

66. 10 teaspoons   _____

67. 6 drops   _____

68. 25 milliequivalents   _____

Convert these measurements to the units shown.

69. 1 oz =   _____ T

70. 16 oz =   _____ lb

71. 4 T =   _____ oz

72. 24 oz =   _____ cups

Write the terms for these abbreviations.

73. 20 mEq   _____

74. 15 lb   _____

75. 50 gtt   _____

76. 8 T   _____

Calculate the amounts to administer and then write them in the blank spaces.

77. Ordered: Lanoxin 0.125 mg PO daily
    On hand: Lanoxin 0.25 mg tablets
    Administer: _____ tablet(s)

78. Ordered: Duricef 1 g PO bid
    On hand: Duricef 500 mg capsules
    Administer: _____ capsule(s)

79. Ordered: Synthroid 0.1 mg PO daily
    On hand: Synthroid 50 mcg tablets
    Administer: _____ tablet(s)

80. Ordered: Diabinese 0.1 g PO daily
    On hand: Diabinese 100 mg tablets
    Administer: _____ tablet(s)

81. Ordered: amoxicillin 100 mg PO qid
    On hand: 80 mL bottle of Amoxil (amoxicillin)
    Oral pediatric suspension 125 mg for 5 mL
    Administer: _____ mL

82. Ordered: Septra-DS suspension 200 mg PO bid
    On hand: Septra-DS suspension 400 mg for 5 mL
    Administer: _____ mL

83. Ordered: Esidrix solution 100 mg PO bid
    On hand: Esidrix solution 50 mg for 5 mL
    Administer: _____ t

84. Ordered: digoxin elixir 0.25 mg PO daily
    On hand: digoxin elixir 50 mcg/mL
    Administer: _____ mL

85. Ordered: Tylenol 0.5 g PO q4h PRN pain
    On hand: Tylenol 500 mg for 5 mL
    Administer: _____ t

86. Ordered: Pathocil 125 mg PO q6h
    On hand: Pathocil suspension 62.5 mg for 5 mL
    Administer: _____ t

87. Ordered: erythromycin 1.2 g PO q8h
    On hand: erythromycin 400 mg per 5 mL
    Administer: _____ mL

88. Ordered: cephalexin 375 mg PO tid
    On hand: cephalexin 250 mg per 5 mL
    Administer: _____ t

89. Ordered: Demerol syrup 75 mg PO q4h PRN pain
    On hand: Demerol syrup 50 mg for 5 mL
    Administer: _____ mL

90. Ordered: Coumadin 7.5 mg PO daily
    On hand: Coumadin 2.5 mg tablets
    Administer: _____ tablet(s)

91. Ordered: Urecholine 50 mg PO tid
    On hand: Urecholine 25 mg tablets
    Administer: _____ tablet(s)

92. Ordered: V-Cillin K 300,000 units PO qid
    On hand: V-Cillin K 200,000 units for 5 mL
    Administer: _____ mL

93. Ordered: codeine gr 1/4 PO daily
    On hand: codeine 30 mg tablets
    Administer: _____ tablet(s)

94. Ordered: Orinase 250 mg PO bid
    On hand: Orinase 0.5 g tablets
    Administer: _____ tablet(s)

95. Ordered: Ceclor suspension 225 mg PO bid
    On hand: Ceclor suspension 375 mg for 5 mL
    Administer: _____ mL

96. Ordered: Aspirin gr v PO daily
    On hand: Aspirin 325 mg tablets
    Administer: _____ tablet(s)

97. Ordered: Levaquin 0.5 g PO daily
    On hand: Levaquin 500 mg tablets
    Administer: _____ tablet(s)

98. Ordered: atropine gr 1/100 IM on call to OR
    On hand: atropine 0.4 mg/mL
    Administer: _____ mL

99. Ordered: lidocaine 50 mg IV Stat
    On hand: lidocaine 2%
    Administer: _____ mL

100. Ordered: heparin 3,500 units subcutaneous q12h
     On hand: heparin 5,000 units/mL
     Administer: _____ mL

101. Ordered: Lasix 60 mg IV Stat
     On hand: Lasix 20 mg for 2 mL ampule
     Administer: _____ mL

Using the formula $D \times Q/H = X$, answer the following:

102. (*D*) represents _____.

103. (*Q*) represents _____.

104. (*H*) represents _____.

105. (*X*) represents _____.

Select terms from your reading to fill in the blanks.

106. The common syringe that is used for intradermal testing is the _____.

107. The volume of solution for IM injection is 0.5 to _____ mL.

108. The most common insulin combining NPH and regular insulin is _____, but 50/50 insulin is also available.

109. The anticoagulant heparin is measured in _____ units.

110. Intravenous fluids and drugs may be administered by intermittent or _____ IV infusion.

111. Body surface area is determined by using a _____ and the child's height and weight.

112. Dosage calculations use such pediatric formulas as Clark's rule, _____ rule, and _____ rule.

113. Clark's rule is based on the _____ of the child.

114. _____ rule is used for children older than 1 year of age.

115. _____ rule is a method of estimating the dose of medication for infants younger than 1 year of age.

116. The most common medication errors occur because of _____ _____.

117. In the hospital, _____ _____ are the most common cause of morbidity and preventable death.

118. Health professionals may report medication errors to the _____.

119. _____ and improvement programs are used by hospitals and other health care facilities to monitor medication errors.

120. Strategies for handling medication errors involve four steps: assessment, planning, implementation, and _____.

Unit 3

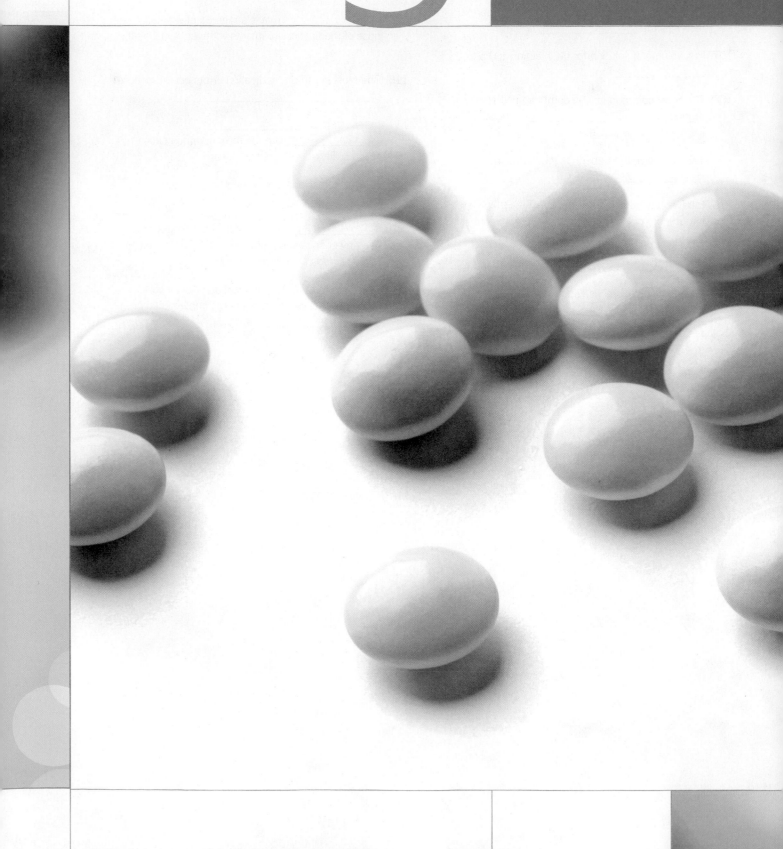

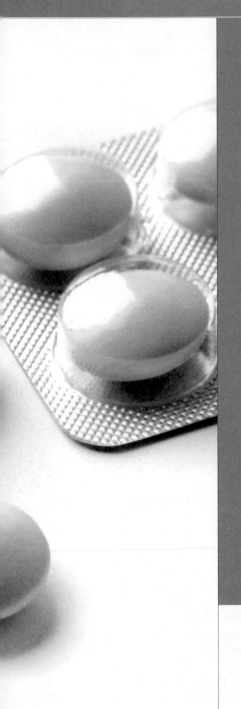

DRUG EFFECTS ON MULTIPLE SYSTEMS

"Antibiotic use has had a tremendous impact on the way microorganisms respond to various agents. Subtherapeutic doses or overuse can affect microorganism resistance."

Chapter 9

Nutritional Aspects of Pharmacology and Herbal Substances

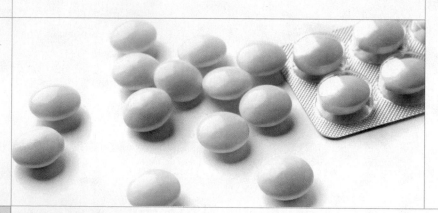

Chapter Objectives

After completing this chapter, you should be able to:

1. Identify the seven basic food components and explain their major functions.
2. Differentiate the classifications of nutrients.
3. Explain the role of calories in the diet.
4. Define the role of essential fatty acids in optimal health.
5. List the water-soluble vitamins.
6. Discuss the toxicity of vitamin A.
7. Indicate the significance of vitamin E deficiency in infants.
8. List the five essential trace minerals and the symptoms of their toxicity.
9. Explain general indications for total parenteral nutrition.
10. Describe the benefits of food additives.

Key Terms

additives (page 147)

alpha tocopherol (AL-fa toh-KAW-ferrol) (page 139)

anemia (uh-NEE-mee-uh) (page 138)

antioxidant (page 140)

ascorbic acid (as-SCOR-bik) (page 136)

beriberi (BEH-ree BEH-ree) (page 137)

calciferol (kal-SIH-fuh-rol) (page 140)

calcitonin (kal-sih-TOE-nin) (page 140)

calcitriol (kal-SIH-tree-ol) (page 140)

carbohydrates (page 134)

carotene (KAH-roh-teen) (page 139)

cholecalciferol (koh-luh-kal-SIH-fehrol) (page 139)

cholesterol (koh-LES-teh-rol) (page 134)

cobalamin (koh-BAL-luh-min) (page 138)

congenital hypothyroidism (page 143)

essential amino acids (page 133)

fatty acids (page 133)

fiber (page 135)

goiter (GOY-ter) (page 143)

hypervitaminosis (hy-per-vy-tuh-mih-NOH-sis) (page 140)

macrominerals (mak-ro-MIH-neh-ruls) (page 133)

macrominerals (page 133)

major minerals (page 142)

nutrition (page 133)

pellagra (peh-LEH-gruh) (page 137)

phylloquinone (fil-loh-KWIH-nohen) (page 139)

recommended dietary allowances (RDAs) (page 145)

rickets (page 140)

spina bifida (SPY-nuh BIFF-ih-duh) (page 138)

total parenteral nutrition (TPN) (page 146)

Introduction

Nutrition is the process of how the body takes in and uses food and other sources of nutrients for growth and repair of tissues. This process has five parts: intake, digestion, absorption, metabolism, and elimination. This chapter gives you an understanding of how a well-planned diet can lead to optimal health and well-being for your patients, and it provides important information about food and drug interactions.

Nutrients

The human body needs a variety of nutrients for energy, growth, repair, and basic processes. Seven basic food components provide these nutrients and work together to help keep the body healthy:

1. Proteins
2. Fatty acids (also called *lipids* or *fats*)
3. Carbohydrates
4. Fiber
5. Vitamins
6. Minerals
7. Water

Only proteins, fats, and carbohydrates contain calories and provide the body with energy. The remaining four food components perform a variety of other essential functions. The nutritional sciences study the nature and distribution of nutrients in food, their metabolic effects, and the consequences of inadequate food intake.

A nutrient is any element or compound from the diet that supports normal metabolism, growth, reproduction, or other normal body functioning. Some nutrients are called *essential* because they are needed by the body for normal functioning. Essential nutrients cannot be synthesized by the body and thus must be derived from the diet. Essential nutrients include vitamins, minerals, amino acids, fatty acids, and some carbohydrates. On the other hand, *nonessential* nutrients are those the body can synthesize from other compounds, although they may also be derived from the diet. Another way that nutrients are subdivided is into *macronutrients* and *micronutrients*.

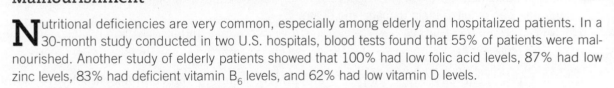

Focus Point

Malnourishment

Nutritional deficiencies are very common, especially among elderly and hospitalized patients. In a 30-month study conducted in two U.S. hospitals, blood tests found that 55% of patients were malnourished. Another study of elderly patients showed that 100% had low folic acid levels, 87% had low zinc levels, 83% had deficient vitamin B_6 levels, and 62% had low vitamin D levels.

Macronutrients

Macronutrients are needed by the body in relatively large amounts and constitute the bulk of the diet. They supply energy as well as essential nutrients needed for growth, maintenance, and activity. Carbohydrates, fats (including essential fatty acids), proteins, **macrominerals** (dietary minerals needed by the human body in high quantities), and water are macronutrients. Carbohydrates are converted to glucose (a simple sugar) and other monosaccharides (carbohydrates that cannot form any simple sugar), fats are converted to fatty acids and glycerol, and proteins are converted to peptides and amino acids. These macronutrients are interchangeable as sources of energy; fats yield 9 kilocalories of energy per 1 g consumed (9 kcal/g); proteins and carbohydrates yield 4 kcal/g.

The macrominerals, such as sodium, chloride, potassium, calcium, phosphorus, and magnesium, are required by humans in relatively large quantities (that is, grams) per day. Water is also considered a macronutrient because it is required in the amount of 1 mL/kcal of energy expended, or about 2,500 mL/day.

ESSENTIAL AMINO ACIDS

Essential amino acids are those components of proteins that cannot be synthesized by the body and must be provided by the diet. Of the 20 amino acids in proteins, nine are essential. The requirement for dietary protein correlates with the growth rate, which varies at different times in the life cycle. The amino acid composition of proteins varies widely.

ESSENTIAL FATTY ACIDS

Essential **fatty acids** (such as linoleic acid and linolenic acid) are required in amounts equaling 6% to 10% of fat intake (5–10 g/day). These fatty acids must be provided by the diet; for example, vegetable oils provide linoleic acid and linolenic acid. Essential fatty acids are required for the formation of prostaglandins (hormone-like substances) and thromboxanes (biochemically related to the prostaglandins). Fatty acids, particularly omega-3 fatty acids, appear to play a role in decreasing the risk of coronary artery disease. Research has shown that consumption of omega-3 fatty acids decreases triglyceride levels and the growth rate of atherosclerotic plaque, slightly lowers blood pressure, and decreases the risk of arrhythmias.

Fatty acids can be either saturated or unsaturated. The chemical structure of a *saturated* fatty acid contains all the hydrogen possible and therefore is dense, heavy, and solid at room temperature. Examples of saturated fats are the fats found in dairy products and meats.

Unsaturated fatty acids can take on more hydrogen and are less heavy and less dense. Unsaturated fats are usually liquid at room temperature. If fatty acids have one unfilled hydrogen bond, the fat is called *monounsaturated*. Olives, olive oil, and peanut oil contain monounsaturated fats. *Polyunsaturated* fats, such as corn, safflower, and soy oils, have two or more unfilled hydrogen bonds. All essential fatty acids are polyunsaturated fatty acids, but not all polyunsaturated fatty acids are essential fatty acids.

Cholesterol, a natural lipid found in cell membranes, is found in highest concentrations in animal muscles and organ cells. Cholesterol does not exist in plants. It is essential for certain cell structures; however, excess cholesterol can deposit in blood vessels, form atherosclerotic plaque, and lead to cardiovascular disease.

CARBOHYDRATES

Carbohydrates in food provide about two-thirds of an individual's fuel for daily energy needs. They aid in fat metabolism and help reserve protein for uses other than supplying energy, such as repairing and building our bodies. The daily requirement for carbohydrates is 50% to 60% of total caloric intake. Carbohydrate deficiency leads to weight loss, protein loss, and fatigue.

Focus Point

Blood Glucose Levels

The central nervous system (CNS) requires a constant minute-to-minute supply of glucose to function properly. Sustained low blood glucose levels, which can be caused by an excessively low intake of carbohydrates, can result in brain damage and death.

There are two basic types of carbohydrates: *simple sugars*, which are found in fruits, some vegetables, milk, and table sugar, and *complex carbohydrates*, which are found in such grain foods as pastas, breads, and rice and such fruits and vegetables as potatoes, broccoli, corn, apples, and pears. The two types of carbohydrates have a function in health and consist of many variations. With the exception of fibers, carbohydrates are easily digested and absorbed into the body. Simple sugars are quickly absorbed, but complex carbohydrates must be processed before they can be absorbed in the intestinal tract. A small amount of glucose is stored in the liver and muscles as glycogen (starch). This stored glucose is available to supplement dietary supplies of carbohydrates. Excess amounts of carbohydrates are stored in the body as fat or *adipose* tissue. Carbohydrates are also needed to regulate protein and fat metabolism.

Focus on Pediatrics

Lactose Sensitivity

Lactose is the sugar contained in human and animal milk. It must be broken down in the body by the enzyme lactase to enable the body to digest dairy products. Many infants and children have trouble digesting foods that contain lactose and must eliminate those foods from their diets. Children who are especially sensitive to dietary lactose are often referred to as being *lactose-intolerant*. Generally, removing milk products from the diet is recommended for lactose-intolerant children. Lactose-free milk can be substituted, as can sources of calcium, such as yogurt, buttermilk, and cheese, which contain less lactose than milk.

FIBER

Fiber is a type of complex carbohydrate that does not supply energy or heat to the body. Fiber is the tough, stringy part of vegetables and grains. It can be classified as soluble or insoluble. *Soluble fiber*, found in foods such as oats, dry beans, barley, and some fruits and vegetables, tends to absorb fluid and swell when eaten. Water-soluble fiber helps to lower blood cholesterol levels. It also may stabilize blood sugar levels in the body by slowing the absorption of carbohydrates into the blood. *Insoluble fiber*, which is found in the bran of whole wheat and brown rice, primarily promotes regular bowel movements by contributing to stool bulk, which stimulates peristalsis. It also helps to prevent colon cancer (the stool bulk scours the intestines of waste matter as it passes through) and seems to reduce the risk of heart attack. Although insoluble fiber is not absorbed by the body, it serves to increase and soften the bulk of the stool, promoting normal defecation. Therapeutically, insoluble fiber can help treat and prevent constipation, diverticular disease, and irritable bowel syndrome. It is linked to reduction in gallstone formation and risks of certain types of cancer, especially colon cancer, and other diseases.

The recommended amount of daily dietary fiber intake for adults is 25 to 40 g/1,000 kcal. Because fiber works with other substances and nutrients, it is advisable to get dietary fiber from a variety of food sources. Adequate water intake is especially important for fiber to work properly. Without adequate water intake, constipation and bloating may occur. Water also stimulates peristalsis in the intestine.

✴ Apply Your Knowledge 9.1

The following questions focus on what you have just learned about macronutrients and their role in health.

CRITICAL THINKING

1. What is an essential nutrient?
2. Name two essential fatty acids and describe the indications of omega-3 fatty acids.
3. Describe cholesterol.
4. What is the indication of water-soluble fiber?
5. Classify carbohydrates and name an example for each.
6. What are macronutrients?
7. Name six macrominerals.
8. What is the effect of insoluble fiber in the human body?

Micronutrients

Vitamins and essential trace minerals comprise *micronutrients*—a group of nutrients that are required in very small amounts by the human body for normal functioning. Foods contain small amounts of these micronutrients. However, if any of these micronutrients is lacking in the diet, biochemical alterations—such as changes in the structure and function of tissues and organs—result and possibly cause deficiency or diseases.

VITAMINS

Vitamins are organic (carbon-containing) compounds required for normal human growth, development, and maintenance of normal body function; however, the amount needed by the body is very small. The total volume of vitamins that a healthy individual normally requires per day would barely fill a teaspoon! Thus, vitamin requirements are measured in milligrams or micrograms—exceedingly small and difficult units to visualize. Deficiencies of vitamins occur when a special condition or disorder creates an increased need in a particular person at a particular time.

Vitamins are classified by their solubility: They are soluble in either water or fat. This difference has importance in bodily storage of vitamins and in vitamin deficiency or toxicity.

Water-Soluble Vitamins (B and C Vitamins)

Water-soluble vitamins include eight members of the vitamin B group (Table 9-1 ■) and vitamin C (**ascorbic acid**). All members of the B-vitamin group act as coenzymes (organic chemicals that must combine with an enzyme in order for the enzyme to function)—usually after being processed. The coenzymes are frequently grouped together because many are found in similar foodstuffs.

Table 9-1 ■ Water-Soluble Vitamins

GENERIC NAME	TRADE NAME	FUNCTIONS	HYPOVITAMINOSIS (*DEFICIENT INTAKE*)	HYPERVITAMINOSIS (*EXCESSIVE INTAKE*)
B_1 (thiamine)	Betalins, Bewon, Biamine	Metabolic reactions coenzyme	Anorexia, depression, dyspnea, loss of muscle strength, memory loss, and peripheral neuritis	Very little toxicity; in extreme overdosage, symptoms include hypotension, neuromuscular or ganglionic blockage, and respiratory depression
B_2 (riboflavin)	Riboflavin	Metabolic reactions coenzyme	Anemia, dermatitis of the face, sore throat and mouth, and swollen tongue	Low toxicity levels, but in extreme overdosage, symptoms include dark urine, nausea, and vomiting
B_3 (nicotinamide, niacin, or nicotinic acid)	Niac, Nicobid, Novoniacin	Metabolic reactions coenzyme	Dementia, diarrhea, dizziness, headache, impaired memory, insomnia, skin eruptions, and sore mouth	Diarrhea, dizziness, dry skin, dysrhythmias, flushing, muscle pain, nausea, pruritus, and vomiting
B_5 (pantothenic acid)	None	Metabolic reactions coenzyme	Induced in humans via a metabolic antagonist; symptoms include cardiac instability, depression, frequent infections, and neurologic disorders	None, except in unusually high doses: diarrhea
B_6 (pyridoxine)	Beesix, Hexa-Betalin, Nestrex	Amino acid metabolic coenzyme	Peripheral neuritis, seborrheic-like skin lesions, seizures, and sore mouth	Low toxicity (except in chronic overuse; then neurotoxicity, including clumsiness, lack of muscle coordination, and numbness)
B_7 (biotin)	None	Metabolic reactions coenzyme	Anorexia, depression, dry skin, fine and brittle hair, fungal infections, hair loss, muscle pain, nausea and vomiting, rashes, and seborrheic dermatitis	No documented cases of overdosage
B_9 (folate, folic acid, or pteroylglutamic acid)	Apo-Folic, Folacin, Folvite	Amino acid and nucleic acid metabolic coenzyme	Megaloblastic anemia	Allergic reactions, fever, pruritus, rashes, and redness of skin
B_{12} (cobalamin, cyanocobalamin, or hydroxocobalamin)	Hydrobexan, Hydroxo-12, LA-12	Nucleic acid metabolic coenzyme	Abnormal blood cell production, confusion, dementia, memory loss, and nervous system damage	No toxic effects; overdosage is extremely rare but may cause a deficiency of the other B vitamins

GENERIC NAME	TRADE NAME	FUNCTIONS	HYPOVITAMINOSIS (*DEFICIENT INTAKE*)	HYPERVITAMINOSIS (*EXCESSIVE INTAKE*)
Choline	None	Metabolic reactions coenzyme	Liver damage in adults, alterations in memory, and increased fetal brain cell death	None listed for choline alone, but when used in combination preparations, symptoms of overdosage include confusion, diarrhea, dizziness, drowsiness, headache, hearing impairment, respiratory changes, sweating, and vomiting
C (ascorbic acid)	Apo-C, Ascorbicap, Cebid	Coenzyme and antioxidant	Anemia, gingivitis, and scurvy	Dizziness, kidney stones; in high doses, diarrhea, nausea and vomiting, and redness of skin

THIAMINE (VITAMIN B₁)

Also called *vitamin B₁*, thiamine is converted into a pyrophosphate, which functions as a coenzyme in some important carbohydrate metabolic processes. For example, the metabolism of alcohol depends on thiamine pyrophosphate. People with alcoholism frequently experience thiamine deficiency because heavy consumption of alcohol interferes with the body's ability to absorb the vitamin from food.

The main natural dietary sources of thiamine are whole grains (especially wheat germ), lean meats, fish, soybeans, and other beans. Processed foods are often fortified with thiamine.

Deficiency of thiamine leads to the disease **beriberi**, which is characterized by edema, cardiovascular abnormalities, and neurologic symptoms.

RIBOFLAVIN (VITAMIN B₂)

Riboflavin—also called *vitamin B₂*—is important in the metabolism of fats, carbohydrates, and proteins. The main dietary sources of riboflavin are dairy products, yeast products, and liver. Almonds are also a good source, and many other plant products contain reasonable amounts.

A deficiency of riboflavin causes cheilosis (fissures on the lips) and stomatitis (cracks in the angles of the mouth). Glossitis (inflammation of the tongue) and seborrheic dermatitis—mainly of the face and scrotum—can occur, as can a decreased resistance to infections. There is no known danger of excessive consumption of riboflavin. However, patients using riboflavin supplements should be warned that their urine may be bright yellow.

Riboflavin is sensitive to light and other foods; therefore, vitamin supplements containing riboflavin should be kept out of direct sunlight.

NICOTINAMIDE (VITAMIN B₃)

Nicotinamide is also known as *niacin*. Humans can actually make some of this vitamin from the amino acid tryptophan. The main food sources of nicotinamide are liver, yeast products, peanuts, whole grain cereals, and fish (tuna is exceptionally high in this vitamin). Deficiency of nicotinamide causes **pellagra**—a condition marked by "the four Ds": dementia, dermatitis, diarrhea, and death.

Nicotinamide is therefore used chiefly in the treatment of patients with pellagra. It also has been found to be useful with thiamine and riboflavin in the treatment of those with nutritional deficiency in chronic alcoholism because these patients also have deficiencies of thiamine and riboflavin. Large doses lower cholesterol, triglycerides, and free fatty acids. Therefore, nicotinamide is used in the treatment of patients with hypercholesterolemia (high blood cholesterol level)—mostly in combination with the cholesterol-lowering drugs cholestyramine, colestipol, or clofibrate (see Chapter 19). Toxicity associated with high doses of niacin includes hepatic impairment, severe hypotension, and various skin conditions.

Focus Point

Pharmacologic Doses of Niacin

At high doses, niacin decreases blood levels of low-density lipoprotein cholesterol (the bad cholesterol) and triglyceride levels—both of which are linked with cardiovascular disease. In addition, pharmacologic doses of niacin improve high-density lipoprotein cholesterol (the good cholesterol) levels. When niacin is used in this sense, it functions more as a drug than a vitamin and should be used only under medical supervision.

PANTOTHENIC ACID (VITAMIN B$_5$)

The term *pantothenic* derives from the Greek, meaning "all over the place." This vitamin is needed for the formation of the important coenzyme A, which is required for numerous biochemical processes. A deficiency syndrome has been experimentally induced in human volunteers and results in vomiting, cramps, abdominal pains, and personality changes. Pantothenic acid is readily available in many plant and animal sources. It is very difficult for individuals to have a deficiency of this vitamin.

PYRIDOXINE (VITAMIN B$_6$)

Vitamin B$_6$ does not denote a single substance but rather is a collective term for a group of naturally occurring pyridines that are metabolically and functionally interrelated: pyridoxine, pyridoxal, and pyridoxamine. The various forms of pyridoxine are widely distributed in animal and plant products, making deficiency rare.

Vitamin B$_6$ reputedly has several therapeutic uses. It is used routinely in patients on isoniazid therapy to prevent neuritis. Pyridoxine is also prescribed to treat women with hyperemesis gravidarum (nausea during pregnancy), particularly when given parenterally, and to suppress lactation when given orally.

BIOTIN

Biotin is widely available in the foods we eat, and deficiency is almost unknown. It is also made by the natural flora of the intestine. Biotin does not seem to produce any toxicity if taken in excess, and abuse of this vitamin does not seem to be common.

FOLATE

The name *folate* comes from the Latin word *falium*, meaning "leaf." The name was given to this vitamin because a major source is from dark green leafy vegetables. *Folate* is now used as the common, generic name for this vitamin that exists in many chemical forms. The most stable form of folate is folic acid, which is rarely found in food but is the form usually used in vitamin supplements and fortified food products. In its basic coenzyme role, folate is essential to the formation of all body cells because it takes part in the creation of DNA, the important cell nucleus material that transmits genetic characteristics. Folate is also essential to the formation of hemoglobin and synthesis of amino acids.

A direct deficiency of folate causes a special type of **anemia** (a deficiency of hemoglobin, red blood cell number, or red blood cell volume) called *megaloblastic anemia*, which is a particular risk during pregnancy because of increased fetal growth demands for folate. Rapidly growing adolescents—especially those following fad diets—and those who smoke develop low levels of folate in the blood, risking anemia.

The role of adequate folate in reducing the serious public health problem of neural defects during pregnancy has received increasing study and public awareness in recent years. Neural tube defects, such as **spina bifida** (a condition wherein the spinal column is imperfectly closed, resulting in protrusion of the meninges or spinal cord) and anencephaly (the congenital absence of most of the brain and spinal cord), are the most common birth defects involving the brain and spinal cord. Therefore, increased folic acid intake is recommended for all women who are capable of becoming pregnant. Adverse effects of excess consumption of folate from foods have not been observed.

COBALAMIN (VITAMIN B$_{12}$)

Vitamin B$_{12}$ is also known as **cobalamin**, which promotes normal function of all cells, especially normal blood formation. It is also necessary for proper nervous system function.

Although it is essential, the amount of dietary vitamin B$_{12}$ needed for normal human metabolism is very small. Vitamin B$_{12}$ deficiency is responsible for pernicious anemia. A component of the digestive gastric secretions called *intrinsic factor* is necessary for absorption of vitamin B$_{12}$ into the bloodstream. Gastrointestinal (GI) disorders that destroy the cell lining can disrupt the secretion of intrinsic factor and thus inhibit vitamin B$_{12}$ absorption. If the vitamin cannot be absorbed to make hemoglobin, pernicious anemia occurs. In such cases, vitamin B$_{12}$ must be given by injection to bypass the absorption defect. Deficiency is much more common in elderly individuals because of a lack of either intrinsic factor or hydrochloric acid in the stomach, not because of insufficient dietary intake.

Although small amounts of vitamin B$_{12}$ are stored in the liver, excess intake of vitamin B$_{12}$ does not produce adverse effects in healthy individuals; therefore, no toxicity has been established. This vitamin is naturally found only in animal products (it is originally made by bacteria in the intestine of herbivores), such as fish, meat, poultry, eggs, milk, and milk products; breakfast cereals often are fortified with vitamin B$_{12}$.

VITAMIN B FACTORS (CHOLINE)

Choline is a water-soluble nutrient associated with the B-complex vitamins. Although it is synthesized in the human body, choline plays an important role as a structural component of cell membranes. Choline is an essential component in the production of acetylcholine, which is a neurotransmitter involved in memory storage, muscle control, and many other functions. A deficiency of choline from food sources appears to be associated with liver damage. This occurs because very-low-density lipoproteins cannot be synthesized, causing fat to accumulate in the liver and resulting in liver damage. Choline deficiency can affect healthy nerve function and may play a role in the development of Huntington's chorea, Parkinson's disease, and Alzheimer's disease.

Choline is found naturally in a wide variety of foods, especially milk, eggs, liver, and peanuts.

Excess choline rarely causes toxicity. Adverse effects have only been observed in cases in which choline intake was several times greater than normal intake from food. Very high doses of choline have been associated with lowered blood pressure, fishy body odor, sweating, excessive salivation, and reduced growth rate.

ASCORBIC ACID (VITAMIN C)

Vitamin C (ascorbic acid) is required for building and maintaining strong tissues for wound healing, resistance to infection, and enhanced iron absorption. Vitamin C has several critical functions in the body. It acts as a protective agent (antioxidant) and plays a role in many metabolic and immunologic activities—perhaps as a preventive agent in many cancers and cardiovascular disease. Ascorbic acid is thought to lower the incidence of atherosclerosis by aiding the conversion of cholesterol to bile acids. It enhances iron bioavailability, promotes calcium absorption, and aids in wound healing and tissue repair. Ascorbic acid is also essential for the body's constant production of collagen in connective tissue as part of normal tissue turnover.

A deficiency of ascorbic acid can result in scurvy—a serious and severe disease caused by the degeneration of connective tissue. Scurvy is marked by anemia, edema of the gums, and bleeding into the skin and mucous membranes.

The two best sources of vitamin C are capsicums and guavas—not citrus fruits, as is commonly believed. Kiwi fruit is also very high in ascorbic acid. If large doses of ascorbic acid are used, plenty of water should be taken at the same time to avoid the formation of kidney stones. Diarrhea and gastritis can occur with large doses.

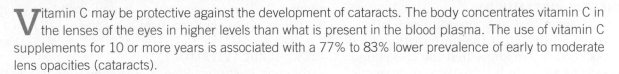

Focus on Geriatrics

Vitamin C and Cataracts

Vitamin C may be protective against the development of cataracts. The body concentrates vitamin C in the lenses of the eyes in higher levels than what is present in the blood plasma. The use of vitamin C supplements for 10 or more years is associated with a 77% to 83% lower prevalence of early to moderate lens opacities (cataracts).

Fat-Soluble Vitamins

Fat-soluble vitamins include retinol (vitamin A), **chole-calciferol** (vitamin D₃), ergocalciferol (vitamin D₃), **alpha tocopherol** (vitamin E), and **phylloquinone** (vitamin K₁) and menaquinone (vitamin K₁). Unlike water-soluble vitamins, fat-soluble vitamins are stored in the body. This storage can create an excess of these vitamins and may lead to toxicities. Excess amounts of vitamin A, in particular, can cause toxicity.

RETINOL (VITAMIN A)

The major function of vitamin A, or retinol, is in the retina of the eye. Retinol is an essential part of rhodopsin, which is a pigment in the eye commonly known as visual purple. A mild deficiency of vitamin A may cause night blindness, slow adaptation to darkness, or glare blindness. Adequate intake of retinol prevents two eye conditions: xerophthalmia (blindness) and xerosis (burning and itching).

Focus on Pediatrics

Vitamin A Deficiency

Dietary vitamin A deficiency is the number one cause of blindness in children worldwide.

Retinol also maintains healthy epithelial tissue (the vital outside layer of protective cells covering open surfaces of the body), such as skin and the inner mucous membranes in the nose, throat, eyes, GI tract, and genitourinary tract. These tissues provide our primary barrier to infection. Retinol is essential to the growth of skeletal and soft tissues and influences the stability of cell membranes and protein synthesis. Vitamin A is also important in the production of immune cells responsible for fighting bacterial, parasitic, and viral attacks.

Fish liver oils, butter, egg yolk, liver, and cream are sources of natural vitamin A. Although vitamin A only occurs naturally in the fat part of milk, the FDA requires that all milk—including nonfat milk—be fortified with vitamin A. **Carotene** is found in dark green and yellow vegetables and fruits. Beta-carotene (one of three carotenes: alpha, beta, and gamma) is important to human nutrition because the body can convert it to vitamin A, thus making it a primary source of the vitamin. Some good sources of beta-carotene are turnip greens, spinach, carrots, sweet potatoes, mangos, pumpkins, and apricots.

The liver can store large amounts of retinol. In healthy individuals, the storage efficiency in the liver of ingested retinol is more than 50%, and the liver contains about 90% of the body's total store. Thus, large amounts of supplemental retinol added to normal dietary sources can cause toxicity. Excess vitamin A intake is called **hypervitaminosis** A. Symptoms of this toxicity include loss of hair, jaundice, joint pain, and thickening of the long bones. Liver injury and ascites (fluid accumulation in the abdominal cavity) may occur.

Focus Point

Overconsumption of a Vitamin or Mineral

Nutrition experts suggest that individuals who suspect they have been taking too much of a vitamin (or mineral) should not stop taking it completely but rather should cut back to about half the current dosage. This is because the body has adjusted itself to the overly large dose, and stopping it altogether could trigger a deficiency. Individuals should consult their doctors or a registered dietician in these cases, especially if they have diabetes or high blood pressure.

CHOLECALCIFEROL (VITAMIN D)

Vitamin D is not actually a true vitamin because it is made in our own bodies with the help of the sun's ultraviolet rays. Today, we know that the compound made in our skin by sunlight is actually a prohormone (an intraglandular chemical substance that can be processed to become a hormone). This compound, when distributed in the skin, has been given the name cholecalciferol—often shortened to **calciferol** (vitamin D$_3$), which controls calcium metabolism in bone building. The initial compound produced in the skin by sunlight is a cholesterol base. Calciferol is activated by cholesterol in the liver and then in the kidney, becoming the active vitamin D hormone called **calcitriol**.

Calcitriol acts physiologically with two other hormones: the parathyroid hormone (PTH), which is critical to calcium and phosphorus balance, and **calcitonin**, a thyroid hormone that lowers blood levels of calcium and phosphate and promotes bone formation. In balance with these two hormones, vitamin D stimulates absorption of calcium and phosphorus in the small intestine. A deficiency of calcitriol causes **rickets**, a condition characterized by malformation of skeletal tissue in growing children. Children with rickets have soft long bones that bend under their own weight.

Only yeast and fish liver oils are natural sources of vitamin D. Therefore, the only regular food sources of vitamin D are those that have been fortified with the vitamin.

Excess intake of vitamin D, especially in infants, can be toxic. Symptoms of toxicity, or hypervitaminosis D, include calcification of soft tissue, such as in the kidneys, lungs, and fragile bones. A deficiency of vitamin D leads to rickets, osteomalacia, and osteoporosis. Hypoparathyroidism may also occur because calcium cannot be absorbed for use by the body without vitamin D. (For a discussion of osteoporosis, see Chapter 22; for hypoparathyroidism, see Chapter 23.)

TOCOPHEROL (VITAMIN E)

Early vitamin studies identified a substance necessary for animal reproduction that was chemically an alcohol. This substance was named *tocopherol*. The most vital function of tocopherol is its action as an antioxidant. An **antioxidant** is an agent that prevents cellular structure from being broken down by oxygen. Vitamin E can protect fragile red blood cell walls (mainly in premature infants) from breaking down—a condition that is termed *hemolytic anemia*.

A deficiency of vitamin E in young infants, especially premature infants who miss the final 1 to 2 months of gestation when tocopherol stores are normally built up, are particularly vulnerable to hemolytic anemia. In older children and adults, a deficiency of tocopherol disrupts the normal synthesis of myelin (the protective fat covering of nerve cells that helps them pass messages along specific tissue, such as spinal cord fibers), and affects physical activity, such as walking and vision.

The richest sources of tocopherol are vegetable oils (wheat germ, soybean, and safflower oil), nuts, fortified cereals, and avocado.

Tocopherol from food sources has no known toxic effect in humans. Supplemental intake of tocopherol that exceeds the normal dose may interfere with vitamin K activity and blood clotting.

VITAMIN K

Vitamin K is composed of a group of substances with similar biologic activity in blood clotting. The major form found in plants and initially isolated from alfalfa is phylloquinone, or vitamin K_1, because of its chemical structure. Whereas phylloquinone is our dietary form of vitamin K, menaquinone, or vitamin K_2, is synthesized by intestinal bacteria.

Vitamin K is known to have two metabolic functions in the body: blood clotting and bone development. Vitamin K is essential for maintaining normal levels of some blood-clotting factors, particularly the factor prothrombin. Phylloquinone can serve as an antidote for the excess effects of anticoagulant drugs, such as warfarin (Coumadin). Phylloquinone is often used in the control and prevention of certain types of hemorrhages.

Because intestinal bacteria synthesize menaquinone, a constant supply is normally available to back up dietary sources. Therefore, deficiency of vitamin K is not usually found in humans. Only some clinical conditions related to blood clotting, malabsorption, or lack of intestinal bacteria to synthesize the vitamin lead to deficiency. Green leafy vegetables are clearly the best dietary sources of vitamin K. Small amounts of phylloquinone are found in milk and dairy products, meats, fortified cereals, fruits, and vegetables.

Toxicity from vitamin K—even when large amounts are taken over extended periods—has not been observed.

Focus on Pediatrics

Vitamin K

Because the intestinal tract of a newborn is sterile, phylloquinone is routinely given to prevent hemorrhage when the umbilical cord is cut. The "vitamin K shot" given at birth has the trade names of AquaMephyton, Mephyton, and Phytonadione.

Focus on Natural Products

Mineral and Vitamin Interactions

Caution patients to adhere to the following guidelines when taking vitamins and mineral supplements:

- Insufficient vitamin D intake hinders the uptake of calcium.
- High amounts of supplemental vitamin C reduce copper levels in the body.
- Vitamin C can increase iron absorption as much as 30%.
- Excessive amounts of vitamin E interfere with iron absorption.
- Vitamin B_6 is required to metabolize magnesium and zinc.

✳ Apply Your Knowledge 9.2

The following questions focus on what you have just learned about vitamins and their role in health.

CRITICAL THINKING
1. What are the classifications of fat-soluble vitamins? List the characteristics of each classification.
2. How does scurvy occur?
3. What is the result of thiamine deficiency?
4. Name the generic forms of vitamins B_1, B_3, B_5, B_6, and B_{12}. Explain the functions of each.
5. Describe pellagra, spina bifida, and pernicious anemia as well as their causes.
6. What is rickets? List its signs and symptoms.
7. Discuss antioxidants and give two examples.

Focus Point

Proper Dosage of Vitamins

A nurse or medical assistant should advise patients about vitamins to prevent deficiency or toxicity. Patients should be told that vitamins are noncaloric essential nutrients found in a wide variety of foods that are needed in very small amounts for specific metabolic control and disease prevention. They should be warned that certain health problems are related to inadequate or excessive vitamin intake.

MINERALS

The body requires stores of minerals in varying amounts. For example, the body stores relatively large quantities of calcium, mostly in bone tissues: Adults who weigh 150 pounds have about 3 pounds of calcium in their bodies. On the other hand, about 3 g of iron is stored in adults of similar weight. In both cases, the amount of each mineral is essential for its specific task. Minerals are inorganic and do not contain carbon.

Major Minerals

Elements called **major minerals**, such as calcium, occur in large amounts in the body. The daily requirements of the major minerals—including calcium, phosphorus, sodium, potassium, magnesium, and chlorine—are more than 100 mg/day.

CALCIUM

Calcium and phosphorus deficiencies are usually caused by metabolic rather than nutritional deficits. Calcium acts in bone formation, impulse conduction, myocardial and skeletal muscle contractions, and blood clotting. The major sources of calcium are milk, cheese, salmon, green leafy vegetables, and whole grains.

Calcium absorption is dependent on vitamin D, the amount of phosphorus in the blood, and PTH. Such bone deformities as rickets, osteomalacia, and osteoporosis occur with calcium deficiency. Excess amounts of calcium in the blood, or hypercalcemia, may cause constipation, hypotension, nausea, vomiting, kidney stones, and cardiac arrhythmias.

PHOSPHORUS

Phosphorus is also needed for bone formation as well as tooth formation and energy. Fat storage and metabolism of other nutrients depend on this mineral. The best sources of phosphorus are milk, cheese, legumes, beef, fish, and pork.

Phosphorus supplements may cause electrolyte imbalances, GI upsets, and bone or joint pain. Phosphorus deficiency can cause anemia, bone brittleness, confusion, and weakness. The toxic effects of excessive phosphorus may cause hypocalcemia and kidney stones.

SODIUM

Sodium is the major electrolyte in the extracellular fluid (ECF). It helps body fluid balance and acid–base balance. Sodium also regulates nerve transmission and cell membrane irritability. The primary source of sodium is table salt. Other sources include meat, milk, celery, and carrots.

Deficiency of sodium may cause headache, confusion, nausea, weakness, anxiety, muscle spasms, and hypotension. Sodium toxicity produces hypertension and edema.

POTASSIUM

Potassium is a major electrolyte of intracellular fluid. It is found in blood, nerve tissue, and muscle fibers. Potassium is necessary for normal cardiac and muscle function. The best sources for potassium are oranges, bananas, red meats, vegetables, yams, milk products, and coffee.

Potassium deficiency can cause loss of muscle tone, weakness, paralysis, cardiac arrhythmias, and digitalis toxicity. Excessive potassium may produce muscle weakness, diarrhea, severe dehydration, abdominal pain, hypotension, and cardiac arrest.

MAGNESIUM

Magnesium is required to form proteins. It stimulates muscle contraction and nerve transmission, activates enzymes, and aids in bone formation. Good sources of magnesium include green leafy vegetables, whole grains, and legumes.

An excess or deficit in magnesium may cause tetany, convulsions, or muscle spasms.

CHLORINE

Chlorine is a major electrolyte, along with sodium, in the ECF. It is a component of gastric hydrochloric acid. Its sources include table salt, meat, milk, and processed foods. A deficiency in chlorine is rare, and toxic levels do not occur.

Essential Trace Minerals

Essential trace minerals, also called *microminerals*, are defined as those having a required intake of less than 100 mg/day. They are not less important than major minerals; rather, they are needed in smaller amounts. These minerals include iron, iodine, fluoride, zinc, chromium, selenium, manganese, molybdenum, and copper. Fluoride forms a compound with calcium (CaF_2) that stabilizes the binding substances in bones and teeth and prevents tooth decay. Except for deficiencies of iron and zinc, other deficiencies of microminerals are uncommon in clinical practice in industrialized countries. Therefore, in the following section, only iron, zinc, fluoride, and copper are discussed.

IRON

Although essential for life, iron is toxic in excess. Thus, the body has developed systems for balancing iron intake and excretion and for efficiently transporting iron into and out of cells to maintain health. Iron functions in the synthesis of hemoglobin and in the body's general metabolism. The human body contains about 45 mg of iron per kilogram of body weight.

Iron is widely distributed in the U.S. food supply, mainly in meat, eggs, vegetables, and cereals. The body absorbs iron more readily when it is ingested with vitamin C.

The major condition caused by iron-deficiency is anemia. Iron-deficiency anemia is the most prevalent nutritional problem in the world today. Women and children are affected more than others. Iron deficiency may result from several causes, including:

✳ Inadequate supply of dietary iron

✳ Excessive blood loss

✳ Inability to form hemoglobin because of the absence of other necessary factors such as vitamin B_{12} (for example, pernicious anemia)

✳ Lack of gastric hydrochloric acid necessary to help liberate iron for absorption

On the other hand, iron toxicity can occur from a single large dose (20 to 60 mg/kg) and can be fatal.

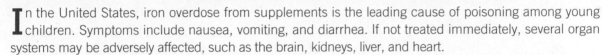

Focus on Pediatrics

Iron Toxicity

In the United States, iron overdose from supplements is the leading cause of poisoning among young children. Symptoms include nausea, vomiting, and diarrhea. If not treated immediately, several organ systems may be adversely affected, such as the brain, kidneys, liver, and heart.

IODINE

In humans, the basic function of iodine is to participate in the thyroid gland's synthesis of the hormone thyroxine, which in turn controls the body's basal metabolic rate. After thyroxine is used to stimulate metabolic processes in cells, it is broken down in the liver, and the iodine portion is excreted in bile as inorganic iodine. The average adult body contains only 20 to 50 mg of iodine.

Seafood provides a good amount of iodine, although the major reliable source is iodized table salt.

A lack of iodine in the diet contributes to several deficiency diseases, such as **goiter** (a swelling of the thyroid gland), **congenital hypothyroidism** (a condition of extreme hypothyroidism characterized by physical deformity, dwarfism, and mental retardation), and myxedema (a life-threatening complication of hypothyroidism, marked by coma, hypothermia, and respiratory depression). Goiter is a classic condition that often occurs in areas where the water and soil contain little iodine.

Intake of iodine through supplementation may result in toxicity for some individuals. Excess iodine may result in acne-like skin lesions or may worsen the pre-existing acne of adolescents or young adults.

Focus on Pediatrics

Congenital Hypothyroidism

Congenital hypothyroidism is a serious condition that occurs in children born to mothers who had limited iodine intake during adolescence and pregnancy. During pregnancy, the mother's iodine need takes precedence over that of the developing child. Thus, the fetus experiences iodine deficiency and continues to do so after birth. These children are retarded in their physical and mental development.

ZINC

Zinc is an essential trace element with wide clinical significance. It is especially important during growth periods, such as pregnancy, lactation, infancy, childhood, and adolescence. Zinc is more abundant in the adult body than any of the other microminerals—about 1.5 g in women and 2.5 g in men. Zinc is present in minute quantities in all body organs, tissues, fluids, and secretions.

Zinc is very important during periods of rapid tissue growth, such as childhood and adolescence. Retarded physical growth (such as dwarfism) and retarded sexual maturation (especially in men) have been observed in some populations in whom dietary intake of zinc is low. Zinc deficiency commonly causes poor wound healing, hair loss, diarrhea, and skin irritation. Impaired taste and smell are improved with increased zinc intake if previous dietary intake has been inadequate.

The greatest source of dietary zinc in the United States is meat, which supplies about 70% of the zinc consumed. Seafood, particularly oysters, is another excellent source of zinc.

Zinc toxicity from food sources is uncommon. However, prolonged supplementation in excess of recommendations can cause such adverse effects as nausea, vomiting, and decreased immune function. Excess zinc inhibits the absorption of copper, resulting in copper deficiency.

FLUORIDE

Fluoride forms a strong bond with calcium, which means that fluoride accumulates in calcified body tissues, such as bones and teeth. Fluoride's main function in human nutrition is to prevent dental caries. Fluoride strengthens the ability of the tooth structure to withstand the erosive effect of bacterial acids. The continuous intake of fluoride throughout life maximizes the protective effect of fluoride on teeth and maintains an adequate level of fluoride in tooth enamel. Fish products and tea contain the highest concentration of fluoride in foods.

Because fluoride stimulates new bone formation, it has become an experimental drug in the treatment of patients with osteoporosis. Presently, no evidence supports fluoride's ability to prevent osteoporosis. There is also no recommendation to increase fluoride intake during pregnancy and lactation.

Focus on Pediatrics

Fluoride

Fluoridated toothpaste and other tooth products containing fluoride should not be swallowed; therefore, children younger than 6 years of age should not use these products because they are unable to avoid swallowing them.

COPPER

This trace element has frequently been called the "iron twin" because the two are metabolized in much the same way and share functions as components of cell enzymes. Both are also related to energy production and hemoglobin synthesis. Severe copper deficiency is rare. However, copper depletion that causes low blood levels has been observed during total parenteral nutrition (TPN) and in cases of anemia. An increase in copper intake is recommended for pregnant or lactating women to meet their increased needs.

The richest food sources of copper are organ meats, especially liver, followed by seafood, nuts, seeds, legumes, and grains.

Wilson's disease is a genetic disorder causing excess storage of copper in the body. Without treatment, Wilson's disease can result in liver and nerve damage.

✱ Apply Your Knowledge 9.3

The following questions focus on what you have just learned about essential trace minerals and their role in health.

CRITICAL THINKING

1. What is the result of iodine deficiency? Explain the disorders it may cause.
2. What are essential trace minerals? Name each of them.
3. Which major minerals exist in the highest quantities in the human body? What are their major functions?
4. Compare the function of zinc with that of fluoride in the human body.
5. What are the causes of iron deficiency?
6. Differentiate between sodium and potassium.
7. What is the cause of Wilson's disease? Explain which organs of the body this disease usually damages.

Nutritional Requirements

The objective of a proper diet is to achieve and maintain a desirable body composition and a high potential for physical and mental work. The daily dietary requirements for essential nutrients, including energy sources, depend on age, sex, height, weight, and metabolic and physical activity. The Food and Nutrition Board of the National Academy of Sciences/National Research Council and the U.S. Department of Agriculture periodically review the scientific literature on human requirements for the 45 essential nutrients. Every 5 years, the Food and Nutrition Board issues **recommended dietary allowances (RDAs)**, which are computed to meet the needs of all healthy individuals. For vitamins and minerals, about which less is known, safe and adequate daily dietary intakes have been estimated.

For good health, body composition must be kept within reasonable limits. This requires balancing energy intake with energy expenditure. If energy intake exceeds expenditure or expenditure decreases, body weight increases, resulting in obesity. Conversely, if energy intake is less than expenditure, body weight decreases.

Female patients need to know about the importance of nutrition during pregnancy. Pregnant women should be advised to gain about 25 to 35 pounds during pregnancy. The rate of weight gain should be 2 to 5 pounds in the first trimester and about 1 pound per week thereafter. Gaining too little weight contributes to the risk of having a small baby; gaining too much weight may cause an early delivery or a very large baby as well as health issues for the woman, such as gestational diabetes, high blood pressure, and varicose veins.

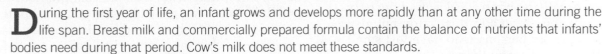

Focus on Pediatrics

Nutritional Requirements

During the first year of life, an infant grows and develops more rapidly than at any other time during the life span. Breast milk and commercially prepared formula contain the balance of nutrients that infants' bodies need during that period. Cow's milk does not meet these standards.

Nutritional Support

Oral supplementation with energy- and protein-rich foods is indicated for patients on modified consistency diets who require continued diet therapy, those with chronic disease and anorexia, and those with chronic inflammatory disease or terminal malignancy. *Modified consistency diets* are those that provide foods in a physically altered form (such as chopped, ground, or pureed). Some conditions that warrant the use of modified consistency diets include tooth problems and gum conditions. Other indications result from head or neck injuries or surgeries.

ENTERAL NUTRITION

Enteral tube nutrition may be used in patients with a functioning GI tract to supplement or completely replace oral feeding. Complete replacement of oral feeding is indicated for patients who require intensive protein

and caloric support and who are unable or unwilling to take oral supplementation. Enteral nutrition is safer and less expensive than TPN and is the preferred route when the integrity of the GI tract is preserved. General indications include severe protein-energy malnutrition, trauma to the head and neck or neurologic disorders preventing satisfactory oral feeding, coma or depressed mental state, hepatic failure, and serious illness (such as burns), in which metabolic requirements are high. Specific indications may include preparation of the bowel for surgery in seriously ill or malnourished patients.

PARENTERAL NUTRITION

Parenteral nutrition is administered intravenously and can be partial or total. Partial parenteral nutrition supplies only part of the patient's daily nutritional requirements to supplement oral intake. Many hospitalized patients receive dextrose or amino acid solutions by this method as part of their routine care.

Focus Point

Cachexia

Cachexia is a specific profound syndrome caused by malnutrition and a disturbance in glucose and fat metabolism. It is usually seen in patients with terminal cancer or AIDS and in patients who are in generally poor health. It is indicated by an emaciated appearance.

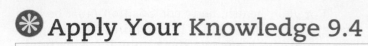

✳ Apply Your Knowledge 9.4

The following questions focus on what you have just learned about nutrition.

CRITICAL THINKING

1. What is cachexia?
2. Compare cow's milk with breast milk.
3. What is total parenteral nutrition?
4. Explain how total parenteral nutrition is administered.
5. What is the normal range of weight gain during pregnancy? Explain the risk of too little weight gain in this period.

TOTAL PARENTERAL NUTRITION

TPN supplies all the patient's daily nutritional requirements. A peripheral vein may be used for short periods, but when concentrated solutions are used for prolonged periods, thrombosis can occur. Therefore, central venous access is usually required. TPN is used not only in the hospital for long-term administration but also at home, enabling many persons who have lost small intestine function to lead useful lives.

Nutrient–Drug Interactions

The concept of drug interaction is often extended to include situations in which food or certain dietary items influence the activity of a drug. For example, drug interactions with foods, herbs, or other natural substances may alter the activity of a drug.

Foods can influence the absorption of a number of drugs. In some situations, absorption may be delayed but not reduced. In other circumstances, the total amount of drug absorption may be the result of slowed gastric emptying. However, food may also affect absorption by binding with a drug, decreasing the access of drugs to sites of absorption, altering the dissolution rate of drugs, or altering the pH of the GI contents.

The presence of food in the GI tract reduces the absorption of many anti-infective agents. However, there are some exceptions, such as penicillin V (Pen-Vee-K), amoxicillin (Amoxil), doxycycline (Doryx, Vibramycin), and minocycline (Dynacin, Minocin). With these drugs, it is generally recommended that they be given at least 1 hour before or 2 hours after meals to achieve optimum absorption.

There have been reports of serious reactions (hypertensive crises) occurring in people being treated with monoamine oxidase inhibitors (MAOIs), such as phenelzine (Nardil) and isocarboxazid (Marplan), after ingesting certain foods containing a high amount of tyramine.

Tyramine is metabolized by MAOIs; normally, enzymes in the intestinal wall and liver protect against the pressor actions of amines in foods. However, when these enzymes are inhibited, large quantities of unmetabolized tyramine can accumulate and act to release norepinephrine from adrenergic neurons. Among the foods having the highest tyramine content are aged cheeses (such as cheddar; in contrast, cottage and cream cheeses contain little or no tyramine and need not be restricted). Other foods with very high amounts of tyramine include certain alcoholic beverages (such as Chianti wine), pickled fish (such as herring), concentrated yeast extracts, and broad bean pods.

The consumption of grapefruit juice has been reported to increase the serum concentration and activity of a number of medications, such as certain calcium channel blockers (such as amlodipine [Norvasc], nisoldipine [Nisocor], and cyclosporine [Neoral]. The bioavailability of most of these agents is generally low, primarily as a result of extensive first-pass metabolism. It has been suggested that components of grapefruit juice reduce the activity of the cytochrome P-450 enzymes (a group of enzymes involved in the metabolism of many drugs).

Certain drugs, such as laxatives, colchicine, cholestyramine (Questran), and colestipol (Colestid), have been reported to cause malabsorption problems that result in decreased absorption of vitamins and nutrients from the GI tract. It should be recognized that these agents also can alter the absorption of other drugs that are administered simultaneously.

Many drugs affect appetite, which in turn can lead to deficiencies of certain nutrients. Drugs may also affect absorption and tissue metabolism (Table 9-2 ■).

Certain drugs affect mineral metabolism. Diuretics, especially thiazide diuretics, and corticosteroids, such as prednisone, hydrocortisone, methylprednisolone, and others, can cause potassium depletion, which increases the risk of digitalis-induced cardiac arrhythmias. Potassium depletion may also

Table 9-2 ■ Drugs That Affect Appetite, Absorption, and Tissue Metabolism

DRUGS OR DRUG CLASSIFICATIONS	DRUG EFFECTS
Alcohol, antihistamines, insulin, some psychoactive drugs, steroids, sulfonylureas, thyroid hormone	Increased appetite
Bulk agents (guar gum, methylcellulose), cyclophosphamide, digitalis, glucagon, indomethacin, morphine	Decreased appetite
Chlortetracycline, indomethacin, kanamycin, methotrexate, neomycin, p-aminosalicylic acid, phenindione	Malabsorption
Warfarin, narcotic analgesics, phenothiazines, phenytoin, probenecid, thiazide diuretics	Hyperglycemia
Aspirin, barbiturates, beta-blockers, monoamine oxidase inhibitors, phenacetin, phenylbutazone, sulfonamides	Hypoglycemia
Aspirin and p-aminosalicylic acid, chlortetracycline, colchicine, dextrans, fenfluramine, glucagon, L-asparaginase, phenindione, sulfinpyrazone, trifluperidol	Reduced plasma lipids
Adrenal corticosteroids, chlorpromazine, ethanol, growth hormone, oral contraceptives (estrogen–progesterone type), thiouracil, vitamin D	Increased plasma lipids
Chloramphenicol, tetracycline	Decreased protein metabolism

result from the regular use of purgatives (agents that promote bowel movements). Corticosteroids and aldosterone cause marked sodium and water retention. Sodium and water retention also occur with estrogen–progestin oral contraceptives (Ortho-Novum, Norinyl) and phenylbutazone (Alka Butazolidin, Azolid). Sulfonylureas (used to treat type 2 diabetes), phenylbutazone, and lithium (Eskalith) can impair the uptake or release of iodine by the thyroid gland; oral contraceptives can lower plasma zinc levels and elevate copper levels. Prolonged use of corticosteroids, which reduces the work of the construction cells in the bones, causing bone loss, can lead to osteoporosis (see Chapters 22 and 26 for more information about osteoporosis).

Vitamin metabolism is also affected by some drugs. Ethanol alcohol impairs thiamine absorption, and isoniazid is a pyridoxine (vitamin B$_6$) antagonist. Ethanol and oral contraceptives inhibit folic acid absorption. Anticonvulsant-induced vitamin D deficiency is well recognized. Vitamin B$_6$ malabsorption has been reported with salicylic acid, potassium iodide (Lugol's solution, Thyro-Block), colchicine, ethanol, and oral contraceptive use.

Food Additives and Contaminants

The addition of chemicals to foods to facilitate their processing and preservation, to enhance their restorative or stimulating properties, and to control natural contaminants is stringently regulated. Only food **additives** that have passed exacting laboratory testing are permitted to be used at specific levels.

Reported health problems suspected to be caused by some food additives have been trivial and largely anecdotal. Adverse health effects of approved additives and contaminants in the long term have not been established.

The benefits of additives, including reducing waste and providing the public with a greater variety of attractive foods than would otherwise be possible, must be weighed against known risks. The issues involved are frequently complex. The use of nitrite in cured meats is an example. Nitrite inhibits the growth of *Clostridium botulinum* and imparts a desired flavor. However, evidence indicates that nitrite is converted in the body to nitrosamines, which are known carcinogens in animals. On the other hand, the amount of nitrite added to cured meat is small compared with the amount that may be ingested from naturally occurring good nitrates that are converted to nitrite by the salivary glands. In addition, dietary vitamin C can reduce nitrite formation in the GI tract.

Patients need to know about the role of nutrition in helping to prevent specific medical conditions. Health-care professionals should emphasize to patients that careful reading of food package is a good habit and that nutrient–drug interactions can create adverse effects. Therefore, patients should always tell their health-care providers what nutrient supplements they are taking on a regular basis and ask about nutrient–drug interactions when prescribed a new medication.

✳ Apply Your Knowledge 9.5

The following questions focus on what you have just learned about nutrient–drug interactions.

CRITICAL THINKING

1. What are the benefits of additives in food?
2. Name two drugs that affect mineral metabolism and can cause potassium depletion.
3. Name five foods that contain the highest amounts of tyramine.
4. What is the concept of drug interaction?
5. What are the adverse health effects of approved food additives in the long term?

Herbal Supplements

An *herbal supplement* may be defined as any mixture of ingredients based on plant sources and designed for the improvement of health or treatment of certain conditions. However, herbal supplements are not considered by the FDA to be drugs but rather food products. They are often used by individuals to supplement traditional medical therapies. This practice has led to undesired medical outcomes, interactions with drugs, and toxicity. Patients must understand that the taking of herbal supplements should not occur without consulting their physician. There should be an open dialogue about which supplements are being taken and in what quantities, especially when prescription drugs are also being used. Because the FDA does not regulate these supplements, there is no independent verification of their quality or effectiveness or the quantity of ingredients they contain.

Herbal supplements are available in many different forms, including capsules, liquids, and powders. Many people believe that herbal supplements—because they are "natural"—contain stronger healing properties than "synthetic" drugs. The lack of real testing of these supplements means that proof of actual effectiveness is not well documented. The term *herb* is defined as a *botanical* product without stems or bark. Botanicals have been used for thousands of years to treat many different conditions. Their popularity has continually increased and decreased over time. *Complementary and alternative medicine (CAM)* involves different healing systems and therapies, including herbal therapies, nutritional supplements, and special diets.

There are many differences between herbal supplements and prescription or over-the-counter drugs. Perhaps most important is that most modern drugs contain only one active ingredient that is standardized and measured with accuracy. However, many herbal supplements contain a variety of active ingredients in widely varying quantities and strengths. It is quite possible that they contain large amounts of active chemicals that may not work well together for a controlled effect.

There have been recent attempts to standardize certain herbal extracts, including ginkgo leaf, ginseng root, and kava kava rhizome.

The Dietary Supplement Health and Education Act (DSHEA) of 1994 attempted to regulate herbal supplements as part of its overall description of *dietary supplements*. These supplements are defined as products that are intended to enhance or supplement the diet. They include botanicals, vitamins, minerals, and other extracts or metabolites not already approved as drugs by the FDA. As a result of this act, the FDA can now remove any supplement that it determines poses a significant or unreasonable risk to the public. Manufacturers of these products must label them clearly as "dietary supplements." However, the act is lacking in its regulatory capacity.

There is still no real standardization in the dietary supplement industry. Manufacturers do not have to demonstrate the effectiveness of these products before they can be sold. They also do not have to prove the safety of these supplements. The labeling of these products is required to state that the product is not intended to diagnose, treat, cure, or prevent any disease, but the labels can still make other claims. For example, it is legal for manufacturers to state that their supplements promote healthy immune systems, reduce anxiety and stress, and help to maintain cardiovascular function and that they may reduce pain and inflammation. The labels may say that the product contains certain substances, but this claim may or may not be correct, and the included amounts of ingredients may or may not be factual.

The Dietary Supplement and Nonprescription Drug Consumer Protection Act took effect in 2007. It required that manufacturers must include contact information on product labels for consumers so they can report adverse effects of the products. If a manufacturer is alerted to such an event, it must inform the FDA of the occurrence within 15 days after receiving a consumer complaint. Manufacturers must keep records of these events for at least 6 years—subject to FDA inspection. The FDA now also requires manufacturers to evaluate the identity, potency, purity, and composition of their products, with labels accurately reflecting this information.

Patient medical histories should always include complete listings of herbal supplements so their effects and interactions can be tracked over time. Also, these products have a potential for causing allergic reactions because of ingredients that may be either not listed on the labels or not noticed by the consumer. Patients taking such medications as insulin, warfarin, or digoxin should be educated about never taking supplements without first discussing them with their physicians because these drugs have a great potential for interactions.

Specialty supplements are nonherbal supplements that may be obtained from a variety of different animal or plant sources. They are usually more specific in their actions than herbal products and are intended to be used only for very specific conditions. Such substances as chondroitin and glucosamine are natural body substances necessary for healthy cartilage and may be taken in supplement form. Amino acids, flaxseed, and fish oils with omega fatty acids are other examples of specialty supplements.

Table 9-3 ■ lists the top 20 herbal supplements, their uses, and potential interactions.

Table 9-3 ■ Top-Selling Herbal Supplements

HERB	USES	POTENTIAL INTERACTIONS
Cranberry	For urinary tract infections	No known interactions
Soy	As protein, vitamin, and mineral supplementation; for menopausal symptoms; to prevent cardiovascular disease; and as an anticancer agent	Thyroid agents (dextrothyroxine, levothyroxine, liothyronine, liotrix, thyroglobulin)
Garlic	To reduce blood cholesterol and blood pressure; as an anticoagulant	Aspirin and other NSAIDs, warfarin, insulin, oral hypoglycemic agents
Saw palmetto	To treat benign prostatic hypertrophy	Anticoagulants, antiplatelet agents, hormones (such as estrogens), oral contraceptives, and androgens, immunostimulants, and NSAIDs
Ginkgo	To improve memory and reduce dizziness	Anticonvulsants, aspirin and NSAIDs, heparin, warfarin, TCAs
Echinacea	To enhance the immune system; as an anti-inflammatory agent	Amiodarone, anabolic steroids, ketoconazole, methotrexate
Milk thistle	As an antitoxin; to protect against liver disease	Drugs that are metabolized by the P-450 enzyme (such as beta-blockers and certain analgesics)
St. John's wort	To reduce depression and anxiety; as an anti-inflammatory agent	CNS depressants, opioid analgesics, cyclosporine, efavirenz, indinavir, protease inhibitors, SSRIs, TCAs, warfarin
Ginseng	To relieve stress, decrease fatigue, and enhance the immune system	CNS depressants, digoxin, diuretics, insulin, oral hypoglycemic agents, warfarin
Black cohosh	To relieve menopausal symptoms	Antihypertensives, hormone replacement therapies, oral contraceptives, and sedative–hypnotics
Green tea	As an antioxidant; to lower LDL cholesterol; to prevent cancer; to relieve various GI problems	Antacids, bronchodilators, MAOIs, xanthines, dairy products, ephedra
Evening primrose (oil)	As a source of essential fatty acids; to relieve premenstrual or menopausal symptoms; to relieve rheumatoid arthritis and other inflammatory conditions	Phenothiazines, such as chlorpromazine

(continued)

Table 9-3 ■ Top-Selling Herbal Supplements (*continued*)

HERB	USES	POTENTIAL INTERACTIONS
Valerian	To relieve stress and promote sleep	Barbiturates, benzodiazepines, and other CNS depressants
Horny goat weed	To enhance sexual function	High blood pressure medications, anticoagulants, antiplatelet agents, NSAIDs, thrombolytics, ticlopidine, tirofiban, warfarin
Grape seed extract	As a source of essential fatty acids; as an antioxidant; to restore microcirculation to body tissues	No known interactions but should never be used during pregnancy and lactation; should also not be given to children
Bilberry	To treat diarrhea, menstrual cramps, vision problems, varicose veins, and circulatory problems	Anticoagulants, antiplatelet agents, aspirin, insulin, iron, NSAIDs, oral antidiabetic agents
Red clover	To treat menopausal symptoms and cancer	Anticoagulants and antiplatelet agents
Yohimbe	To increase male sexual potency; as an aphrodisiac; for weight loss	ACE inhibitors, antihypertensives, beta-blockers, calcium channel blockers, alpha-adrenergic blockers, CNS stimulants, MAOIs, phenothiazines, SSRIs, sympathomimetics, TCAs, caffeine-containing products, and high-tyramine foods (such as wine, beer, aged cheese, liver)
Horse chestnut seed extract	To treat circulatory problems, varicose veins, edema, itching, cramping, and hemorrhoids	Anticoagulants, antidiabetic agents, aspirin and other salicylates, iron salts
Ginger	To treat GI problems, for menstrual cramps, and as an anti-inflammatory agent	Aspirin and other NSAIDs, heparin, warfarin

ACE = angiotensin-converting enzyme; CNS = central nervous system; GI = gastrointestinal; LDL = low-density lipoprotein; MAOI = monoamine oxidase inhibitor; NSAID = nonsteroidal anti-inflammatory drug; SSRI = selective serotonin reuptake inhibitor; TCA = tricyclic antidepressant.

✳ Apply Your Knowledge 9.6

The following questions focus on what you have just learned about herbal supplements.

CRITICAL THINKING

1. What are herbal supplements?
2. Which laws regulate herbal supplements?
3. Name three examples of specialty supplements.
4. Why was the Dietary Supplement and Nonprescription Drug Consumer Protection Act passed?
5. Name the seven top-selling herbal supplements in the United States.
6. Why has the use of herbal and dietary supplements increased in the United States?

Alternative Therapies

CAM therapies are those that are "outside" of mainstream health care. They focus on treating each person individually, considering the health of the whole person. CAM emphasizes the integration of mind and body, promoting disease prevention, self-care, and self-healing. It also recognizes spirituality as part of health and healing.

Research continues to determine if CAM therapies are totally, partially, or not at all effective. Most likely, some CAM therapies have merit, but others do not. CAM therapies include homeopathy, chiropractic, acupuncture, massage, yoga, meditation, hypnotherapy, biofeedback, prayer, and detoxification therapies, among many others. The value of CAM therapies realistically lies in their ability to reduce the need for medications. When drug doses are reduced, this leads to fewer potential adverse effects.

Health-care professionals should be sensitive to patients' beliefs about CAM therapies. Advantages and limitations of these therapies should be explained to patients so they can make accurate choices about their health-care treatments. Often, alternative therapies can work together with pharmacotherapy to achieve the proper treatment and healing of patients.

PRACTICAL SCENARIO 1

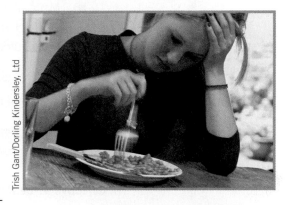

Trish Gant/Dorling Kindersley, Ltd

Kate, an abnormally thin 15-year-old girl, is taken to the emergency room by her mother, who reports that the girl is dizzy and shaky, complaining of a pounding heartbeat, and has been having crying spells for the past 2 weeks. Medical records indicate that Kate was diagnosed at age 12 years with bulimia nervosa, an eating disorder associated with emotional distress that is characterized by frequent episodes of binge eating (eating an amount of food within 1 hour that is significantly larger than normal for most people) and purging (self-induced vomiting and abuse of diuretics or laxatives). For the past 6 months, Kate has been eating small quantities of only a few foods and exercising excessively because she believes she is still too fat. Her mother fears that Kate's illness has evolved into anorexia nervosa, a common progression. The medical examination finds that Kate has lost 30% of her body weight in 1 year, her electrolytes are seriously imbalanced, and she is hypoglycemic and has protein energy malnutrition. She is admitted to the hospital for immediate treatment.

Critical Thinking Questions

1. Assuming Kate's gastrointestinal tract is functional, what would be the most efficient method of reversing her physiologic and nutritional starvation?
2. Which of Kate's nutritional deficits is the probable cause of her cardiac arrhythmia?

PRACTICAL SCENARIO 2

A 3-year-old child was brought to his pediatrician's office. While the medical assistant was taking the history of the patient from his mother, she noticed that the child's legs appeared to be "bowing." His mother asked the medical assistant about the cause of this condition in her child.

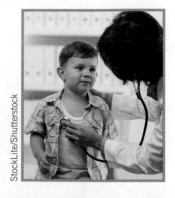

StockLite/Shutterstock

Critical Thinking Questions

1. What is the most common cause of deformity of the leg bones in children?
2. What is the most appropriate treatment for a patient with this condition?

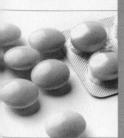

Chapter Capsule

This section repeats the objectives from the beginning of the chapter and then provides a summary of the most important concepts for that objective. Use this section as a quick review and to check your knowledge.

Objective 1: Identify the seven basic food components and explain their major functions.

- Proteins, lipids (fats), carbohydrates, fiber, vitamins, minerals, and water
- Provide energy, promote growth and repair of the body, and ensure the basic processes for life by keeping the body healthy

Objective 2: Differentiate the classifications of nutrients.

- Generally classified as macronutrients and micronutrients
- Macronutrients (needed by the body in relatively large amounts): carbohydrates, fats, proteins, macrominerals, and water
- Micronutrients (required by the body in small amounts): vitamins and essential trace minerals

Objective 3: Explain the role of calories in the diet.

- Supply the body with energy
- About two-thirds of total calories come from carbohydrates

Objective 4: Define the role of essential fatty acids in optimal health.

- Linoleic and linolenic acid (provided by vegetable oils): required for the formation of prostaglandins (hormone-like substances) and thromboxanes (biochemically related to the prostaglandins)

Objective 5: List the water-soluble vitamins.

- B and C vitamins

Objective 6: Discuss the toxicity of vitamin A.

- Called *hypervitaminosis A*
- Marked by loss of hair, jaundice, joint pain, and thickening of the long bones
- May also cause liver injury and fluid accumulation in the abdominal cavity (ascites)

Objective 7: Indicate the significance of vitamin E deficiency in infants.

- Causes infants to be particularly vulnerable to hemolytic anemia

Objective 8: List the five essential trace minerals and the symptoms of their toxicity.

- Iron: nausea, vomiting, and diarrhea
- Iodine: acne-like skin lesions, worsening of pre-existing acne
- Zinc: nausea, vomiting, and decreased immune function
- Fluoride: discolored teeth, brittle tooth enamel and bones, brain damage, heartburn, and pain in the extremities
- Copper: liver and nerve damage

Objective 9: Explain general indications for total parenteral nutrition.

- Inability to use the oral route
- Coma or depressed mental state
- Severe burns or serious illness, with high metabolic requirements
- Severe protein-energy malnutrition

Objective 10: Describe the benefits of food additives.

- Reduce waste.
- Provide greater variety of attractive foods.
- Inhibit bacterial growth.
- Impart desired flavor.
- Enhance restorative or stimulating properties.
- Control natural contaminants.

Internet Sites of Interest

- Medline Plus, a service of the U.S. National Library of Medicine and the National Institutes of Health (NIH), provides information about the latest vitamin- and mineral-related studies at **http://www.nlm.nih.gov/medlineplus/vitamins.html**.

- For general information and resources regarding dietary supplements, search the Food and Nutrition Information Center at the website of the U.S. Department of Agriculture at **http://www.nal.usda.gov/**.

- The American Dietetic Association provides a wealth of nutrition fact sheets at **http://www.eatright.org/**.

- Nutritional tips for pregnant women are available at the website of the Weight-Control Information Network, a service of the National Institute of Diabetes and Digestive and Kidney Diseases, at **http://win.niddk.nih.gov/publications/two.htm**.

- The National Heart, Lung, and Blood Institute (NHLBI) provides a tip sheet for reading food labels at **http://www.nhlbi.nih.gov**. Search for "food labels."

- Guidelines for good nutrition for older adults is available at the website of the National Institute on Aging at **http://www.niapublications.org**. Search for "nutrition."

- The Office of Dietary supplements of the National Institutes of Health offers information on dietary supplement decision making, claims and labeling, research, consumer safety, and nutritional recommendations at **http://ods.od.nih.gov/Health_Information**.

Chapter 10

Toxicology

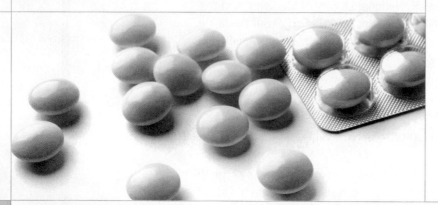

Chapter Objectives

After completing this chapter, you should be able to:

1. Explain the importance of poisons and antidotes.
2. Describe the detection of poisons.
3. List the most common poisonings seen today in the United States.
4. Explain important factors that are related to risks of poisoning.
5. Describe poison prevention programs.
6. Explain how the most common poisonings occur.
7. Compare lead poisoning and mercury poisoning.
8. Name the antidotes for cyanide, methanol, opiates, and organophosphates.
9. Describe arsenic, atropine, and cyanide poisonings.
10. Differentiate between digitalis toxicity and lithium toxicity.

Key Terms

acetaminophen (page 157)
acids (page 158)
alkalies (page 158)
antihistamines (page 158)
arsenic (page 159)
atropine (page 159)
benzene (page 159)
carbon monoxide (CO) (page 159)
cyanide (page 160)

detergents (page 160)
ethylene glycol (page 157)
fluorides (page 160)
formaldehyde (page 157)
iodine (page 161)
isopropyl alcohol (page 161)
lead (page 156)
magnesium sulfate (page 161)
mercury (page 157)

methyl alcohol (page 157)
opioids (page 161)
petroleum distillates (page 162)
phenol (page 162)
phosphorus (page 162)
salicylism (page 158)
soaps (page 160)
toluene (page 159)

Introduction

Identifying cases of poisoning and correctly assessing the potential toxicity of the poison in each case are essential in preserving life. Poisons should always be considered in young children, especially when their symptoms are not specific for any disease. Children commonly eat or drink substances found in the home that may be dangerous. Other high-risk individuals include elderly adults, hospitalized patients, workers on the job, and people exposed to environmental pollutants. A thorough drug history should be obtained if the patient is conscious. Blood and urine samples should be collected as quickly as possible because the type and speed of onset of symptoms will substantiate whether the patient's condition is due to poisons. Poison control centers keep a wealth of information that may be accessed when poisoning is suspected.

Poisoning

A poison is defined as any agent that (in relatively small amounts) can cause death or serious bodily harm. All drugs are potential poisons when used improperly or in dosages that are greater than normal. Accidental poisoning by chemicals causes more than 5,000 deaths each year in the United States. In comparison, suicides by using chemicals number more than 6,000 annually. However, a much greater number of persons are made seriously ill by chemical agents than are actually killed by them. Unfortunately, some of these people are left with permanent adverse effects.

Accidental poisonings occur far more often at home than through industrial exposure, and the effects are usually acute. Industrial intoxication is more often the result of chronic exposure. Accidental poisoning usually results from the ingestion of toxic substances, with the majority of occurrences involving children. In most instances, accidental poisonings should be preventable. This is especially true in accidental poisonings of young children via drugs and chemicals found in the home. Pharmacists can play a key role in preventing accidental poisonings, especially those caused by drugs.

Focus On Accidental Poisonings

Childhood Poisonings

Accidental poisonings in the home occur most commonly in children younger than the age of 5 years. Widespread use of child-resistant containers with safety caps has reduced poisoning deaths in this age group.

DETECTION OF POISONS

Optimal treatment of poisoned patients requires correct diagnosis. Although some chemical substances have very characteristic toxic effects, most adverse effects from poisonings can simulate other diseases. Poisoning is often included in the diagnoses of coma, convulsions, acute psychosis, acute hepatic or renal insufficiency, and bone marrow depression. Poisoning is usually not considered when the major manifestation is a mild psychiatric disturbance or neurologic disorder, abdominal pain, bleeding, fever, hypotension, pulmonary congestion, or skin eruption. Furthermore, patients may be unaware that they have been exposed to a poison, as seen in cases of chronic intoxications or after attempted suicide or abortion. If they are aware, they may be unwilling to admit it.

In every poisoning case, identification of the toxic agent should be attempted. Specific antidotal therapy is obviously impossible without the poison being correctly identified. Some poisons can produce clinical features that are characteristic enough to strongly suggest the diagnosis. Careful examination may reveal the unmistakable odor of cyanide; a cherry-colored flushing of carboxyhemoglobin in skin and mucous membranes; or the pupillary constriction, salivation, and gastrointestinal (GI) hyperactivity produced by insecticides. Chemical analysis of body fluids provides the most accurate identification of the intoxicating agent. Some common poisons, such as aspirin and barbiturates, can be identified and their amounts ascertained by relatively simple laboratory procedures. Others require more complex toxicologic tests. Chemical analyses of body fluids or tissues are of high importance in the diagnosis and evaluation of chronic intoxications.

INFLUENTIAL FACTORS

Factors that are important in the consideration of poisoning risk and prevention include:

* **Age:** Most poisonings occur in children and are accidental. When poisonings occur in teenagers and adults, they may be suicide related or often caused by overdosage or taking various substances concurrently that are contraindicated for such use. Patients should be educated about carefully reading prescription labels and following the prescriber's guidelines exactly as written.

✳ **Location:** Most children experience poisonings in the home, including areas such as the garage, where many dangerous substances may be stored. Also, products actually kept inside cars and other vehicles are usually capable of causing poisonings.

✳ **Access:** Locked medicine cabinets, cupboards, and other areas where poisonous substances are kept offer good protection against children gaining access. At the very least, medications and chemicals should not be stored within reach of children. In the majority of accidental childhood poisonings, poisonous materials are left in easy reach of children (Figure 10-1 ■).

✳ **Containers:** By storing chemicals and medications in their original containers, labeling is usually effective in helping to reduce the risk of poisoning. Dangerous substances should never be stored in containers, such as used soft drink bottles. A child might understandably assume that what is inside is still soda. Drinking glasses, dishes, and bowls should never be used to measure or transfer dangerous substances into other containers.

✳ **Supervision:** The best way to ensure that children do not accidentally poison themselves is to keep them in sight. Allowing children to play in areas where substances are stored without adult supervision accounts for the majority of at-home poisonings. When substances are being discarded, they should never be left out in sight, especially near areas where children play.

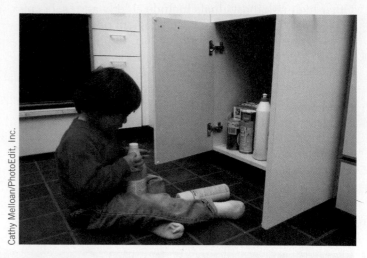

Figure 10-1 ■ In the majority of accidental childhood poisonings, poisonous materials are left in easy reach of children.

Cathy Melloan/PhotoEdit, Inc.

✴ Apply Your Knowledge 10.1

The following questions focus on what you have just learned about accidental poisonings.

CRITICAL THINKING

1. Why do accidental poisonings occur more often at home?
2. How can pharmacists play a key role in preventing accidental poisonings?
3. What are the most important signs and symptoms of cyanide poisoning?
4. List influential factors of poisoning risks.
5. How can poisons be detected?
6. How many people are poisoned annually in the United States?
7. Why can child-resistant packaging reduce accidental poisoning?
8. Why should identification of toxic agents always be attempted?

Common Poisons

The most common poisonings seen today involve non-prescription drugs, household products, solvents, pesticides, and poisonous plants. The following sections discuss specific poisons and their actions as well as clinical poisonings.

LEAD

Lead poisoning can occur where there is old paint or lead pipes. Vegetable gardens can also be sources of lead. In adults, lead poisoning is rare. However, it is one of the most common yet preventable childhood health problems today. Children may ingest flakes of old paint containing lead, mistaking it for "candy" because of attractive colors. Lead can also contaminate water flowing through older lead pipes, slowly poisoning those who drink it. Lead poisoning causes severe damage to the brain, nerves, red blood cells, and digestive system.

Symptoms of acute poisoning include a metallic taste in the mouth, abdominal pain, vomiting, diarrhea, collapse, and coma. Large amounts directly affect the nervous system and cause headache, convulsions, coma, and death. Treatment usually includes the administration of *chelating agents* to help the body rid itself of lead by binding to lead so it can be excreted. For mild poisoning, the chelating agent penicillamine may be used alone. For chronic poisoning, penicillamine may be used in combination with edetate calcium disodium and dimercaprol. For acute poisoning, gastric lavage is performed.

MERCURY

Acute **mercury** poisoning often occurs by the ingestion of inorganic mercuric salts or the inhalation of metallic mercury vapor. Ingestion of mercuric salts causes a metallic taste, salivation, thirst, burning in the throat, discoloration and edema of oral mucous membranes, abdominal pain, vomiting, bloody diarrhea, and shock. Direct nephrotoxicity causes acute renal failure. Acute chemical pneumonia may be caused by the inhalation of high concentrations of metallic mercury vapor. There is no effective specific treatment for mercury vapor pneumonitis. Ingested mercuric salts can be removed by lavage, with activated charcoal also administered.

For acute ingestion of mercuric salts, dimercaprol can be given unless the patient has severe gastroenteritis. In treating chronic poisoning, the person must be removed from exposure. Neurologic toxicity is not reversible by using chelation. With the advent of many alternate types of thermometers made for home use, the use of mercury thermometers should cease. Mercury in all its forms is toxic and can result in permanent brain and kidney damage. A broken thermometer easily releases the toxic substance. For reference purposes, it takes only 1 g of mercury to contaminate all the fish in a 20-acre lake.

There is approximately 0.7 g of mercury in the average home thermometer—an amount that is surely toxic to an individual exposed to it. Many major retailers have already stopped selling mercury thermometers as a result. The medical instrument industry recommends the use of digital thermometers. Old mercury thermometers should be disposed of by contacting local environmental health or public works departments. (Disposal sites for household hazardous wastes are often listed in the city or county government section of the white pages of a local telephone directory.)

ACETAMINOPHEN

Acetaminophen is a popular alternative to salicylates as an analgesic and antipyretic and a common cause of poisoning. Although toxic and lethal doses of acetaminophen may vary from patient to patient, hepatic damage will most likely occur if an adult has taken more than 8 g as a single dose. Clinical signs of acetaminophen poisoning are nonspecific. In the first few hours after ingestion, lethargy, nausea, vomiting, and diaphoresis may occur. Hepatic damage is the most important manifestation of acetaminophen toxicity and becomes evident 1 to 2 days after ingestion. Treatment should begin with the induction of emesis or gastric lavage, followed by the administration of activated charcoal. Treatment with acetylcysteine is most effective if started within 10 hours after ingestion.

METHYL ALCOHOL AND ETHYLENE GLYCOL

Methyl alcohol is also called *wood alcohol* or *methanol*. Ingestion of methanol and **ethylene glycol** results in the production of metabolic acids and causes metabolic acidosis. A dose as small as 30 mL can be fatal. Ingestion of only 15 mL of methanol has caused permanent blindness by producing severe optic nerve and central nervous system (CNS) toxicity. Symptoms of methanol poisoning usually do not appear until 12 to 24 hours after ingestion, when toxic metabolites have accumulated in sufficient quantities. Methanol is converted to **formaldehyde** and *formic acid*. Manifestations include headache, dizziness, nausea, vomiting, CNS depression, and respiratory failure. In the treatment of patients with methyl alcohol intoxication, emesis and gastric lavage are of use only within the first 2 hours after ingestion. Intravenous (IV) administration of large amounts of sodium bicarbonate combats acidosis. IV ethanol therapy should be used.

Ethylene glycol is a solvent found in products ranging from antifreeze and de-icing solutions to carpet and fabric cleaners. It has a sweet taste and is intoxicating—factors that contribute to its abuse potential. A lethal dose is approximately 100 mL. Gastric lavage with syrup of ipecac is ineffective because the syrup is rapidly absorbed by the intestine. Acidosis occurs as ethylene glycol is converted to oxalic and lactic acid. Toxicity manifests in three stages: neurologic symptoms (ranging from drunkenness to coma), which appear within 12 hours; cardiorespiratory disorders (such as tachycardia and pulmonary edema); and flank pain and renal failure (caused by the plugging of the tubules with oxalate crystals).

The enzyme known as *alcohol dehydrogenase* metabolizes methanol and ethylene glycol into toxic metabolites. This enzyme is also used in the metabolism of ethanol. Because alcohol dehydrogenase has an affinity for ethanol that is 10 times greater than its affinity for methanol or ethylene glycol, IV or oral ethanol is used as an antidote for methanol and ethylene glycol poisoning.

FORMALDEHYDE

Formaldehyde is a gas available as a 40% solution (formalin), which is used as a disinfectant, fumigant, or deodorant. Poisoning may be diagnosed by the characteristic odor of formaldehyde. This agent reacts chemically with cellular components and depresses cellular functions, with a fatal dose of formalin being about 60 mL. Ingestion of formalin immediately causes severe abdominal pain, nausea, vomiting, and diarrhea. This may be followed by collapse, coma, severe metabolic acidosis, and anuria. Death is usually caused by circulatory failure. Because any organic material can inactivate formaldehyde, milk, bread, and soup should be administered immediately unless activated charcoal is available.

SALICYLATES

Each year, 30 million pounds of aspirin are consumed in the United States, and salicylates can be found in most American households. Aspirin is found as an ingredient in many compound analgesic tablets. The ingestion of 10 to 30 g of aspirin or sodium salicylates may be fatal to adults. However, survival has been reported after an oral dose of 130 g of aspirin. Salicylate intoxication may result from the cumulative effect of therapeutic administration of high doses. Toxic symptoms may begin at dosages of 3 g/day or may not appear when 10 g/day is given. Therapeutic salicylate intoxication is usually mild and is called **salicylism**. The earliest symptoms are vertigo and impairment of hearing.

Further overdosage causes nausea, vomiting, sweating, diarrhea, fever, drowsiness, and headache. Effects on the CNS may progress to hallucinations, convulsions, coma, cardiovascular collapse, pulmonary edema, hyperthermia, and death. Treatment of patients with salicylate poisoning consists of first inducing emesis or using gastric lavage, after which activated charcoal and then an osmotic cathartic are administered. Respiratory depression may require artificial ventilation with oxygen. Convulsions may be treated with diazepam or phenobarbital. Peritoneal dialysis and hemodialysis are also highly effective in removing salicylates from seriously poisoned patients.

Focus Point

Ingestion of Methanol

Methanol can be absorbed through the skin or GI tract or inhaled through the lungs.

ACIDS

Corrosive **acids** are used in many types of industry and laboratories. They are almost always ingested with suicidal intent. Their toxic effects are attributable to direct chemical action. Ingestion of acids may cause irritation; bleeding; severe pain; and severe burns in the mouth, esophagus, and stomach. Profound shock often develops, which may be fatal. Ingested acid should be immediately diluted with large amounts of water or milk. The emesis or gastric lavage is contraindicated because of the danger of perforation. Diagnostic esophagoscopy, if performed, should be done within the first 24 hours after ingestion.

ALKALIES

Strong **alkalies** are used throughout various industries as well as in cleansers and drain cleaners. They include ammonium hydroxide, potassium hydroxide (potash), potassium carbonate, sodium hydroxide (lye), and sodium carbonate (washing soda). The toxic effects of alkalies are attributable to irritation and destruction of local tissues. After ingesting any of these agents, the patient will experience severe pain in the mouth, pharynx, chest, and abdomen. Vomiting of blood and diarrhea is common. The esophagus or stomach may become perforated immediately or after several days. Treatment consists of immediate administration of large amounts of water or milk. Esophagoscopy should be done within the first 24 hours. Steroids are usually administered for about 3 weeks to decrease the incidence of stricture formation.

ANTIHISTAMINES

There is a wide variation among patient tolerance to **antihistamines** and in the symptoms of poisoning. When poisoned by antihistamines, patients may experience CNS excitement or depression. In adults, drowsiness, stupor, and coma may occur. Treatment is supportive, focused on the removal of the unabsorbed drug and the maintenance of vital functions. Convulsions may be controlled with phenobarbital or diazepam.

ARSENIC

Arsenic is a cellular toxin that is readily absorbed through the GI tract and lungs. It has a metallic taste and garlic-like odor, causing extreme GI irritation. Signs and symptoms include nausea, vomiting, hemorrhagic gastroenteritis, cardiogenic shock, ventricular tachyarrhythmias, pulmonary edema, pancytopenia, hemolytic anemia, convulsions, coma, polyneuropathy, renal dysfunction, skin lesions, and others. Arsenic poisoning is treated with advanced life support, endotracheal intubation, fluid therapy, gastric lavage, gastrotomy, chelation therapy, hemodialysis, and blood transfusions. Arsenic poisoning may cause neurotoxic effects and multisystem organ failure.

ATROPINE

Atropine is a widely prescribed drug. Young children are very susceptible to poisoning with this agent. Older persons appear to be more sensitive to the CNS effects of atropine. The most characteristic symptoms of atropine poisoning are dryness of mouth, thirst, dysphasia, hoarseness, dilated pupils, blurring of vision, flushing, tachycardia, hypertension, and urinary retention. Treatment includes emesis or gastric lavage, followed by the administration of activated charcoal. Physostigmine salicylate should be given IV if symptoms are severe.

BENZENE AND TOLUENE

Benzene and **toluene** are solvents used in paint removers, dry cleaning solutions, and rubber and plastic cements. Benzene is also present in most types of gasoline. Poisoning may result from ingestion or from breathing the concentrated vapors of these agents. Toluene is an ingredient present in some cements that is "sniffed" or "huffed" as a recreational drug. Acute poisoning with these compounds causes CNS manifestations. Restlessness, excitement, euphoria, and dizziness, progressing to coma, convulsions, and respiratory failure, are common. The treatment of acute and chronic poisoning with benzene or toluene is symptomatic.

Focus Point

Gastric Lavage Tubing

Gastric lavage should be performed with the largest tube appropriate for the patient.

BENZODIAZEPINES

Benzodiazepines are easily absorbed, exhibiting 85% to 99% protein binding the plasma. They are lipid-soluble, weak acids. Benzodiazepines are mainly eliminated by the liver. CNS depressant effects materialize within 30 minutes of acute overdose. Respiratory depression and coma can occur with ultra-short-acting agents and when benzodiazepines are combined with other CNS depressants. Early in the course of poisoning, excitation may occur. Benzodiazepines are absorbed by activated charcoal, which is the method of choice for GI decontamination. Respiratory support should be provided as necessary.

BLEACHES

Whereas industrial strength bleaches contain 10% or more sodium hypochlorite, household products (e.g., Clorox, Purex, and Sanichlor) contain 3% to 6%. For reference, the solution used for chlorinating swimming pools contains 20%. The corrosive action of bleaches in the mouth, pharynx, and esophagus is similar to that of sodium hydroxide. Treatment consists of dilution of the ingested bleach with water or milk.

CARBON MONOXIDE

Carbon monoxide (CO) is a colorless, odorless, tasteless, and nonirritating gas present in the exhaust of internal combustion engines in concentrations of 3% to 7%. CO is responsible for about 3,500 accidental deaths and suicides every year in the United States. The toxic effects of CO are the result of tissue hypoxia. The most characteristic sign of severe CO poisoning is a cherry color of the skin and mucous membranes. Treatment requires effective ventilation in the presence of high oxygen (O_2) concentrations and the absence of CO. If necessary, ventilation should be supported artificially. Pure O_2 should be administered. Cerebral edema should be treated with diuretics and steroids.

COCAINE

Cocaine is rapidly metabolized by the liver, and its effects are seen quickly—in less than 5 minutes. Peak response occurs in 8 to 12 minutes, lasting for approximately 30 minutes. Signs and symptoms of acute cocaine poisoning include elevated blood pressure, pulse, respirations, and temperature. Other symptoms include anxiety, headache, tremors, nausea, vomiting, confusion, hallucinations, and abdominal cramps. Treatment involves benzodiazepines, oxygen therapy, dextrose, thiamine, barbiturates, fluid replacement, activated charcoal, and advanced life support. Severe cocaine abuse often results in long-term cardiovascular complications, cerebrovascular accidents, and other conditions.

CYANIDE

Cyanide is an exceedingly potent and rapid-acting poison but one for which specific and effective antidotal therapy is available. Cyanide poisoning may result from the inhalation of hydrocyanic acid or from the ingestion of soluble inorganic cyanide salts. Parts of many plants also contain substances such as amygdaline, which release cyanide when they are digested.

Cyanide poisoning is a true medical emergency; however, treatment is highly effective if given rapidly. Chemical antidotes should be immediately available wherever emergency medical care is dispensed. Diagnosis is made by the characteristic "bitter almond" odor on the breath of the victim. Treatment involves the administration of nitrite, which produces methemoglobin

in the body. Supportive measures, especially artificial respiration with 100% oxygen, should be instituted as soon as possible.

DETERGENTS AND SOAPS

Detergents and soaps fall into three groups: anionic, nonionic, and cationic. The first group contains common **soaps** and household **detergents**. They may cause vomiting and diarrhea but have no serious effects, and no treatment is required. However, some laundry compounds contain phosphate water softeners. If ingested, these agents may cause hypocalcemia, but the ingestion of nonionic detergents also does not require treatment.

Cationic detergents are commonly used for bactericidal purposes in hospitals and homes. These compounds are well absorbed in the GI tract and interfere with cellular functions. The fatal oral dose is approximately 3 g. Ingestion produces nausea, vomiting, shock, coma, and convulsions. It may cause death within a few hours. The treatment consists of minimizing GI absorption by emesis and gastric lavage with ordinary soap solution, which rapidly inactivates cationic detergents. Activated charcoal should also be administered.

Focus Point

The Potency of Cyanide

Cyanide poisoning may cause cardiac arrest and death within 1 to 15 minutes.

DIGITALIS

Digitalis contains *digoxin*, which is used for the treatment of heart failure. Increased digoxin levels may result from concomitant therapy with such drugs as amiodarone, erythromycin, quinidine, tetracycline, and other drugs. Signs and symptoms of digitalis poisoning include cardiac arrhythmias, tachycardia, nausea, vomiting, seizures, visual abnormalities, dizziness, altered serum potassium levels, and others. The treatment includes activated charcoal, atropine, antiarrhythmics, electrical cardioversion, fragment antigen-binding (Fab fragment) therapy, and advanced life support. Digitalis poisoning may result in multiple-organ failure and recurrence of toxicity after treatment has ended.

FLUORIDES

Fluorides are used in insecticides. The gas called "fluorine" is used in industry. Fluorine and fluorides are cellular poisons. Fluorides also interact with

calcium to cause hypocalcemia. Ingestion of 1 to 2 g of sodium fluoride may be fatal. Inhalation of fluorine or hydrogen fluoride produces coughing and choking. After 1 or 2 days, fever, cough, cyanosis, and pulmonary edema may develop. The ingestion of fluoride salts is followed by nausea, vomiting, diarrhea, and abdominal pain.

The federal safe standard for the ingestion of fluoride is 4 parts per million (ppm) per day. However, each recommended dose of most brands of toothpaste contains 500 to 1,500 ppm. Toothpaste should never be swallowed for this reason. The fluoride content of fluoridated water is lower—usually only 0.1 ppm (per serving). With a fluoride overdose, death results from respiratory paralysis or circulatory collapse. The treatment for acute fluoride poisoning consists of immediate administration of milk, limewater (calcium hydroxide solution), or calcium lactate solution. Gastric lavage or emesis can be used, and charcoal can be given.

IODINE

The traditional antiseptic **iodine** tincture is an alcoholic solution of 2% iodine and 2% sodium iodide. A strong iodine solution (Lugol's solution) is an aqueous solution of 5% iodine and 10% potassium iodide. The fatal dose of tincture of iodine is approximately 2 g. Iodides are less toxic, with no reported fatalities. The diagnosis of iodine poisoning is indicated by a brown discoloration of the oral mucous membranes. Iodine has corrosive effects on the GI tract. Burning abdominal pain, nausea, vomiting, and bloody diarrhea may occur soon after ingestion. Fever, delirium, stupor, and anuria have also been observed. The treatment consists of the immediate administration of milk, starch, bread, or activated charcoal.

ISOPROPYL ALCOHOL AND ACETONE

Isopropyl alcohol is used as a sterilizing agent or as rubbing alcohol. Ingestion produces gastric irritation and raises the danger of vomiting with aspiration. The systemic effects of isopropyl alcohol are similar to those of ethyl alcohol, but isopropyl alcohol is twice as potent. Emesis should be induced or gastric lavage should be performed. Acetone is used in cleaners, nail polish removers, and solvents. Isopropyl is actually metabolized to acetone in the liver via the enzyme alcohol dehydrogenase. Acetone is excreted in the kidneys and lungs, and both of these agents are CNS depressants. Hemodialysis is effective for removing isopropyl alcohol and acetone. It should be considered in patients with high serum levels who do not respond to conservative therapy.

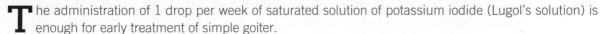

Focus Point

Treatment of Simple Goiter

The administration of 1 drop per week of saturated solution of potassium iodide (Lugol's solution) is enough for early treatment of simple goiter.

LITHIUM

Lithium is primarily used for bipolar and unipolar depression. It is absorbed, distributed, and eliminated slowly. Acute toxicity usually causes initial GI symptoms followed by CNS complications. Signs and symptoms include nausea, vomiting, memory impairment, delirium, hypertension, tachycardia, tremors, seizures, coma, and hypothermia. The treatment includes advanced life support, fluid therapy, benzodiazepines, whole-bowel irrigation, hemodialysis, amiloride, and other treatments. Complications of lithium poisoning may include permanent encephalopathy, nystagmus, ataxia, and choreoathetosis (the occurrence of involuntary movements).

MAGNESIUM SULFATE

Magnesium sulfate is used IV as a hypotensive agent and orally as a cathartic. Magnesium is a profound depressant of the CNS. With normal renal function, poisoning after oral or rectal administration is unlikely. In the presence of impaired renal function, an oral dose

of 30 g may be fatal. Oral ingestion of magnesium sulfate may cause GI irritation. Systemic poisoning can cause paralysis, hypotension, hypothermia, coma, and respiratory failure. The treatment of patients with magnesium poisoning includes the IV administration of 10 mL of a 10% solution of calcium gluconate.

OPIOIDS

Opioids include morphine, heroin, and codeine. These drugs have widely varying potencies and durations of action. All these agents decrease CNS and sympathetic nervous activity. Mild intoxication is characterized by euphoria, drowsiness, and constricted pupils. More severe intoxication may cause hypotension, bradycardia, hypothermia, coma, and respiratory arrest. Death is usually caused by apnea or pulmonary aspiration of gastric contents. If the patient arrives for medical care shortly after ingestion, the stomach should be emptied by emesis or gastric lavage, and activated charcoal should be administered. Naloxone is an opioid antagonist that can rapidly reverse signs of narcotic intoxication.

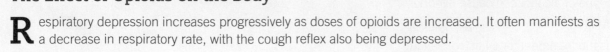

Focus Point

The Effect of Opioids on the Body

Respiratory depression increases progressively as doses of opioids are increased. It often manifests as a decrease in respiratory rate, with the cough reflex also being depressed.

ORGANOPHOSPHATE AND CARBAMATE INSECTICIDES

Organophosphate and carbamate insecticides are compounds that irreversibly inhibit acetylcholinesterase and are absorbed through the skin, lungs, and GI tract. They become widely distributed throughout the tissues and are only slowly eliminated by the liver. Toxicity may be achieved between 30 minutes and 2 hours after absorption. The treatment of patients with organophosphate poisoning includes removing contaminated clothing, washing the skin with soap and water, and using activated charcoal to decontaminate the GI tract. Additional treatment may involve oxygen administration, ventilatory assistance, and treatment of seizures.

PETROLEUM DISTILLATES

Diesel oil, gasoline, kerosene, and paint thinner are all liquid **petroleum distillates**. Kerosene is widely used as a fuel and as a component of cleaning agents, furniture polishes, insecticides, and paint thinners. Petroleum distillates are CNS depressants; they damage cells by dissolving cellular lipids. Pulmonary damage manifested by pulmonary edema or pneumonitis is a common and serious complication.

Inhalation of gasoline or kerosene vapors induces symptoms that resemble those of alcoholic intoxication. Headache, nausea, and a burning sensation in the chest may be present. Oral ingestion of petroleum distillates causes irritation of the mucous membranes of the upper part of the intestinal tract. During treatment, extreme care must be used to prevent aspiration. When large amounts have been ingested, gastric emptying is indicated. Emesis may be induced if the patient is alert. Oxygen therapy should also be given.

PHENOL

Phenol and related compounds (creosote, cresols, hexachlorophene, Lysol, and tannic acid) are used as antiseptics, caustics, and preservatives. The approximate fatal oral dose ranges from 2 mL for phenol and cresols to 20 mL for tannic acid. Ingestion of these agents produces the erosion of mucosa from the mouth to the stomach. Vomiting of blood as well as bloody diarrhea may occur. Other adverse effects include hyperpnea, pulmonary edema, stupor, coma, convulsions, and shock. Emesis and lavage are indicated for treatment when there is no significant corrosive injury to the esophagus. Activated charcoal should be administered.

PHOSPHORUS

Phosphorus occurs in two forms: a red, nonpoisonous form, and a yellow, fat-soluble, highly toxic form. The yellow form of phosphorus is used in rodent and insect poisons and in fireworks. Yellow phosphorus causes fatty degeneration and necrosis of tissues, particularly of the liver. The lethal ingested dose of yellow phosphorus is approximately 50 mg. The ingestion of yellow phosphorus may cause pain in the upper part of the GI tract, vomiting, diarrhea, and a garlic odor to the breath. Patients may also develop hepatomegaly, jaundice, hypocalcemia, hypotension, and oliguria. The treatment includes emesis or gastric lavage and the administration of activated charcoal and an osmotic cathartic.

✳ Apply Your Knowledge 10.2 ▬▬▬▬▬

The following questions focus on what you have just learned about common poisons.

CRITICAL THINKING

1. Describe the treatment for acetaminophen poisoning.
2. Differentiate the signs and symptoms of corrosive acid poisonings from alkali poisonings.
3. Discuss the treatment for carbon monoxide poisoning.
4. What is ethylene glycol? Describe the treatment for ethylene glycol poisoning.
5. What are the signs and symptoms of the ingestion of formalin?
6. What is Lugol's solution?
7. What are the complications of lead poisoning?
8. Discuss systemic poisoning with magnesium sulfate.
9. What are three methods used to remove ingested substances?
10. What are the most common sources of poisons affecting the general population?
11. What is the effect of alcohol on the CNS?
12. Which type of alcohol can cause blindness?
13. What are the signs of poisoning by digoxin?
14. What is the treatment for ingested bleach?

Antidotes

Specific antidotal therapy is available for only a few poisons. Some systemic antidotes exert their therapeutic effect by reducing the concentration of the toxic substance. They may do this by combining with the poison or by increasing its rate of excretion.

Other systemic antidotes compete with the poison for its receptor site. Specific antidotes are listed in Table 10-1 ■.

Table 10-1 ■ Poisons and Antidotes

POISON	ANTIDOTES
Acetaminophen	N-Acctylcysteine
Benzodiazepines	Flumazenil
Carbon monoxide	Oxygen
Cyanide	Amyl nitrate
Iron	Deferoxamine
Methanol	Ethanol
Opiates	Naloxone
Organophosphates	Atropine or pralidoxime

CYANIDE ANTIDOTE KIT

Most cyanide antidote kits consist of the following:

✻ Two ampules of sodium nitrate injection (USP 300 mg in 10 mL of sterile water)

✻ One vial of sodium thiosulfate injection (intraperitoneal; 25 g in 50 mL of sterile water)

✻ Twelve gauze-covered ampules of amyl nitrate inhalant (0.3 mL)

✻ One sterile 10-mL plastic disposable syringe with a 22-gauge needle

✻ One sterile 50 mL plastic disposable syringe with a 22-gauge needle

✻ One stomach tube

✻ One nonsterile 50-mL syringe

✻ One set of instructions for the treatment of cyanide poisoning

Sodium nitrite reacts with hemoglobin to form methemoglobin, which removes cyanide ions from various tissues and couples with them to become cyanmethemoglobin, which has a relatively low toxicity. Sodium thiosulfate converts cyanide to thiocyanate. The combination of sodium nitrite and sodium thiosulfate is the best therapy against cyanide and hydrocyanic acid poisoning. The two substances are injected IV—one after the other (the nitrite followed by the thiosulfate). They are capable of detoxifying approximately 20 lethal doses of sodium cyanide and are effective even after respiration has stopped. As long as the heart is still beating, the chances of recovery after using this method are very good.

Prevention

Quality, in-depth education about poisons and poisonings is the best method to address the problem. Directions and steps for poison prevention should be clear and determinate. Accurate lists of all potential poisons should be supplied. Often, parents are unaware that a specific product is actually poisonous. Naming actual locations to store specific products in the household does far more than generalizing about how many children are poisoned at home each year. Person-to-person counseling about specific medications and other substances, detailing their poisoning potential, is invaluable. The use of safety containers and child-resistant packaging must be stressed to parents and family members (Figure 10-2 ■). Certain medications sold over the counter are not currently required to have child-resistant packaging even though, if taken in large quantities, they could cause severe harm and even death.

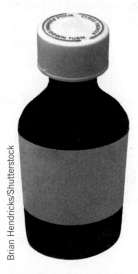

Brian Hendricks/Shutterstock

Figure 10-2 ■ Child-resistant packaging.

Poison Control Centers

A network consisting of more than 600 poison control centers exists in the United States. Poison treatment information is available free of charge 24 hours a day. The first poison control center was established in Chicago, led by the Illinois chapter of the American Academy of Pediatrics. Shortly afterward, the Duke University Poison Control Center was established in North Carolina. The idea of poison control centers then spread across the country.

In 1957, the FDA established the National Clearinghouse for Poison Control Centers to coordinate activities at poison control centers across the United States. This clearinghouse collected and standardized product toxicology data, reproduced this information on large file cards, and distributed them nationwide to poison control centers.

✳ Apply Your Knowledge 10.3

The following questions focus on what you have just learned about antidotes, cyanide poisoning, and poison control centers.

CRITICAL THINKING

1. What are the antidotes for methanol poisoning, opiate overdose, and benzodiazepine overdose?

2. Why is the administration of nitrite preferred to treat cyanide poisoning?

3. What are the reasons that poison control centers are available 24 hours a day in the United States?

PRACTICAL SCENARIO 1

A 76-year-old grandmother with a history of angina pectoris and heart attacks went to Florida to visit her daughter and granddaughter. She had medications in her purse that did not have childproof lids because she lived alone and there was no danger of a child being poisoned. A few hours after she arrived at her daughter's house, her granddaughter wouldn't awaken from her nap and had a nosebleed. The child's mother called 911, and the child was taken to the emergency room in an ambulance. It was soon discovered that she had swallowed half of the bottle of one of her grandmother's medications, presumably taking them from her grandmother's purse while she was taking a shower and the child's mother was cooking.

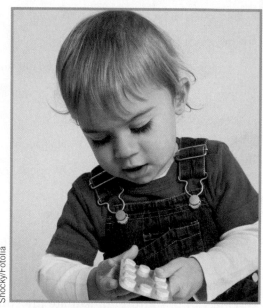

Shocky/Fotolia

Critical Thinking Questions

1. What could have been done to prevent this type of accident?
2. If the medication the child consumed was aspirin, what treatments would be indicated?

PRACTICAL SCENARIO 2

On a cold winter evening, a family lit its fireplace to help warm up the house. One of the family's children was using his laptop near the fire. A while later, as his father was working in his office, he noticed that the air in the house smelled of smoke. He entered the family room and noticed that his son was asleep. He tried to get him to go to bed, but he was unresponsive. He quickly opened all the house's windows and got his children and wife, who was in the back bedroom, outside. He then went back in and found that the chimney flue had not been opened.

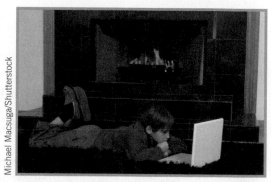

Michael Macsuga/Shutterstock

Critical Thinking Questions

1. What gas had most likely overcome the family?
2. Why did the father open the windows and take the family outside?

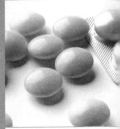

Chapter Capsule

This section repeats the objectives from the beginning of the chapter and then provides a summary of the most important concepts for that objective. Use this section as a quick review and to check your knowledge.

Objective 1: Explain the importance of poisons and antidotes.

- A poison is any agent that in relatively small amounts can cause death or serious bodily harm. All drugs are potential poisons when used improperly or in dosages that are greater than normal.

- Specific antidotal therapy is available for only a few poisons. Some systemic antidotes exert their therapeutic effect by reducing the concentration of the toxic substance. They may do this by combining with the poison or by increasing its rate of excretion. Other systemic antidotes compete with the poison for its receptor site.

Objective 2: Describe the detection of poisons.

- The optimal treatment of poisoned patients requires correct diagnosis. Most adverse effects from poisonings can simulate other diseases. In every poisoning case, the identification of the toxic agent should be attempted. Specific antidotal therapy is obviously impossible without the poison begin correctly identified. Some poisons can produce clinical features that are characteristic enough to strongly suggest the diagnosis. Chemical analysis of body fluids provides the most accurate identification of the intoxicating agent.

Objective 3: List the most common poisonings seen today in the United States.

- The most common poisonings in the United States involve lead, mercury, acetaminophen, methyl alcohol, ethylene glycol, formaldehyde, salicylates, acids, alkalies, antihistamines, arsenic, atropine, benzene, toluene, benzodiazepines, bleaches, carbon monoxide, cocaine, cyanide, detergents, soaps, digitalis, fluorides, iodine, isopropyl alcohol, acetone, lithium, magnesium sulfate, opioids, organophosphate and carbamate insecticides, petroleum distillates, phenol, and phosphorus.

Objective 4: Explain important factors that are related to risks of poisoning.

- Factors that are important in the consideration of poisoning risk and prevention include age (most poisonings occur in children and are accidental), location (usually at home), access (locked medicine cabinets, cupboards, and other areas are helpful in protecting against poisonings), containers (using original containers with proper labeling), and supervision (keep children in sight at all times).

Objective 5: Describe poison prevention programs.

- The best method of poison prevention is quality, in-depth education. All directions and steps should be clear and determinate, and accurate lists of all potential poisons should be supplied. Naming actual locations to store specific products in the household does far more than generalizing about how many children are poisoned at home each year. Person-to-person counseling about specific medications and other substances, detailing their poisoning potential, is invaluable. The use of safety containers and child-resistant packaging must be stressed to parents and family members. Lack of the use of child-resistant packaging can lead to severe harm and even death.

Objective 6: Explain how the most common poisonings occur.

■ Most common poisonings occur at home, with acute effects. These mostly accidental poisonings usually result from the ingestion of toxic substances—most often by children. These examples are usually preventable if proper measures are taken. Common cases of poisoning are usually caused by unlocked storage areas, repackaging poisons into containers that do not bear warning labels or other accurate labeling, and the lack of proper supervision of children.

Objective 7: Compare lead poisoning and mercury poisoning.

■ Lead poisoning usually affects children and may involve old paint containing lead, pipes made of lead, and vegetable gardens. Lead poisoning causes severe damage to the brain, nerves, red blood cells, and digestive system. Symptoms include a metallic taste, abdominal pain, vomiting, diarrhea, collapse, coma, headache, convulsions, and death. Treatment usually involves such chelating agents as penicillamine, edetate calcium disodium, and dimercaprol. Gastric lavage may also be indicated.

■ Mercury poisoning often occurs by the ingestion of inorganic mercuric salts or the inhalation of metallic mercury vapor. Symptoms include a metallic taste, salivation, thirst, burning in the throat, discoloration and edema of oral mucous membranes, abdominal pain, vomiting, bloody diarrhea, shock, acute renal failure, and acute chemical pneumonia. There is no specific treatment for mercury vapor pneumonitis. Ingested mercuric salts can be removed by lavage, with activated charcoal also administered. Dimercaprol can be given, and if poisoning is chronic, the patient must be removed from exposure to mercury.

Objective 8: Name the antidotes for cyanide, methanol, opiates, and organophosphates.

■ Cyanide—antidote: amyl nitrate
■ Methanol—antidote: ethanol
■ Opiates—antidote: naloxone
■ Organophosphates—antidote: atropine or pralidoxime

Objective 9: Describe arsenic, atropine, and cyanide poisonings.

■ Arsenic poisoning: Arsenic is a cellular toxin readily absorbed through the GI tract and lungs; it has a metallic taste and garlic-like odor, and it causes extreme GI irritation. Signs and symptoms include nausea, vomiting, hemorrhagic gastroenteritis, cardiogenic shock, ventricular tachyarrhythmias, pulmonary edema, pancytopenia, hemolytic anemia, convulsions, coma, polyneuropathy, renal dysfunction, and skin lesions. Patients are treated with advanced life support, endotracheal intubation, fluid therapy, gastric lavage, gastrotomy, chelation therapy, hemodialysis, and blood transfusions.

■ Atropine poisoning: Although young children are very susceptible to atropine poisoning, older persons appear to be more sensitive to its CNS effects; symptoms include dryness of mouth, thirst, dysphasia, hoarseness, dilated pupils, blurred vision, flushing, tachycardia, hypertension, and urinary retention. The treatment includes emesis, gastric lavage, activated charcoal, and physostigmine salicylate.

■ Cyanide poisoning: A potent, rapid-acting poison, cyanide may exert its effects via the inhalation of hydrocyanic acid or from the ingestion of soluble inorganic cyanide salts.

Many plants also release cyanide when they are digested. In a true medical emergency, patients with cyanide poisoning respond to rapid treatment. Chemical antidotes should be readily available at emergency care facilities. A distinct "bitter almond" odor will be present on the breath of the victim, and the treatment involves the administration of nitrite. Supportive measures include artificial respiration with 100% oxygen.

Objective 10: Differentiate between digitalis toxicity and lithium toxicity.

■ Digitalis toxicity: Digitalis poisoning may result in multiple-organ failure and recurrence of toxicity after treatment with activated charcoal, atropine, antiarrhythmics, electrical cardioversion, fragment antigen-binding therapy, and advanced life support.

■ Lithium toxicity: Acute lithium toxicity causes initial GI symptoms, followed by CNS complications. It is absorbed, distributed, and eliminated slowly.

Internet Sites of Interest

■ Symptoms of mercury poisoning, mercury prognosis, and detoxification guide: **http://heartspring.net/mercury_poison_symptoms.html**.

■ American Association of Poison Control Centers: **http://www.aapcc.org/dnn/default.aspx**.

■ Alcohol poisoning symptoms: **http://www.about-alcoholism-info.com/Alcohol_Poisoning_Symptoms.html**.

■ Poisoning causes, symptoms, diagnosis, and treatment: **http://www.emedicinehealth.com/poisoning/article_em.htm**.

■ Lead poisoning: **http://www.mayoclinic.com/health/lead-poisoning/FL00068**.

■ Aspirin and other salicylate poisoning: **http://www.emedicinehealth.com/aspirin_poisoning/article_em.htm**.

■ The Poison Center: common poisons at home and work: **http://www.ncpoisoncenter.org/body.cfm?id=87**.

■ Household poisons: **http://poison.org/prevent/house.asp**.

Chapter 11

Substance Abuse

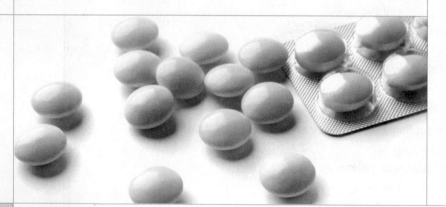

Key Terms

additive effect (page 169)
benzodiazepines (page 170)
cannabinoids (page 170)
delirium tremens (DT) (page 176)
detoxification (page 174)

hallucinogens (page 170)
opioids (page 170)
polysubstance abuse (page 169)
psychological treatment (page 174)
sedatives (page 170)

substance abuse (page 169)
substance-dependent (page 169)
tetrahydrocannabinol (THC) (page 170)
tobacco dependence (page 174)
withdrawal (page 170)

Introduction

Substance abuse is a major issue in today's society. Throughout history, natural and prescription drugs have been used to increase physical or mental performance. These substances cause a relaxed feeling and a change in psychological state. The most commonly abused substances include alcohol, prescription medications, over-the-counter (OTC) medications, and illegal drugs. Addiction is very prevalent and refers to any physical or psychological dependence on any substance. It is a psychological and biological problem. Many drug takers use more than one drug, which is referred to as *polysubstance abuse*. Drug abuse is generally associated with anxiety and depression. The most common addiction today does not involve any of the previously mentioned substances; rather, the most common addiction is to nicotine, as found in cigarettes and other tobacco products.

Substance Abuse

Substance abuse may affect every level of a person's life. People are described as having a substance abuse problem when they experience significant distress in their lives and when any four of the following things occur:

1. Failure to fulfill parenting, school, or work obligations
2. Hazardous behavior, such as driving under the influence
3. Recurrent related legal problems, such as driving under the influence (DUI)
4. Continued use of substances despite continuing social or interpersonal problems

People are termed to be **substance-dependent** when they exhibit any three of the following signs:

1. Tolerance
2. Withdrawal
3. Increasing consumption
4. Desire to quit
5. Excessive time spent on abuse
6. Fewer occupational, recreational, or social activities
7. Continued use while understanding the physiologic and psychological effects

A *substance abuse disorder* is one that includes substance abuse and dependence. Addiction is defined as progressive, chronic abuse of a substance that causes a person to use the substance repeatedly despite serious health and social consequences. It depends on varying factors based on the drug or drugs used. These include cost, availability, dose, and method of administration. Other factors that may influence addiction include experience with drugs, risk-taking behaviors, certain diseases that require scheduled drugs to be taken, educational opportunities, and peer influences.

Sedatives and hypnotics are used to promote relaxation in small doses but can induce sleep and confusion when used in higher doses. Very high doses can induce coma and even death. Any combination of these agents can be lethal; this is known as the **additive effect**.

ADDICTIVE DRUGS

Addictive drugs include cannabinoids such as hashish and marijuana, depressants such as barbiturates and benzodiazepines, such dissociative anesthetics as ketamine and phenylcyclohexylpiperidine (PCP), such hallucinogens as lysergic acid diethylamide (LSD) and mescaline, such opioids and morphine derivatives as codeine and morphine, such stimulants as amphetamine and cocaine, and such other compounds as anabolic steroids and dextromethorphan. Misuse of prescription drugs exceeds the combined use of *all* street drugs except marijuana. Currently, about 9% of Americans are dependent on drugs or alcohol. Use of two or more different substances of abuse is referred to as **polysubstance abuse**.

Recent studies have shown the following percentages and numbers of users of abused drugs:

* Marijuana: 5.8% of Americans or 14.4 million people
* Sedatives: 2.8% of Americans or 6.9 million people
* Opioids: 2.1% of Americans or 5.2 million people
* Cocaine: 0.8% of Americans or 2.1 million people
* Hallucinogens: 0.4% of Americans or 1 million people
* Methamphetamine: 0.2% of Americans or 500,000 people

Out of all substance abusers, only 6.4% on average believe they need treatment. Drug addiction can start early. Of people older than 18 who first tried marijuana before age 14, a total of 13% are now substance abusers. Apparently, the earlier in life the person begins using drugs, the higher the chance he or she will have a long-term substance use disorder.

Focus Point

Withdrawal Syndrome

Withdrawal syndrome is defined as the unpleasant symptoms that are experienced when a physically dependent client discontinues the use of an abused drug.

Central Nervous System Depressants

Central nervous system (CNS) depressants cause relaxation or sedation and include barbiturates, nonbarbiturate sedative–hypnotics, benzodiazepines, opioids, and alcohol. The CNS depressants allowed for medical use are controlled because of their abuse potential. The following paragraphs explain these agents in detail. Alcohol and alcoholism are explained later in this chapter.

BARBITURATES AND NONBARBITURATE SEDATIVE–HYPNOTICS

There are two major types of **sedatives** (tranquilizers): barbiturates and nonbarbiturate sedative–hypnotics. They are used for sleep disorders and certain forms of epilepsy. These agents have similar actions to each other and may cause physical or psychologic dependence as well as tolerance when taken at high doses or for extended periods. Sedatives are often combined with alcohol and other CNS stimulants. Those who become addicted often vary between these drugs and amphetamines in an attempt to control their wakefulness and sleep patterns.

Some sedatives last for as long as an entire day, with higher doses causing similar effects to those of alcohol intoxication. Commonly abused barbiturates include amobarbital (Amytal), secobarbital (Seconal), pentobarbital (Nembutal), and the combination of amobarbital and secobarbital (known as Tuinal). Medical use of these agents has decreased greatly in the past 20 years. Overdoses of these agents are very dangerous, potentially causing respiratory arrest, coma, and death.

BENZODIAZEPINES

Benzodiazepines are CNS depressants that are widely prescribed, largely replacing barbiturates for various conditions. They are usually used to treat anxiety but also for muscle relaxation and the prevention of seizures. Commonly used benzodiazepines include alprazolam (Xanax), diazepam (Valium), midazolam (Versed), temazepam (Restoril), and triazolam (Halcion). Frequently abused, these agents may cause

patients to appear remote from others, giddy, disoriented, or sleepy. Although these agents seldom cause death because of overdose, users frequently combine them with alcohol and illegal drugs to increase their effects. In these cases, the outcome may be fatal. **Withdrawal** from benzodiazepines is not as severe compared with withdrawal from alcohol or barbiturates. However, drug levels of benzodiazepines, remain higher in the body for several weeks, making abuse of these agents extremely dangerous.

OPIOIDS

Opioids (narcotic analgesics) are used for severe pain, diarrhea, and persistent cough. This class of drugs includes natural substances derived from unripe poppy seeds (codeine, morphine, and opium). Synthetic forms of these agents are available, including fentanyl (Duragesic or Sublimaze), meperidine (Demerol), methadone (Dolophine), oxycodone (OxyContin), propoxyphene (Darvon), and the illegal drug *heroin*. Orally administered opioids take effect within 30 minutes and can last for more than 1 day. Parenteral forms, including *heroin*, cause a euphoric rush, intense sedation, and abnormally slow body functions. Signs of use include constricted pupils, respiratory depression, and the ability to tolerate increased amounts of pain. Overdose is extremely dangerous and potentially fatal.

Opioid addiction may develop rapidly, and withdrawal is very unpleasant (although not life threatening compared with barbiturate withdrawal). Methadone is often used to treat patients with addiction to other opioids because it does not produce the same degree of euphoria and has longer lasting effects. It may also be addictive—but to a lesser degree—and helps those who are addicted to heroin to withdraw from that drug without unpleasant withdrawal symptoms. Methadone is an orally administered opioid, which helps to remove further risks (via parenteral injection) of contact with such diseases as AIDS and hepatitis. Methadone may be used throughout a patient's lifetime (in certain cases), with withdrawal taking longer than that of heroin or morphine but with less intense symptoms.

✳ Apply Your Knowledge 11.1

The following questions focus on what you have just learned about substance abuse and addictive drugs.

CRITICAL THINKING

1. What are the effects of substance abuse on an individual?
2. What is polysubstance abuse?
3. What are six examples of CNS system depressants?
4. What are the indications of benzodiazepines?
5. What are the indications of opioids for various conditions?

Cannabinoids

Cannabinoids are obtained from the hemp plant (*Cannabis sativa*) and are usually smoked to obtain their effects. Cannabinoids include marijuana, hashish, and hash oil, with the most psychoactive agent being delta-9-**tetrahydrocannabinol (THC)**.

MARIJUANA

Marijuana is a natural substance that is the most commonly used illicit drug in the United States. It is regularly referred to as *dope*, *grass*, *pot*, *reefer*, or *weed*. The effects of marijuana include decreased coordination and motor activity, confusion, paranoia, euphoria, increased thirst, increased hunger, and bloodshot eyes. Effects occur within a few minutes and last for up to 24 hours. Marijuana smoke is generally inhaled more deeply than cigarette smoke, introducing four times the particulates of tar into the lungs. Daily use increases the risks of lung cancer and respiratory conditions and leads to a lack of motivation.

However, marijuana produces very little physical dependence or tolerance, with withdrawal symptoms being nearly nonexistent. Because THC metabolites remain in the body for many months (or years depending on usage), tests can easily show that a person has been using marijuana or has quit before the tests. THC is detectable in the urine for several days after using marijuana. Although 13 states currently have medical marijuana usage laws, the drug is still federally classified as a Schedule I drug. Its medical value is still controversial, but legalized use of the drug is growing. Recently, in California, marijuana extract has been approved for sale as an additive to ice cream for patients who are approved to use medical marijuana.

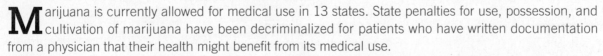

Focus Point

The Use and Legalization of Marijuana

Marijuana is currently allowed for medical use in 13 states. State penalties for use, possession, and cultivation of marijuana have been decriminalized for patients who have written documentation from a physician that their health might benefit from its medical use.

HALLUCINOGENS

Hallucinogens are quite diverse but produce similar effects, including altered consciousness that may appear "dreamlike." They are all Schedule I drugs with no approved medical use. The prototype hallucinogen is LSD.

LSD

Hallucinogens such as LSD have widely variable effects that are based on the user's mood, expectations, and environment. Repeated use may bring about entirely different effects. However, common effects, include laughter, hallucinations or "visions," deep personal insight, afterimages (trailing images of other people as they move), or religious "revelations." Users often mention that colors, lights, sounds, and other sensations are greatly intensified. However, hallucinogens also have the potential to bring about terrifying experiences, which may include anxiety, confusion, panic attacks, paranoia, and severe depression.

Commonly referred to as "acid," LSD was originally derived from a fungus growing on the grain known as rye and can also be obtained from fungal growths on other grains. It is usually administered orally as a liquid, capsule, or tablet. LSD is often placed, in droplet form, onto paper that contains cartoon images related to the drug culture. After drying, the user may ingest a piece of the paper to experience the drug's effects. LSD is immediately distributed through the body, with effects usually beginning within 1 hour. These effects may last for up to 12 hours, increasing blood pressure and heart rate, raising body temperature, and dilating the pupils. Repeated use can lead to impaired memory and reasoning ability as well as psychoses. Flashbacks occur in some users, wherein the drug's effects reoccur without further administration. Tolerance to LSD may occur, but little or no dependence has been seen.

OTHER HALLUCINOGENS

Other hallucinogens with similar effects to LSD include:

✱ DOM or STP (2,5 dimethoxy-4-methylamphetamine): often used at "rave" parties recreationally

✱ Ketamine (also known as "special coke" or the "date rape drug"): legally used as an anesthetic but also produces unconsciousness and amnesia

✱ MDA (3,4-methylenedioxyamphetamine; also known as the "love drug"): believed to increase sexual desires

✱ MDMA (3,4-methylenedioxymethamphetamine; also known as "Ecstasy" or "XTC"): an amphetamine originally used for research but has become very popular among young adults and teenagers for recreational use

✱ Mescaline: found in the peyote cactus of Mexico and Central America

✱ PCP (also known as angel dust or phencyclidine): produces a long, trancelike state that can cause severe brain damage

CENTRAL NERVOUS SYSTEM STIMULANTS

CNS stimulants increase the activity of the CNS and are legally available (by prescription) to treat narcolepsy, attention deficit hyperactivity disorder (ADHD), and obesity. These drugs produce improved mental and physical performance, a sense of exhilaration, prolonged wakefulness, and are often used illegally to "get high." CNS stimulants have similar effects to norepinephrine by activating neurons in the *reticular formation* of the brain. Most of them affect cardiovascular and respiratory activity to increase blood pressure and respiration, dilate the pupils, and cause sweating and tremors. Overdoses of certain CNS stimulants may cause seizures and cardiac arrest.

Stimulants include amphetamines, methylphenidate, cocaine, and caffeine.

AMPHETAMINES

In high doses and short-term use, amphetamines cause feelings of euphoria, self-confidence, alertness, and empowerment. Long-term use usually results in feelings of anxiety, restlessness, and rage (especially when "coming down" from the ultimate effects of the drug). After years of prescribing amphetamines and dextroamphetamines, it became understood that their risks outweighed their medical uses. Newer agents that are much safer have replaced these agents except for certain conditions. However, illegally produced amphetamines continue to be popular drugs in substance abuse.

Dextroamphetamine (Dexedrine) is used for short-term weight loss after other methods have failed and for narcolepsy. Methamphetamine (commonly known as *ice*) is a common recreational drug administered in powdered or crystallized form that gives users a "rush." It may also be smoked and is a Schedule II drug (marketed as Desoxyn). Most abusers obtain methamphetamine from illegal "meth" laboratories. Another variant—methcathinone (known as *cat*)—is a Schedule I agent that is illegally made for injection, inhalation, or oral administration.

METHYLPHENIDATE

Methylphenidate (Ritalin) is a CNS stimulant used for children diagnosed with ADHD. For those who are hyperactive or inattentive, Ritalin has a calming effect, helping the patient to focus on specific tasks for longer periods of time than he or she normally can. When taken by adults, Ritalin usually causes the opposite effects. It is a Schedule II drug with similar effects to amphetamines and cocaine. Illegally, the drug is administered by inhalation or injection—sometimes being mixed with heroin (known as a *speedball*).

COCAINE

Cocaine is obtained from the leaves of the South American coca plant and has been used since 2,500 BC. Users who chew coca leaves or make teas from them only receive slow absorption of the drug, and only tiny amounts of cocaine are present in the leaves. However, in the United States, cocaine is a Schedule II drug that is used entirely differently. It produces rapid and intense effects that are similar to but greater than the effects of amphetamines. It is usually inhaled, smoked, or injected to produce intense euphoria, analgesia, decreased hunger, increased sensory perception, and illusions of physical strength. Large doses heighten these effects and also cause rapid heartbeat, pupil dilation, elevated body temperature, and sweating. When the euphoric feelings diminish, the user experiences insomnia, irritability, depression, and extreme distrust of others. A "crawling" skin sensation may occur, and chronic use (by inhalation) results in many nasal problems. These include continual running of the nose, a reddened "crusting" around the nostrils, and nasal cartilage deterioration. Overdose may lead to convulsions, dysrhythmias, stroke, and death from respiratory arrest. Withdrawal from amphetamines and cocaine is usually less intense than from barbiturates or alcohol.

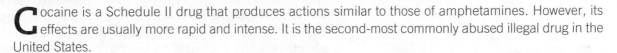

Focus Point

Cocaine

Cocaine is a Schedule II drug that produces actions similar to those of amphetamines. However, its effects are usually more rapid and intense. It is the second-most commonly abused illegal drug in the United States.

CAFFEINE

Caffeine occurs naturally in the seeds, fruits, or leaves of more than 63 different plants. Coffee, chocolate, ice cream, soft drinks, and tea contain significant amounts of caffeine. It increases the effectiveness of OTC pain relievers and is commonly added to their formulations. The body metabolizes caffeine after several hours, and the drug causes pronounced diuresis. It produces increased mental alertness, restlessness, irritability, nervousness, and insomnia. Physical effects include bronchodilation, increased blood pressure and production of stomach acid, and blood glucose level alteration. Repeated use results in physical dependence and tolerance. Withdrawal from caffeine produces fatigue, headaches, depression, and impaired physical and mental performance.

EFFECTS OF SUBSTANCE ABUSE

The mental states that often encourage drug abuse include anxiety and depression. Abuse often prevents users from seeking proper treatment for the reason they chose to abuse drugs in the first place. Anxiety, panic disorder, and insomnia are all increased by the use of stimulants. Although depression is numbed by alcohol, opioids, and sedatives initially, they cause depression over longer periods of time. Psychoses can be precipitated by hallucinogens and stimulants. Results of drug abuse include imprisonment, unemployment, cognitive dysfunction, family disharmony, financial loss, poor decisions, and sexual relationships that otherwise would not have occurred.

The physical effects of substance abuse may include diseases caused by sexual intercourse. These may include hepatitis B and C, human immunodeficiency virus (HIV), and sexually transmitted diseases. Drug use is shown more in victims of sexual assault, and intravenous drug abuse may be associated with hepatitis, HIV, and *Staphylococcal endocarditis*. Smoking and alcohol have been linked to more serious drug abuse. Heart attacks and strokes are commonly linked to the use of cocaine. Drug overdoses can lead to respiratory depression, seizures, confusion, pneumonia, coma, and death. Drugs can also cause auto accidents, fetal impairment, suicide, and violence.

* Apply Your Knowledge 11.2

The following questions focus on what you have just learned about cannabinoids, hallucinogens, and CNS stimulants.

CRITICAL THINKING

1. Which substance is the most commonly used illicit drug in the United States?
2. What are the adverse effects of repeated use of LSD on the CNS?
3. What are the most commonly used CNS stimulants?
4. What are the adverse effects of cocaine overdose?
5. What are the symptoms of withdrawal from caffeine?

PREVENTION AND TREATMENT

Schools can receive grants for drug testing and education of parents, students, and teachers through the Office of National Drug Control Policy (ONDCP). More than 4,000 schools across the United States used random student drug testing programs to provide early intervention for those students labeled "at risk." Risk factors for drug abuse include:

✳ Absent or problem parents

✳ Substance-abusing peers or parents

✳ Permissive parents

✳ Poor parental discipline

✳ Access to prescriptions

✳ Student absenteeism

✳ Aggressive behavior in adolescents

✳ Poor social skills

✳ Poor academic performance

✳ Transition periods in adolescent life

✳ Early drug use

✳ The method of drug administration

When treating patients with addiction, **detoxification** must first take place. Withdrawal may cause physical and psychological symptoms and can require hospitalization or other inpatient treatment. Detoxification is the period of getting over physical withdrawal when an addict stops taking a drug, and medical management may be required to prevent serious health problems. Medications used for ongoing management of withdrawal include methadone or Suboxone. However, most treatment is psychological in nature.

Psychological treatment uses motivational interviewing. The most popular treatment programs are Narcotics Anonymous (NA) and Alcoholics Anonymous (AA) (Figure 11-1 ■). Often, members attend both programs' meetings because of their combined use of narcotics and alcohol. These programs use group therapy with addicts, family members, and peers. Additional individual psychotherapy and drug counseling may be used. Continuous urine tests are used to prevent the addict from relapsing, and recovering addicts are sometimes given financial or other incentives to stay clean.

Pharmacologic treatment involves substances that are used in lieu of the addictive substances, although this type of treatment is not used for hallucinogen or stimulant addicts. Methadone eliminates the physical cravings for heroin; Suboxone does the same but also makes the user ill if he or she tries to use heroin while taking this drug. Again, frequent urine toxicology screens are used to find if the addict is occasionally using his or her addictive substances.

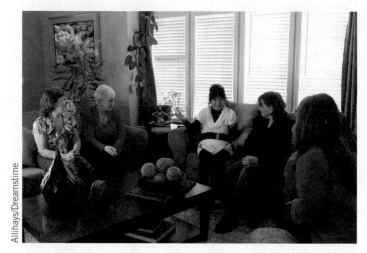

Figure 11-1 ■ Alcoholics Anonymous is one of the most popular treatment programs available for substance abusers.

✳ Apply Your Knowledge 11.3

The following questions focus on what you have just learned about the prevention and treatment of substance abuse.

CRITICAL THINKING

1. What are the risk factors for drug abuse?

2. What is the drug of choice to treat heroin addiction?

3. What is the role of schools regarding the prevention of addiction to substances?

CIGARETTE SMOKING

The single-largest cause of preventable death and illness in the United States is smoking. It is the most common addiction of all, and nicotine is highly addictive (Figure 11-2 ■). Continued consumption of tobacco despite significant physical, economic, or social side effects is termed **tobacco dependence**. The physical adverse effects of smoking are usually serious later in life and include cancer, emphysema, and heart attacks. Smoking-related cancers often attack certain people in their early 30s and often result in death. Nearly 20% of Americans smoke. Because it is legal, smoking is not perceived to be an addiction by many.

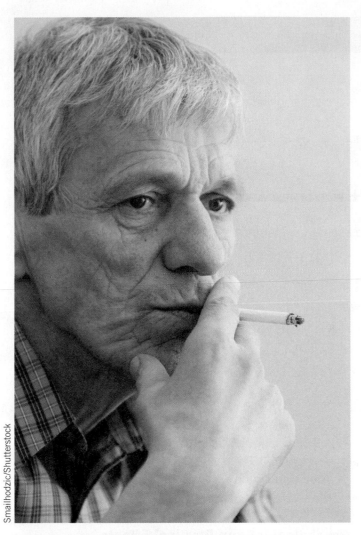

Smailhodzic/Shutterstock

Figure 11-2 ■ Smoking is the single-largest preventable cause of death and illness in the United States.

Nicotine is sometimes considered to be a CNS stimulant, but it is unique because of its legality, high potential for addiction, and carcinogenic effects. It affects most body systems, increasing alertness, ability to focus, and relaxation and causing lightheadedness. Directly stimulating the CNS, nicotine accelerates the heart rate and increases blood pressure and may result in muscular tremors in certain people. It also increases the basal metabolic rate, leading to weight loss and appetite reduction. Physical and psychologic dependence occur relatively quickly.

Withdrawal from nicotine causes anxiety, cravings, impaired attention, insomnia, continual thoughts about smoking, gastrointestinal disturbances, and headaches. Nicotine has been proven to be a psychoactive substance. The adverse effects of nicotine are caused by carbon monoxide levels, its addictive properties, irritants in the tar found in tobacco, and passive smoke inhalation.

Nearly 443,000 people die annually in the United States from various effects of smoking. Half of all Americans who continue to smoke will die from a smoking-related disease. Tobacco smoking affects all body systems but primarily the respiratory, cardiovascular, and nervous systems. Smoking is the major cause of lung cancer deaths. Lung cancer risk is 23 times greater in male smokers than in lifelong nonsmokers. Cancers throughout the body are much greater in occurrence as a result of smoking.

Those who do not die from smoking-related illnesses experience pneumonia, being chronically short of breath and sometimes having to be on a respiratory for much of their lives. Chronic smoking leads to heart disease and chronic obstructive pulmonary disorder. Statistically, one cigarette shortens the smoker's life by 5 minutes. Stopping smoking has many long-term health benefits. Because every body system is affected (in varying degrees) by the use of tobacco products, morbidity and mortality are greatly affected by the cessation of smoking.

Passive smoking involves sidestream smoke (from the end of the cigarette) and mainstream smoke (that which has been exhaled by the smoker). Passive smoking can affect a fetus via the mother's respiratory system, causing low birthweight, which can lead to neonatal death, stillbirth, and intellectual disabilities. Children of smokers have a higher incidence of bronchitis, pneumonia, asthma, middle ear problems, growth retardation, and sudden infant death syndrome.

On average, smoking reduces life expectancy by 14 years. For an average five-person family, smoking adds $4,213 to its budget per year. However, a total of 90% of smokers say they would like to quit. A further reason to quit is that insurance premiums of all types are lower for nonsmokers. The following reasons help to convince a person to quit:

✳ Those with familial history of cancers may have a higher risk level for contracting the disease themselves.

✳ Heart disease is greatly increased by smoking.

✳ Chronic lung disease will shorten the smoker's life.

✳ Lower back pain is greatly increased by smoking.

✳ Smoking repels many potential dates, girlfriends or boyfriends, wives or husbands, and so on.

✳ Smoking increases wrinkling and premature aging.

Smoking cessation techniques include:

✳ Smoking cessation clinics

✳ Literature about quitting techniques

✳ Nicotine replacements

✳ The drug bupropion

✳ The drug varenicline (Chantix)

✳ Drug counseling

✳ Hypnotherapy

✳ Acupuncture

✳ Progressive filters

✳ Employer-offered financial incentives

Focus Point

Cigarette Smoking

Tobacco smoke contains about 4,000 chemical agents, including more than 60 carcinogens (agents that cause cancer).

✳ Apply Your Knowledge 11.4

The following questions focus on what you have just learned about cigarette smoking.

CRITICAL THINKING

1. What are the serious complications of cigarette smoking later in life?
2. What are the effects of nicotine on the cardiovascular system?
3. What are the symptoms of withdrawal from nicotine?
4. What techniques are used for smoking cessation?
5. What are the benefits of stopping cigarette smoking?

ALCOHOLISM

Ethyl alcohol (commonly known as *alcohol*) is a widely abused drug that is legal and readily available. Alcohol has enormous economic, health, and social consequences. In small quantities, alcohol has been shown to reduce the risk of heart attack and stroke, but long-term abuse can have devastating effects. Alcohol is a CNS depressant that easily crosses the blood–brain barrier to cause effects within 5 to 30 minutes. Effects are based on the amount consumed and include relaxation, memory impairment, sedation, loss of coordination, decreased inhibition, and reduced judgment. Alcohol affects the breath of the user and increases blood flow to the face and cheeks as well as other parts of the body. It mimics the effects of many antidepressants, antianxiety agents, and sedatives, and health care personnel should verify which drugs a patient has consumed before any treatment. Also, mouthwashes containing alcohol can make the patient's breath smell from the drug—similar to the effects of drinking.

Alcohol is absorbed more slowly when there is food in the stomach. Detoxification of alcohol by the liver (*metabolism*) occurs slowly at a constant rate of about 15 mL per hour. This is essentially the same as one serving of alcohol per hour, which is based on the following:

* 12 fl oz of regular beer (about 5% alcohol)
* 8 to 9 fl oz of malt liquor (about 7% alcohol)
* 5 fl oz of wine (about 12% alcohol)
* 3 to 4 fl oz of fortified wine (sherry or port) (about 17% alcohol)
* 2 to 3 fl oz of an aperitif, cordial, or liqueur (about 24% alcohol)
* 1.5 fl oz of brandy or "hard liquor" (about 40% alcohol or more)

Psychological and Physical Effects of Alcoholism

Acute overdoses of alcohol cause vomiting, severe hypotension, respiratory failure, and coma. More than 85,000 Americans die every year due to alcohol use and related behaviors. High rates of alcohol consumption produce increased depressant effects on the brain. Alcohol should never be combined with other CNS depressants because effects are cumulative, resulting in profound sedation or coma. Withdrawal from alcohol is severe and potentially life threatening, causing anxiety, insomnia, or seizures. Long-term alcoholics may experience **delirium tremens (DT)**, commonly referred to as "the DTs." Symptoms include confusion, disorientation, agitation, hallucinations, anxiety, panic, a "crawling" sensation of the skin, and paranoia.

The liver is the most affected organ when chronic alcohol abuse occurs. *Cirrhosis* is the debilitating and potentially fatal failure of the liver to function normally. When the liver becomes impaired, blood clotting and nutritional states are affected. Liver impairment makes the organ more sensitive to all substances that it metabolizes. Patients should be honest with their physicians and nurses about their use of alcohol because dosage levels must be determined based on this information. When a patient does not admit his or her alcohol consumption correctly, dosage levels of medications may be too high to be processed and may harm the patient.

Treatment of Alcoholism

Patients with acute alcohol withdrawal are treated with such benzodiazepines as Valium or Librium as well as antiseizure medications. Additional treatments for

alcohol abuse include behavioral counseling, self-help groups (such as AA), and the drug disulfiram (Antabuse), which discourages relapses of alcohol use. Antabuse works by stopping the metabolism of alcohol, bringing about headache, nausea, and vomiting within 5 to 10 minutes after alcohol is consumed. After it is discontinued, the patient will be sensitive to alcohol consumption for an additional 2 weeks. Other agents used to treat patients with alcoholism include acamprosate calcium (Campral) and naltrexone (ReVia).

Focus Point

Consumption of Alcohol

Consuming more than one alcoholic drink per hour will usually result in blood alcohol levels above the legal limit for operating a vehicle.

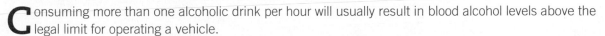

✳ Apply Your Knowledge 11.5

The following questions focus on what you have just learned about alcoholism.

CRITICAL THINKING

1. What are the benefits of small quantities of alcohol in the human body?
2. What are the symptoms of acute overdoses of alcohol?
3. Why should alcohol never be combined with other CNS depressants?
4. Which organ is most affected by chronic alcoholism?
5. What is the treatment of acute alcohol withdrawal?.

PRACTICAL SCENARIO 1

A 17-year-old female student begins to demonstrate signs of depression and irritability. She begins to spend more and more time alone in her room. She continually comes home later than she is supposed to. Several weeks later, her mother receives a phone call from the school when her daughter is found having convulsions on the restroom floor. The mother is instructed to go to the local hospital, where her daughter has been transported by ambulance. After several tests and verifying that the patient has had no history of epilepsy, the physician acknowledges that the girl has been using cocaine.

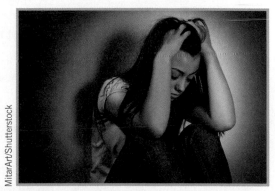

MitarArt/Shutterstock

Critical Thinking Questions
1. Why is substance abuse common amongst teenagers?
2. What are the common symptoms of an overdose of cocaine?

PRACTICAL SCENARIO 2

Suzanne was hired as a medical assistant at a family practice office. At the time she was hired, the office manager told her that the facility conducted random drug screening tests, and Suzanne signed an agreement indicating her compliance. After being employed for a few months, the physician noticed that Suzanne was occasionally behaving suspiciously while at work. She was sometimes late or did not show up to work without calling to let the office know. One day, she asked her physician if he could order a urine test for her because she suspected she was pregnant. He ordered the pregnancy test, and because he was suspicious of her recent behavior, also ordered tests for the presence of any drugs in her system. After 48 hours, the results came back. Suzanne was indeed pregnant, and the physician noticed that the drug test indicated the presence of nicotine and cocaine.

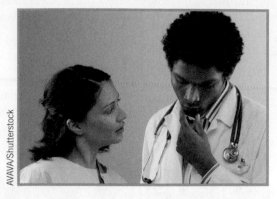

AVAVA/Shutterstock

Critical Thinking Questions

1. What do you think were the consequences of these events?
2. What are the adverse effects of nicotine and cocaine on a developing fetus?

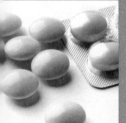

Chapter Capsule

Objective 1: Define *addiction* and list several factors on which it may be based.

- Addiction is defined as a progressive and chronic abuse of a substance that causes a person to use it repeatedly despite serious health and social consequences.
- Addiction may be based on the cost, availability, dose, and method of administration as well as risk-taking behavior, prior drug experience, certain diseases requiring the use of scheduled drugs, educational opportunities, and peer influences.

Objective 2: Identify the most commonly abused drugs in the United States.

- The most commonly abused drugs in the United States include alcohol, marijuana, sedatives, opioids, cocaine, hallucinogens, and methamphetamine.

Objective 3: List five substances that cause relaxation or sedation.

- Five substances that cause relaxation or sedation are barbiturates, nonbarbiturate sedative–hypnotics, benzodiazepines, opioids, and alcohol.

Objective 4: Explain opioid addiction and its withdrawal.

- Opioid addiction may develop rapidly. Methadone is often used to treat an addiction to other opioids because it does not produce the same degree of euphoria and has longer lasting effects.
- Opioid withdrawal is very unpleasant (although not life threatening compared with barbiturate withdrawal). Methadone is used, in part, to help heroin addicts withdraw with less unpleasant symptoms. Withdrawal from methadone itself—if a person becomes addicted—takes longer that that from heroin or morphine but with less intense symptoms.

Objective 5: Discuss cannabinoids and their effects on the central nervous system.

- Cannabinoids are obtained from the hemp plant (*Cannabis sativa*) and are usually smoked to obtain their effects. They include marijuana, hashish, and hash oil, with the most psychoactive agent being delta-9-tetrahydrocannabinol (THC).

- The effects of cannabinoids on the central nervous system include decreased coordination and motor activity, confusion, paranoia, and euphoria. Effects occur within a few minutes and last for up to 24 hours. The most commonly used cannabinoid—marijuana—produces very little physical dependence or tolerance, with withdrawal symptoms being nearly nonexistent.

Objective 6: Compare hallucinogens and opioid drugs.

- Hallucinogens produce altered, "dreamlike" consciousness and are all Schedule I drugs with no approved medical use. The prototype hallucinogen is LSD. Common effects include laughter, hallucinations or "visions," deep personal insight, afterimages, and religious "revelations." Other common effects include greatly intensified colors, lights, sounds, and other sensations.

- Opioid drugs are used for severe pain, diarrhea, and persistent cough. They are derived from unripe poppy seeds and include codeine, morphine, opium, and heroin. Oral opioids take effect within 30 minutes and can last for more than 1 day. Signs of use include a euphoric rush, intense sedation, abnormally slow body functions, constricted pupils, respiratory depression, and the ability to tolerate increased amounts of pain.

Objective 7: Explain the effects of substance abuse.

- Substance abuse may affect every level of a person's life. It is signified by a failure to fulfill parenting, school, or work obligations; hazardous behavior, such as driving under the influence; recurrent related legal problems, such as DUI; and continued use of substances despite continuing social or interpersonal problems.

- A person is "substance dependent" when he or she exhibits any three of these signs: tolerance; withdrawal; increasing consumption; desire to quit; excessive time spent on abuse; fewer occupational, recreational, or social activities; and continued use while understanding the physiologic and psychological effects.

Objective 8: Describe withdrawal from nicotine.

- Withdrawal from nicotine causes anxiety, cravings, impaired attention, insomnia, continual thoughts about smoking, gastrointestinal disturbances, and headaches.

Objective 9: Explain the psychological and physical effects of alcoholism.

- Psychological effects of alcoholism include increased depressant effects on the brain, sedation, confusion, disorientation, agitation, hallucinations, anxiety, panic, and paranoia.

- Physical effects of alcoholism include vomiting, severe hypotension, respiratory failure, potential coma, severe withdrawal symptoms, insomnia, seizures, delirium tremens, a crawling sensation of the skin, liver cirrhosis and liver failure, impaired blood clotting, and an impaired nutritional state.

Objective 10: Discuss signs and symptoms of withdrawal from alcohol.

■ Withdrawal from alcohol is severe and potentially life threatening, causing anxiety, insomnia, or seizures. Long-term alcoholics may experience "the DTs" (delirium tremens), which causes confusion, disorientation, agitation, hallucinations, anxiety, panic, crawling of the skin, and paranoia.

 Internet Sites of Interest

■ Hallucinogens: **http://emedicine.medscape.com/article/293752-overview**.

■ Cigarette smoking: **http://www.cancer.org/Cancer/CancerCauses/TobaccoCancer/ CigaretteSmoking/cigarette-smoking-toc**.

■ Marijuana Infofacts: **http://www.drugabuse.gov/infofacts/marijuana.html**.

■ The most addictive drugs: **http://www.michaelshouse.com/drug-addiction/most-addictive-drugs-world/**.

■ Substance abuse: **http://www.emedicinehealth.com/substance_abuse/article_em.htm**.

■ CNS stimulants: **http://www.faqs.org/health/topics/38/Central-nervous-system-stimulants.html**.

■ Prescription drug abuse and addiction: **http://www.nida.nih.gov/researchreports/prescription/prescription3.html**.

■ Alcoholism: **http://www.mayoclinic.com/health/alcoholism/DS00340**.

■ The Substance Abuse and Mental Health Services Administration: **http://www.samhsa.gov**.

PEARSON
myhealthprofessionskit™

Go to www.myhealthprofessionskit.com to access the Companion Website created for this textbook. Simply select "Basic Health Science" from the choice of disciplines. Find this book and then log in using your username and password to access interactive learning games, assessment questions, animations, and more.

Chapter Objectives

After completing the chapter, you should be able to:

1. Identify the major types of antibiotics by drug class.
2. Describe the principal mechanisms of action of cephalosporins, vancomycin, and isoniazid.
3. Outline the main adverse effects of macrolides, aminoglycosides, and chloramphenicol.
4. Contrast bactericidal and bacteriostatic actions.
5. List the first-line antituberculosis agents and two characteristic adverse effects of each drug.
6. Explain the classifications of cephalosporins.
7. Discuss the contraindications, precautions, and interactions of the penicillins and tetracyclines.
8. List three antiviral drugs for HIV- and AIDS-related secondary viral infections and explain their mechanisms of action.

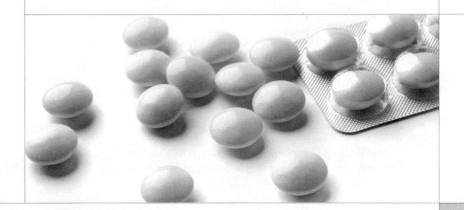

Key Terms

antibacterial spectrum (an-tie-bak-TEE-ree-ul SPEK-trum) (page 188)

antibiotics (an-tie-by-AW-tiks) (page 183)

antimicrobial (an-tie-my-KRO-bee-ul) (page 184)

bacteria (page 183)

bactericidal (bak-tee-ree-SY-dul) (page 184)

bacteriostatic (bak-tee-ree-oh-STAH-tik) (page 184)

broad-spectrum (page 190)

candidiasis (kan-dih-DIE-uh-sis) (page 194)

fungi (FUN-guy) (page 183)

gram-negative (page 188)

gram-positive (page 186)

immunocompromised (im-myoo-no-KOM-pro-miezd) (page 204)

nucleoside (NEW-clee-oh-sied) (page 203)

parasites (PAH-rah-syts) (page 183)

pathogenic (pah-thoh-JEH-nik) (page 182)

serum sickness (page 186)

subtherapeutic doses (page 183)

viruses (page 183)

Introduction

Infection is the most common cause of death for many people afflicted with a chronic or critical illness, with the very young and the very old being particularly susceptible. Infections are caused by microorganisms that gain entry into the body. After a microorganism invades the human body, the signs and symptoms generally associated with infection are generated, including fever and an elevated white blood cell (WBC) count. The microorganisms that cause infection and disease are called *pathogens*, and the major types of microorganisms that can cause infection include bacteria, viruses, fungi, and parasites, which are defined further in this chapter.

Different pathogens inhabit various environments, such as hospitals, the food supply, water, and animals or humans. Globalization of the world's population and faster air travel to nearly every spot on Earth have major implications for the worldwide spread of infectious agents. Rapidly spreading infections may be particularly dangerous to populations when infected individuals are asymptomatic for long periods or the infection itself is difficult to identify for other reasons.

Infection with **pathogenic** (disease-causing) microorganisms has become a tool of war and terrorism throughout the world. Weapons of mass destruction may be nuclear, chemical, or biological in nature. Whether the situation involves anthrax spores sent through the mail or the threat of smallpox being introduced to a nonimmunized population, the various methods of preventing infections have key roles in the defense of humanity. Health-care professionals play a vital part in the prevention, early detection, and management of infections.

Transmission of Infection

Transmission of disease requires a chain of events that must occur unbroken to allow one human to infect another. The pathogenic organism must live and reproduce in a reservoir (Figure 12-1 ■). The reservoir may be a human being, as with the influenza virus; an animal, as in bats with rabies; or soil, as in enterobiasis (pinworm infection).

The pathogen must have a portal of exit, with a mode of transmission from the reservoir to a susceptible victim. For example, *Neisseria gonorrhoeae*—the organism that is responsible for gonorrhea—usually resides in the urethra of the male and the vaginal canal of the female. The microorganism is transmitted by sexual contact.

Control of infectious disease occurrence depends on breaking this chain of transmission in one or more places (Figure 12-2 ■). A pathogen can be vulnerable

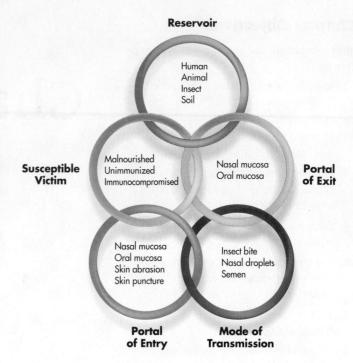

Figure 12-1 ■ Chain of transmission of microorganisms from host to victim.

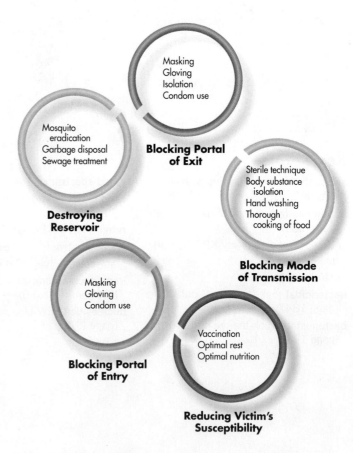

Figure 12-2 ■ Breaking the chain of transmission of microorganisms from host to victim.

in one or more links of the transmission chain. Some pathogens, such as bacteria, are susceptible to direct attack with antibiotics. Antibiotics are designed to directly kill the pathogen or hold it in check so the body's defenses can eradicate it. Some microorganisms have developed resistance to **antibiotics** (substances produced by microorganisms that in low concentrations are able to inhibit or kill other microorganisms) through repeated exposure to **subtherapeutic doses** (doses that are below the level used to treat diseases) and use of antibiotics for nonbacterial infections. This *antibiotic resistance* is a major threat to the success of the management of bacterial infections.

Destroying nonhuman reservoirs and vectors of the pathogen can also break the chain of transmission. For example, controlling the number of mosquitoes with insecticides is a method used to curb the spread of malaria and West Nile virus (see Chapter 13). Blocking the portal of exit can also block transmission of the pathogen. Having patients with tuberculosis (TB) wear masks as they move through the hospital and implementing respiratory isolation techniques to stop droplet transmission are interventions aimed at blocking the portal of exit.

Finally, host susceptibility is an important aspect of the transmission of a pathogen. Such factors as age, gender, ethnic group, and genetic makeup affect the susceptibility of the host. Although these factors cannot be changed, improving the host's immune system by improving his or her nutritional status, decreasing stress, and limiting fatigue can decrease the host's susceptibility to infection. Immunization of the host also has a key role in blocking the transmission of infection and provides active immunity, thus allowing the creation of host antibodies to help prevent future infections. In contrast, immunoglobulin given to the host can provide passive immunity to some infections, allowing for short-term prevention of disease transmission or infection.

Antibiotic use has had a tremendous impact on the way microorganisms respond to various agents. Using subtherapeutic doses of or overusing antibiotics can affect the resistance that microorganisms have to them. Resistance may be altered because of mutation (a change in gene chemistry that continues in subsequent cell divisions) or by the continuous exposure of a microbe to an antibiotic.

Focus Point

Handwashing Reduces Transmission

Frequent handwashing with soap, friction, and warm running water is one of the most effective ways to reduce pathogenic transmission.

Types of Microorganisms

The four basic types of microorganisms that can be helpful or pathogenic to the host are:

1. **Bacteria:** single-celled organisms with a cell wall and cellular organelles that allow them to live independently in the environment

2. **Viruses:** tiny genetic parasites that require the host cell to replicate and spread

3. **Fungi:** nonphotosynthetic, eukaryotic single- or multicellular organisms that are found throughout the environment; fungi have a cell wall containing sterol

4. **Parasites:** protozoa, roundworms, flatworms, and arthropods

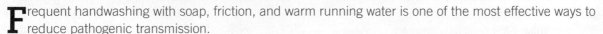

✳ Apply Your Knowledge 12.1

The following questions test your understanding of the transmission of infection and the types of microorganisms.

CRITICAL THINKING

1. How can infectious disease be controlled?
2. What are "weapons of mass destruction"? Name two examples.
3. What is the chain of transmission of infectious diseases?
4. What are pathogens? Name four classes of these microorganisms.
5. What are subtherapeutic doses?

Antibacterial Agents

Little distinction exists today between the terms *antibiotic* and **antimicrobial** (referring to an agent that tends to destroy microbes, prevent their multiplication or growth, or prevent their pathogenic action). The most common sources of natural antibiotics are molds and bacteria. Antibiotics are produced by one microorganism and inhibit the growth of others. However, many antibiotics are now partially or wholly synthesized in commercial laboratories. Included in this group are the penicillins, cephalosporins, aminoglycosides, tetracyclines, and macrolides. Important synthetic antibacterial agents, including nitrofurantoin and the quinolones, are also used clinically.

Antibiotics inhibit the growth of or kill microorganisms when given in sufficient concentrations—ideally, low enough to exert their effect but remain harmless to the host. Systemic antibacterial agents can be **bactericidal** (capable of killing microbes) or **bacteriostatic** (capable of inhibiting microbial growth) but also rely on host defenses to aid in eliminating bacterial pathogens.

Antibiotics were discovered in 1928 when Sir Alexander Fleming was performing research on influenza. One year later, he found penicillin by culturing the mold *Penicillium notatum*. In 1938, British researchers studied the effects of natural penicillins on infectious disease. In 1941, natural penicillins were used clinically for the treatment of infections.

Factors to consider when selecting antibiotics for therapy in patients should include identification of:

✳ Likely or specific microorganisms
✳ Antimicrobial susceptibility
✳ Bactericidal versus bacteriostatic properties
✳ Host status, such as allergy history, age, pharmacokinetic factors, renal and hepatic function, pregnancy status, anatomic site of infection, and host defenses

Focus On

Sulfonamides

Sulfanilamides (sulfa drugs) are antibacterial agents that were first synthesized in 1908, but it was many years before their therapeutic value was discovered. In 1937, researchers in England synthesized sulfapyridine, which was the first sulfonamide used with great success in combating pneumonia. After that, a large number of other sulfonamides, such as sulfathiazole and sulfadiazine, were synthesized. Today, sulfamethoxazole is the most commonly used sulfonamide and is usually combined with trimethoprim and abbreviated SMZ/TMP.

The sulfonamides and trimethoprim act by inhibiting the folic acid synthesis that most bacteria require. Although humans rely on dietary sources for the folic acid they need, most bacteria must synthesize it on their own. Sulfonamides were the first antimicrobial agents, but their clinical use has been greatly restricted as a result of the development of resistant bacteria, their significant side effects, and the availability of other drugs. The sulfonamides are no longer preferred for the treatment of urinary tract infections (UTIs) but are still important and effective for some infections. This is particularly true for new sulfa drugs. Table 12-1 ■ lists the various sulfa drugs.

How do they work?

The mechanism of the antimicrobial action of the sulfonamides has been analyzed extensively. These agents block a specific step in the biosynthetic pathway of folic acid. They are primarily bacteriostatic, meaning that they slow the multiplication of bacteria. Bacteria cannot absorb folic acid; therefore, it is made from precursors, specifically para-aminobenzoic acid (PABA). The sulfonamides interfere with PABA and folic acid formation, thereby destroying the bacteria. The efficacy of sulfonamides is generally enhanced when the drugs are used in combination with trimethoprim, which inhibits the conversion of dihydrofolate to folinic acid.

How are they used?

Sulfonamide therapy alone has a minor place in the treatment of patients with infectious diseases. Major advantages of sulfonamides are their low cost and ease of administration. The combination of trimethoprim with sulfamethoxazole is the treatment of choice for most UTIs, otitis media (especially in children), sinusitis, some lower respiratory infections, and ulcerative colitis.

What are the adverse effects?

Major disadvantages of sulfonamides are their untoward effects (blood dyscrasias, crystalluria, hematuria, and life-threatening hepatitis). However, the new sulfa drugs in use today cause fewer allergic reactions than do the older drugs. Sulfonamides may cause several adverse effects, such as aplastic anemia, leukopenia, thrombocytopenia, and even agranulocytosis. Loss of appetite is a common mild adverse effect, with nausea, vomiting, diarrhea, fever, stomatitis (inflammation of the mouth), and photosensitivity also being seen. Crystalluria may occur during use of older sulfonamides but may be helped by increased fluid intake on the part of patients throughout therapy.

What are the contraindications and interactions?

Sulfonamides must be avoided in patients with known hypersensitivity, during lactation, and in children younger than 2 years of age. These drugs are contraindicated near the end of pregnancy.

Sulfonamides may interact with oral anticoagulants and cause increased anticoagulant effects. Sulfonamides accompanied by methotrexate may increase the risk of bone marrow suppression. These agents may prevent the metabolism of oral hypoglycemic drugs, resulting in an increase of hypoglycemic reaction. When a sulfonamide is administered with a hydantoin, the serum hydantoin level may be increased.

What are the important points patients should know?

Instruct patients to take sulfonamide drugs on an empty stomach either 1 hour before or 2 hours after a meal with a full glass of water (at least eight to ten 8-oz glasses of water should be consumed every day). Instruct patients to complete the full course of therapy and avoid prolonged exposure to sunlight, which may result in a skin reaction that is similar to severe sunburn.

Table 12-1 ■ Various Sulfa Drugs

GENERIC NAME	TRADE NAME	AVERAGE DOSAGE IN ADULTS	ROUTE OF ADMINISTRATION
mafenide	Sulfamylon	Apply to burned area 1–2 times/d	Topical
silver sulfadiazine	Silvadene, Thermazene, SSD (cream)	Apply to burned area 1–2 times/d	Topical
sulfadiazine	Sulfadiazine	Loading dose: 2–4 g; maintenance dose: 2–4 g/d in 4–6 divided doses	PO
sulfamethizole	Thiosulfil Forte	0.5–1 g tid–qid	PO
sulfamethoxazole	Gantanol	Initial dose: 2 g; maintenance dose: 1 g bid–tid	PO
sulfasalazine	Azulfidine	Initial dose: 1–4 g/d in divided doses; maintenance dose: 2 g/d in evenly spaced doses of 500 mg qid	PO
sulfisoxazole	Gantrisin	Loading dose: 2–4 g; maintenance dose: 4–8 g/d in 4–6 divided doses	PO
trimethoprim (TMP) and sulfamethoxazole (SMZ)	Bactrim, Septra	160 mg TMP/800 mg SMZ q12h	PO
		8–10 mg/kg/d (based on TMP) in 2–4 divided doses	IV

IV, intravenous; PO, oral; qid, four times a day; tid, three times a day.

Focus On

Penicillins

The name *penicillin* now designates a number of antibiotic substances produced by the growth of various *Penicillium spp.* or by other means. The penicillins are listed in Table 12-2 ■.

How do they work?

Penicillin interferes with the synthesis of peptidoglycans—important building blocks of bacterial cell walls. The penicillins may be bactericidal or bacteriostatic.

(Continued)

Focus On (Continued)

. . . .

There are four classes of penicillins: (1) natural penicillins, (2) penicillinase-resistant penicillins, (3) aminopenicillins, and (4) extended-spectrum penicillins.

How are they used?

Although penicillin G is the original penicillin, it remains the drug of choice for the treatment of almost all infections caused by nonpenicillinase-producing and non–methicillin-resistant **gram-positive** bacteria (those that have the ability to resist decolorization with alcohol after being treated with Gram's crystal violet stain that imparts a violent color to the bacterium when viewed by microscope). Penicillin is the drug of choice against infections by gram-positive, nonpenicillinase-producing *cocci*, such as *Staphylococcus aureus, Staphylococcus epidermidis*, and *Streptococcus* group B. Therefore, penicillins can be used for UTIs, gonorrhea, syphilis, septicemia, meningitis, pneumonia, and other respiratory infections. Because of penicillinase-producing organisms, many skin and other types of infections must be treated with an extended-spectrum penicillin—sometimes along with another drug.

What are the adverse effects?

Penicillin is a very safe drug in most cases, with low toxicity. However, hypersensitivity reactions may occur in a low percentage of patients. The most common manifestation of this allergic response is a raised, itchy skin rash, **serum sickness** (a reaction to a foreign serum), angioedema and difficulty breathing, and nephropathy.

Side effects of oral administration of penicillins are nausea, vomiting, diarrhea, and a black "hairy" tongue (temporary overgrowth of harmless bacteria or yeast in the mouth). A nonallergic and harmless rash may also occur during amoxicillin therapy and is differentiated from a true hypersensitivity reaction based on the absence of a raised or itchy rash. Very high concentrations of penicillin are neurotoxic, and nerve damage has resulted from intramuscular (IM) administration.

What are the contraindications and interactions?

Penicillins are contraindicated in patients with a history of hypersensitivity to penicillin or the cephalosporins. The drugs should be used cautiously in patients with renal disease or during pregnancy and lactation. Some penicillins, such as penicillin V and ampicillin, may interfere with the effectiveness of birth control pills that contain estrogen. The effectiveness of penicillin decreases when it is used with the tetracyclines because penicillin is bactericidal and requires actively producing bacteria for full effect (whereas the tetracyclines are bacteriostatic). Absorption of most penicillins is affected by food. They should be given 1 hour before or 2 hours after meals.

What are the important points patients should know?

Advise patients to take penicillin on an empty stomach (1 hour before or 2 hours after meals) to facilitate absorption. Note that amoxicillin may be taken with meals to decrease gastric upsets. Hypersensitivity may occur after oral administration of penicillin, so advise the patient to discontinue the medication and immediately contact his or her physician.

Table 12-2 ◼ Penicillins

GENERIC NAME	TRADE NAME	AVERAGE DOSAGE IN ADULTS	ROUTE OF ADMINISTRATION
Natural Penicillins			
penicillin G (aqueous)	Pfizerpen	≤20–30 million units/d; dosage may also be based on weight	IV or IM
penicillin G benzathine	Bicillin L-A	≤2.4 million units/d	IM
penicillin G procaine, IM	Wycillin	600,000–2.4 million units/d	IM
penicillin V	Beepen VK, Pen-Vee-K	125–500 mg q6h or q8h	PO

GENERIC NAME	TRADE NAME	AVERAGE DOSAGE IN ADULTS	ROUTE OF ADMINISTRATION
Semisynthetic Penicillins, Penicillinase-Resistant Penicillins			
cloxacillin	Cloxapen, Tegopen	250–500 mg q6h	PO
dicloxacillin	Dynapen, Dycill, Pathocil	125–250 mg q6h	PO
nafcillin	Unipen, Nallpen	250 mg–1,250 mg/d	PO
		500 mg q4–6h	IM
		3–6 g/d for 24–48h only	IV
oxacillin	Bactocill	500 mg–1 g q4–6h	PO
		250 mg–1 g q4–6h	IM, IV
Aminopenicillins			
amoxicillin	Amoxil, Trimox, Wymox	250–500 mg q8h or 875 mg bid	PO
amoxicillin and clavulanate acid	Augmentin	250–500 mg q8h or 875 mg q12h	PO
ampicillin (oral)	Omnipen, Principen, Totacillin	250–500 mg q6h	PO
ampicillin (parenteral)	Omnipen-N	1–12 g/d in divided doses q4–6h	IM, IV
ampicillin/sulbactam	Unasyn	0.5–1 g sulbactam with 1–2 g ampicillin q6–8h	IM, IV
bacampicillin	Spectrobid	400–800 mg q12h; dosage may also be based on weight	PO
Extended-Spectrum Penicillins			
mezlocillin	Mezlin	200–300 mg/kg/d in 4–6 divided doses; ≤350 mg/kg/d	IM, IV
piperacillin and tazobactam	Zosyn	12 mg /1.5 g given as 3.375 g q6h	IV
piperacillin	Pipracil	3–4 g q4–6h; maximum dosage, 25 g/d	IM, IV
ticarcillin	Ticar	150–300 mg/kg/d q3h, q4h, or q6h; 24 g/d	IM
		150–300 mg/kg/d q3h, q4h, or q6h; maximum dosage, 2 g/d	IV
ticarcillin and clavulanate	Timentin	3.1 g q4–6h or 200–300 mg/kg/d in divided doses q4–6h	IV

bid, twice a day; IM, intramuscular; IV, intravenous; PO, oral.

Focus Point

Penicillin Allergy

An allergic reaction to penicillin is an immediate life-threatening systemic reaction that typically occurs after exposure to penicillin injection. The patient must be closely observed for this reaction after injection.

Focus On

Cephalosporins

The cephalosporins are a group of antibiotics closely related to the penicillins. Currently, they are classified into four generations based on their **gram-negative** spectrum and stability in the presence of beta-lactamases (agents that retard the action of enzymes). Gram-negative bacteria cannot resist decolorization with alcohol after being treated with Gram's crystal violet. After decolorization, they can be readily counterstained with safranin, which gives them a pink or red color when viewed under a microscope. However, this classification scheme is becoming less reliable because newer agents have led to more exceptions and less precise criteria for differences in the **antibacterial spectrum** (the range of bacteria against which an agent is effective). Whereas those with a broad spectrum are effective against many different kinds of bacteria, those with a narrow spectrum may be effective against only a single type or a few (Table 12-3 ■).

The different generations of cephalosporins are explained below:

✳ First generation: Exhibit highest activity against gram-positive bacteria and lowest activity against gram-negative bacteria
✳ Second generation: Are more active against gram-negative bacteria and less active against gram-positive bacteria than first-generation cephalosporins
✳ Third generation: Are considerably less active than first-generation agents against gram-positive bacteria (especially staphylococci), have a much expanded spectrum of activity against gram-negative organisms, and are more resistant to gram-negative beta-lactamases
✳ Fourth generation: Have improved gram-positive spectrum and expanded gram-negative activity of third-generation cephalosporins

How do they work?

The cephalosporins have a mechanism of action that is very similar to that of the penicillins. They affect the bacterial cell wall and are bactericidal, resulting in the destruction of bacteria.

How are they used?

The cephalosporins are effective against a wide variety of infections because they have a broad spectrum. The first- and second-generation cephalosporins are used frequently for prophylaxis during certain surgical procedures to reduce the risk of postoperative wound infections. Cefazolin is preferred because it has a higher serum concentration and longer elimination half-life. A number of second- and third-generation cephalosporins are effective alternatives as prophylactic agents for various surgical procedures. Cephalosporins are generally not the first drugs of choice for any bacterial infections because equally effective and less expensive alternatives are available.

What are the adverse effects?

Hypersensitivity occurs in about 5% to 10% of patients taking cephalosporins; manifestations are drug fever, skin rash, urticaria (hives), serum sickness, anaphylaxis, neutropenia, and nephritis. Other adverse effects of cephalosporins include pain, sterile abscess, nausea, vomiting, glossitis, diarrhea, and abdominal pain. Cephalosporins have a 5% to 10% cross-sensitivity with penicillins.

What are the contraindications and interactions?

Cephalosporins should not be used in combination with other antibiotics that cause nephrotoxicity or ototoxicity. Such diuretics as furosemide and ethacrynic acid also enhance nephrotoxicity and make certain cephalosporins ototoxic. Estrogen-containing oral contraceptives and cephalosporins taken concurrently may result in therapeutic failure.

What are the important points patients should know?

Instruct patients to take cephalosporins on an empty stomach. If gastric irritation occurs, patients may take these drugs with food.

Table 12-3 ■ Cephalosporins

GENERIC NAME	TRADE NAME	AVERAGE DOSAGE IN ADULTS	ROUTE OF ADMINISTRATION
First Generation			
cefadroxil	Duricef	500 mg–1 g/d	PO
cefazolin	Ancef, Kefzol, Zolicef	250 mg–1 g/d	IM or IV
cephalexin	Keflex	25 mg–1 g/d	PO
cephalothin	Cephalonia	50 mg–2 g/d	IV
cephapirin	Cefadyl	25 mg–4 g/d	PO
cephradine	Velosef	250 mg/d	PO, IM, or IV
Second Generation			
cefaclor	Ceclor	125–500 mg/d	PO
cefonicid	Monocid	50 mg–12 g/d	IM or IV
cefoxitin	Mefoxin	2 g/d	IV
cefuroxime	Ceftin	125–500 mg/d	PO
Third Generation			
cefixime	Suprax	100–400 mg/d	PO
cefoperazone	Cefobid	1–6 g/d	IM or IV
cefotaxime moxalactam	Claforan	75 mg–4 g/d	IV
cefprozil	Cefzil	250–500 mg/d	PO
ceftriaxone	Rocephin	1–2 g/d	IV
Fourth Generation			
cefepime	Maxipime	500 mg–2 g/d	IM or IV

IM, intramuscular; IV, intravenous; PO, oral.

✳ Apply Your Knowledge 12.2

The following questions focus on what you have just learned about sulfonamides, penicillins, and cephalosporins.

CRITICAL THINKING

1. Define the terms *bacteriostatic* and *bactericidal*.
2. What is the mechanism of action of the sulfonamides?
3. What are the characteristics of gram-positive bacteria?
4. What are the characteristics of the four generations of cephalosporins?

Superinfections

Superinfections may be caused by a disruption of the nonpathogenic microorganisms within the human body (also known as *normal flora*) that is often attributed to the use of antibiotics. When antibiotics destroy large numbers of normal flora, the chemical environment of the body is altered and a new infection is "superimposed" on an original infection (hence the term *superinfection*). The altered chemical environment allows for the uncontrolled growth of microorganisms (fungal or bacterial) that are not affected by the antibiotic in use. Superinfections may occur with any antibiotic—most often when antibiotics are used for long periods or over repeated therapy courses.

Superinfections can develop rapidly and become very serious or even life threatening. Oral penicillins and cephalosporins often cause bacterial superinfections in the bowel, characterized by diarrhea (or bloody diarrhea), abdominal cramping, fever, and rectal bleeding. A common bacterial superinfection is *pseudomembranous colitis*. Penicillins and cephalosporins are commonly associated with vaginal yeast infections.

Focus on Geriatrics

The Risk of Superinfection among Elderly Patients

Older patients taking penicillin over a long period and those who are chronically ill or debilitated are more likely to contract a superinfection such as pseudomembranous colitis. This condition is potentially life threatening and produces a toxin that affects the lining of the colon. Signs and symptoms include abdominal cramping and severe diarrhea containing visible blood and mucus. Use of antibiotics should be discontinued, and severe cases may require treatment with intravenous (IV) fluids and electrolytes, oral vancomycin, and protein supplements.

Focus On

Aminoglycosides

Aminoglycosides have been very important antibiotics for the treatment of infections caused by gram-negative bacilli. They are **broad-spectrum** antibiotics (effective against a wide range of organisms). The clinically important aminoglycosides are amikacin (Amikin), gentamicin (Garamycin), kanamycin (Kantrex), neomycin (Mycifradin), netilmicin (Netromycin), streptomycin, and tobramycin (Nebcin). Table 12-4 ■ lists various aminoglycosides.

How do they work?

The aminoglycosides combine with bacterial (not human) ribosomes to arrest protein synthesis. This interference prevents cell reproduction, resulting in death of the bacteria.

How are they used?

Large doses of aminoglycosides are given orally before abdominal surgery to reduce the number of intestinal bacteria. The usual route of administration for systemic effects is either IM or IV. Aminoglycosides are also commonly administered via the ophthalmic or otic route in the form of eye or ear drops to treat localized infections.

What are the adverse effects?

The serious adverse effects of aminoglycosides include ototoxicity and nephrotoxicity. Nephrotoxicity may occur, depending on renal function, the age of the patient, and the drug dose. Careful drug dosing is very important with younger and older patients. Prolonged use of aminoglycosides may cause a superinfection.

What are the contraindications and interactions?

Aminoglycosides should not be used during pregnancy because they may cause fetal harm, particularly hearing loss and deafness in newborn babies. When aminoglycosides are used concurrently with penicillins, the desired effects of the aminoglycosides may be greatly decreased. Still, these drugs are often used in combination, especially in the treatment of bacterial endocarditis. These drugs should be given several hours apart. The drug action of warfarin (an oral anticoagulant) can increase if taken simultaneously with aminoglycosides. The risk of ototoxicity increases when ethacrynic acid and aminoglycosides are given.

What are the important points patients should know?

Instruct patients to increase fluid intake while taking aminoglycosides. This measure assists in preventing renal failure from nephrotoxicity. To minimize toxicity problems, short treatment periods (7–10 days) and once-daily administration should be used.

Table 12-4 ■ Aminoglycosides

GENERIC NAME	TRADE NAME	AVERAGE DOSAGE IN ADULTS	ROUTE OF ADMINISTRATION
amikacin	Amikin	15 mg/kg/d in 2–3 divided doses	IV or IM
gentamicin	Garamycin	3–5 mg/kg/d (standard dose)	IM
		6–7 mg/kg/d (once daily)	IV PO
kanamycin	Kantrex	15 mg/kg/d q8–12h	PO, IM, or IV
neomycin	Mycifradin	50–100 mg/kg/d	PO
		10–15 mg/d	Topical
netilmicin	Netromycin	3–6 mg/kg/d	IV or IM
streptomycin	Streptomycin	0.5–1 g q12–24h	IM
tobramycin	Nebcin	3–5 mg/kg/d (standard dose)	IV, IM, or ophthalmic
vancomycin	Vancocin	6–7 mg/kg/d (once daily)	PO or IV

IM, intramuscular; IV, intravenous; PO, oral.

Focus On

Macrolides

The term *macrolide* refers to the large chemical ring structure characteristic of these antibiotics. The macrolides include erythromycin (E-mycin, others), azithromycin (Zithromax), clarithromycin (Biaxin), troleandomycin (Tao), and dirithromycin (Dynabac). Erythromycin is produced by *Streptomyces erythreus*. Macrolides are bacteriostatic at normal doses and bactericidal at higher doses. They are also commonly used as alternative drugs in patients who are allergic to penicillin because they are effective against many of the same organisms. Table 12-5 ■ lists common macrolides. The macrolides are active against gram-positive and gram-negative aerobic bacteria and atypical organisms, including chlamydiae, mycoplasmae, legionellae, rickettsia, and spirochetes.

How do they work?

The mechanism of action of the macrolides is inhibition of bacterial protein synthesis by binding to the bacterial ribosome, which stops bacterial growth. Macrolides bind equally to ribosomes from gram-positive and gram-negative bacteria.

How are they used?

Macrolides are indicated for treatment of bacterial-related exacerbations of chronic obstructive pulmonary disease, skin structure infections, pharyngitis, tonsillitis, sinusitis, bronchitis, other respiratory tract infections, pneumonia, acute otitis media, duodenal ulcers, pelvic inflammatory disease, intestinal amebiasis, rheumatic fever, soft tissue infections, urethritis, syphilis, Legionnaires' disease, UTIs, and rectal infections.

What are the adverse effects?

In general, the macrolides are considered safe agents. Gastrointestinal (GI) effects, such as abdominal pain, nausea, and vomiting, are the most common adverse effects. The newer macrolides cause fewer GI side effects. Hepatotoxicity related to the use of the macrolides is rare but may be serious. Extremely high doses of IV erythromycin and oral clarithromycin have been associated with ototoxicity. Phlebitis may occur with IV administration of the macrolides.

What are the contraindications and interactions?

Macrolides are contraindicated in patients with hypersensitivity to them. They must be avoided in individuals who have a history of erythromycin-associated hepatitis

(Continued)

Focus On (Continued)

or liver dysfunction. Erythromycin inhibits the hepatic metabolism of theophylline. It may interfere with the metabolism of digoxin, corticosteroids, and cyclosporine. In fact, drug interaction between macrolides and cyclosporine and the resulting toxicity has led to the removal of several drugs from the market in the United States.

What are the important points patients should know?

Instruct patients to take oral macrolides with a full glass of water on an empty stomach (1 hour before or 2 hours after meals) to get the maximum effect. Enteric-coated, sustained-release preparations can be administered with food and are often prescribed for patients with a GI intolerance.

Table 12-5 ■ Commonly Used Macrolides

GENERIC NAME	TRADE NAME	AVERAGE DOSAGE IN ADULTS	ROUTE OF ADMINISTRATION
azithromycin	Zithromax	5–2,000 mg	PO
clarithromycin	Biaxin	7.5–500 mg	PO
dirithromycin	Dynabac	250 mg	PO
erythromycin base	Eryc, E-mycin	250 mg	PO
erythromycin estolate	Ilosone	30 mg–1 g	IM, IV, or PO
erythromycin stearate	Erythrocin	30 mg–1 g	IV or PO
troleandomycin	Tao	125–500 mg	PO

IM, intramuscular; IV, intravenous; PO, oral.

❊ Apply Your Knowledge 12.3

The following questions focus on generic and trade names of antibacterial and antiviral drugs.

CRITICAL THINKING
1. How do aminoglycosides work?
2. What are the trade names of gentamicin, kanamycin, netilmicin, and tobramycin?
3. What are the mechanisms of action of the macrolides?
4. What are the generic names of Biaxin, Ilosone, and Zithromax?
5. What are the important points patients should know about macrolides?

Focus On

Fluoroquinolones

The antibacterial drugs known as quinolones have been in use since 1964, when nalidixic acid was released. Since 1990, the fluoroquinolones have become a dominant class of bactericidal antimicrobial agents.

In general, the fluoroquinolones possess activity against gram-positive, gram-negative, and atypical organisms. The older fluoroquinolones (ciprofloxacin [Cipro], norfloxacin [Noroxin], and ofloxacin [Floxin]) are highly active against gram-negative pathogens, but their activity against gram-positive pathogens is limited. The newer fluoroquinolones have enhanced activity against the gram-positive pathogens while maintaining similar gram-negative activity (Table 12-6 ■).

How do they work?

The fluoroquinolones exert their bactericidal effect by interfering with an enzyme (DNA gyrase) that is required by bacteria for the synthesis of DNA. This action inhibits cell reproduction, resulting in the death of the bacteria.

How are they used?

The fluoroquinolones have a broad spectrum of antimicrobial activity. They are used to treat UTIs, prostatitis, gonorrhea, anthrax, pneumonia and other respiratory tract infections, and infections of bones and joints.

What are the adverse effects?

Adverse effects are usually mild and transient. They include nausea, vomiting, diarrhea, flatulence, abdominal discomfort, skin rashes, photosensitivity (especially severe with sparfloxacin), and some nephrotoxicity. Rare but severe reactions that have also been reported include neuropsychiatric effects, cardiac abnormalities, and liver dysfunction. In children, fluoroquinolones may damage developing cartilage.

What are the contraindications and interactions?

Fluoroquinolones should be avoided in children younger than 18 years and in pregnant or lactating women. When fluoroquinolones are used with caffeine, such symptoms as insomnia and hyperactivity may occur. Antacids decrease the absorption of the drug and should not be given for 2 hours after the administration of the antibiotic.

What are the important points patients should know?

Advise patients that fluoroquinolones should not be taken with milk or other dairy products, antacids, magnesium laxatives, or iron supplements. Advise patients to drink adequate fluids to maintain a high urine output, thereby preventing crystalluria. Instruct patients to report visual disturbances, dizziness, lightheadedness, or depression that may indicate potential early central nervous system (CNS) toxicity. If these manifestations occur, advise patients to avoid driving and operating heavy machinery and to report the effects immediately. Alcohol may worsen these effects and should be avoided.

Table 12-6 ■ Fluoroquinolones

GENERIC NAME	TRADE NAME	AVERAGE DOSAGE IN ADULTS	ROUTE OF ADMINISTRATION
Classical Fluoroquinolones			
ciprofloxacin	Cipro	500–750 mg q12h (PO) 400 mg q12h (IV)	PO, IV
enoxacin	Penetrex	200–400 mg q12h for 1–2 wk	PO
levofloxacin	Levaquin	PO: 250–500 mg/d; IV: 25 mg/mL	PO, IV
lomefloxacin	Maxaquin	400 mg/d for 2 wk	PO
nalidixic acid	NegGram	500 mg (tablet form) and 300 mg/5 mL (suspension form)*	PO
norfloxacin	Noroxin	400 mg q12h for 3 d	PO
ofloxacin	Floxin	200–400 mg q12h	PO
Newest Fluoroquinolones			
gatifloxacin	Tequin	PO: 400 mg/d for 7–14 d; IV: 400 mg/40 mL	PO, IV
moxifloxacin	Avelox	400 mg/d for 5–10 d	PO
sparfloxacin	Zagam	Loading dose: 400 mg on day 1; then 200 mg/d for 10 d	PO
trovafloxacin	Trovan	100 mg	PO

*Most antibiotic suspensions such as this example should be refrigerated after constitution.

IM, intramuscular; IV, intravenous; PO, oral.

Focus on Pediatrics

Avoid Fluoroquinolones in Children

Fluoroquinolones should be avoided in children because studies in young animals have documented the erosion of cartilage. However, these agents have been used safely in children with cystic fibrosis without harm.

Focus On

Tetracyclines

The tetracyclines are all very much alike with respect to their antimicrobial spectra and the untoward effects they elicit. They differ mainly in their absorption, duration of action, and suitability for parenteral administration (Table 12-7 ■).

How do they work?

The tetracyclines are broad-spectrum antibiotics and are mainly bacteriostatic. They bind to the bacterial ribosomes and prevent protein synthesis. The tetracyclines have activities against gram-positive and gram-negative bacteria, mycobacteria, rickettsia, and chlamydiae.

How are they used?

The tetracyclines are used in the treatment of infections caused by a wide range of microorganisms. They are effective against *Rickettsia spp.* (Rocky Mountain spotted fever and typhus fever). These drugs are also indicated for therapy of chlamydial infections, cholera, brucellosis, tularemia, and amebiasis. Tetracyclines are prescribed as an alternative to penicillin for the treatment of gonorrhea, syphilis, Lyme disease, anthrax, and *Haemophilus influenzae* respiratory infections. Doxycycline (Vibramycin) is highly effective in the prophylaxis of "traveler's diarrhea."

What are the adverse effects?

The tetracyclines cause a number of untoward effects. GI toxicity is common with oral use; it is probably caused by the combined effect of local irritation and alteration of the intestinal flora. Manifestations are heartburn, nausea, vomiting, and diarrhea. They are also associated with photosensitivity reactions, predisposing patients to severe sunburn.

The broad-spectrum antibacterial activity of the tetracyclines may cause superinfections, as can that of penicillins, cephalosporins, and sulfa drugs. This occurs most commonly in the bowel, but it may also readily occur in the mouth, lungs, and vagina. The most common superinfection is **candidiasis**, which is an infection or disease caused by *Candida spp.*, especially *Candida albicans*—usually resulting from debilitation, physiologic change, prolonged administration of antibiotics, and barrier breakage. Overgrowth from staphylococci may also occur. Staphylococcal enteric superinfections are frequently fatal.

Various hypersensitivity reactions or hepatotoxicity may occur. Tetracyclines may cause a darker pigment (graying) in developing teeth in children younger than 8 years old and may impair bone growth.

What are the contraindications and interactions?

The tetracyclines should be avoided in patients with hypersensitivity or liver diseases and in children younger than 8 years old. These drugs are also contraindicated in pregnant and lactating women.

Certain foods (such as dairy products) and drugs (such as laxatives, antacids that contain aluminum and calcium, and iron preparations) may reduce the absorption of tetracyclines. Therefore, it is recommended that tetracyclines be taken on an empty stomach. Phenytoin and barbiturates can decrease the effectiveness of tetracyclines.

What are the important points patients should know?

Instruct patients that tetracyclines should be taken on an empty stomach (1 hour before or 2 hours after meals) to facilitate absorption. The absorption of tetracyclines is strongly influenced by the presence of food and other drugs. Advise patients that because tetracyclines can cause photosensitivity reactions, they should avoid the sun during the warmest time of day (10 AM to 2 PM), use a sunblock, and wear a hat as well as protective clothing. Tetracyclines should be stored away from light and extreme heat because the effects of light and heat cause tetracyclines to decompose and produce toxic breakdown products. Expired tetracyclines should be disposed of immediately.

Table 12-7 ■ Tetracyclines

GENERIC NAME	TRADE NAME	AVERAGE DOSAGE IN ADULTS	ROUTE OF ADMINISTRATION
chlortetracycline	Aureomycin	250–500 mg q6h	PO
demeclocycline	Declomycin	150 mg q6h	PO
doxycycline	Vibramycin	100–200 mg initially; then 100 mg bid	PO
minocycline	Minocin	200 mg initially and then 100 mg bid	PO, IV
oxytetracycline	Terramycin	250 mg/d	PO
tetracycline	Achromycin, Sumycin Panmycin, Steclin	250–500 mg q6h; 100 mg bid–tid	PO, IM

bid, twice a day; IM, intramuscular; IV, intravenous; PO, oral; tid, three times a day.

✳ Apply Your Knowledge 12.4

The following questions focus on what you have just learned about fluoroquinolones and tetracyclines.

CRITICAL THINKING
1. What is the mechanism of action of the fluoroquinolones?
2. What are the contraindications of fluoroquinolones?
3. What are the main indications of tetracyclines?
4. Why are tetracyclines contraindicated in pregnant women and in children younger than 8 years of age?
5. What are the trade names of minocycline, doxycycline, and chlortetracycline?

MISCELLANEOUS ANTIBACTERIAL AGENTS

These antibacterial agents are principally second-line drugs because of emerging resistance, concerns with toxicity, or special activity against selected organisms (Table 12-8 ■). Discussion of chloramphenicol, clindamycin, vancomycin, and other miscellaneous antibacterial agents follows (in several of the following tables).

Table 12-8 ■ Miscellaneous Antibacterial Agents

GENERIC NAME	TRADE NAME	AVERAGE DOSAGE IN ADULTS	ROUTE OF ADMINISTRATION
chloramphenicol	Chloromycetin, others	12.5 mg/kg qid	PO
clindamycin	Cleocin	500 mg–2 g/d in 3–4 divided doses	IV
		500 mg q6h	PO
		8–20 mg/kg/d in 3–4 equal doses	IM
		15–40 mg/kg/d in 3–4 equal doses	Topical
linezolid	Zyvox	600 mg bid	PO
spectinomycin	Trobicin	2 g as single dose	IM
vancomycin	Vancocin	500 mg qid–1 g bid	IV

bid, twice a day; IM, intramuscular; IV, intravenous; PO, oral; qid, four times a day.

Focus On

Chloramphenicol

Chloramphenicol (Chloromycetin, others) is highly effective against rickettsial diseases (such as Rocky Mountain spotted fever), chlamydial diseases, and many bacterial infections.

How does it work?

Chloramphenicol is primarily bacteriostatic and a secondary bactericidal medication against a few bacterial strains. This agent interferes with protein synthesis.

How is it used?

Because of serious toxic reactions, the systemic use of chloramphenicol should be limited only to very serious infections that cannot be managed by other drugs. It is still the drug of choice for typhoid fever.

What are the adverse effects?

Bone marrow injury is the major toxic effect of chloramphenicol. Thrombocytopenia, granulocytopenia, and aplastic anemia are the most serious blood cell formation disturbances observed and have resulted in a number of fatalities. In neonates, its use may cause gray-baby syndrome.

What are the contraindications and interactions?

Chloramphenicol must be avoided in patients with known hypersensitivity to the drug. It must be used cautiously in patients with severe liver or kidney disease, in elderly patients, and during pregnancy and lactation.

Chloramphenicol may inhibit the metabolism of dicoumarol, tolbutamide, and phenytoin, leading to prolonged action and increased effects of these drugs. Phenobarbital can reduce the effect of chloramphenicol levels and may cause toxicity.

What are the important points patients should know?

Advise patients to take oral chloramphenicol with a full glass of water on an empty stomach and to avoid driving or operating heavy machinery if confusion or visual disturbances occur. Instruct patients to report any manifestation of blood dyscrasias, such as sore throat, weakness, unexplained bruising or bleeding, and fever, to their physician promptly.

Focus on Pediatrics

Gray-Baby Syndrome

Gray-baby syndrome is a fatal cyanosis. Its symptoms include vomiting; abdominal distension; and loose green stools owing to the inability of infants to metabolize the drug.

Focus On

Clindamycin

Clindamycin (Cleocin) is an antibacterial agent used as an alternate drug for treating infections caused by penicillin-resistant *S. aureus*.

How does it work?

Clindamycin is bacteriostatic and inhibits bacterial protein synthesis. This agent is active against most gram-positive and many anaerobic organisms.

How is it used?

Clindamycin is the drug of choice for the treatment of GI infections caused by *Bacteroides fragilis*. It is perhaps the best drug for the topical treatment of acne vulgaris. Lincomycin has marked toxicity. It is used only against infections for which it has been determined to be the most effective drug, including joint, bone, abdominal, and female genitourinary tract infections.

What are the adverse effects?

Clindamycin may cause abdominal pain, nausea, vomiting, and diarrhea. It may also result in antibiotic-associated (pseudomembranous) colitis.

What are the contraindications and interactions?

The contraindications include previous hypersensitivity to lincomycin and clindamycin and impaired liver function. This agent should be avoided in newborn babies. It is not safe for use in pregnant or lactating women. Clindamycin must be used cautiously in patients with impaired kidney function, a history of GI disease (particularly colitis), a history of liver disease, or asthma. It may potentiate the effects of neuromuscular blocking agents.

What are the important points patients should know?

Advise patients to take lincomycin with a full glass of water on an empty stomach. Because the medicine works best when the dose is constant, remind patients to take doses as scheduled.

Spectinomycin

Spectinomycin (Trobicin) is an antibiotic produced by *Streptomyces spectabilis*. This agent is bacteriostatic. It has variable activity against a wide variety of gram-negative and gram-positive organisms.

How does it work?

Spectinomycin suppresses protein synthesis in gram-negative bacteria, especially *Neisseria gonorrhoeae*.

How is it used?

Spectinomycin is used only for the treatment of uncomplicated gonorrhea in patients sensitized or resistant to penicillin.

What are the adverse effects?

The common adverse effects of spectinomycin include headache, dizziness, chills, fever, insomnia, nervousness, nausea, and vomiting. It also causes pain and soreness at the injection site.

What are the contraindications and interactions?

The safety of spectinomycin during pregnancy, lactation, and in infants or children is not established. This drug is also contraindicated in known cases of hypersensitivity to spectinomycin. No significant drug or food interactions for this agent are known.

What are the important points patients should know?

Advise patients to use condoms to prevent transmission of gonorrheal infection. It may be necessary to treat patients' partners to prevent reinfection. Instruct patients to avoid driving or operating heavy machinery if dizziness occurs after administration.

Vancomycin

Vancomycin (Vancocin) is the drug of choice for severe infections caused by drug-resistant *Staphylococcus* and *Clostridium* infections.

How does it work?

Vancomycin suppresses cell wall synthesis and is bactericidal. This drug is eliminated unchanged by the kidneys.

How is it used?

Vancomycin is usually reserved for serious infections, especially those caused by methicillin-resistant staphylococci. It is useful in patients who are allergic to penicillin or cephalosporins. Typical uses include osteomyelitis, endocarditis, and staphylococcal pneumonia. When given orally, vancomycin is useful in the treatment of pseudomembranous colitis.

What are the adverse effects?

The most serious side effects of vancomycin are ototoxicity and nephrotoxicity. Additional adverse effects include chills, fever, nausea, skin rashes, and urticaria. Local pain and phlebitis at the site of IV injection have been reported as well as a flushing sensation that can occur if the agent is infused too rapidly.

What are the contraindications and interactions?

Vancomycin must be avoided in patients with known hypersensitivity to this drug. It is also contraindicated in patients with previous hearing loss. Vancomycin should be administered with caution in neonates, children, older adults, pregnant women, and patients with impaired kidney function or renal failure. Vancomycin increases the neuromuscular blockade of the muscle relaxants atracurium, pancuronium, tubocurarine, and vecuronium.

What are the important points patients should know?

Advise patients to notify their health-care providers if they experience ringing in the ears while taking this medicine.

Focus Point

Red-Man Syndrome and Vancomycin

Vancomycin may cause "red-man syndrome," a condition that is manifested by facial flushing and hypotension caused by very rapid infusion of the drug. A 1-g dose should be infused over at least 60 minutes.

Focus On

Linezolid

Linezolid (Zyvox) is one of the oxazolidinones, a class of totally synthetic antibiotics first investigated in the late 1980s as antidepressant drugs. Later, these agents were discovered to have excellent antibacterial activity. The main reason for their development has been the increased resistance of gram-positive pathogens. The FDA approved the first agent of this class in April 2000. The initial drug was linezolid (Zyvox), which is the only oxazolidinone commercially available to date.

How does it work?

Linezolid is a protein synthesis–inhibiting compound that usually produces a bacteriostatic effect. The principal activity is against gram-positive aerobic organisms, including staphylococci, streptococci, and enterococci.

How is it used?

Linezolid is used for gram-positive drug-resistant microorganisms that are highly virulent.

What are the adverse effects?

In general, linezolid is well tolerated. The most common adverse effects are nausea, vomiting, diarrhea, and leukopenia.

What are the contraindications and interactions?

Linezolid is contraindicated in patients who are hypersensitive to the drug or its components. The use of linezolid with such adrenergic drugs as dopamine, epinephrine, or pseudoephedrine may cause hypertension. Blood pressure and heart rate should be monitored. Other items that may cause interactions include serotoninergic drugs and foods and beverages high in tyramine (including aged cheeses, air-dried meats, chocolate, fish, sauerkraut, red wines, tap beers, and soy sauce).

What are the important points patients should know?

Advise patients to avoid foods that contain tyramine while taking oxazolidinones.

✳ Apply Your Knowledge 12.5

The following questions focus on what you have just learned about the miscellaneous antibacterial agents.

CRITICAL THINKING

1. What is the drug of choice for typhoid fever?
2. What is the mechanism of action of spectinomycin?
3. How does vancomycin work?
4. What is the drug of choice for the treatment of GI infections caused by *Bacteroides fragilis*?
5. What are the most serious side effects of vancomycin?

ANTITUBERCULOSIS AGENTS

TB is a worldwide disease caused by *Mycobacterium tuberculosis*, an acid-fast aerobic bacillus. Any organ system can be affected by the disease, but the most common sites are the lungs and lymph nodes.

Worldwide, 3 million people die of TB each year. An estimated 10 to 15 million people in the United States have TB. Ninety percent of cases involve the reactivation of prior infection; the remainder of cases are new infections. The majority of new cases occur in malnourished individuals, those living in overcrowded conditions, immunosuppressed individuals, incarcerated persons, immigrants, and elderly persons.

The twentieth century was characterized by a decline in the incidence of TB in most developed countries. This was largely because of antibiotic drugs, active immunization, screening of people and livestock, and better living conditions. More recently, a disturbing increase in occurrence of this infection has been seen. This increase appears to be attributable to immigration patterns, drug-resistant strains of TB, and a prevalence of conditions that impair immunity (for example, HIV/AIDS and organ transplant therapy).

As many as four different drug combinations may be required to treat TB. These combinations are divided into the first- and second-line antituberculotics on the basis of their efficacy, activity, and adverse effects. Therapy is usually started with ethambutol (Myambutol), isoniazid (INH), rifampin (Rifadin, Rimactane), and pyrazinamide (PZA) for the first 2 months, followed by INH and rifampin for a further minimum of 4 months. This regimen is suitable if bacteriology shows fully sensitive acid-fast bacilli (which may include *Mycobacteria* or *Nocardia spp.*) on culture (Table 12-9 ■).

Table 12-9 ■ Most Commonly Used Antituberculotics

GENERIC NAME	BRAND NAME	AVERAGE DOSAGE IN ADULTS	ROUTE OF ADMINISTRATION
capreomycin	Capastat	1 g/d	IM
ciprofloxacin	Cipro	100–750 mg q12h	PO
		200–400 mg 8–q12h	IV
cycloserine	Seromycin	250 mg q12h	PO
ethambutol	Myambutol	400 mg/d	PO
ethionamide	Trecator-SC	500–750 mg/d	PO
isoniazid (INH)	Laniazid, Nydrazid	5–10 mg/kg/d (≤300 mg/d)	PO, IM
isoniazid-pyrazinamide-rifampin	Rifater	300 mg/d	PO, IV
ofloxacin	Floxin	200–400 mg q12h	PO
pyrazinamide	PZA	15–35 mg/kg/d in 3–4 divided doses (≤2 g/d)	PO
rifampin	Rifadin, Rimactane	600 mg/d with other antitubercular agents	PO, IV
rifapentine	Priftin	600 mg twice weekly for 2 mo and then 600 mg/wk for 4 mo	PO
streptomycin	Streptomycin	15 mg/kg (≤1 g) as a single dose	IM

IM, intramuscular; IV, intravenous; PO, oral;

Focus On

Isoniazid

INH is the most potent and selective of the known tuberculostatic antibacterial agents. It is tuberculocidal to growing bacteria and the most effective agent in the therapy of TB. The drug is never used alone because of the rapid emergence of resistance.

How does it work?

INH acts by interfering with the biosynthesis of bacterial proteins, nucleic acid, and lipids.

How is it used?

INH is used in the treatment of all forms of active TB caused by susceptible organisms and as a preventive agent in high-risk persons, such as household members and persons with positive tuberculin skin test reactions.

What are the adverse effects?

The common adverse effects include restlessness, insomnia, convulsions, optic neuritis, and psychoses. The drug also may cause nausea, vomiting, aplastic anemia, fever, and skin rashes.

What are the contraindications and interactions?

INH-associated hypersensitivity reactions, liver damage, and pregnancy are contraindications for its use. This drug should be used cautiously in patients with chronic liver disease, renal dysfunction, history of convulsive disorders, and chronic alcoholism.

What are the important points patients should know?

Advise patients that INH is absorbed better on an empty stomach. Instruct patients to avoid driving or operating heavy machinery if dizziness or drowsiness occurs and to contact their physicians if tinnitus (ringing in the ears), visual changes, dizziness, or ataxia (an inability to coordinate muscle activity) occurs. Patients must notify their physicians if symptoms of hepatotoxicity occur, including fever, liver tenderness, loss of appetite, malaise, or jaundice.

Focus on Geriatrics

Risk of Fatal Hepatitis with Isoniazid Therapy

Older patients taking INH are very susceptible to a potentially fatal hepatitis, especially if they regularly drink alcohol. Careful monitoring for signs of liver impairment is necessary. Good patient observation alerts the caregiver to the warning signs, which include increased serum alanine transferase and increased serum aspartate transaminase (liver enzymes), increased serum bilirubin (a substance released into the blood when red blood cells break down), and jaundice. Liver dysfunction in older adults may also be caused by the antitubercular drugs PZA and rifampin.

Focus On

Ethambutol

Ethambutol (Myambutol) is a tuberculostatic drug that is effective against tubercle bacilli that are resistant to INH or streptomycin.

How does it work?

Ethambutol's mechanism of action is not completely understood, but it appears to inhibit RNA synthesis and arrest multiplication of tubercle bacilli. The emergence of resistant TB strains is delayed by administering ethambutol in combination with other antituberculosis drugs.

How is it used?

Ethambutol can be used in conjunction with at least one other antituberculotic in the treatment of pulmonary TB.

What are the adverse effects?

Ethambutol occasionally causes optic neuritis, with blurred vision and diminished visual acuity to green light. Although these effects disappear on discontinuation, the drug should be discontinued at the first indication of a loss in visual acuity. Eye tests should be made before and at monthly intervals after the onset of therapy.

Other adverse effects include pruritus, anorexia, nausea, vomiting, abdominal pain, headache, vertigo, fever, hallucinations, and abnormal liver function.

What are the contraindications and interactions?

Ethambutol is contraindicated in patients with optic neuritis or a history of hypersensitivity to the drug. It is also contraindicated in children younger than 6 years. Ethambutol should be used cautiously in patients with renal impairment, hepatic disease, gout, cataracts, or diabetic retinopathy and in those who are pregnant or lactating. Ethambutol absorption is decreased with aluminum salts.

What are the important points patients should know?

Instruct patients about the importance of regular eye examinations while taking ethambutol. If the patient experiences problems with vision, the drug should be stopped immediately.

Advise patients to take ethambutol with meals to lessen gastric irritation and to avoid driving or operating heavy machinery if drowsiness or dizziness occurs.

Rifampin

Rifampin (Rifadin, Rimactane) is a broad-spectrum antibiotic that is effective against most gram-positive bacteria and variably active against gram-negative organisms. *M. tuberculosis* is very susceptible to this drug.

How does it work?

Rifampin inhibits the activity of DNA-dependent RNA polymerase (an enzyme responsible for creating different RNA molecules) in susceptible bacterial cells, thereby suppressing RNA synthesis.

How is it used?

Rifampin is used primarily with other antituberculosis agents for the initial treatment and retreatment of clinical TB and as short-term therapy to eliminate meningococci from the nasopharynx of an asymptomatic carrier of *Neisseria meningitides* when the risk of meningococcal meningitis is high.

What are the adverse effects?

Fatigue, drowsiness, headache, confusion, dizziness, nausea, vomiting, heartburn, skin rashes, and renal insufficiency may be observed with rifampin administration. This drug may also cause a reddish-orange discoloration of such body fluids as tears, urine, sweat, and saliva.

What are the contraindications and interactions?

Rifampin must be avoided in patients with a history of hypersensitivity to the drug. It should be used with caution in patients with hepatic disease or a history of alcoholism and in those who are pregnant or lactating.

Rifampin decreases concentrations of alfentanil (Alfenta, an opioid analgesic), alosetron (Lotronex, which is used to treat irritable bowel syndrome), barbiturates, benzodiazepines, and many other drugs. The use of rifampin with oral anticoagulants or oral hypoglycemics may decrease the effects of these drugs.

What are the important points patients should know?

Inform patients that rifampin may cause urine, feces, saliva, sputum, sweat, and tears to develop a red-orange appearance. This effect is harmless. Advise patients not to wear soft contact lenses because they may become permanently stained. Instruct patients to take rifampin on an empty stomach and to avoid driving or operating heavy machinery if drowsiness or dizziness occurs. Instruct patients to notify their physicians if manifestations of hepatotoxicity, including fever, loss of appetite, liver tenderness, malaise, or jaundice, occur.

Pyrazinamide

PZA is an antituberculosis drug used for initial treatment in combination with INH and rifampin. It generally is administered with INH, which it potentiates. However, it is quite toxic and should be held in reserve until other therapies fail.

How does it work?

PZA is bacteriostatic against *M. tuberculosis.* When used alone, resistance may develop in 6 to 7 weeks. Therefore, administration with other effective agents is recommended.

(Continued)

Focus On (Continued)

How is it used?

PZA is used for short-term therapy of advanced TB before surgery and to treat patients unresponsive to such primary agents as INH and streptomycin.

What are the adverse effects?

Hepatotoxicity is the principal adverse effect reported with PZA use. Other adverse effects include nausea, vomiting, diarrhea, skin rashes, and myalgia.

What are the contraindications and interactions?

PZA should be avoided in patients with a history of hypersensitivity to the drug. It is contraindicated in patients who have severe liver damage and patients who are pregnant or lactating. PZA must be used cautiously in patients with gout or diabetes mellitus, a history of peptic ulcer, and impaired kidney function. PZA decreases the effects of allopurinol, colchicine, and probenecid. This drug increases liver toxicity when used with rifampin.

What are the important points patients should know?

Instruct patients to notify their physician if manifestations of hepatotoxicity, including fever, liver tenderness, loss of appetite, malaise, or jaundice, occur.

✳ Apply Your Knowledge 12.6

The following questions focus on what you have just learned about the antituberculosis agents.

CRITICAL THINKING

1. What are the characteristics of *Mycobacterium tuberculosis*?
2. What are the first-line antituberculotics?
3. What is the most effective agent in the therapy of tuberculosis?
4. What are the adverse effects of rifampin?
5. How is pyrazinamide used in the treatment of tuberculosis?

Antiviral Agents

Viruses cause much of the morbidity and mortality in populations worldwide, but the number of drugs available to treat such viruses is still quite low. Antiviral drug development has become very active in the past decade, especially with the challenges of the AIDS epidemic.

Only a few antiviral drugs have been successfully used in the United States. However, several viral diseases, including measles, mumps, rubella, polio, chicken pox, smallpox, and rabies, are prevented by vaccines. The antiviral agents reviewed here are acyclovir (Zovirax), amantadine (Symmetrel), didanosine, ribavirin (Virazole), zanamivir (Relenza), ganciclovir (Cytovene), and zidovudine (AZT, Retrovir). Table 12-10 ■ shows the classification of various antiviral drugs.

Table 12-10 ■ Antiviral Drugs

GENERIC NAME	TRADE NAME	AVERAGE DOSAGE IN ADULTS	ROUTE OF ADMINISTRATION
acyclovir	Zovirax	5–10 mg/kg over 1h q8h for ≤7 d	IV
		200–800 mg q4–8h for 5–10 d	PO
amantadine	Symmetrel	200 mg/d single dose or 100 mg/d bid	PO
cidofovir	Vistide	5 mg/kg over 1 h/wk for 2 consecutive wk; then once every 2 wk	IV

GENERIC NAME	TRADE NAME	AVERAGE DOSAGE IN ADULTS	ROUTE OF ADMINISTRATION
didanosine	Videx, Videx EC	125–300 mg bid	PO
famciclovir	Famvir	125–500 mg q8–12h for 5–7 d	PO
foscarnet	Foscavir	Initial: 40–90 mg/kg over 1h q8–12h for 2–3 wk	IV
		Maintenance: 90–120 mg/kg/d	
ganciclovir	Cytovene	Induction: 5 mg/kg q12h for 7–21 d	
		Maintenance: 5–6 mg/kg/d for 5–7 d	IV
		Maintenance: 1,000 mg tid with food or 500 mg q3h while awake up to 6 times/d	PO
oseltamivir	Tamiflu	75 mg daily for 5 d–6 wk	PO
rimantadine	Flumadine	100 mg bid (usually for 1 wk)	PO
ribavirin	Virazole	For infants and children with RSV: solution 20 mg/mL delivered in mist at 12.5 L/m for 12–18 h, 3–7 d	Inhalation
tenofovir disoproxil fumarate	Viread	300 mg/d with a meal	PO
valacyclovir	Valtrex	500 mg–2 g/d bid–tid for 3–10 d	PO
valganciclovir	Valcyte	900 mg bid with food for 21 d; maintenance: 900 mg/d with food	PO
zanamivir	Relenza	5 mg blister bid via Diskhaler	Inhaler
zidovudine	AZT, Retrovir	200 mg q4h ×1 mo; then 100 mg q4h	PO

bid, twice a day; IV, intravenous; PO, oral; tid, three times a day.

HIV INFECTIONS

Human immunodeficiency virus (HIV), which results in acquired immunodeficiency syndrome (AIDS), is caused mainly by two viruses: HIV-1 and HIV-2. HIV-1 is found worldwide, but HIV-2 infections are most common in parts of Africa and India. The antiviral drugs used to suppress HIV are effective mostly against the HIV-1 strain. The virus infects a group of helper T lymphocytes, which are called *CD4 cells*. This results in the individual with AIDS becoming more susceptible to other infections, such as bacteria, fungi, protozoans, and other viruses. Most AIDS patients die from these secondary infections. It is important to remember that not all individuals infected with HIV develop AIDS, but they continue to be carriers of the virus.

Antiviral drugs are used alone or in combinations for the treatment of HIV infection. Highly active antiretroviral therapy (HAART) has been shown to reduce viral load, increase CD4 lymphocyte counts in individuals infected with HIV, delay the onset of AIDS, and prolong the survival of patients with AIDS. The incidence of and mortality from AIDS have declined substantially since 1996 because of HAART. The benefits of HAART, which involve the combination of three to four drugs effective against HIV, have been widely publicized. Two distinct categories of drugs are combined: **nucleoside** analogues (derived from nucleic acid) and protease inhibitors.

The use of HAART presents formidable challenges, including harsh side effects and the potential for rapid development of drug resistance. Protease inhibitors do not work as well with a third category of HIV drugs—the nonnucleoside analogues—which should not be taken alone. Presently, because of the limited number of HAART medications available in the United States, only a few drug combinations are possible. HAART regimens can also fail because of the lack of viral load response (the body's reaction to antiviral agents) or the patient's poor adherence to treatment. Missing a single dose of HAART even twice a week can cause the development of drug-resistant HIV.

This is a real danger because adherence to the drug regimen is difficult. The simplification of HIV antiretroviral therapy regimens has been shown to improve adherence. One combination antiviral agent approved for the treatment of HIV infection and AIDS is 2′,3′-dideoxycytidine (ddC, also called *zalcitabine*), which is to be used only with the popular drug zidovudine (AZT, Retrovir).

Focus On

Acyclovir

Acyclovir (Zovirax) is an antiviral agent used for initial and recurrent mucosal and cutaneous herpes simplex virus types 1 and 2. It is also used for herpes zoster infections in **immunocompromised** (weakened immune system) patients. Valacyclovir (Valtrex), which is a chemically modified version of acyclovir, is used for the suppression and treatment of mucosal herpes infections.

How does it work?

Acyclovir interferes with DNA synthesis and inhibits viral multiplication.

How is it used?

Acyclovir is also used to treat herpes simplex, herpes simplex encephalitis in patients older than 6 months, acute herpes zoster (shingles), and chicken pox.

What are the adverse effects?

Adverse effects of acyclovir include vertigo, headache, tremors, depression, hair loss, and phlebitis at injection sites. It may also cause nausea, vomiting, anorexia, and diarrhea.

What are the contraindications and interactions?

Acyclovir is contraindicated in patients who are allergic to this agent. It should not be used in patients with renal disease or seizures or during lactation.

What are the important points patients should know?

Instruct patients to report adverse effects of therapy, including decreased urination, CNS changes (such as confusion, anxiety, or depression), and gastric irritation.

- -

Amantadine

Amantadine (Symmetrel) is used to prevent or treat symptoms of influenza A viral infections (also known as the *flu* or *grippe*) as well as respiratory tract illnesses.

How does it work?

Amantadine inhibits replication of the influenza A virus by interfering with viral attachment and by the uncoating (disassembly or disintegration) of the virus.

How is it used?

Amantadine is used to treat a wide variety of patients of all ages who have symptoms of influenza, but it may also be used to treat some patients with parkinsonism.

What are the adverse effects?

The most pronounced adverse effects of amantadine are insomnia, nightmares, confusion, ataxia (loss of muscular control), headache, dizziness, dyspnea, hypotension, edema, urine retention, constipation, nausea, and dry mouth.

What are the contraindications and interactions?

Amantadine is contraindicated in patients with hypersensitivity to the drug and should be used cautiously in elderly patients and patients with seizure disorders, peripheral edema, heart failure, hepatic disease, eczema-type rash, mental illness, orthostatic hypotension, renal impairment, and cardiovascular disease. Amantadine interacts with anticholinergics and CNS stimulants. It also should not be used with the herb known as jimsonweed or with alcohol.

What are the important points patients should know?

Advise patients to report adverse effects of therapy, including CNS changes (such as confusion, insomnia, nightmares) and urine retention. Instruct patients to rise slowly from sitting and lying positions to avoid experiencing dizziness caused by postural hypotension.

Didanosine

Didanosine (Videx, Videx EC) is an antiretroviral and nucleoside reverse transcriptase inhibitor.

How does it work?

Didanosine can inhibit the replication of the HIV virus that has become resistant to zidovudine (AZT). Its mechanism of action is similar to that of zidovudine.

How is it used?

Didanosine is used in advanced HIV infection in patients who are intolerant to AZT or who demonstrate significant clinical or immunologic deterioration during zidovudine therapy.

What are the adverse effects?

The major adverse effects of didanosine are peripheral neuropathies and pancreatitis, which may be fatal. These effects are more likely in high doses of the drug. This drug is minimally toxic to bone marrow. Common adverse effects include headache, dizziness, insomnia, seizures, abdominal pain, nausea, vomiting, diarrhea, constipation, and dry mouth.

What are the contraindications and interactions?

Contraindications for didanosine include hypersensitivity to the drug and pregnancy or lactation. It must be administered cautiously to individuals with peripheral vascular disease, history of neuropathy, chronic pancreatitis, renal impairment, or liver disease.

Aluminum and magnesium-containing antacids may increase the aluminum- and magnesium-associated adverse effects. The effectiveness of dapsone may be reduced by didanosine. Absorption of didanosine is significantly decreased by food.

What are the important points patients should know?

Instruct patients to maintain an adequate fluid intake to increase urine output, thereby preventing renal problems.

. . . .

Ribavirin

Ribavirin (Virazole) is a synthetic nucleoside analogue with broad-spectrum antiviral activity against both DNA and RNA viruses.

How does it work?

Its exact mechanism of action is not fully understood, but it is believed to involve multiple mechanisms, including selective interference with viral ribonucleic protein synthesis.

How is it used?

Ribavirin given by aerosol into an infant oxygen hood has been effective for the treatment of respiratory syncytial virus pneumonia.

What are the adverse effects?

The adverse effects of ribavirin include abdominal cramps, jaundice, anemia, and hypotension.

What are the contraindications and interactions?

Ribavirin is contraindicated in patients with severe cardiovascular disease, congestive heart failure, angina, pancreatitis, and hepatitis. It is also contraindicated in patients with renal failure, sickle-cell disease, pregnancy, and lactation. No specific drug interactions have been identified, but clinical experience with the systemic administration of ribavirin is limited.

What are the important points patients should know?

Advise patients to report adverse effects of hepatotoxicity, including fever, liver tenderness, loss of appetite, and jaundice.

. . . .

Ganciclovir

Ganciclovir (Cytovene) is a synthetic purine (crystalline, organic base) nucleoside analogue that is approved for the treatment of cytomegalovirus (CMV) infections but not for HIV itself.

How does it work?

After conversion to ganciclovir triphosphate, ganciclovir is incorporated into viral DNA and inhibits viral DNA polymerase. By this action, it can terminate viral replication.

How is it used?

Ganciclovir is used for the prophylaxis and the treatment of systemic CMV infections in immunocompromised patients, including HIV-positive and transplant patients. It is also prescribed for CMV retinitis.

(Continued)

Focus On (Continued)

What are the adverse effects?

Ganciclovir's black box warnings include increased potential for dose-limited neutropenia, thrombocytopenia, and anemia. Other adverse effects are fever, headache, disorientation, ataxia, confusion, tremor, edema, and phlebitis.

What are the contraindications and interactions?

Ganciclovir is contraindicated in patients with hypersensitivity to the drug or to acyclovir (Zovirax). It must be avoided in lactating women. Ganciclovir should be used cautiously in patients with renal impairment, older adults, and pregnant women. Its safety and efficacy in children are not established. No specific drug interactions have been identified.

What are the important points patients should know?

Instruct patients to report adverse effects of therapy, including such CNS changes as confusion, depression, ataxia, and tremor.

Zidovudine

Zidovudine (AZT, Retrovir) is often known by the abbreviation AZT, which stands for *azidothymidine* (its simplified chemical name).

How does it work?

Zidovudine is a major nucleoside in DNA. On entering host cells, this drug is converted to a triphosphate by endogenous (grown from within) cellular enzymes. It appears to act by being incorporated into growing DNA chains by viral reverse transcriptase, thereby terminating viral replication.

How is it used?

Zidovudine is used for patients who have asymptomatic HIV infection and early or late symptomatic HIV disease. It can also be prescribed for prevention of perinatal transfer of HIV during pregnancy.

What are the adverse effects?

Common adverse effects of zidovudine include fever, dyspnea, malaise, weakness, myalgia, and myopathy. In some patients, headache, insomnia, dizziness, anxiety, or bone marrow depression may be seen.

What are the contraindications and interactions?

Acetaminophen (Tylenol), ganciclovir (Cytoven), and interferon α-2A (Roferon-A) may enhance bone marrow suppression. Interaction of aspirin, dapsone (DDS), indomethacin (Indocin), methadone (Dolophine, Methadone), vincristine (Oncovin, VCR), and valproic acid (Depakene) may increase the risk of AZT toxicity.

Zidovudine is contraindicated in patients who are hypersensitive to the drug; in severe bone marrow depression, hepatomegaly, hepatitis, or other liver disease risk factors; and in those with renal insufficiency. It interacts with a wide variety of drugs, including atovaquone (Malarone), fluconazole (Diflucan), probenecid (Benemid, others), doxorubicin (Adriamycin, Rubex), ribavirin, stavudine (Zerit), and phenytoin (Dilantin).

What are the important points patients should know?

Advise patients to avoid taking such nonsteroidal anti-inflammatory drugs as aspirin or indomethacin or paracetamol while taking zidovudine. These drugs may inhibit the metabolism of zidovudine, therefore increasing the possibility of toxicity.

✳ Apply Your Knowledge 12.7

The following questions focus on what you have just learned about antiviral agents and HIV infections.

CRITICAL THINKING

1. Differentiate between HIV and AIDS.
2. What are the trade names of acyclovir, ganciclovir, oseltamivir, and zidovudine?
3. What are the indications of amantadine (Symmetrel)?
4. What is the mechanism of action of acyclovir?
5. Why do patients with AIDS become more susceptible to other infections?

PRACTICAL SCENARIO 1

A physician orders penicillin for a 15-year-old patient without closely checking the patient's chart. While the medical assistant prepares to explain to the patient and her mother how she should take the medication, he notices that the chart indicates that the patient has an allergy to penicillin.

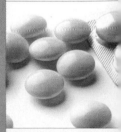

Brian Warling/PH College

Critical Thinking Questions

1. What is the first thing the medical assistant should do?
2. How might the medical assistant ensure that the physician sees information about drug allergies in a patient's chart?
3. When taking a patient history, what important question should *always* be asked each time the patient is seen in the office or clinic?

PRACTICAL SCENARIO 2

Kasey, a 34-year-old woman who tested positive for Lyme disease, went to a family practice office. The physician ordered tetracycline, which is the drug of choice for Lyme disease. After 2 weeks of taking antibiotics, at a routine gynecologic examination, the nurse practitioner asked Kasey if she knew she was pregnant. Kasey was surprised, and as they discussed her health, the nurse practitioner asked if she was on any medication. Kasey told her about the Lyme disease and the prescription for tetracycline.

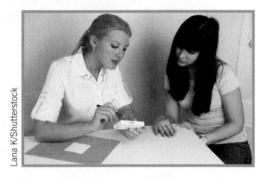

Lana K/Shutterstock

Critical Thinking Questions

1. What are the contraindications of tetracycline related to pregnant women?
2. Does Lyme disease cause any harm to a developing fetus?

Chapter Capsule

This section repeats the objectives from the beginning of the chapter and then provides a summary of the most important concepts for that objective. Use this section as a quick review and to check your knowledge.

Objective 1: Identify the major types of antibiotics by drug class.

■ Sulfa drugs, penicillins, cephalosporins, aminoglycosides, tetracyclines, macrolides, synthetic antibacterial agents (such as nitrofurantoin and the quinolones)

Objective 2: Describe the principal mechanisms of action of cephalosporins, vancomycin, and isoniazid.

■ Cephalosporins—bactericidal, affecting the bacterial cell wall
■ Vancomycin—bactericidal, suppressing cell-wall synthesis
■ Isoniazid—interfering with biosynthesis of bacterial proteins, nucleic acid, and lipids

Objective 3: Outline the main adverse effects of macrolides, aminoglycosides, and chloramphenicol.

- Macrolides—abdominal pain, nausea, and vomiting
- Aminoglycosides—ototoxicity and nephrotoxicity
- Chloramphenicol—bone marrow injury, blood cell formation disturbances, and gray-baby syndrome

Objective 4: Contrast bactericidal and bacteriostatic actions.

- Bactericidal—kills bacteria
- Bacteriostatic—inhibits growth of bacteria

Objective 5: List the first-line antituberculosis agents and two characteristic adverse effects of each drug.

- Isoniazid—restlessness, insomnia
- Ethambutol—optic neuritis, blurred vision
- Rifampin—fatigue, drowsiness
- Pyrazinamide—hepatotoxicity, nausea

Objective 6: Explain the classifications of cephalosporins.

- First generation: highest activity against gram-positive bacteria and lowest activity against gram-negative bacteria
- Second generation: more active against gram-negative bacteria and less active against gram-positive bacteria than the first-generation cephalosporins
- Third generation: considerably less active than first-generation agents against gram-positive bacteria; much expanded spectrum of activity against gram-negative organisms
- Fourth generation: improved gram-positive spectrum of activity; expanded gram-negative activity of third-generation cephalosporins

Objective 7: Discuss the contraindications, precautions, and interactions of the penicillins and tetracyclines.

- Penicillins—contraindications: hypersensitivity, renal disease, pregnancy, lactation; precautions: give 1 hour before or 2 hours after meals; interactions: estrogen-containing birth control pills, tetracyclines
- Tetracyclines—contraindications: hypersensitivity, liver diseases, children younger than 8 years, pregnancy, lactation; precautions: take tetracyclines on an empty stomach; interactions: dairy products, laxatives, antacids containing aluminum and calcium, iron preparations, phenytoin, barbiturates

Objective 8: List three antiviral drugs for HIV- or AIDS-related secondary viral infections and explain their mechanisms of action.

- Didanosine—enters host cells and is incorporated into growing DNA chains by viral reverse transcriptase, thereby terminating viral replication
- Ganciclovir—after conversion to ganciclovir triphosphate, incorporated into viral DNA, inhibiting viral DNA polymerase and then terminating viral replication
- Zidovudine—mechanism of action similar to didanosine

Internet Sites of Interest

- AIDSLINE contains abstracts on AIDS topics compiled by the U.S. National Library of Medicine. Abstracts are arranged by year at **http://www.aegis.com/aidsline**.

- A wealth of information on treatments for infectious diseases is available at the website of the National Foundation for Infectious Diseases at **http://www.nfid.org/publications**.

- The appropriate use of antibiotics is a topic of great concern for the public and health-care providers. See the website of the Alliance for the Prudent Use of Antibiotics at **http://www.tufts.edu/med/apua** for consumer and professional information on this topic.

- Reports and news articles on HIV/AIDS in children around the world are available on the UNICEF website at **http://www.unicef.org/aids**.

PEARSON
myhealthprofessionskit™

Go to www.myhealthprofessionskit.com to access the Companion Website created for this textbook. Simply select "Basic Health Science" from the choice of disciplines. Find this book and then log in using your username and password to access interactive learning games, assessment questions, animations, and more.

Chapter 13

Antifungal, Antimalarial, and Antiprotozoal Agents

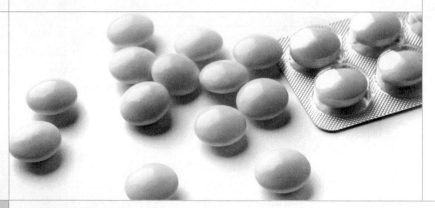

Key Terms

fungicidal (fun-jih-SY-dul) (page 215)

mycoses (my-KOH-seez) (page 211)

porphyria (por-FEE-ree-uh) (page 215)

protozoan (pro-toh-ZO-un) (page 211)

radical cure (page 215)

thrush (page 211)

Introduction

Most healthy human beings are resistant to fungal infections but may become infected when overwhelming numbers of fungi infiltrate their systems. Fungi may enter the body in routes that include the skin, mucous membranes, and respiratory tract. Because of the common use of antibiotics and drugs, such as oral contraceptives, more and more patients are at risk for fungal infections.

Malaria is a serious disease that is caused by a **protozoan**, a single-celled highly mobile microorganism. *Plasmodium* protozoans, which cause malaria, are transmitted to humans by mosquitoes. Malaria can become a long-term condition and can kill affected persons because of its severity.

Other infections caused by protozoans include dysentery, amebiasis, and a sexually transmitted disease known as *trichomoniasis*. The number of severe protozoan infections is large, and many of these infections do not exhibit specific symptoms.

Fungal Infections

Molds and yeasts are so widely distributed in air, dust, contaminated objects, and normal flora that humans are constantly being exposed to them. More than 1 million species of fungi have been identified. Only about 20 of these are associated with systemic infections and cause opportunistic infections. Normal healthy individuals are resistant to most fungal infections, called **mycoses**, and are infected only when faced with overwhelming numbers of the fungi. In other cases, opportunistic pathogens may invade an individual whose natural resistance is low because of other illnesses or even some medications.

Mycoses involve complex interactions among the portal of entry into the human body, the number of infecting organisms generally required to cause disease, the virulence of the fungus, and the host's resistance. Fungi enter the body mainly via respiratory, mucous, and cutaneous routes. In general, the agents of primary mycoses have a respiratory portal (spores inhaled from the air). Subcutaneous agents enter through compromised skin, and cutaneous and superficial agents enter through the contamination of the skin surface. Spores and yeasts can all be infectious, but spores are most often involved because of their durability and abundance.

The human body is extremely resistant to fungi. Among its numerous antifungal defenses are the normal integrity of the skin, mucous membranes, and respiratory cilia, but the most important defenses are cell-mediated immunity, phagocytosis (a process in which cells, called *phagocytes*, consume foreign material), and the inflammatory reaction.

A common opportunistic infection is candidiasis (also called *moniliasis* or *thrush*). **Thrush** is a yeast infection in the mouth caused by *Candida albicans*, a normal resident of the gastrointestinal tract and vagina (Figure 13-1 ■). Thrush can occur during the use of broad-spectrum antibiotics or by the alteration of the environmental conditions in the female reproductive system because of pregnancy or oral contraceptive use. This disease usually results from debilitation (immunosuppression, especially AIDS).

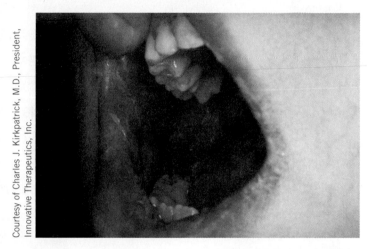

Courtesy of Charles J. Kirkpatrick, M.D., President, Innovative Therapeutics, Inc.

Figure 13-1 ■ Oral *Candida albicans*. Courtesy of Charles J. Kirkpatrick, M.D., president, Innovative Therapeutics, Inc.

The incidence of human fungal infections has increased in recent years because more patients are now at risk for these pathogens. Causes include increased exposure resulting from more frequent surgeries, use of broad-spectrum antimicrobials, immunosuppressive drug therapy for cancer and organ transplantation patients, and HIV.

Antifungal Agents

Antifungal drugs are classified into three categories:

1. Drugs for systemic mycoses
2. Oral drugs for mucocutaneous infections
3. Topical drugs for mucocutaneous infections (Table 13-1 ■)

The major drugs for systemic mycoses include amphotericin B (Amphocin), flucytosine (Ancobon), ketoconazole (Nizoral), and griseofulvin (Fulvicin, Grifulvin V). Nystatin (Mycostatin) and fluconazole (Diflucan) are used for local *C. albicans* infections of the skin and mucous membranes. Overall, the "azole" antifungals are the most commonly prescribed antifungals in the United States.

Table 13-1 ■ Antifungal Agents

GENERIC NAME	TRADE NAME	AVERAGE DOSAGE IN ADULTS	ROUTE OF ADMINISTRATION
Systemic Antifungal Drugs			
amphotericin B	Amphocin	0.25–1.5 mg/kg/d	IV
caspofungin	Cancidas	70 mg on day 1; then 50 mg/d; infuse doses over 1 h	IV
fluconazole	Diflucan	100–200 mg/d	PO, IV
flucytosine	Ancobon	12.5–37.5 mg/kg q6h	PO
griseofulvin	Fulvicin, Grifulvin V	500 mg/d	PO
itraconazole	Sporanox	200 mg/d	PO
ketoconazole	Nizoral	200–400 mg/d	PO
nystatin	Mycostatin (suspension)	400,000–600,000 mg qid	PO
	Nilstat (tablets)	1,000,000 mg bid	PO
Topical Antifungal Drugs			
amphotericin B	Fungizone	Apply to lesions 2–4 times/d for 1–4 wk	Topical
ciclopirox	Loprox, Penlac	Massage cream into affected area and surrounding skin in the morning and evening	Topical
clotrimazole	Lotrimin	Apply small amount to affected areas in the morning and evening	Topical
econazole	Spectazole	Apply sufficient amount to affected areas in the morning and evening	Topical
haloprogin	Halotex	Apply liberally to affected area bid for 2–3 wk	Topical
naftifine	Naftin	Apply cream once daily or apply gel twice daily; may use up to 4 wk	Topical
oxiconazole	Oxistat	Apply to affected area once daily in the evening	Topical

bid, twice a day; IV, intravenous; PO, oral; qid, four times a day.

Focus on Pediatrics

Thrush in Babies

In babies, thrush causes difficulty in breastfeeding and chronic diaper rash (which may appear as slightly raised ulcers or skin lesions of a creamy white color). Oral thrush (white patches in the mouth or throat) in babies may infect the nipples of the mother, causing drying or cracking.

Focus On

Amphotericin B

Amphotericin B (Amphocin) has the widest spectrum of antifungal activity of any systemic antifungal drug.

How does it work?

Most antifungal drugs act by interfering with the synthesis of ergosterol, a chemical found in fungal cell membranes. This results in a change in the permeability of the fungal cell membrane and either slowed growth or destruction of the fungal organism.

How is it used?

Administration of amphotericin B by the intravenous (IV) route is extremely useful for therapy of systemic fungus diseases. It is also used by nasal spray in the prophylaxis of aspergillosis in immunocompromised patients and orally for treatment of oral candidiasis.

What are the adverse effects?

Amphotericin B may induce chills and fever, nausea and vomiting, diarrhea, abdominal cramps, dyspepsia, headache, vertigo, thrombophlebitis, anemia, cardiac arrest, and skin rashes. The most serious adverse effect of amphotericin B is renal damage. This drug is also able to cause blood dyscrasias and loss of hearing.

What are the contraindications and interactions?

Amphotericin B is contraindicated in patients hypersensitive to the drug and should be used cautiously in patients with impaired renal function. It interacts with many other drugs, including antineoplastics, cardiac glycosides, corticosteroids, nephrotoxic drugs (including antibiotics and pentamidine), thiazides, and flucytosine (Ancobon); it should not be used with leukocyte transfusions.

What are the important points patients should know?

Inform patients that when given IV, this drug may cause fever, chills, headache, and nausea in the first few hours of therapy, but these adverse reactions usually decrease as therapy continues. Advise patients to notify their physicians if improvement does not occur within 1 to 2 weeks and to report loss of hearing, dizziness, cloudy or pink urine, or greatly increased urination. The treatment of cutaneous infections, such as nail infections, usually requires several months or longer of therapy. Advise patients to wash towels and clothing that were in contact with affected areas after each treatment. Topical cream slightly discolors the skin when rubbed in, and nail lesions may be stained. Instruct patients to drink plenty of fluids.

Focus on Geriatrics

Amphotericin B and Kidney Damage

Amphotericin B (Amphocin) is a very toxic agent that in most cases should be administered intravenously. Elderly patients who use this drug must be very careful because kidney damage is the most serious toxic effect of amphotericin B. Elderly patients who have renal impairment must be tested for creatinine clearance.

Focus on Natural Products

Interactions Between Gossypol and Amphotericin B

The herb gossypol, which is derived from cottonseed oil, may be used to treat endometriosis in women. It may also be used by men and women to prevent pregnancy. Gossypol used with amphotericin B (Amphocin) may increase the risk of renal toxicity.

Focus On

Flucytosine

Flucytosine (Ancobon) is an antifungal agent used for a wide variety of severe fungal infections.

How does it work?

Flucytosine is converted in the fungus to 5-fluorouracil, which is incorporated into RNA and interferes with normal protein synthesis.

How is it used?

Certain fungal organisms are more sensitive to interference from the drug than are human cells, so flucytosine is useful in the treatment of some fungal infections. It is the drug of choice to treat chromomycosis and of second choice to treat systemic candidiasis. It may be combined with amphotericin B (Amphocin) for first-choice treatment of aspergillosis or cryptococcosis (a fungal disease of the lungs), especially in patients with meningitis.

What are the adverse effects?

Flucytosine commonly causes nausea, vomiting, diarrhea, and skin rashes. Bone marrow suppression, manifest by anemia, leukopenia, and thrombocytopenia, has been reported. Sedation, confusion, hallucinations, headache, and vertigo occur infrequently.

What are the contraindications and interactions?

Flucytosine is contraindicated in patients who are hypersensitive to the drug and should be used with extreme caution in patients who have impaired hepatic or renal function or who have bone marrow suppression. It interacts with amphotericin B, causing synergistic effects and increasing toxicity.

What are the important points patients should know?

Instruct patients to report fever, sore mouth or throat, and a tendency for unusual bleeding or bruising to their physicians. They must be aware that the general duration of therapy is 4 to 6 weeks, but it may need to be continued for several months. Instruct patients not to breastfeed while taking this drug without consulting their physicians.

Ketoconazole

Ketoconazole (Nizoral) is an antifungal used to treat many varieties of candidiasis infections as well as coccidioidomycosis, blastomycosis, histoplasmosis, chromomycosis, paracoccidioidomycosis, and severe cutaneous dermatophyte infections that resist griseofulvin (Fulvicin, Grifulvin V) therapy.

How does it work?

Ketoconazole blocks the fungal synthesis of ergosterol, which is essential to the integrity of the cell membranes of nearly all pathogenic fungi.

How is it used?

Ketoconazole has a broad spectrum of antifungal activity. This drug, or amphotericin B, is the drug of choice for the treatment of blastomycosis, coccidioidosis, and histoplasmosis. It is an alternative drug for candidiasis. Successful treatment sometimes requires months.

What are the adverse effects?

The most common adverse effects of ketoconazole include nausea and vomiting, diarrhea, pruritus (severe itching), abdominal cramps, headache, photophobia, fever, and impotence.

What are the contraindications and interactions?

Ketoconazole should not be used in patients with hypersensitivity to this drug or in patients with chronic alcoholism or fungal meningitis. Safety during pregnancy and lactation and in children younger than 2 years has not been established. Ketoconazole should be used cautiously in patients with a history of liver disease or with HIV infection.

Cimetidine (Tagamet) inhibits and rifampin (Rifadin) induces the metabolism of ketoconazole. Rifadin decreases the biosynthesis of androgens and estrogens.

What are the important points patients should know?

Instruct patients to promptly report the signs and symptoms of hepatotoxicity to their physician. Advise them to avoid over-the-counter (OTC) drugs for gastric distress (such as Rolaids, Tums, and Alka-Seltzer) and to check with their physicians before taking any other nonprescription medications. Tell patients to not alter the dose or dose interval before consulting their physicians.

Griseofulvin

Griseofulvin (Fulvicin, Grifulvin V) is an effective agent in the treatment of superficial fungal infections.

How does it work?

Griseofulvin is fungistatic and not **fungicidal** (having a killing action on fungi). Its action involves deposition in newly formed skin and nail beds, where it binds to keratin, protecting these sites from new infection.

How is it used?

Griseofulvin is used systemically and is highly effective in the management of dermatophyte infections of the skin, hair, and nails. Because it does not kill but only arrests reproduction of the organism, it is necessary to continue medication long enough for the entire epidermis to be replaced, thereby removing reinfecting organisms.

What are the adverse effects?

Griseofulvin may cause hypersensitivity, skin rashes, pruritus, serum sickness, severe headache, insomnia, fatigue, mental confusion, psychotic symptoms, and vertigo. This agent also causes heartburn, nausea, vomiting, diarrhea, flatulence, dry mouth, and unpleasant taste sensations. Nephrotoxicity and hepatotoxicity may occur.

What are the contraindications and interactions?

Griseofulvin is contraindicated in patients with **porphyria** (a group of diseases affecting heme, the oxygen- binding portion of hemoglobin) or liver disease. Safe use of this drug during pregnancy, lactation, or in children younger than 2 years has not been established.

Griseofulvin with alcohol may cause flushing and tachycardia. Barbiturates may decrease hypoprothrombinemic effects of oral anticoagulants. Griseofulvin may increase estrogen metabolism and decrease contraceptive efficacy of oral contraceptives.

What are the important points patients should know?

Advise patients to continue treatment as prescribed to prevent relapse. Instruct them to avoid exposure to intense natural or artificial sunlight because photosensitivity reactions may occur. Advise women to not breastfeed while taking this drug without consulting their physicians.

✳ Apply Your Knowledge 13.1

The following exercises focus on what you have just learned about antifungal agents.

CRITICAL THINKING

1. How do fungi enter the body and cause infection?
2. Compare molds with yeasts.
3. What are mycoses and what factors are required to cause a disease?
4. Describe moniliasis and describe which patients are more susceptible to this condition.
5. What are the classifications of antifungal agents?
6. What are the trade names of amphotericin B, fluconazole, ketoconazole, and clotrimazole?
7. What are the indications of amphotericin B?
8. What is the mechanism of action for griseofulvin?

Malarial Infections

Malaria is caused by several species of the protozoan *Plasmodium*, of which *Plasmodium vivax* and *Plasmodium falciparum* are the most common. The most serious infections involve *P. falciparum*, which causes a higher incidence of complications and deaths. These protozoans all have complex life cycles involving the anopheles mosquito and the red blood cells of the human host. The infection caused by *P. vivax* is a persisting tissue phase that continues to infect the blood at intervals for many years. Thus, the ideal drug to combat malarial infections should eradicate the *microzoan* from not only the blood but from the tissue as well to effect what is termed a **radical cure**.

Antimalarial Agents

Several antimalarials differ in their points of interruption of the cycle of the parasite (an organism that lives on or in another and draws its nourishment from the host organism) and in the type of malaria affected. In addition, parasite resistance (especially that of *P. falciparum*) to these drugs is an important therapeutic problem.

Antimalarial drugs include chloroquine (Aralen), primaquine (Primaquine), quinine (Quinamm), and hydroxychloroquine (Plaquenil). Some agents are used for the actual prevention of malaria. They include mefloquine (Lariam); quinacrine (Mepacrine); and folic acid antagonists, such as pyrimethamine (Daraprim) (Table 13-2 ■).

Table 13-2 ■ Antimalarial Drugs

GENERIC NAME	TRADE NAME	AVERAGE DOSAGE IN ADULTS	ROUTE OF ADMINISTRATION
chloroquine	Aralen	300–700 mg/wk, 2 wk before exposure and for ≤4 wk after leaving endemic area	PO
doxycycline (tetracycline)	Vibramycin	100 mg daily 1–2 days before, continuously during, and 4 wk after travel	PO
hydroxychloroquine	Plaquenil	400 mg/wk	PO
mefloquine	Lariam	5 tablets with water as a single oral dose, and then 250 mg/wk and then every other wk	PO
primaquine	Primaquine	15 mg/d for 14 d	PO
pyrimethamine	Daraprim	25 mg once/wk up to 10 wk	PO
quinine	Quinamm	260–650 mg q8h for 6–12 d	PO

PO, oral.

Focus On

Chloroquine

Chloroquine (Aralen) is one of the most commonly used drugs for prophylaxis and the treatment of acute malarial attacks that are caused by *P. vivax, Plasmodium malariae, Plasmodium ovale*, and susceptible strains of *P. falciparum*.

How does it work?

Chloroquine is a protozoacidal drug. The agent destroys *Plasmodia* organisms by interfering with their metabolism or inhibiting normal replication of the protozoan.

How is it used?

Chloroquine is used for the control of acute attacks of *P. vivax* malaria and for suppression against all plasmodia except chloroquine-resistant *P. falciparum*. The drug is neither a prophylactic nor a radical curative agent in *P. vivax* malaria. In regions where *P. falciparum* is generally sensitive to chloroquine, it is markedly effective in terminating acute attacks of nonresistant *P. falciparum* malaria and usually brings about a complete cure in this type of malaria.

Chloroquine is the drug of choice for the oral treatment of all malaria except that caused by resistant *P. falciparum*.

What are the adverse effects?

The adverse effects include pigmentation of the skin and nail beds, pruritus, fatigue, toxic psychosis, and ototoxicity. Chloroquine may also cause corneal opacities (clouding of the corneas of the eyes) and retinopathy.

What are the contraindications and interactions?

Chloroquine is contraindicated in patients with liver disease, hypersensitivity to 4-aminoquinolines, psoriasis, porphyria, and renal disease. This drug should also not be used by children or by pregnant or lactating women.

Certain antacids and laxatives decrease chloroquine absorption, and chloroquine may interfere with the response to rabies vaccine.

What are the important points patients should know?

Advise patients to promptly report visual or hearing disturbances, muscle weakness, loss of balance, and symptoms of blood dyscrasia (fever, sore mouth or throat, unexplained fatigue, easy bruising, or bleeding). Instruct them to wear dark glasses in sunlight and bright light (because of photophobia) to reduce the risk of ocular damage and to avoid driving or other potentially hazardous activities until a reaction to the drug is known. Inform patients that this drug may cause rusty yellow or brown discoloration of the urine.

Primaquine

Primaquine (Primaquine) is an antimalarial agent that is very important for the radical cure of relapsing *P. vivax* or *P. ovale* malaria. It is not used for suppressive therapy or for the control of the acute clinical attacks of the disease.

How does it work?

Primaquine acts directly on the preformed nucleic acid DNA in the microorganisms. It is also gametocidal against the four human malaria species. The mechanism of antimalarial action is unknown.

How is it used?

Primaquine is indicated for the cure of relapsing *P. vivax* malaria. It eliminates symptoms and the infection as well as prevents relapse.

What are the adverse effects?

Primaquine in recommended doses is generally well tolerated. It infrequently causes nausea, vomiting, abdominal cramps, and headache. More serious (but rare) adverse effects include leukopenia, agranulocytosis, and cardiac arrhythmias.

What are the contraindications and interactions?

Primaquine is contraindicated in patients with rheumatoid arthritis and lupus erythematosus. Primaquine should be avoided in pregnancy.

What are the important points patients should know?

Instruct patients to examine their urine after each voiding and report darkening or a red tinge or a decrease in urine volume. Advise them to report chills, fever, pain in the region of the diaphragm, and cyanosis (all of which suggest a hemolytic reaction). Instruct patients to not breastfeed while taking this drug.

Quinine

Quinine (Quinamm) remains the first-line therapy for *P. falciparum* malaria, especially severe disease. A chemically related drug—quinidine gluconate (Quinaglute Duratabs)—is an antidysrhythmic drug that is used off-label to treat severe malaria via IV administration.

How does it work?

Quinine is an agent that is destructive to *gametes*, or germ cells, and acts rapidly against all *Plasmodium* malaria except *P. falciparum*. The actual mechanism of action of quinine is unknown.

How is it used?

Quinine is the treatment of choice for severe *P. falciparum*. It is not generally used in chemoprophylaxis owing to its toxicity.

What are the adverse effects?

The adverse effects of quinine include visual and hearing disturbances, fever, headache, flushing, syncope (fainting), and cardiovascular collapse. It may also cause vomiting, diarrhea, and abdominal pain.

What are the contraindications and interactions?

Quinine should be discontinued if signs of hypersensitivity occur. It should be avoided in those with visual or auditory problems. It must be used with great caution in those with underlying cardiac abnormalities. Aluminum-containing antacids may block absorption. Quinine can raise plasma levels of warfarin and digoxin. Dosage must be reduced in renal insufficiency.

What are the important points patients should know?

Instruct patients to report feelings of faintness to their physicians and to eat a balanced diet with no excesses of fruit juices or milk. Advise patients to not self-medicate with OTC drugs without advice from their physicians and to not increase, decrease, skip, or discontinue doses without consulting their physicians.

(Continued)

Focus On (Continued)

. . . .

Hydroxychloroquine

Hydroxychloroquine (Plaquenil) suppresses malaria attacks that are caused by *P. vivax*, *P. malariae*, *P. ovale*, and susceptible strains of *P. falciparum*.

How does it work?

The mechanism of action of hydroxychloroquine is based on its ability to form complexes with the DNA of parasites, thereby inhibiting replication and transcription to RNA and DNA synthesis of the parasites.

How is it used?

Hydroxychloroquine is a suppressive prophylaxis agent that is also used for the treatment of acute malarial attacks caused by all forms of susceptible malaria. This drug is used adjunctively with primaquine (Primaquine) for the eradication of *P. vivax* and *P. malariae*. Hydroxychloroquine is commonly prescribed for the treatment of rheumatoid arthritis and lupus erythematosus.

What are the adverse effects?

Hydroxychloroquine may cause nausea, vomiting, anorexia, diarrhea, abdominal cramps, and weight loss. This agent may also produce fatigue, vertigo, headache, anxiety, retinopathy, blurred vision, and mood changes. The serious adverse effects (which are rare) include aplastic anemia, agranulocytosis, thrombocytopenia, and alopecia.

What are the contraindications and interactions?

Hydroxychloroquine should be avoided in patients with known hypersensitivity to the drug or in patients with visual field changes associated with quinoline compounds. It is also contraindicated in patients who have psoriasis or porphyria. Safe use of hydroxychloroquine for juvenile arthritis or in lactating women is not established. It must be used cautiously in patients with liver disease, alcoholism, and impaired renal function.

Aluminum- and magnesium-containing antacids and laxatives decrease hydroxychloroquine absorption. This agent may interfere with the response to the rabies vaccine.

What are the important points patients should know?

Inform patients about adverse effects and related symptoms when receiving prolonged therapy with this drug. Advise them to follow the drug regimen exactly as prescribed by their physician and to keep this drug out of the reach of children. Instruct women to not breastfeed while taking this drug without first consulting their physicians.

Focus on Pediatrics

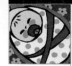

Antimalarial Drugs and Children

Children who will be traveling to countries that require antimalarial vaccinations should be vaccinated 4 to 6 weeks before embarking to ensure full protection. Also, for antimalarial prescription drugs, infants' and children's dosages must usually be specially prepared; thus, adequate time also needs to be allowed for this. Guidelines must be followed exactly because *overdosage can be fatal*. One agent in particular—hydroxychloroquine (Plaquenil)—is particularly toxic to infants and children, and extra care must be taken in administration. Taking as few as 3 to 4 tablets (250–mg strength) of chloroquine (Aralen), which is similar to hydroxychloroquine, has resulted in the death of small children.

✳ Apply Your Knowledge 13.2

The following questions focus on what you have just learned about antimalarials.

CRITICAL THINKING

1. What are the causes of malaria and its mode of transmission?
2. List seven generic names of antimalarial drugs.
3. What is the indication of primaquine?
4. What is the actual mechanism of action of quinine?
5. Who should be vaccinated against malaria?

Protozoal Infections

Although protozoal infections are very common, they are actually caused by only a small number of species often restricted geographically to the tropics and subtropics. Two protozoal organisms—*Entamoeba histolytica* and *Giardia lamblia*—are frequently responsible for causing dysentery (an inflammatory disease of the lower intestinal tract) in humans. Infection caused by the protozoan *E. histolytica* is also called *amebic dysentery* or *amebiasis* and is relatively rare in the United States. The third important protozoal infection is *Trichomonas vaginalis*, which causes a sexually transmitted disease (common in the United States) called *trichomoniasis* (Figure 13-2 ■).

Amebic infections generally remain confined to the intestines, where they may give rise to dysentery, or they may locate elsewhere, especially in the liver. The chemotherapy of amebiasis must provide drugs to treat the intestinal and extraintestinal forms of the disease and be capable of eliminating amebic cysts from the intestine.

The most commonly reported intestinal protozoal infection in the United States is giardiasis, caused by the flagellated protozoan *G. lamblia*. Most patients are asymptomatic. However, these organisms cause diarrhea that can be transient or persistent. Infection results from the ingestion of *G. lamblia* cysts, which may exist in water that is contaminated with fecal matter.

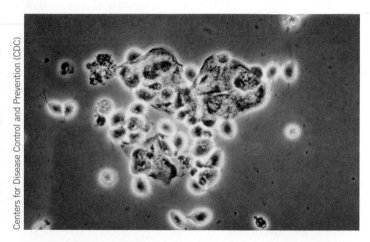

Centers for Disease Control and Prevention (CDC)

Figure 13-2 ■ Vaginal discharge with microorganisms caused by trichomoniasis.

Antiprotozoal Agents

Drugs that are used for the treatment of *E. histolytica* include metronidazole (Flagyl), iodoquinol (Yodoxin), tetracyclines, and paromomycin (Humatin). No safe drug exists that will eradicate all the motile forms, cysts, and extraintestinal amoebas in amebic infections, but combination drug therapy can eliminate parasites from all sites. Chemotherapy with metronidazole is usually successful in cases of giardiasis (Table 13-3 ■).

Table 13-3 ■ Antiprotozoal Agents

GENERIC NAME	TRADE NAME	AVERAGE DOSAGE IN ADULTS	ROUTE OF ADMINISTRATION
iodoquinol	Yodoxin	630–650 mg tid for 20 d; may repeat after a 2–3 wk drug-free interval	PO
		For trichomoniasis, giardiasis: 2 g once or 250 mg tid for 7 d	PO
metronidazole	Flagyl	1 dose of 2 g, or 500 mg bid for 7 d	PO, IV
paromomycin	Humatin	25–35 mg/kg divided in 3 doses for 5–10 d	PO

IV, intravenous; PO, oral; tid, three times a day.

Focus On

Metronidazole

Metronidazole (Flagyl) is an amebicide that is used to treat liver abscess, intestinal amebiasis, trichomoniasis, anaerobic infections, vaginosis, diarrhea, colitis, and pelvic inflammatory disease and prevent postoperative infection after colorectal surgery.

How does it work?

Metronidazole is a direct-acting trichomonacide and amebicide that works at intestinal and extraintestinal sites. It apparently enters cells of microorganisms that contain the enzyme nitroreductase, forming unstable compounds that bind to DNA, inhibiting synthesis and causing cell death.

How is it used?

Metronidazole is prescribed for asymptomatic and symptomatic trichomoniasis in female and male patients. It is also used for acute intestinal amebiasis and amebic liver abscess. Metronidazole is usually indicated for preoperative prophylaxis in colorectal surgery, elective hysterectomy or vaginal repair, and emergency appendectomy.

What are the adverse effects?

The adverse effects of metronidazole include nausea, vomiting, anorexia, abdominal cramps, metallic or bitter taste, skin rashes, pruritus, flushing, fever, vertigo, headache, confusion, depression, restlessness, and insomnia. The urine sometimes turns a dark color.

What are the contraindications and interactions?

Metronidazole should not be used in patients with diseases of the central nervous system. The drug has been found to be carcinogenic in mice and rats. It has been used in pregnancy without consequence, but it is advisable to withhold it during pregnancy if possible. Metronidazole interacts with cimetidine, disulfiram, lithium, oral anticoagulants, phenobarbital, phenytoin, and alcohol. For safety, alcohol should be completely avoided while taking metronidazole and for 3 days after stopping administration of the medication. Interaction between metronidazole and alcohol may result in tachycardia, skin warmth or redness, tingling sensations, nausea, and vomiting.

What are the important points patients should know?

Instruct patients to adhere closely to the established regimen without schedule interruptions or dose change. They must refrain from intercourse during therapy for trichomoniasis unless a condom is used to prevent reinfection. Inform patients that sexual partners should receive concurrent treatment. Asymptomatic trichomoniasis in men is a frequent source of reinfection in their female partners. Also, instruct patients to avoid alcohol while taking this drug.

Focus Point

Fungal Superinfections

Usually occurring in the anal and genital areas or in the vagina or mouth, fungal superinfections cause anal or vaginal itching, vaginal discharge, and lesions on the tongue or mouth. A common type of fungal superinfection is known as *candidiasis* or *moniliasis*. This superinfection may occur because of an overgrowth of yeast-like fungi in the vagina. Normally, multiplication of these microorganisms is controlled because of a strain of vaginal bacteria known as *Doderlein bacillus*. Penicillin therapy may destroy these bacteria, causing the fungi to multiply at a rapid rate. Symptoms include vaginal discharge and itching.

Focus On

Iodoquinol

Iodoquinol (Diquinol, Yodoxin) is an anti-infective, anti-amebicide, and antiprotozoal agent.

How does it work?

Iodoquinol is a direct-acting amebicide that works in the intestinal lumen. When it enters the cells of protozoa, it affects the DNA, inhibiting synthesis and causing cell death.

How is it used?

Iodoquinol is used only as a luminal amebicide and has no effect against extraintestinal amebic infections. It is commonly prescribed either concurrently or in alternating courses with another intestinal amebicide.

What are the adverse effects?

Infrequent adverse effects of iodoquinol include diarrhea—which usually stops after several days—nausea, vomiting, abdominal pain, anorexia, headache, rash, and pruritus. Iodoquinol can cause blurred vision, optic atrophy, permanent loss of vision, and thyroid hypertrophy.

What are the contraindications and interactions?

Iodoquinol is contraindicated in patients with hypersensitivity to any iodine-containing preparations or foods and those with hepatic or renal damage. Safe use during pregnancy or lactation is not established.

What are the important points patients should know?

Instruct patients to report skin rash and symptoms of a sudden decrease in their leukocyte count, such as chills, fever, weakness, and fatigue, and to complete the full course of treatment. Their stools need to be examined at 1, 3, and 6 months after the termination of treatment to ensure the infection has not returned.

✳ Apply Your Knowledge 13.3

The following questions focus on what you have just learned about antiprotozoal infections and agents.

CRITICAL THINKING

1. Compare *Entamoeba histolytica* with *Giardia lamblia*.
2. What are the trade names of metronidazole, paromomycin, and iodoquinol?
3. What are the contraindications of metronidazole?
4. What is the classification of iodoquinol?
5. What are the main adverse effects of iodoquinol?

PRACTICAL SCENARIO 1

A 62-year-old woman with lung cancer is exhibiting symptoms of an infection. She is admitted to her local hospital, and after testing, her physician diagnoses her as having aspergillosis, a fungal disease of the lungs. He prescribes amphotericin B by intravenous injection.

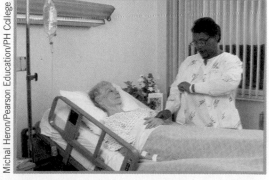

Michal Heron/Pearson Education/PH College

Critical Thinking Questions

1. The patient asks the nurse what adverse effects she can expect from the drug. What would be the appropriate answer for the nurse to give the patient?
2. Can you think of any adverse reactions the nurse needs to monitor this patient for?
3. What patient education should the nurse provide to this patient?

PRACTICAL SCENARIO 2

A medical assistant called a patient named Laila to tell her about her recent examination and laboratory test results. Laila had a vaginal infection and needed a specific medication. The medical assistant said she would call in the prescription for the medication to Laila's local pharmacy. Laila asked what type of vaginal infection she had and was told that it was caused by a type of protozoa. The medical assistant also told her the medication should be taken twice daily for a maximum of 7 days.

Andrey Kiselev/Fotolia

Critical Thinking Questions

1. What is the drug of choice for this type of protozoal infection?
2. If the physician ordered this drug of choice, what are its potential adverse effects?

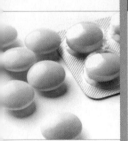

Chapter Capsule

This section repeats the objectives from the beginning of the chapter and then provides a summary of the most important concepts for that objective. Use this section as a quick review and to check your knowledge.

Objective 1: Identify the risk factors that will most likely cause patients to acquire systemic and serious fungal infections.

- Constant exposure to systemic-causing infections present in the air, dust, fomites, and even among the normal flora in the environment of humans
- Exposure to overwhelming numbers of fungi
- Immunosuppression (especially HIV and AIDS) and immunosuppressive drug therapies (including those used for cancer and organ transplantation patients)
- Frequent surgeries
- Use of broad-spectrum antimicrobials

Objective 2: List four different pharmacotherapies for the treatment of systemic and superficial fungal infections.

- Amphotericin B (Amphocin)
- Flucytosine (Ancobon)
- Ketoconazole (Nizoral)
- Griseofulvin (Fulvicin, Grifulvin V)

Objective 3: Explain how fungi and protozoans may gain access to a human host.

- Fungi: via respiratory, mucous, and cutaneous routes
- Protozoans: via creatures such as mosquitoes that attack the red blood cells; other protozoans are transmitted by sexual activity or the consumption of contaminated foods or water

Objective 4: Describe the general drug actions, uses, and contraindications of antifungal agents.

■ Actions: interference with the synthesis of ergosterol, a chemical found in fungal cell membranes

■ Uses: systemic fungal diseases; superficial moniliasis infections; in the prophylaxis of aspergillosis in immunocompromised patients; cryptococcosis (a fungal disease of the lungs often occurring in patients with meningitis); blastomycosis; histoplasmosis; candidiasis; dermatophyte infections of the skin, hair, and nails

■ Contraindications: hypersensitive patients—those with impaired hepatic or renal function, bone marrow suppression, chronic alcoholism, and porphyria; ketoconazole (Nizoral) should not be used for patients with fungal meningitis or HIV infection; the safety of use for ketoconazole and griseofulvin (Fulvicin, Grifulvin V) during pregnancy or lactation and in children younger than 2 years old has not been established

Objective 5: Describe the general drug indications of antimalarial agents.

■ Chloroquine (Aralen): control of acute attacks of vivax malaria; suppression against all *Plasmodia spp.* except chloroquine-resistant *P. falciparum*; oral treatment of all malaria except that caused by resistant *P. falciparum*

■ Primaquine (Primaquine): cure of relapsing vivax malaria

■ Quinine (Quinamm): treatment of severe *P. falciparum*

■ Hydroxychloroquine (Plaquenil): suppressive prophylaxis agent; treatment of acute malarial attacks caused by all forms of susceptible malaria; used adjunctively with primaquine for the eradication of *P. vivax* and *P. malariae*

Objective 6: Identify the three common protozoans that cause dysentery, trichomoniasis, and giardiasis.

■ Dysentery: *E. histolytica* and *G. lamblia*

■ Trichomoniasis: *T. vaginalis*

■ Giardiasis: *G. lamblia*

Objective 7: Explain the drugs that are most frequently used in the treatment of intestinal amebiasis and their contraindications.

■ Metronidazole (Flagyl)—a direct-acting trichomonacide and amebicide that works at intestinal and extraintestinal sites; contraindicated in patients with central nervous system diseases and should be withheld during pregnancy

■ Iodoquinol (Yodoxin)—a direct-acting amebicide that works in the intestinal lumen; contraindicated in patients with hypersensitivity to any iodine-containing preparations or foods and those with hepatic or renal damage; safe use during pregnancy or lactation is not established

Objective 8: Discuss drugs used to treat protozoal infections.

■ Metronidazole (Flagyl): for *E. histolytica*, amebiasis, and trichomoniasis

■ Other drugs that treat *E. histolytica* are iodoquinol (Yodoxin), tetracyclines, and paromomycin (Humatin)

■ Adverse effects: nausea, vomiting, anorexia, abdominal cramps, metallic or bitter taste, skin rashes, pruritus, flushing, fever, vertigo, headache, confusion, depression, restlessness, insomnia, darkening of urine; found to be carcinogenic in mice and rats

Internet Sites of Interest

- For information on nail fungus, including diagnosis and treatments, check out the Mayo Clinic website at **http://www.mayoclinic.com**. Search "nail fungus."

- Patients with HIV and those who are immunocompromised are more susceptible to fungal infections than healthy individuals. Information on opportunistic fungal infections in HIV-positive individuals can be found at **http://www.thebodypro.com/treat/candida.html**, a website provided by the HIV/AIDS Resources for Healthcare Professionals.

- The Centers for Disease Control and Prevention (CDC) offers tips for travelers who may visit areas where malaria is a concern: **http://www.cdc.gov/malaria**.

- At **http://healthresources.caremark.com/topic/protodrugs**, you can find information provided by Caremark on protozoal infections and the drugs used to treat them, including patient education tips.

- A fact sheet on trichomoniasis is provided by the CDC at **http://www.cdc.gov/std/Trichomonas/STDFact-Trichomoniasis.htm** and contains reliable patient education information.

PEARSON myhealthprofessionskit™

Go to www.myhealthprofessionskit.com to access the Companion Website created for this textbook. Simply select "Basic Health Science" from the choice of disciplines. Find this book and then log in using your username and password to access interactive learning games, assessment questions, animations, and more.

Chapter Objectives

After completing this chapter, you should be able to:

1. State the names and functions of blood cells involved in immunity.

2. List the major components of the lymphatic system.

3. Discuss and contrast the various types of immunities.

4. Explain the differences between active and passive immunity.

5. State the main action of immunizing agents.

6. Contrast inactivated and attenuated vaccines.

7. List the most common adverse effects associated with vaccinations.

8. Describe the most common childhood immunizations.

9. List the most common adult immunizations.

10. Explain how immunoglobulins work to provide immunity.

Chapter 14

Vaccines and Immunoglobulins

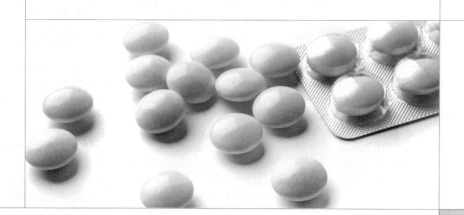

Key Terms

active immunity (ih-MYOO-nih-tee) (page 228)

antibodies (AN-tih-bah-deez) (page 226)

antigens (AN-tih-jenz) (page 226)

asplenia (as-PLEN-ee-yuh) (page 233)

attenuated (ah-TEN-yoo-ay-ted) (page 228)

booster (page 232)

cell-mediated immunity (page 226)

globulins (GLOB-yoo-linz) (page 235)

humoral (HYOO-moh-rul) **immunity** (page 226)

immune response (page 226)

immunity (page 226)

immunogen (ih-MYOO-no-jen) (page 228)

immunoglobulins (ih-myoon-o-GLOB-yoo-linz) (page 228)

isotypes (EYE-so-typz) (page 235)

lymph (limf) (page 226)

lymphatic (lim-FAH-tik) **vessels** (page 226)

lymphocytes (LIM-foh-sites) (page 226)

lymphoid (LIM-foyd) **organs** (page 226)

macrophages (MAK-ro-fah-jez) (page 226)

passive immunity (page 228)

pathogens (PAH-tho-jenz) (page 226)

toxin (TOKS-in) (page 229)

toxoids (TOX-oyds) (page 229)

vaccination (vak-sih-NAY-shun) (page 228)

vaccine (vak-SEEN) (page 228)

Introduction

Immunizing agents and allergenic extracts are two of the main groups of drugs that are classified as *biologics* by the FDA. Biologics are chemical agents that produce biological responses in the body. As a group, particularly the active immunizing agents, biologics possibly have prevented more morbidity and mortality than all other drugs combined. *Vaccina vaccine* may be considered the most effective drug to date because it has virtually eradicated smallpox from our world. A similar success for the *poliomyelitis virus vaccines* appears imminent.

The Immune System

The human immune system is a truly amazing constellation of responses to attacks from outside the body. The immune system is part of the lymphatic system, which is composed of the lymph vessels; lymph nodes; and other organs, such as the thymus gland, spleen, and tonsils. This system rids foreign substances from the blood and lymph, combats infectious diseases, maintains tissue fluid balance, and absorbs fats.

When microorganisms or foreign substances invade the body, the body responds by producing more white blood cells, or **lymphocytes**. The body continues to fight the invaders by forming special proteins manufactured by the lymphocytes, called **antibodies**. The dominant cells of the lymphatic system, lymphocytes are vital to our ability to resist or overcome infection and disease. They respond to the presence of (1) invading **pathogens**, such as bacteria or viruses; (2) abnormal body cells, such as cancer cells; and (3) foreign proteins, such as the toxins released by some bacteria. Lymphocytes attempt to eliminate these threats or render them harmless by a combination of physical and chemical attack.

Lymphocytes respond to specific threats, such as a bacterial invasion of a tissue, by organizing a defense against that specific type of bacterium. Such a *specific defense* of the body is known as an **immune response**. **Immunity** is the ability to resist infection and disease through the activation of specific defenses.

The lymphatic system, shown in Figure 14-1 ■, includes the following three components:

1. **Vessels:** A network of **lymphatic vessels** begins in peripheral tissues and ends at connections to the venous system
2. **Fluid:** A fluid called **lymph** flows through the lymphatic vessels
3. **Lymphoid organs: Lymphoid organs** are connected to the lymphatic vessels and contain large numbers of lymphocytes; examples of the organs are the lymph nodes, spleen, and thymus

The blood contains three classes of lymphocytes:

1. T cells (thymus-dependent)
2. B cells (bone marrow–derived)
3. Natural killer (NK) cells

T cells comprise approximately 80% of circulating lymphocytes. *Cytotoxic* T cells directly attack foreign cells or body cells infected by viruses. These lymphocytes are the primary cells that provide **cell-mediated immunity**.

B cells constitute 10% to 15% of circulating lymphocytes. B cells can differentiate into *plasma cells*, which are responsible for the production and secretion of *antibodies*. Antibodies are globular proteins that are often called *immunoglobulins (Igs)*. Antibodies react with specific chemical targets called **antigens**. Antigens are usually pathogens, parts or products of pathogens, or other foreign compounds.

NK cells make up the remaining 5% to 10% of circulating lymphocytes. These lymphocytes attack foreign cells, normal cells infected with viruses, and cancer cells that appear in normal tissues.

Cell-Mediated Immunity and Humoral Immunity

Cell-mediated immunity depends on the functions of the T cells, which are responsible for a delayed type of immune response. The T lymphocyte becomes sensitized by the first contact with a specific antigen. T cells and **macrophages** (immune cells derived from monocytes) work together in cell-mediated immunity to destroy the antigen. T cells attack the antigens directly rather than producing antibodies. Cell-mediated immunity may also occur without macrophages. T cells defend the body against viral, fungal, and some bacterial infections. If cell-mediated immunity is lost, as in the case of acquired immunodeficiency syndrome (AIDS), the body is unable to protect itself against many viral, bacterial, and fungal infections.

Humoral immunity is based on the antigen–antibody response. B cells, which are responsible for humoral immunity, produce circulating antibodies to act against an antigen. B cells arise from a separate population of stem cells of the bone marrow than that which produces T cells. These cells undergo multiplication and processing in lymphoid tissue elsewhere than in the thymus gland. B cells, similar to T cells, have surface receptors that enable them to recognize the appropriate antigen. But unlike T cells, B cells do not themselves interact to neutralize or destroy the antigen. On recognition of the antigen, they take up residence in secondary lymphoid tissue and proliferate to form daughter lymphocytes. These B cells then develop into plasma cells. The plasma cells produce antibodies and release them into the circulation at the lymph nodes. Some of the activated B cells do not become plasma cells. Instead, they turn into memory cells, which continue to produce small amounts of the antibody long after the infection has been overcome.

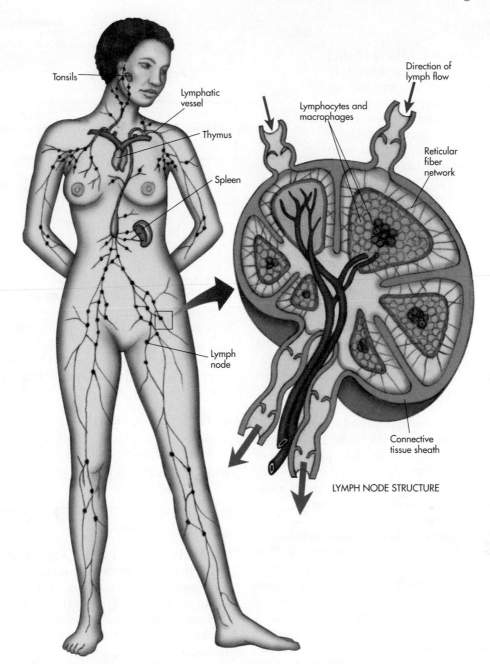

Figure 14-1 ■ The lymphatic system includes the tonsils, lymph nodes, spleen, and lymphatic vessels. Within the lymph nodes are the macrophages and lymphocytes.

✳ Apply Your Knowledge 14.1

The following questions focus on what you have just learned about white blood cells and immunity.

CRITICAL THINKING

1. What are natural killer cells? Describe their functions.
2. What types of lymphocytes are responsible for humoral immunity?
3. What is cell-mediated immunity?
4. Differentiate between antigens, antibodies, and macrophages.
5. What are cytotoxic T cells?

Immunity

Immunity is the state or condition of being resistant to invading microorganisms. It is normally acquired either by contracting a disease and then developing immunity to it or by being vaccinated with proteins from the causative agent. For example, a person with a normal immune system who contracts rubella (German measles) develops a lifelong immunity to the disease. Alternatively, a person may be vaccinated with dead rubella viruses to acquire immunity. In both cases, the immune system responds to proteins in the virus and develops a *memory* for it. The next time the person is exposed to the live virus, the immune system *remembers* its past exposure and attacks and kills the virus before it can cause an infection.

Immunizing agents are broadly classified on the basis of the type of immunity they induce. Knowing the properties of the different types of immunity is fundamental to understanding immunizing agents and their applications. There are two main types of immunity: active and passive.

Active immunity is a form of acquired immunity that develops in an individual in response to an **immunogen** (antigen). This may be naturally acquired by exposure to an infectious disease or artificially acquired by receiving active immunizing agents (*vaccines*). The term **vaccination** is used as a synonym for active immunization.

Passive immunity involves the transfer of the effectors of immunity, which are called **immunoglobulins** or antibodies, from an immune individual to another. This occurs naturally by the active transport across the placental barrier of IgG antibodies from mother to fetus and, to a lesser extent, by the transfer of IgA antibodies in the mother's milk to the nursing infant. The onset of passive immunity is much quicker than that of active immunity, but the duration is much shorter because there is no active immune response to the immunogen (Figure 14-2 ■).

IMMUNIZING AGENTS

Immunizing agents are among the oldest of modern drugs and can be traced to the beginning of immunology in 1798, when Edward Jenner introduced his

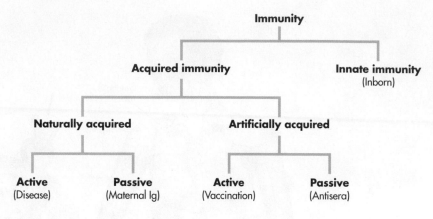

Figure 14-2 ■ Types of immunity.

vaccine for smallpox. A **vaccine** is a preparation of killed microorganisms, living **attenuated** (their virulence has been reduced) organisms, or living virulent organisms that are administered to produce or artificially increase immunity to a particular disease. They are the most successful and powerful drugs yet developed. Active immunizing agents have these advantages:

✳ Their main action is to *prevent* rather than to treat disease; most of the commonly used vaccines are highly effective.

✳ They have been proven to be remarkably *safe* in actual practice.

✳ Active immunizing agents are generally available at a relatively *low cost*.

Active immunizing agents are immunogenic drugs that are usually administered to patients before their being exposed to diseases to provide long-term, even permanent protection against the diseases. Perhaps active immunization will one day be used for a variety of conditions, ranging from cancer to drug abuse.

Passive immunizing agents date to the early part of the twentieth century after the discovery of Igs (antibodies). Various antitoxins derived from animals held an important place in therapy before the development of antibiotics, but these products—in contrast to the vaccines—had a number of problems with respect to efficacy and safety.

Focus on Pediatrics

Routine Immunization Reduces Disease

Immunization for diphtheria, tetanus, and pertussis (DTP) has been routinely given in the United States since the late 1940s, resulting in dramatic reductions in the incidence of all these diseases.

Focus On

Vaccines

Most vaccines consist of entire microorganisms that may be either *inactivated* (killed) or *attenuated* (live). One way to attenuate a virus is through laboratory manipulation, in which a bacterium is developed that lacks a **toxin** (a chemical produced by a microorganism that can be harmful), an enzyme, or some other normal constituent that causes symptoms of disease. The bacterium's virulence is thereby lessened.

Most bacterial vaccines contain killed bacteria or their components. It is important to understand that the live vaccines contain less immunogen than the killed vaccines and must actually cause an infection within the patient to induce a protective immune response.

Another type of vaccine contains **toxoids**, which are protein toxins that have been modified to reduce their hazardous properties without significantly altering their antigenic properties. The oldest and best-known active immunizing agents are diphtheria toxoid and tetanus toxoid, which protect against the bacterial exotoxins.

Whereas a *simple vaccine* is one that protects against a single disease, a *combined vaccine* is a combination product that protects against two or more diseases.

How do they work?

The principle underlying vaccination is that exposure to an antigen (a virus or bacterium) in a relatively harmless form sensitizes immune cells for a possible subsequent exposure to the organism. On re-exposure, the memory of the previous challenge triggers an immune response more quickly. Because the person's own immune processes are stimulated by this agent, this is a form of active immunity. Usually, more than one dose of the vaccine is required to trigger a rapid and full immune response. The number of doses needed reflects the potency of the vaccine.

How are they used?

The indications and recommendations for the use of vaccines depend on several factors, such as safety and efficacy, as with other drugs. The FDA approves the indications for each licensed product. Vaccines are used against a range of bacterial infections, including diphtheria, tetanus, pertussis, pneumonia, tuberculosis, typhoid, cholera, meningitis, plague, and Q fever. Vaccines are also available against such viral infections as measles, mumps, and rubella (MMR); poliomyelitis; hepatitis A and B; influenza; rabies; and yellow fever (see Tables 14-1 ■ and 14-2 ■).

What are the adverse effects?

The most common adverse effects associated with vaccinations include localized inflammation at the site of injection, a mild fever, headache, malaise, nausea, and dizziness. Convulsions resulting in permanent brain damage have been reported after administration of pertussis vaccine, but these reactions are rare. In some individuals, an allergic reaction may occur immediately after vaccination. The recipient should be observed for a short time after the vaccine is administered, and adrenaline should always be available in case anaphylaxis occurs.

What are the contraindications and interactions?

Immunizations are contraindicated in people with acute febrile illness, during pregnancy and lactation, and in those who are known to have developed anaphylactoid reactions with previous vaccines.

When several vaccines are given at the same time, the potential for drug interaction is increased. An example of this situation would be when typhoid, cholera, and plague vaccines are administered together.

What are the important points patients should know?

Instruct patients to monitor the injection site for reactions. Advise women to avoid breastfeeding until checking with their physicians.

✳ Apply Your Knowledge 14.2 ━━━━

The following exercise focuses on what you have just learned about various types of immunities, vaccines, and toxoids.

CRITICAL THINKING

1. What are inactivated and attenuated vaccines? Name two examples of each.

2. Compare active immunity and passive immunity.

3. What is immunity?

4. What are toxoids? Name two examples.

5. Name four vaccines that are administered subcutaneously.

Table 14-1 ■ Bacterial Vaccines

VACCINE	ROUTES OF ADMINISTRATION
Live Attenuated Vaccines	
Bacillus Calmette Guérin (BCG) vaccine*	PC
Typhoid vaccine	PO or subcutaneous
Inactivated Vaccines	
Anthrax vaccine, adsorbed	Subcutaneous
Cholera vaccine	Intradermal, subcutaneous, IM
Haemophilus influenzae type b (Hib)	IM
Lyme disease vaccine	IM
Meningococcal polysaccharide vaccine	Subcutaneous
Pertussis vaccine, adsorbed	IM
Pneumococcal conjugate vaccine	Subcutaneous or IM
Tetanus toxoid, adsorbed	IM

*Bacillus Calmette Guerin (BCG) vaccine is not generally recommended for use in the United States because of a low risk of infection with *Mycobacterium tuberculosis* and other reasons. It should be considered only for people who meet specific criteria determined by a tuberculosis expert.

IM, intramuscular; PC, percutaneous; PO, oral.

Table 14-2 ■ Inactivated Virus Vaccines

VACCINE	ROUTES OF ADMINISTRATION
Hepatitis A vaccine	IM
Hepatitis B vaccine	IM
Influenza virus vaccine (types A and B)	IM
Poliovirus vaccine, inactivated	Subcutaneous
Rabies virus vaccine	IM

*The measles, mumps, and rubella (MMR) vaccine contains live attenuated viruses and must be administered subcutaneously.

IM, intramuscular.

Standards for Childhood Immunization

The Advisory Committee on Immunization Practices (ACIP) currently recommends that children be immunized against eight infectious diseases as well as against hepatitis A in areas of high incidence (Table 14-3 ■). Childhood immunization remains one of the most important public health measures in the United States.

Haemophilus influenzae type b (Hib) was the leading cause of invasive bacterial disease (e.g., meningitis) among children until pediatric immunization was introduced in 1988. The vaccine contains inactivated bacteria (HibTiter, PedvaxHIB).

The Salk inactivated vaccine (IPV, IPOL; 1954) and the Sabin live vaccine (1961) are two types of polio immunizations that have been very effective against

Table 14-3 ■ Recommended Immunization Schedule for Persons Ages 0 to 6 Years—United States, 2011

Recommended Immunization Schedule for Persons Aged 0 Through 6 Years—United States • 2011
For those who fall behind or start late, see the catch-up schedule

Vaccine ▼ Age ►	Birth	1 month	2 months	4 months	6 months	12 months	15 months	18 months	19–23 months	2–3 years	4–6 years
Hepatitis B[1]	HepB	HepB			HepB						
Rotavirus[2]			RV	RV	RV[2]						
Diphtheria, Tetanus, Pertussis[3]			DTaP	DTaP	DTaP	see footnote[3]	DTaP				DTaP
Haemophilus influenzae type b[4]			Hib	Hib	Hib[4]	Hib					
Pneumococcal[5]			PCV	PCV	PCV	PCV				PPSV	
Inactivated Poliovirus[6]			IPV	IPV		IPV					IPV
Influenza[7]						Influenza (Yearly)					
Measles, Mumps, Rubella[8]						MMR		see footnote[8]			MMR
Varicella[9]						Varicella		see footnote[9]			Varicella
Hepatitis A[10]						HepA (2 doses)				HepA Series	
Meningococcal[11]										MCV4	

Range of recommended ages for all children

Range of recommended ages for certain high-risk groups

This schedule includes recommendations in effect as of December 21, 2010. Any dose not administered at the recommended age should be administered at a subsequent visit, when indicated and feasible. The use of a combination vaccine generally is preferred over separate injections of its equivalent component vaccines. Considerations should include provider assessment, patient preference, and the potential for adverse events. Providers should consult the relevant Advisory Committee on Immunization Practices statement for detailed recommendations: **http://www.cdc.gov/vaccines/pubs/acip-list.htm**. Clinically significant adverse events that follow immunization should be reported to the Vaccine Adverse Event Reporting System (VAERS) at **http://www.vaers.hhs.gov** or by telephone, **800-822-7967**. Use of trade names and commercial sources is for identification only and does not imply endorsement by the U.S. Department of Health and Human Services.

These recommendations must be read along with the footnotes, which can be found in Appendix D.

Courtesy of Centers for Disease Control and Prevention: *Recommended Immunization Schedule for Persons Aged 0 Through 6 Years—United States, 2011*. Available at http://www.cdc.gov/vaccines/recs/schedules/downloads/child/0-6yrs-schedule-pr.pdf.

poliomyelitis. There has been no poliomyelitis in the Americas in recent years except for vaccine-associated disease and a few importation cases.

Measles, mumps, and rubella (German measles) are three important viral diseases that can potentially be eradicated by mass active immunization. The combined vaccine (MMR) was licensed in 1971 and has been recommended for routine immunizations since 1977.

Hepatitis B infection is a major worldwide health problem with many facets, including acute and chronic disease, liver failure and cirrhosis, hepatic carcinoma, and chronic carriers. Neonates born to mothers who are positive for hepatitis B should be immunized immediately with the vaccine (Energix B, Heptava B) and hepatitis B Ig.

Varicella (*chicken pox*) is a highly communicable disease that is generally benign but also causes herpes and sometimes may be accompanied by serious complications, such as encephalitis and bacterial superinfection. Varicella is more serious in adults, particularly in immunodeficient individuals, in whom it can cause devastating disease. The varicella vaccine (Varivax) was licensed in 1995 and appears to be very effective in protecting against chicken pox, but it is much too early to completely evaluate the impact of the immunization program on the epidemiology of varicella-zoster.

The ACIP recommends hepatitis A vaccination (Havrix, VAQTA) for children residing in communities where the incidence of hepatitis A is high and common.

In June 2006, the FDA licensed the first vaccine developed to prevent cancer and other diseases in women that are caused by certain types of the genital human papillomavirus (HPV). This vaccine (trade name Gardasil) protects against four HPV types (6, 11, 16, and 18) that are responsible for cervical cancer and 90% of genital warts. This vaccine is recommended for girls and women between the ages of 9 and 26 years.

The best time for girls to receive this vaccine is ages 10 to 11 years (this age group is used because, ideally, the vaccine should be administered before the onset of sexual activity). The recommendations for HPV vaccine are: three intramuscular injections over a 6-month period, with the second dose given 2 months after the first dose and the third dose given 6 months after the first dose.

The HPV vaccine has been tested in more than 11,000 women in many countries throughout the world, including the United States. It has been found to be safe and without any serious side effects. The vaccine appears to be effective for at least 5 years. Efficacy studies for this vaccine in men are ongoing, but currently, no data support its use in men.

❋ Apply Your Knowledge 14.3

The following questions focus on what you have just learned about the various childhood immunizations.

CRITICAL THINKING

1. What are five examples of viral vaccines?

2. What are five examples of bacterial vaccines?

3. What vaccine should be given to toddlers every year?

4. What vaccine can be given at birth? Explain why.

5. What is varicella and what is the name of its vaccine?

6. What is the best time for girls to receive HPV vaccine? Explain how many vaccines should be received.

Standards of Immunization for Adults Younger Than Age 65 Years

Pertussis vaccine is not recommended for adults, but the other nine vaccines (see Table 14-3) are commonly indicated under certain circumstances if there is not evidence of immunity, such as a reliable history of having the disease or positive serologic tests. Three circumstances in which it is particularly important that the pediatric immunizations are up to date are:

1. Individuals who travel internationally because some of these diseases remain prevalent in other parts of the world

2. Women of childbearing age who may become pregnant because the immunity (such as IgG) women transfer to the fetus depends on their immune status

3. Individuals with chronic illnesses because they may be more susceptible to a disease or its adverse effects

The only routine immunization recommended for all normal adults between the ages of 18 and 65 years is a **booster** dose (a dose given to increase the effectiveness of the original medication) of adult diphtheria and tetanus toxoid every 10 years. Unfortunately, many adults in this country do not comply with this recommendation and may not even be aware of it. Sometimes, patients with traumatic injury are given a tetanus booster in the emergency room or physician's office at the time of injury.

Annual influenza immunization (Fluzone, FluShield) is recommended for those at high risk for influenza complications as well as those capable of *nosocomial* (hospital) transmission of influenza to high-risk patients (for example, physicians, nurses, pharmacists, and others who provide inpatient, outpatient, and home health-care services as well as nonprofessional caregivers).

Pneumococcal vaccine (Pneumovax 23, Pnu-Immune 23) should be administered to people with any major immunosuppression condition, such as human immunodeficiency virus (HIV) infection, organ transplant, and some cancers. This vaccine should also be administered to patients with pulmonary or cardiovascular diseases, chronic hepatic or renal disorders, and diabetes mellitus. Meningococcal vaccine (Menomune A/C/Y/W) is recommended for some travelers and some closed populations in which outbreaks may occur.

The only disease for which an *International Certificate of Vaccination* may still be required is yellow fever. Travelers to underdeveloped countries (and some developed countries) may find other vaccines recommended. Hepatitis A vaccine (Havrix, VAQTA) is most likely, but cholera, typhoid, and plague vaccines may occasionally be suggested.

Hepatitis B vaccine (Energix B, Heptavax B) is essential for health-care workers with exposure to human blood and tissues, and a number of other immunizations are recommended for those in high-risk occupations.

Bacillus Calmette Guérin (BCG) vaccine is recommended only in extremely high-risk individuals in whom other controls are impractical. Besides for tuberculosis, BCG vaccine is also used to treat bladder cancer by direct instillation into the bladder. This is sometimes called nonspecific immunotherapy, but the precise mechanism is unknown. The vaccine does promote a local inflammatory response that may be responsible for the antitumor effects.

In 2009, H1N1 influenza A first appeared in Mexico, spreading to many countries all over the world. The World Health Organization named H1N1 (which was initially referred to as the "swine flu") a pandemic virus.

A vaccine against H1N1 became available in October 2009. It is available in killed and inactivated forms—either by injection or as a nasal spray. For children younger than age 10 years, the vaccine is administered in two separate doses—given 21 to 28 days apart. In those age 10 years and older, it is administered as a single dose. Severe infections and even deaths have occurred in every age group contracting the disease.

In the first quarter of 2010, approximately 57 million cases of H1N1 occurred in the United States alone, causing nearly 12,000 deaths. Most of these deaths occurred in people younger than age 65 years. Pregnant woman should receive this vaccine, which will also help their babies to be more resistant to developing symptoms of the flu. For the 2010 to 2011 flu season, the H1N1 vaccine was combined with the seasonal flu vaccine.

✳ Apply Your Knowledge 14.4

The following questions focus on what you have just learned about immunizations for adults younger than age 65 years.

CRITICAL THINKING

1. How many boosters of adult diphtheria should a person receive between ages 20 and 70 years?
2. Who should receive the BCG vaccine?
3. What is the name of the cancer vaccine in women?
4. When is hepatitis B immunoglobulin required in infants?
5. What is another name for German measles?

Standards of Immunization for Adults Older Than Age 65 Years

Evaluation of immune status and appropriate vaccination at age 65 years is important to the quality of the later years of life. Every individual should continue to receive adult *diphtheria* and *tetanus toxoid* boosters every 10 years. If this has not been done, it is important to update these vaccinations at age 65 years. Unfortunately, many older Americans are susceptible to these diseases. Those at highest risk of fatal pneumococcal disease, such as individuals with **asplenia** (loss of the spleen), should receive a booster dose 5 years after the initial dose of the *pneumococcal vaccine* (Pneumovax 23, Pnu-Immune 23) (Table 14-4 ■).

The herpes zoster (shingles) vaccine causes an acute, inflammatory eruption of very painful vesicles, which affect the nerves in the skin. Shingles is caused by the varicella-zoster virus (VZV), which also causes chicken pox. The virus lies dormant in the dorsal root ganglia and is usually reactivated after age 65 years. Stress appears to play a role in its reactivation, but the full reason is not understood. The relatively new *Zostavax* vaccine for shingles, licensed in 2006, is still under study. The subcutaneous vaccine is effective in approximately 50% of patients over age 60. Serious adverse reactions to the vaccine include chills, fever, breathing problems, sore throat, flu-like symptoms, severe or painful skin rash, and weakness. The patient's physician should be contacted if any of these serious reactions occur. This vaccine is contraindicated in hypersensitive patients, with allergies to gelatin or neomycin, with immune system disorders, with use of immunosuppressants, and in women who have any possibility of becoming pregnant. Zostavax is also used to reduce the severity and incidence of post-therapeutic neuralgia.

Focus on Geriatrics

Influenza and Pneumonia Immunization

All individuals age 65 years and older should receive annual influenza immunization and a single dose of pneumococcal vaccine. Those who received pneumococcal vaccine before age 65 years should receive a booster dose if it has been 5 or more years since the first dose.

Table 14-4 ■ Recommended Adult Immunization Schedule, 2011

Recommended Adult Immunization Schedule – United States, 2011

Note: These recommendations _must_ be read with the footnotes that follow; the notes contain the number of doses, intervals between doses, and other important information.

Figure 1. Recommended adult immunization schedule, by vaccine and age group

Vaccine ▼　Age group ▶	19–26 years	27–49 years	50–59 years	60–64 years	≥65 years
Influenza[1],*	1 dose annually				
Tetanus, diphtheria, pertussis (Td/Tdap)[2],*	Substitute one-time dose of Tdap for Td booster; then boost with Td every 10 yrs				Td booster every 10 yrs
Varicella[3],*	2 doses				
Human papillomavirus (HPV)[4],*	3 doses (females)				
Zoster[5]				1 dose	
Measles, mumps, rubella (MMR)[6],*	1 or 2 doses		1 dose		
Pneumococcal (polysaccharide)[7,8]	1 or 2 doses				1 dose
Meningococcal[9],*	1 or more doses				
Hepatitis A[10],*	2 doses				
Hepatitis B[11],*	3 doses				

*Covered by the Vaccine Injury Compensation Program.

Figure 2. Vaccines that might be indicated for adults, based on medical and other indications

Vaccine ▼ / Indication ▶	Pregnancy	Immunocompromising conditions (excluding human immunodeficiency virus [HIV])[3,5,6,13]	HIV infection[3,6,12,13] CD4+ T lymphocyte count <200 cells/μL	HIV infection ≥200 cells/μL	Diabetes, heart disease, chronic lung disease, chronic alcoholism	Asplenia[12] (including elective splenectomy and persistent complement component deficiencies)	Chronic liver disease	Kidney failure, end-stage renal disease, receipt of hemodialysis	Healthcare personnel
Influenza[1],*	1 dose TIV annually								1 dose TIV or LAIV annually
Tetanus, diphtheria, pertussis (Td/Tdap)[2],*	Td	Substitute one-time dose of Tdap for Td booster; then boost with Td every 10 yrs							
Varicella[3],*	Contraindicated			2 doses					
Human papillomavirus (HPV)[4],*	3 doses for females through age 26 yrs								
Zoster[5]	Contraindicated			1 dose					
Measles, mumps, rubella (MMR)[6],*	Contraindicated			1 or 2 doses					
Pneumococcal (polysaccharide)[7,8]	1 or 2 doses								
Meningococcal[9],*	1 or more doses								
Hepatitis A[10],*	2 doses								
Hepatitis B[11],*	3 doses								

*Covered by the Vaccine Injury Compensation Program.

☐ For all persons in this category who meet the age requirements and who lack evidence of immunity (e.g., lack documentation of vaccination or have no evidence of previous infection)

☐ Recommended if some other risk factor is present (e.g., on the basis of medical, occupational, lifestyle, or other indications)

☐ No recommendation

These schedules indicate the recommended age groups and medical indications for which administration of currently licensed vaccines is commonly indicated for adults ages 19 years and older, as of January 1, 2011. For all vaccines being recommended on the adult immunization schedule: a vaccine series does not need to be restarted, regardless of the time that has elapsed between doses. Licensed combination vaccines may be used whenever any components of the combination are indicated and when the vaccine's other components are not contraindicated. For detailed recommendations on all vaccines, including those used primarily for travelers or that are issued during the year, consult the manufacturers' package inserts and the complete statements from the Advisory Committee on Immunization Practices (www.cdc.gov/vaccines/pubs/acip-list.htm).

The recommended adult immunization schedule has been approved by the Advisory Committee on Immunization Practices (ACIP), the American Academy of Family Physicians (AAFP), the American College of Obstetricians and Gynecologists (ACOG), and the American College of Physicians (ACP).

Courtesy of Centers for Disease Control and Prevention: *Recommended Adult Immunization Schedule—United States, 2011.* Available at http://www.immunize.org/shop/views/adultsched_pg2.pdf.

Focus On

Immunoglobulins

Globulins are proteins that contain antibodies and are present in blood. Igs are derived from human plasma containing antibodies that have been formed by the body to specific antigens. The antibody content is primarily IgG (90%–98%) and their **isotypes** (atoms of a chemical element that have the same atomic number with nearly identical chemical properties but different physical properties). There are two types of Igs: one that should be administered intramuscularly and one that should be administered intravenously.

The Ig intramuscular (IGIM) products are aqueous solutions containing 15% protein, of which more than 90% is IgG. They are standardized for antibodies to measles, diphtheria, and poliovirus to ensure reasonable uniformity of product, but they contain antibodies specific for numerous bacteria, viruses, and fungi. Ig is given by injection into a muscle.

How do they work?

The Igs are given to provide passive immunity to one or more infectious diseases. Individuals receiving Igs receive antibodies only to the diseases to which the donor blood is immune. The onset of protection is rapid but of short duration (1–3 months).

How are they used?

The main indications of IGIM are for IgG replacement therapy in disorders where there is a deficiency of IgG antibodies and for the passive prevention or modification of hepatitis A and measles in susceptible persons when given shortly after exposure. Passive immunization for measles is particularly important in children younger than 1 year of age because they are prone to measles complications and have not yet been vaccinated. IGIM is not standardized for hepatitis B, and the specific Ig should be used in this case. IGIM can be used for the prevention of varicella in immunocompromised patients if varicella-zoster Ig is not available. It has also been used to prevent fetal damage in women who are exposed to rubella during the first trimester of pregnancy. Igs (intramuscular [IM] or intravenous [IV]) are recommended to HIV-positive patients who are exposed to measles regardless of their immunization status.

What are the adverse effects?

Few adverse reactions are associated with IGIM except for local pain and tenderness at the injection site. As with all Ig products, serious anaphylactic reactions occur occasionally and are the most common selective Ig deficiency.

What are the contraindications and interactions?

IGIM must not be injected intravenously because it can cause serious anaphylactic reactions.

What are the important points patients should know?

Instruct patients to report signs and symptoms of hypersensitivity and infusion symptoms of nausea, chills, headache, or chest tightness. Advise women to avoid breastfeeding without consulting a physician.

Focus Point

Site of Injection

The dosage and the site for the injection vary according to the amount of Ig required and the size of the person (typically, the site is in the buttocks for adults and the leg or arm for children).

✳ Apply Your Knowledge 14.5

The following questions focus on what you have just learned about immunoglobulins.

CRITICAL THINKING
1. What are the classifications of immunoglobulins?
2. What is the route of administration of immunoglobulins?
3. What type of immunity may be provided by the immunoglobulins?
4. What are the contraindications of immunoglobulin?
5. Why is the shingles vaccine recommended more commonly after age 65 years?

PRACTICAL SCENARIO 1

A young mother of an infant is seen at the pediatrician's office for the child's first visit. While you are taking a history of the infant, the mother confides that she does not want her infant to receive any vaccinations because she has heard that immunizations cause autism, diabetes, and seizures. She asks you why her infant needs to be vaccinated.

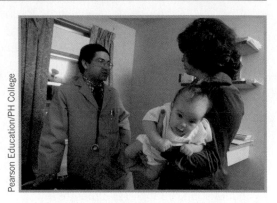

Pearson Education/PH College

Critical Thinking Questions
1. What would you tell her is the purpose of vaccinations?
2. Are there reasons why her child should not be vaccinated?
3. What questions would you suggest she ask the pediatrician to allay her concerns?

PRACTICAL SCENARIO 2

A mother brought her 2-month-old baby to the pediatrician's office to receive her first vaccines. She asked the medical assistant how many vaccines the baby should receive at this time.

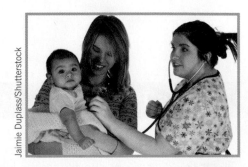

Jaimie Duplass/Shutterstock

Critical Thinking Questions
1. What is the appropriate answer that the medical assistant should give?
2. Which are the vaccines that should be administered at this time?

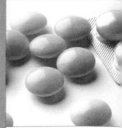

Chapter Capsule

This section repeats the objectives from the beginning of the chapter and then provides a summary of the most important concepts for that objective. Use this section as a quick review and to check your knowledge.

Objective 1: State the names and functions of blood cells involved in immunity.

- White blood cells (lymphocytes)—manufacture antibodies to overcome infection and disease
- T cells, B cells, and natural killer cells—attack viruses, fungi, bacteria, and other foreign cells that invade the body

Objective 2: List the major components of the lymphatic system.

- Lymphatic vessels, lymph fluid, lymph nodes, the thymus gland, spleen, and tonsils

Objective 3: Discuss and contrast the various types of immunities.

- Humoral immunity—B cells produce circulating antibodies to act against an antigen
- Cell-mediated immunity—T cells attack the antigens directly rather than producing antibodies

Objective 4: Explain the differences between active and passive immunity.

- Active immunity—a form of acquired immunity that develops in response to an antigen either naturally acquired by exposure to an infectious disease or artificially acquired by receiving active immunizing agents (*vaccines*)
- Passive immunity—the transfer of immunoglobulins (antibodies) from an immune individual to another, occurring naturally in the active transport across the placental barrier of immunoglobulin G (IgG) antibodies from mother to fetus or by the transfer of IgA antibodies in the mother's milk

Objective 5: State the main action of immunizing agents.

- Prompt the body's immune system to become resistant to a specific disease or several diseases
- Sensitize immune cells for a possible subsequent re-exposure to the organism, thus triggering an immune response

Objective 6: Contrast inactivated and attenuated vaccines.

- Inactivated vaccines—microorganisms in the vaccine are killed, prompting immunity in the injected individual; most bacterial vaccines are inactivated
- Attenuated (live) vaccines—these vaccines cause an infection within the patient to induce a protective immune response; they contain less immunogen than killed vaccines

Objective 7: List the most common adverse effects associated with vaccinations.

- Localized inflammation at the site of injection, mild fever, headache, malaise, nausea, and dizziness

Objective 8: Describe the most common childhood immunizations.

- *Haemophilus influenzae* type b (Hib) (meningitis, other bacterial diseases), Salk inactivated vaccine and the Sabin live vaccine (poliomyelitis), MMR (measles, mumps, rubella), diphtheria, tetanus, pertussis, hepatitis B, varicella-zoster (chicken pox)

Objective 9: List the most common adult immunizations.

- Influenza vaccine annually; booster dose of adult diphtheria and tetanus toxoid every 10 years; after the initial dose of pneumococcal vaccine, a booster dose should be given 5 years later (adults older than age 65 years need only one vaccine without a booster)

Objective 10: Explain how immunoglobulins work to provide immunity.

- Derived from human plasma containing antibodies against specific antigens, immunoglobulins provide passive immunity

Internet Sites of Interest

- The Immunization Action Coalition provides numerous articles offering vaccination information for health-care professionals at **http://www.immunize.org**.
- Safe injections are discussed on this World Health Organization's website at **http://www.who.int/immunization_safety/safe_injections/en**.
- The National Immunization Program of the Centers for Disease Control and Prevention offers a quick reference chart, including frequently asked questions, a list of side effects, and current news related to various types of vaccines at **http://www.cdc.gov/vaccines/vpd-vac/vaccines-list.htm**.
- All that you need to know about getting vaccinated for travel to other countries can be found at **http://www.cdc.gov/travel/vaccinat.htm**.
- The Johns Hopkins Bloomberg School of Public Health provides independent assessment of studies related to vaccine safety at **http://www.vaccinesafety.edu**.
- More information from Facts & Comparison's ImmunoFacts' website is available at **http://www.immunofacts.com**. This website covers laws and regulations and government databases in addition to fact sheets, vaccine monographs, and bioterrorism information.

PEARSON myhealthprofessionskit™

Go to www.myhealthprofessionskit.com to access the Companion Website created for this textbook. Simply select "Basic Health Science" from the choice of disciplines. Find this book and then log in using your username and password to access interactive learning games, assessment questions, animations, and more.

Chapter Objectives

After completing this chapter, you should be able to:

1. List the antipyretic properties of anti-inflammatory and analgesic drugs.
2. Describe the role of prostaglandins in inflammation.
3. Outline the dangers of aspirin use.
4. List the uses and side effects of anti-inflammatory drugs.
5. Identify the different types of analgesics.
6. Describe the function of naturally occurring opioids and their receptors.
7. Explain the rationale behind the use of narcotic analgesics.
8. Describe the problems associated with the use of narcotic analgesics.

Chapter 15

Analgesic, Antipyretic, and Anti-Inflammatory Drugs

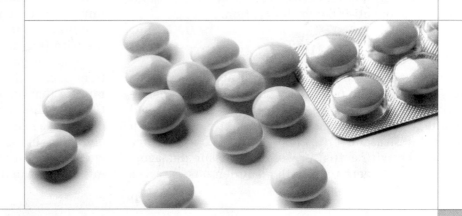

Key Terms

acute (page 240)
analgesic (ah-nul-JEE-zik) (page 240)
antipyretics (an-tih-pye-REH-tiks) (page 240)
bradykinin (brah-dee-KYE-nin) (page 240)
chronic (page 240)

cyclooxygenase (sye-klo-OKS-ih-jehnase) (page 245)
endogenous (en-DAH-jeh-nus) (page 247)
endorphins (en-DOR-finz) (page 240)
enkephalins (en-KEH-fuh-linz) (page 240)
narcotic (page 247)

neurotransmitters (noo-roh-TRANZ-mihters) (page 240)
opiates (OH-pee-uts) (page 247)
opioid (OH-pee-oyd) (page 247)
prostaglandins (prah-stuh-GLAN-dinz) (page 240)

Introduction

Analgesics are agents that relieve pain without significantly disturbing consciousness or altering the actions of the sensory nerves, which carry impulses to the brain. Therefore, many drugs that are used to relieve pain are not truly analgesics. For example, general anesthetics reduce pain but interfere with consciousness (see Chapter 19), local anesthetics reduce pain by blocking peripheral nerve fibers that carry other sensory input (see Chapter 19), antispasmodics indirectly relieve certain types of pain by relaxing smooth muscle (see Chapter 29), and steroids relieve pain associated with rheumatoid arthritis via their anti-inflammatory action (see Chapter 29). The two types of analgesics are nonopioid analgesics and opioid analgesics.

Antipyretics are drugs that reduce elevated body temperature (fever) to normal levels. Certain analgesics and antipyretics also possess anti-inflammatory properties; such agents are used in the treatment of patients with arthritis and other inflammatory conditions. The drugs considered in this chapter have demonstrated **analgesic**—or pain-relieving—action, with or without antipyretic or anti-inflammatory action.

What Is Pain?

Pain is considered to be the central nervous system's (CNS's) reaction to potentially harmful stimuli characterized by physical discomfort. It has been described by the International Association for the Study of Pain as an "unpleasant sensory and emotional experience associated with actual or potential tissue damage." **Acute** pain (severe pain with a sudden onset) serves as an early warning alert to seek medical help for preventing any further damage to our bodies. Although pain can play a beneficial role as a warning system and aid in diagnosis, some pain (such as that associated with the postoperative period or cancer patients) and types of **chronic** pain (lasting a long time or marked by frequent recurrence) have very few positive effects.

Pain stimuli may result from the process of inflammation that causes tissue injury and the release of such different substances as histamine, **prostaglandins** (hormone-like substances that control blood pressure, contract smooth muscle, and modulate inflammation), serotonin, and **bradykinin** (a polypeptide that mediates inflammation, increases vasodilation, and contracts smooth muscle). Such chemical substances initiate an action potential along a sensory nerve fiber or sensitize pain receptors. These pain receptors, called *nociceptors*, are free nerve endings strategically located throughout the body. The pain enters from a pain receptor and sensory fibers, moving into the spinal cord and the brain. After being perceived, interpretation of the pain impulse occurs in the brain cortex, and appropriate autonomic and reflex responses occur to deal with the pain (Figure 15-1 ■).

The transmission of pain impulses relates to the actions of certain chemical substances called **neurotransmitters** that are concentrated in various parts of the CNS and allow communication from nerve cell to nerve cell. These neurotransmitters are known as **endorphins** and **enkephalins** and are capable of binding with opiate receptors in the CNS and thereby inhibit the transmission of pain impulses, providing an analgesic effect.

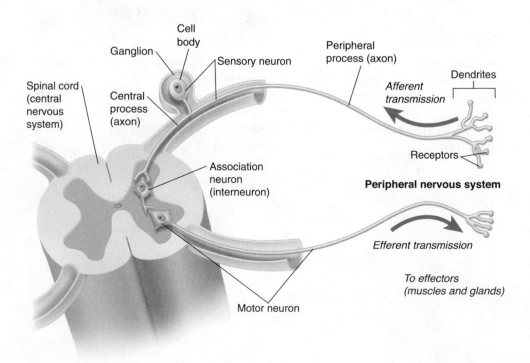

Figure 15-1 ■ Reflex responses to pain.

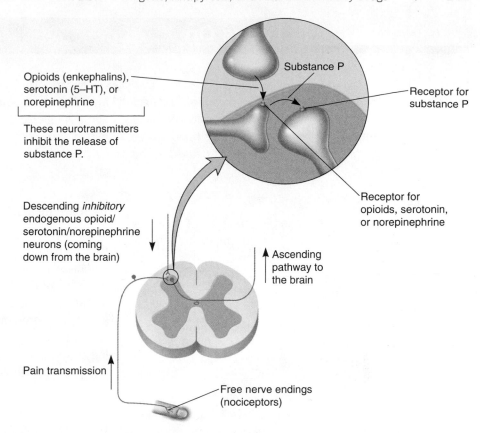

Opioids (enkephalins), serotonin (5–HT), or norepinephrine

These neurotransmitters inhibit the release of substance P.

Substance P

Receptor for substance P

Receptor for opioids, serotonin, or norepinephrine

Descending *inhibitory* endogenous opioid/serotonin/norepinephrine neurons (coming down from the brain)

Ascending pathway to the brain

Pain transmission

Free nerve endings (nociceptors)

Figure 15-2 ■ Endogenous analgesic compounds released after pain stimuli.

These analgesic compounds are released when painful stimuli affect the body (Figure 15-2 ■).

It is believed that a gating mechanism exists within the dorsal horn of the spinal cord. Small nerve fibers (pain receptors) and large nerve fibers ("normal" receptors) synapse on projection cells, which go up the spinothalamic tract to the brain, and inhibitory interneurons within the dorsal horn.

The interplay among these connections determines when painful stimuli go to the brain:

1. When there is no input, the inhibitory neuron prevents the projection neuron from sending signals to the brain (the gate is closed).

2. Normal somatosensory input happens when there is more large-fiber stimulation (or only large-fiber stimulation). The inhibitory neuron and the projection neuron are stimulated, but the inhibitory neuron prevents the projection neuron from sending signals to the brain (the gate is closed).

3. Nociception (pain reception) happens when there is more small-fiber stimulation or only small-fiber stimulation. This inactivates the inhibitory neuron, and the projection neuron sends signals to the brain, informing it of pain (the gate is open).

Descending pathways from the brain close the gate by inhibiting the projector neurons and diminishing pain perception. This theory does not tell us everything about pain perception, but it does explain some things. If you rub or shake your hand after you bang your finger, you stimulate normal somatosensory input to the projector neurons. This opens the gate and reduces the perception of pain.

Nonsteroidal Anti-Inflammatory Drugs

Nonsteroidal anti-inflammatory drugs (NSAIDs) are used to relieve some symptoms caused by arthritis, such as inflammation, swelling, stiffness, and joint pain. However, these medicines do not cure arthritis and help patients only as long as they continue to take them. Some of these drugs are also used to relieve other kinds of pain or to treat other painful conditions, such as menstrual cramps, gout attacks, bursitis, tendonitis, sprains, and muscle strains.

The salicylate group of analgesics and antipyretics is a subset of NSAIDs and are commonly used. These agents are consumed at a rate in excess of 10,000 tons annually, primarily for antiplatelet effects. Aspirin and other salicylate products should not be used in children younger than 12 years of age because of the potential for developing Reye's syndrome.

Focus On

Aspirin

Of all the salicylate drugs, aspirin—or acetylsalicylic acid (Bayer, Ecotrin, St. Joseph's)—is the most commonly used. All commercially available salicylates have similar pharmacologic properties, so aspirin is discussed as the prototype for this group.

How does it work?

Aspirin's mechanism of action is unknown. It may produce analgesia and block pain impulses by inhibiting synthesis of prostaglandin in the CNS. It is thought to relieve fever by central action in the hypothalamic heat-regulating center. In low doses, aspirin also appears to impede clotting in the blood by blocking prostaglandin synthesis, which prevents formation of the platelet-aggregating substance, thus helping to prevent strokes and heart attacks.

How is it used?

Aspirin is used as an antipyretic and analgesic in a variety of conditions. It is used for the relief of pain from simple headache, discomfort, and fever associated with the common cold and minor muscular aches and pains. When aspirin is used for lowering a fever, it is one of the most effective and safest drugs. Aspirin is also used for anti-inflammatory conditions, such as rheumatoid arthritis.

What are the adverse effects?

Although uncommon, adverse effects of aspirin taken in usual doses may include dyspepsia, nausea, vomiting, and occult bleeding (blood in the stool). Prolonged administration of large doses (3.6 g/day or higher) results in occult bleeding and anemia. Massive gastrointestinal (GI) hemorrhage can also occur, particularly in elderly clients.

What are the contraindications and interactions?

In general, salicylates are contraindicated in hypersensitive people and in patients who have GI disturbances, particularly hemorrhaging ulcers. Salicylates should also be used with caution in patients on anticoagulant therapy and avoided in patients who are taking *uricosurics*—agents that promote excretion of uric acid in the urine. Salicylates interact with a wide variety of agents, including antidiabetic drugs (causing increased hypoglycemia) and oral anticoagulants (causing increased anticoagulant effects).

What are the important points patients should know?

Any condition involving bleeding may be worsened by taking aspirin. Advise menstruating women to avoid aspirin if menstrual bleeding is heavy, during the last 3 months of pregnancy, and while breastfeeding. Instruct patient to discontinue aspirin use 1 week before or after surgery, including oral surgery. Advise patients not to use aspirin if symptoms of meningitis exist and to avoid alcohol when taking large doses of aspirin.

Focus on Pediatrics

Aspirin and Reye's Syndrome

The use of aspirin in the treatment of fever in children who have varicella (chicken pox), a common cold, influenza virus infections, or who are younger than 12 years of age may result in the development of Reye's syndrome. The current opinion is that aspirin should not be prescribed for children who have upper respiratory viral infections. If the control of fever, aches, and pains is necessary, alternative measures should be used.

Focus on Geriatrics

Salicylates and Gastrointestinal Bleeding

Administration of salicylates to elderly patients who are vulnerable to GI bleeding may cause this bleeding to become severe. Emergency help should be requested if any of the following symptoms occurs: bloody urine, loss of hearing or vision, confusion, convulsions, diarrhea, difficulty swallowing, dizziness, severe drowsiness, severe excitement, abnormal respiration, change in skin color, hallucinations, sweating, increased thirst, nausea or vomiting, stomach pain, swelling, fever, or a flapping movement of the hands.

Focus On

Nonsalicylate Nonsteroidal Anti-Inflammatory Drugs

Little distinguishes the clinical profile of this group of NSAIDs from the others. In this chapter, only two of these drugs are discussed (ibuprofen and indomethacin) as examples of NSAIDs.

Ibuprofen

Ibuprofen (Motrin, Advil) is an NSAID that possesses analgesic, anti-inflammatory, and antipyretic activities.

How does it work?

Ibuprofen, similar to other NSAIDs, has a mechanism of action that is likely related to its inhibition of prostaglandin synthesis.

How is it used?

Ibuprofen is used for rheumatoid arthritis, osteoarthritis, and arthritis. It is also indicated for patients with mild to moderate pain, dysmenorrhea, and fever.

What are the adverse effects?

Ibuprofen may cause headache, dizziness, nervousness, peripheral edema, fluid retention, and tinnitus. Common adverse effects of ibuprofen include nausea, occult blood loss, peptic ulceration, diarrhea, constipation, abdominal pain, dyspepsia, flatulence, heartburn, and decreased appetite. Severe adverse effects from ibuprofen are azotemia (abnormally high nitrogen-type wastes in the bloodstream), cystitis, hematuria, aplastic anemia, hypoglycemia, and hyperkalemia.

What are the contraindications and interactions?

Ibuprofen is contraindicated in patients who are hypersensitive to the drug and in those with angioedema, nasal polyps, or bronchospastic reaction to aspirin or other NSAIDs. Pregnant women should avoid ibuprofen. Individuals with GI disorders, history of peptic ulcer, hepatic or renal disease, hypertension, and pre-existing asthma should use ibuprofen cautiously. Ibuprofen may interact with antihypertensives, furosemide, and thiazide diuretics and may decrease the effectiveness of diuretics or antihypertensive drugs.

What are the important points patients should know?

Advise patients to notify their physicians if blood appears in the stool, vomitus, or urine or if there is onset of skin rash, pruritus, or jaundice. Driving a vehicle is not advised until the individual patient response to ibuprofen has been assessed. Instruct patients to not take ibuprofen with aspirin, alcohol, or NSAIDs. Breastfeeding women should not take ibuprofen.

Focus On

Indomethacin

Indomethacin (Indocin) is a nonsteroidal drug with anti-inflammatory, antipyretic, and analgesic properties. It is not a simple analgesic because of its potential serious adverse effects and should not be used for minor pain.

How does it work?

Indomethacin produces anti-inflammatory, analgesic, and antipyretic effects by inhibiting prostaglandin synthesis.

How is it used?

Indomethacin is indicated for the treatment of patients with rheumatoid arthritis, rheumatoid spondylitis, osteoarthritis, bursitis, tendonitis, gouty arthritis, and *patent ductus arteriosus* (abnormal fetal connection of the left pulmonary artery and the descending aorta) in premature neonates.

What are the adverse effects?

The most common adverse effects of indomethacin include GI ulcerations, hemorrhage, GI bleeding, increased pain in ulcerative colitis, gastritis, nausea, and vomiting. Indomethacin may also cause blurred vision, hepatic toxicity, aplastic anemia, hemolytic anemia, asthma, pruritus, urticaria, and skin rashes. Depression, mental confusion, coma, and convulsions are also reported.

What are the contraindications and interactions?

Indomethacin is contraindicated in patients who are hypersensitive to the drug and in those with a history of aspirin- or NSAID-induced asthma, rhinitis, or urticaria (hives). It must be avoided by pregnant and breast-feeding women and by neonates with untreated infection, active bleeding, and significant renal impairment. Indomethacin should be used cautiously in patients with epilepsy, parkinsonism, and hepatic or renal disease. Aminoglycosides, cyclosporine, and methotrexate may enhance the toxicity of indomethacin. Antihypertensives, furosemide, and thiazide diuretics may impair response to both drugs.

What are the important points patients should know?

Advise patients taking NSAIDs to notify their physicians promptly if they develop signs of skin rash, breathing problems, or visual disturbances. These are signs of hypersensitivity to NSAIDs.

Focus Point

Allergy to Analgesics

If the patient is allergic to one analgesic, be cautious in giving another over-the-counter (OTC) analgesic.

✳ Apply Your Knowledge 15.1

The following questions focus on what you have just learned about pain and NSAIDs.

CRITICAL THINKING

1. What are neurotransmitters?
2. Describe the process of inflammation.
3. Define *prostaglandins*.
4. What are endorphins and enkephalins?
5. Compare analgesics with antipyretics.
6. Define *NSAIDs*.
7. What is Reye's syndrome?
8. What is the mechanism of action of aspirin?
9. What are the indications of ibuprofen?
10. What is the mechanism of action of indomethacin?

Focus On

Selective Cyclooxygenase-2 Inhibitors

NSAIDs play a major role in the management of inflammation and pain caused by arthritis. A new class of NSAIDs that selectively inhibits the **cyclooxygenase-**2 (COX-2) enzyme has been developed. COX is the name for a group of enzymes required to produce prostaglandins from arachidonic acid. Two subtypes of COX have been identified: COX-1 and COX-2. COX-1 is available in all cells, especially in the platelets, GI tract, and kidneys, and helps maintain homeostasis in these cells. On the other hand, COX-2 appears to be made in macrophages in response to damage to local tissues. One of the first COX-2 inhibitors—celecoxib (Celebrex)—is said to provide therapeutic benefit with less toxicity than traditional NSAIDs. Another COX-2 selective inhibitor—meloxicam (Mobic)—has recently been introduced. COX-2 inhibitors and traditional NSAIDs do not appear to differ significantly in their effectiveness in alleviating pain or inflammation. They have similar GI side effects. However, short-term studies show fewer GI ulcers in patients treated with COX-2 inhibitors compared with traditional NSAIDs. On the other hand, at least one COX-2 inhibitor—rofecoxib (Vioxx)—was voluntarily removed from the market by its manufacturer because of safety concerns: There was an increased risk of cardiovascular events (including heart attack and stroke).

How do they work?

COX-2 inhibitors affect the synthesis of prostaglandins by selectively targeting only the COX-2 enzymes. These agents have similar anti-inflammatory activity without the adverse GI effects associated with COX-1 inhibition. COX-2 inhibitors exert anti-inflammatory and analgesic effects through the inhibition of prostaglandin synthesis by blocking COX activity. The isoenzyme COX-2 is primarily associated with inflammation. Cytokines increase the expression of COX-2—mainly at inflammatory sites—producing prostaglandins that mediate inflammation, pain, and fever.

How are they used?

The FDA has labeled celecoxib (Celebrex) for the treatment of osteoarthritis and rheumatoid arthritis in adults. This agent is recommended in the lowest effective dosage for the shortest duration possible. Meloxicam (Mobic)—the newest COX-2 inhibitor—has been labeled by the FDA for the treatment of osteoarthritis (see Table 15-1 ■).

What are the adverse effects?

Similar to traditional NSAIDs, the COX-2 inhibitors commonly cause abdominal pain, dyspepsia, and diarrhea. There is an increased risk of serious cardiovascular thrombotic events and even myocardial infarction and stroke, which can be fatal. This risk may increase with a longer duration of use. COX-2 inhibitors have been linked to cardiovascular problems, especially in elderly adults, and rofecoxib (Vioxx) was removed from the market for this reason. However, many believe that the other COX-2 inhibitors should be used cautiously in patients with a history of heart disease.

What are the contraindications and interactions?

Treatment with COX-2 inhibitors is contraindicated in patients who have hypersensitivity to these drugs, asthma, urticaria, or previous anaphylactic reactions after taking aspirin or NSAIDs. Because of the potential aggravation of hypertension and lower extremity edema, caution should be exercised in prescribing COX-2 inhibitors to patients with congestive heart failure, fluid retention, or hypertension. COX-2 inhibitors are contraindicated in elderly patients, patients younger than 18 years, and pregnant (third trimester) or lactating women. These agents should be avoided in patients with severe hepatic impairment or advanced renal disease. COX-2 inhibitors may diminish effectiveness of angiotensin-converting enzyme inhibitors. Fluconazole (Diflucan), an antifungal, can increase celecoxib concentrations. COX-2 inhibitors may increase lithium (Eskalith) concentrations.

What are the important points patients should know?

Advise patients to tell their physicians immediately if they experience unexplained weight gain, skin rash, nausea, fatigue, lethargy, jaundice, flu-like symptoms, black tarry stool, or upper GI distress and to avoid alcohol, tobacco, and aspirin and other NSAIDs when taking meloxicam. Instruct women to avoid celecoxib during the third trimester of pregnancy. Neither celecoxib nor meloxicam should be used by women who are breastfeeding.

Table 15-1 ■ Selective COX-2 Inhibitors

GENERIC NAME	TRADE NAME	AVERAGE DOSAGE FOR ADULTS	ROUTE OF ADMINISTRATION
celecoxib	Celebrex	100–200 mg bid	PO
meloxicam	Mobic	7.5 mg/d	PO

bid, twice a day; PO, oral.

Focus On

Acetaminophen

The analgesic efficacy of acetaminophen (Tylenol) is essentially equivalent to that of NSAIDs, but acetaminophen is not anti-inflammatory. Similar to aspirin, acetaminophen has analgesic and antipyretic actions.

How does it work?

The mechanism of action of acetaminophen is unknown. As with most nonopioid analgesics, the mechanism of action is thought to be the inhibition of prostaglandin in the peripheral nervous system, making the sensory neurons less likely to receive pain signals. Acetaminophen blocks the peripheral pain impulses to a lesser degree than other NSAIDs. It lacks the anti-inflammatory action of the salicylates; hence, it is of only limited usefulness in inflammatory rheumatic disorders and is often not considered to be an NSAID agent.

How is it used?

Acetaminophen is effective in the treatment of a wide variety of arthritic and rheumatic conditions involving musculoskeletal pain as well as headache, dysmenorrhea, myalgias, and neuralgias. This agent is also useful in diseases accompanied by fever, discomfort, and pain, such as the common cold and other viral infections. Acetaminophen is particularly useful as an analgesic and antipyretic agent in patients who experience adverse reactions to aspirin.

What are the adverse effects?

The adverse effects of acetaminophen are rare in therapeutic doses, and the drug is usually well tolerated by aspirin-sensitive patients. Sensitivity reactions may occur; in this case, the drug should be stopped. Over long-term use, adverse effects include skin eruptions and urticaria, hypotension, and hepatotoxicity. Acetaminophen frequently is combined with other drugs, such as caffeine, aspirin, and such opiates as codeine and oxycodone. An overdose can cause hepatotoxicity, coma, and internal bleeding. If overdose occurs, the antidote for acetaminophen is acetylcysteine (Mucomyst).

What are the contraindications and interactions?

Acetaminophen is contraindicated in patients with a history of hypersensitivity to this drug. It must be used cautiously in children younger than 3 years of age unless directed by a physician. Repeated administration to patients with anemia or hepatic disease or to children younger than 12 years of age who are affected by rheumatoid conditions should be avoided. Acetaminophen should be avoided in patients with alcoholism, malnutrition, or thrombocytopenia (a platelet deficiency often caused by anticancer drugs). Safety during pregnancy or lactation is not established.

What are the important points patients should know?

Acetaminophen may cause acute liver damage or failure in patients who consume three or more alcoholic drinks per day, but a person does not have to be a chronic drinker to experience damage. Taking acetaminophen after a weekend of drinking can prove fatal. Advise patients to avoid this combination of drugs if possible. The use of acetaminophen with barbiturates (Nembutal, Seconal), carbamazepine (Tegretol), phenytoin (Dilantin), and rifampin (Rifadin, Rimactane) may increase potential hepatotoxicity. With other drugs, such as cholestyramine (Questran), the absorption of acetaminophen is decreased. The maximum dose of acetaminophen should never exceed 4 grams per day.

Focus Point

Differences Among Over-the-Counter Analgesics

OTC analgesics include salicylates, acetaminophen, and NSAIDs. All are antipyretics, but acetaminophen does not have an anti-inflammatory effect. Salicylates are also used to prolong clotting time by preventing platelets from binding together.

✳ Apply Your Knowledge 15.2

The following questions focus on what you have just learned about selective COX-2 inhibitors and acetaminophen.

CRITICAL THINKING

1. Explain selective COX-2 inhibitors.
2. What is the connection between COX-2 inhibitors and cardiovascular risks?
3. Differentiate between COX-1 and COX-2. Where are these substances especially found in the body?
4. Compare aspirin with acetaminophen.
5. What are the adverse effects of long-term overuse of acetaminophen?

Opiates

The analgesic properties of opium and its derivatives have been known for centuries. **Opiates** are drugs derived from opium poppies and include morphine and codeine. **Opioid** is a general term referring to natural, synthetic, or **endogenous** (related to internal structures of function) morphine-related substances. Narcotics are drugs of certain legal status and in general are considered Schedule II drugs. They are controlled substances (see Chapter 2) and are used to treat patients with moderate to severe pain. Narcotics obtained from the raw opium plant include opium, morphine, and codeine.

Raw opium consists of the air-dried milky exudates obtained by the incision of unripe capsules of *Papaver somniferum*, which contains approximately 9.5% morphine. As a medicinal drug, opium has been known for many centuries.

Traditionally, the principal opium-exporting countries have been Iran, Turkey, India, and Yugoslavia. Drugs derived from opium, called *opiates*, owe their activity to the opioid alkaloids. Opium's chief pharmacologic effects are attributable to its morphine content and the presence of other alkaloids in amounts insufficient to significantly modify the morphine type of action. Thus, opium has many of the same uses as morphine, but morphine is nearly always preferred. Opiates have analgesic and other opioid effects.

Focus On

Focus on Morphine

Morphine (Astramorph PF, Duramorph) can be treated chemically to produce such semisynthetic narcotics as hydromorphone, oxycodone, oxymorphone, and heroin. These are classified as Schedule II drugs, except for heroin, which is a Schedule I drug (see Chapter 2) that is an illegal **narcotic** (a medication that induces sleep or stupor and alters mood and behavior) in the United States and is not used in medicine. The properties and actions of synthetic opioids are similar to those of the natural opiates. Synthetic narcotic analgesics include meperidine (Demerol), methadone (Dolophine), remifentanil (Ultiva), and levorphanol (Levo-Dromoran). Natural, synthetic, and semisynthetic narcotics are listed in Table 15-2 ■.

(Continued)

Focus On (*Continued*)

. . . .

How does it work?

Morphine produces its effects by binding to the opioid receptors. Opioid receptors are located presynaptically and postsynaptically along the pain transmission pathways. High densities of receptors are found in the dorsal horn of the spinal cord and higher CNS. Opioid receptors in the brain stem are responsible for the respiratory depressant effects produced by opioid analgesics. Opioid receptors in the higher CNS probably account for the effect of opioid analgesics on pain perception.

There are three major types of opioid receptors: mu, kappa, and delta. Most of the currently used opioid analgesics act primarily at mu receptors; some have varying degrees of activity at the other types of receptors.

How is it used?

Morphine is used in the management of almost all types of moderate to severe pain. Derivatives of morphine are also prescribed for cough inhibition, for treatment of GI pain, and for relieving pain associated with myocardial infarction.

What are the adverse effects?

Morphine causes nausea, vomiting, constipation, dry mouth, biliary tract spasms, dizziness, sedation, and pruritus. The major adverse effect of opioid analgesics, such as morphine, is respiratory depression. Physical and psychological dependence can occur with opioid analgesics. For this reason, health-care providers often hesitate to administer the proper doses, fearing the patient will become dependent or respiratory depression will occur. When used as directed, these drugs are safe and do not cause dependent or adverse effects. Patients should always be properly medicated for pain alleviation.

What are the contraindications and interactions?

Opioid analgesics are contraindicated in patients with known hypersensitivity. They are also contraindicated in patients who have asthma, emphysema, or head injury. Opioid analgesics must be avoided in patients with increased intracranial pressure, severe liver or kidney dysfunction, acute ulcerative colitis, or convulsive disorders. Opioid analgesics must be used cautiously in patients with prostatic hypertrophy because urine retention can occur.

Opioids or opiates can interact with alcohol, causing CNS depression with subsequent respiratory depression. Meperidine (Demerol) undergoes a potentially fatal reaction with monoamine oxidase inhibitors (MAOIs) (antidepressants). Morphine (Astramorph PF, Duramorph) and meperidine should not be mixed because they potentiate each other and are physically incompatible.

What are the important points patients should know?

Inform patients that the most serious adverse effect of narcotic analgesics is respiratory depression. Narcotic analgesics should not be taken if respirations are less than 12 per minute or systolic blood pressure is less than 110 mm Hg in adults. Narcotic analgesics may cause constipation, so advise patients to request symptomatic relief from their health-care providers.

Table 15-2 ■ Classifications of Opioid Analgesics

GENERIC NAME	TRADE NAME	ADULT COMMON DOSAGE RANGE	ROUTE OF ADMINISTRATION
Natural Opioid Analgesics			
codeine	Codeine	15–60 mg analgesic	PO, IM, subcutaneously
morphine	Duramorph, Avinza	10–30 mg q4h PRN or 15–30 mg sustained release of 8–12 h	PO
		2.5–15 mg q4h or 0.8–10 mg/h by continuous infusion	IV
		5–20 mg q4h	IM or subcutaneously
		10–20 mg q4h PRN	By rectum
opium tincture	Laudanum	0.6–1 mL qid (maximum, 6 mL/d)	PO

GENERIC NAME	TRADE NAME	ADULT COMMON DOSAGE RANGE	ROUTE OF ADMINISTRATION
Semisynthetic Opioid Analgesics			
hydrocodone	Hycodan, Robindone A	5–10 mg q4–6h PRN (maximum, 15 mg/d)	PO
hydrocodone with acetaminophen	Lortab, Vicodin	500–1000 mg q4–6h PRN	PO
levorphanol	Levo-Dromoran	2–3 mg q6–8h PRN	PO
		1–2 mg q6–8h PRN	Subcutaneously, IM
		Up to 1 mg q3–6h PRN	IV
oxycodone	OxyContin, Percolone	5–10 mg q6h PRN (OxyContin can be dosed q8h)	PO
oxycodone acetaminophen	Endocet, Percocet	Combination drug: 325–650 mg q4–6h PRN	PO
oxycodone–aspirin	Endodan, Percodan	Combination drug: 325–650 mg q6h PRN	PO
Synthetic Opioid Agonists			
fentanyl	Duragesic, Sublimaze	50–100 mcg q1–2h PRN	IV
		25 mcg/h patch q3d	Transdermal
meperidine	Demerol	50–150 mg q3–4h PRN	PO, subcutaneously, IM, IV
methadone	Dolophine, Methadone	2.5–20 mg q3–8h PRN	PO, subcutaneously, IM
Synthetic Opioid Antagonists			
naloxone	Narcan	0.1–2 mg q2–3 min up to three doses if necessary	IV
naltrexone	Trexan, ReVia	25 mg, followed by another 25 mg in 1 h if no withdrawal response (maximum: 800 mg/d)	PO
Synthetic Opioid Agonist/Antagonists			
buprenorphine	Buprenex, Subutex	0.3 q6h up to 0.6 mg q4h or 25–50 mcg/h by IV infusion	IV, IM
butorphanol	Stadol, Stadol NS	1–4 mg q3–4h PRN (maximum: 4 mg/dose)	IM
		0.5–2 mg q3–4h PRN	IV
pentazocine	Talwin	50–100 mg q3–4h (maximum: 600 mg/d)	PO
pentazocine with naltrexone	Talwin NX	30 mg q3–4h (maximum: 360 mg/d)	IM, IV, subcutaneously

IM, intramuscular; IV, intravenous; PO, oral; PRN, as needed; qid, once a day.

Focus Point

Age Differences in Narcotic Metabolism

The metabolism of narcotics is slower in elderly patients. Therefore, opioid use may have undesirable effects, such as confusion and respiratory depression. In pediatric patients, dosing is difficult because elimination occurs at a different rate. Premature infants with chronic lung disease often have depressed hypoxic drive and require careful monitoring after the administration of opioids.

Focus On

Codeine

Although some codeine is obtained from opium directly, the quantity is not sufficient to meet the extensive use of this alkaloid as a valuable medicinal agent. Much more codeine is used than morphine. This need is met by producing it via partial synthesis from morphine. Codeine does not produce proportionately greater analgesia as the dose is increased.

How does it work?

Similar to morphine and all other opiates, codeine binds to opioid receptors in the brain and spinal cord, thereby relieving pain.

How is it used?

Codeine is useful for inducing sleep in the presence of mild pain. Similar to morphine, this drug is used as an analgesic, sedative, hypnotic, antiperistaltic, and antitussive agent. It is commonly given in combination with aspirin, acetaminophen, or other agents. Administered alone, codeine is a Schedule II drug. In combination with aspirin-like drugs, it is classified as a Schedule III drug (see Chapter 2).

What are the adverse effects?

Codeine is less apt than morphine to cause nausea, vomiting, constipation, and miosis (contraction of the pupils). Tolerance, dependence, and addiction can occur. Similar to morphine, codeine produces cortical and respiratory depression, but serious degrees of either are practically unknown. Patients may also have postural hypotension.

What are the contraindications and interactions?

Codeine is contraindicated in advanced respiratory insufficiency, bronchial asthma, and patients with raised intracranial pressure. Its effects are increased by use with other drugs that have centrally suppressing effects, including alcohol, or with cimetidine (Tagamet). Antidepressive agents and neuroleptics can completely halt the analgesic effects of codeine.

What are the important points patients should know?

Instruct patients to comply with the physician-ordered drug regimen because overuse may lead to dependence and to avoid alcohol and other CNS depressants. Advise patients to report urine retention or severe constipation and to rise slowly from a lying position to prevent postural hypotension.

✳ Apply Your Knowledge 15.3

The following questions focus on what you have just learned about opioid analgesics.

CRITICAL THINKING

1. What is the difference between opioids and opiates? Give an example of each.
2. List four generic names and trade names of synthetic opioids.
3. What are three major types of opioid receptors?
4. What are three classes of opioid analgesics?
5. What are the major adverse effects of opioid analgesics?

Semisynthetic Opioid Analgesics

Semisynthetic opioid analgesics are modifications of the natural alkaloids of opium. These agents have the same advantages of morphine or codeine without their disadvantages. Examples of semisynthetic opioids include hydrocodone, oxycodone, and oxymorphone (see Table 15-2).

Focus On

Hydrocodone

Hydrocodone (Hycodan) is a morphine derivative similar to codeine but is more addicting and has slightly greater antitussive activity and analgesic effects. This CNS depressant relieves moderate to severe pain. Hydrocodone is a Schedule III drug. Hydrocodone is combined with other drugs, such as aspirin-like analgesics, antihistamines, expectorants, and sympathomimetics (drugs that increase cardiac output, dilate bronchioles, and constrict blood vessels).

How does it work?

Hydrocodone suppresses the cough reflex by direct action on the cough center in the medulla of the brain. It also acts as a CNS depressant, which relieves moderate to severe pain.

How is it used?

Hydrocodone is used for relief of nonproductive cough and for moderate to severe pain.

What are the adverse effects?

The most common adverse effects include dry mouth, nausea, vomiting, constipation, sedation, dizziness, and drowsiness. Other adverse effects are euphoria, dysphoria, respiratory depression, pruritus, and skin rashes.

What are the contraindications and interactions?

Hydrocodone is contraindicated in patients with a history of hypersensitivity to this drug and in women who are lactating. It should be used cautiously in patients with asthma, emphysema, a history of drug abuse, and respiratory depression. This drug can be prescribed with caution in children younger than 1 year and in pregnant women. Hydrocodone with alcohol and other CNS depressant compounds may interact and cause severe CNS depression.

What are the important points patients should know?

Instruct patients taking hydrocodone to avoid hazardous activities until response to the drug is determined. Advise patients to drink plenty of liquids to ensure adequate hydration. Because the abuse potential of hydrocodone is high, advise patients to take only the dose prescribed. Patients should never breastfeed while taking this drug.

Oxycodone

Although oxycodone (OxyContin) has less analgesic capability than morphine, it possesses comparable addiction potential and is a Schedule II drug. It frequently is used in combination with aspirin or acetaminophen.

How does it work?

The most prominent actions of oxycodone affect the CNS and organs composed of smooth muscle. Oxycodone binds with specific receptors in various sites of the CNS to alter perception of pain and emotional response to pain, but its precise mechanism of action is not clear. Oxycodone is as potent as morphine and 10 to 12 times more potent than codeine.

How is it used?

This agent is used for relief of moderate to severe pain, such as the type that may occur with bursitis, dislocations, simple fractures, and other injuries. Oxycodone is also indicated to relieve postoperative and postpartum pain.

What are the adverse effects?

The adverse effects of oxycodone include euphoria, dysphoria, lightheadedness, dizziness, sedation, anorexia, nausea, vomiting, constipation, jaundice, hepatotoxicity, and respiratory depression.

What are the contraindications and interactions?

Oxycodone is contraindicated in patients with hypersensitivity to this drug and during pregnancy and lactation. It is also contraindicated in children younger than 6 years of age. It must be used cautiously in people with alcoholism, renal or hepatic disease, and viral infections. Oxycodone is also prescribed with caution in patients with chronic ulcerative colitis, gallbladder disease, head injury, acute abdominal conditions, hypothyroidism, prostatic hypertrophy, and respiratory disease.

What are the important points patients should know?

Instruct patients to take oxycodone in the form prescribed without crushing, chewing, or breaking the medication—it is formulated to be released into the blood slowly. Advise patients to avoid driving, operating heavy machinery, and performing other hazardous activities because oxycodone causes drowsiness and dizziness. Alcohol must also be avoided. This drug may increase the effects of antidepressants, antihistamines, pain relievers, anxiety medications, seizure medications, and muscle relaxants. Instruct patients to take only the dose that was prescribed; taking too much of this drug could result in serious adverse effects and even death.

Synthetic Opioid Antagonists

The term *antagonist*, as used in this section, applies to naloxone and naltrexone, which are antagonists with little or no agonist actions. These competitive opioid antagonists are effective in the management of severe respiratory depression induced by opioid drugs, of asphyxia neonatorum (respiratory distress in the newborn) caused by administration of these drugs to the expectant mother, and for the diagnosis or treatment of opioid addiction.

Focus On

Naloxone

Naloxone (Narcan) is a synthetic opioid antagonist essentially devoid of opioid-agonist properties. Hence, it does not possess morphine-like properties, such as respiratory depression, psychotomimetic effects, and pupillary constriction, which are characteristic of other opioid antagonists.

How does it work?

Available evidence suggests that naloxone antagonizes these opioid effects by competing for the same receptor sites.

How is it used?

Naloxone is prescribed for narcotic overdose and complete or partial reversal of narcotic depression, including respiratory depression induced by natural and synthetic narcotics. Naloxone is a drug of choice when the nature of a depressant drug is not known and for the diagnosis of suspected acute opioid overdose.

What are the adverse effects?

Naloxone may cause reversal of analgesia, tremors, slight drowsiness, hyperventilation, sweating, nausea, vomiting, hypertension, and tachycardia.

What are the contraindications and interactions?

Naloxone is contraindicated in patients with respiratory depression caused by nonopioid drugs. Safety during pregnancy or lactation is not established. Naloxone must be used cautiously in neonates and children. It must be avoided in patients who are suspected to be dependent on narcotics and for those with cardiac irritability.

What are the important points patients should know?

Naloxone reverses the analgesic effects of narcotic agents and may cause withdrawal symptoms or the patient may experience a return of the pain that the narcotic agents were originally prescribed to treat. Instruct patients to tell their physician about postoperative pain that emerges after naloxone is administered.

Naltrexone

Naltrexone (Trexan, ReVia) generally has little or no agonist activity. Its opioid antagonist activity is reported to be two to nine times that of naloxone.

How does it work?

The mechanism of action of naltrexone is not clearly known, but it appears that its competitive binding at opioid receptor sites reduces euphoria.

How is it used?

Naltrexone is used as an adjunct to the maintenance of an opioid-free state in detoxified addicts who are and desire to remain narcotic-free. It is also used in the management of alcohol dependence as an adjunct to social and psychotherapeutic methods.

What are the adverse effects?

Naltrexone causes dry mouth, anorexia, nausea, vomiting, constipation, abdominal cramps, and hepatotoxicity. This agent may also cause muscle and joint pains, headache, nervousness, irritability, dizziness, and depression.

What are the contraindications and interactions?

Naltrexone is contraindicated in patients receiving opioid analgesics and in acute opioid withdrawal and opioid-dependent patients. It must be avoided in patients with acute hepatitis and liver failure. Naltrexone is also contraindicated in any individual who has a positive urine screen for opioids. Safety during pregnancy, lactation, or in children younger than age 18 years is not established.

Phenothiazines (antipsychotics such as Thorazine and Mellaril) may interact with the administration of naltrexone and cause increased somnolence and lethargy. Naltrexone reverses the analgesic effects of narcotic agonists and narcotic agonist–antagonists.

What are the important points patients should know?

Naltrexone may put patients in danger of fatally overdosing if they are using opiates. Advise patients to check with their physicians before taking OTC drugs with naltrexone because opioids are present in many OTC preparations, including cough medicines. Instruct patients to tell their physicians or dentists that they are taking naltrexone before undergoing treatment and to wear medical alert jewelry to indicate naltrexone use. Warn female patients to avoid breastfeeding while using naltrexone without first consulting their physicians. Patients taking methadone (Dolophine) for treatment of opioid dependency or addiction may be able to transfer from methadone to naltrexone after gradual withdrawal and final discontinuation of methadone.

✳ Apply Your Knowledge 15.4

The following questions focus on what you have just learned about synthetic and semisynthetic opioid antagonists.

CRITICAL THINKING

1. What are synthetic opioid antagonists? Name two examples.
2. What are three examples of semisynthetic opioids?
3. What is the most prominent action of oxycodone?
4. Are there any adverse effects of naloxone? Explain.
5. What are the trade names of naltrexone, oxycodone, hydrocodone, and naloxone?

Synthetic Opioid Analgesics

Synthetic opioid analgesics have the properties of morphine as analgesics but have fewer undesirable effects and less addiction potential. Currently available synthetic agents have valuable analgesic and pharmacologic properties that are described in this section.

Focus On

Buprenorphine

Buprenorphine (Buprenex) is a centrally acting synthetic and narcotic analgesic. This opiate agonist–antagonist has agonist activity approximately 30 times that of morphine and antagonist activity equal to or up to three times greater than that of naloxone.

How does it work?

Dose-related analgesia results from a high affinity of buprenorphine for mu-opioid receptors and an antagonist at the kappa-opiate receptors in the CNS.

How is it used?

Buprenorphine is used principally for patients with moderate to severe postoperative pain. It is also administered for pain associated with cancer, accidental trauma, urethral calculi, and myocardial infarction.

What are the adverse effects?

Buprenorphine may cause sedation, drowsiness, vertigo, dizziness, headache, amnesia, euphoria, and insomnia. This agent can also cause hypotension, miosis, nausea, vomiting, diarrhea, and constipation.

(Continued)

Focus On (*Continued*)

What are the contraindications and interactions?

Buprenorphine is contraindicated in known hypersensitivity to this agent or to naloxone. Safely during pregnancy, lactation, and in children younger than 13 years is not established. Buprenorphine may interact with alcohol and cause CNS depression. Diazepam (Valium) may cause respiratory or cardiovascular collapse.

What are the important points patients should know?

Instruct patients to avoid driving or engaging in hazardous activities until response to this drug is known and to avoid alcohol and other CNS depressants. Advise female patients to avoid breastfeeding while using this drug without consulting their physicians.

Fentanyl

Fentanyl (Duragesic, Sublimaze) is a potent and synthetic narcotic agonist analgesic agent with pharmacologic actions similar to those of morphine and meperidine.

How does it work?

The principal mechanism of action of fentanyl is analgesia and sedation, but its action is more prompt and less prolonged than that of morphine or meperidine.

How is it used?

Fentanyl is a short-acting analgesic drug used during operative and perioperative periods. This agent is prescribed as a narcotic analgesic supplement in general and as a regional anesthesia with diazepam (Valium) or droperidol (Inapsine) to produce neuroleptanalgesia (a form of analgesia accompanied by the general quieting of the patient and indifference to environmental stimuli without loss of consciousness). Fentanyl is also given with oxygen and a skeletal muscle relaxant to select high-risk patients, such as those undergoing open-heart surgery.

What are the adverse effects?

The adverse effects of fentanyl include sedation, euphoria, dizziness, delirium (excitement and mental confusion with hallucinations), and convulsions with high doses. This agent may also cause hypotension, bradycardia, cardiac arrest, and respiratory arrest. In some patients, blurred vision and miosis are reported. Other common adverse effects of fentanyl include nausea, vomiting, and constipation.

What are the contraindications and interactions?

Fentanyl is contraindicated in the management of acute or postoperative pain and in mild or intermittent pain that can be otherwise managed by less potent agents. It is also contraindicated at high doses at the initiation of opioid therapy and in patients with hypersensitivity to this agent. This agent may interact with alcohol and other CNS depressants, increasing their effects. Fentanyl may also interact with MAOIs to cause hypertensive crisis.

What are the important points patients should know?

Instruct patients to report muscle rigidity or weakness; unusual postoperative muscle movement of the extremities, eyes, or neck; and any problems breathing after taking this drug.

Meperidine

Meperidine (Demerol) is a synthetic opioid agonist analgesic with multiple actions qualitatively similar to those of morphine.

How does it work?

The most prominent of drug actions are on the CNS and on organs composed of smooth muscle. It acts principally to induce analgesia and sedation.

How is it used?

Meperidine is indicated for preoperative use, relief of moderate to severe pain, supportive anesthesia, and obstetric analgesia.

What are the adverse effects?

Major adverse effects include respiratory depression or arrest, circulatory depression, shock, and cardiac arrest.

The most common untoward effects include dizziness, sedation, nausea, vomiting, and sweating. Other adverse effects include euphoria, headache, weakness, agitation, tremor, seizures, disorientation, and hallucinations.

What are the contraindications and interactions?

Meperidine is contraindicated in patients taking MAOIs; it has inconsistently precipitated severe and occasionally fatal reactions within 14 days. The drug should be used with caution and in reduced dosage in patients taking other opioid analgesics, general anesthetics, phenothiazines, sedatives, tricyclic antidepressants, and other CNS depressants.

What are the important points patients should know?

Advise patients to ambulate carefully and to avoid smoking. Instruct patients to avoid driving or engaging in hazardous activities until drowsiness and dizziness have passed. CNS depressants and alcohol should be avoided. Female patients should not breastfeed while using this drug.

Focus on Geriatrics

Oversedation in Elderly Patients

Sedatives and narcotics must be given with extreme caution to elderly people who may easily become oversedated.

Focus On

Methadone

Methadone (Dolophine) is a synthetic opioid agonist with multiple analgesic actions quantitatively similar to morphine.

How does it work?

Methadone binds with opiate receptors in the CNS, altering the perception of and emotional response to pain.

How is it used?

Methadone is indicated for the relief of moderate to severe chronic pain. It is also used for the detoxification of opioid addiction and for temporary or sometimes long-term maintenance treatment of opioid addiction.

What are the adverse effects?

The adverse effects of methadone are similar to those for other opioid analgesics, especially meperidine (Demerol).

What are the contraindications and interactions?

Methadone is contraindicated in patients with known hypersensitivity. The drug should be used with caution and in reduced dosage in patients taking other opioid analgesics, general anesthetics, phenothiazines and other tranquilizers, sedative–hypnotics, tricyclic antidepressants, MAOIs, and other CNS depressants. The safe use of methadone in pregnancy has not been established. It is not recommended for obstetric analgesia because its long duration may induce respiratory depression in newborns.

What are the important points patients should know?

Instruct patients to make position changes slowly, especially from a supine to an upright position, and to sit or lie down if they feel dizzy or faint. Advise patients to avoid driving or engaging in potentially hazardous activities until the response to this drug is known. Female patients should not breastfeed while taking this drug without consulting their physician.

Focus On

Pentazocine

Pentazocine (Talwin) is a synthetic narcotic agonist–antagonist analgesic that is classified as a controlled substance (Schedule IV drug).

How does it work?

Pentazocine has a similar mechanism of action to that of morphine but with only one-third the strength. Large doses of pentazocine may increase blood pressure and heart rate. When given in usual parenteral doses, it is as effective in relieving moderate to severe pain as the usual parenteral doses of morphine, meperidine, butorphanol, or nalbuphine.

How is it used?

Pentazocine is indicated for the control of moderate to severe pain. It is also used for preoperative analgesia or sedation and as a supplement to surgical anesthesia.

What are the adverse effects?

Pentazocine causes nausea, vomiting, diarrhea, constipation, dry mouth, and alterations of taste. This agent may also cause dizziness, lightheadedness, sedation, euphoria, headache, disturbed dreams, insomnia, syncope (fainting), and visual blurring. Hypotension, tachycardia, and respiratory depression have also been included among its adverse effects.

What are the contraindications and interactions?

Pentazocine is contraindicated in patients with a history of hypersensitivity. This agent must be avoided in patients with head injuries or increased intracranial pressure, in emotionally unstable patients, and in those with a history of drug abuse. Safety during pregnancy or lactation or in children younger than age 12 years is not established. Pentazocine must be used cautiously in patients with impaired kidney or liver function, respiratory depression, biliary surgery, and myocardial infarction with nausea and vomiting. Alcohol and other CNS depressants add to CNS depression with the use of pentazocine.

What are the important points patients should know?

Instruct patients to avoid driving and other hazardous activities until the response to this drug is known. Pentazocine should not be discontinued abruptly after extended use, and female patients should not breastfeed while taking this drug.

✳ Apply Your Knowledge 15.5

The following questions focus on what you have just learned about synthetic opioid analgesics.

CRITICAL THINKING

1. What are the characteristics of buprenorphine?
2. What is the principal mechanism of action of fentanyl?
3. What are the most prominent actions of meperidine?
4. What are the effects of large doses of pentazocine on the cardiovascular system?
5. What are the trade names of meperidine, pentazocine, methadone, and fentanyl?

PRACTICAL SCENARIO 1

Janet is a 4-year-old girl who is found unconscious. Her grandmother calls the physician's office and speaks to the medical assistant, who instructs her to call 911 immediately, which she does. When emergency help arrives, the grandmother states that she put her granddaughter down for a nap around 1:00 PM in the grandmother's bedroom. At about 2:30 PM, she checked on Janet and found her on the floor of the bedroom, unconscious and unresponsive, with an open bottle of acetaminophen beside her. The grandmother says the bottle of 60 tablets was empty, and there were seven to 10 tablets on the floor.

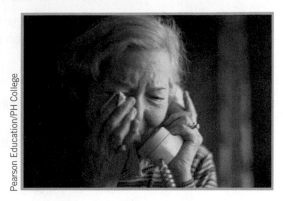

Pearson Education/PH College

Critical Thinking Questions

1. In counseling the grandmother about this incident, what teaching information should be provided by health-care personnel?
2. What are some of the complications of an overdose of acetaminophen?

PRACTICAL SCENARIO 2

A 39-year-old man had back surgery for disc herniations. His physician prescribed oxycodone for pain relief. Two weeks after surgery, he was released on his 40th birthday. To celebrate, he drank several glasses of wine at the party. Upon going to bed, he took several oxycodones for his back pain. The next morning, his wife could not wake him.

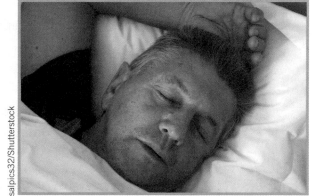

salpics32/Shutterstock

Critical Thinking Questions

1. What was the cause of his death?
2. Why should oxycodone never be taken with alcohol?

Chapter Capsule

This section repeats the objectives from the beginning of the chapter and then provides a summary of the most important concepts for that objective. Use this section as a quick review and to check your knowledge.

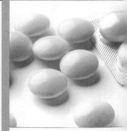

Objective 1: List the antipyretic properties of anti-inflammatory and analgesic drugs.

- Inhibition of prostaglandin synthesis in the CNS
- Central action in the hypothalamic heat-regulating center

Objective 2: Describe the role of prostaglandins in inflammation.

- Prostaglandins are hormone-like substances that modulate inflammation. They initiate an action potential along a sensory nerve fiber or sensitize pain receptors.

Objective 3: Outline the dangers of aspirin use.

- Possible massive GI hemorrhage, dyspepsia, nausea and vomiting, and occult bleeding

Objective 4: List the uses and side effects of anti-inflammatory drugs.

- Used for rheumatoid arthritis, osteoarthritis, arthritis, moderate pain, and fever
- Side effects—dizziness, nervousness, occult blood loss, peptic ulceration, GI bleeding, and others

Objective 5: Identify the different types of analgesics.

- Nonopioid analgesics
- Opioid analgesics

Objective 6: Describe the function of naturally occurring opioids and their receptors.

- Naturally occurring opioids bind to opioid receptors to block pain transmission

Objective 7: Explain the rationale behind the use of narcotic analgesics.

- Effective for almost all types of moderate and severe pain and for cough inhibition
- Mimic endogenous opioids to block pain transmission

Objective 8: Describe the problems associated with the use of narcotic analgesics.

- Can cause respiratory depression
- Can produce physical and psychological dependence

Internet Sites of Interest

- The International Association for the Study of Pain (IASP) offers a discussion about tolerance to opioids at **http://www.iasp-pain.org/PCU01-5.html**.
- The Pain Management: Series is a continuing education program on pain offered by the American Medical Association at **http://www.ama-cmeonline.com**.
- The National Institutes of Health offer information on drugs and other medical conditions at its MedLine Plus website at **http://www.nlm.nih.gov/medlineplus**. Search for NSAIDs.

- An explanation of antipyretics can be found on Wikipedia at **http://en.wikipedia.org/wiki/Antipyretic**. However, always be aware that Wikipedia sites are written by numerous people, not all of whom may be experts in the topic. Therefore, double-check information you find there with other reputable sources.

- The World Health Organization (WHO) has developed a widely recognized protocol for use of pain medications, called the WHO Pain Ladder. An example can be found at **http://www.who.int/cancer/palliative/painladder/en**.

PEARSON myhealthprofessionskit™

Go to www.myhealthprofessionskit.com to access the Companion Website created for this textbook. Simply select "Basic Health Science" from the choice of disciplines. Find this book and then log in using your username and password to access interactive learning games, assessment questions, animations, and more.

Chapter 16

Antineoplastic Agents

Chapter Objectives

After completing this chapter, you should be able to:

1. List the seven warning signs of cancer.
2. Summarize the basic cell cycle and its importance in the use of antineoplastic agents.
3. List commonly used antineoplastic agents in each class.
4. Explain the mechanism of action of each class of antineoplastic agents.
5. Discuss how steroids, estrogens, progestins, antiestrogens, and antiandrogens work in the treatment of cancer.
6. Explain how biologic response modifiers are created and how they work.
7. Describe the advantages of using monoclonal antibodies in the treatment of cancer.
8. Identify the common side effects of chemotherapy treatment.

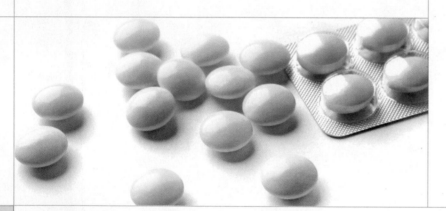

Key Terms

adenocarcinoma (ah-deh-no-kar-sih-NO-muh) (page 261)

adjuvant (AJ-eh-vant) (page 261)

alkylating agents (AL-kih-lay-ting) (page 266)

alopecia (al-o-PEE-shuh) (page 266)

antimetabolites (an-tee-meh-TAH-bo-liytz) (page 267)

antitumor antibiotics (page 270)

benign (beh-NYN) (page 261)

carcinogenic (kars-ih-no-JEN-ik) (page 261)

hybridomas (hy-brih-DOH-muhz) (page 271)

hyperplasia (hy-per-PLAY-shuh) (page 261)

malignant (mah-LIG-nent) (page 261)

metastasis (meh-TAS-tuh-sis) (page 261)

mitosis (my-TOH-sis) (page 262)

monoclonal antibodies (mah-no-KLO-nul) (page 271)

nucleotides (NOO-klee-oh-tiedz) (page 262)

oncogenes (ON-ko-jeenz) (page 261)

palliative (PAH-lee-uh-tiv) (page 261)

partial response (page 263)

plant alkaloids (page 268)

sarcomas (sar-KO-muhs) (page 261)

stable disease (page 263)

teratogenic (teh-rah-toh-JEN-ik) (page 266)

tumor suppressor genes (page 261)

Introduction

Cancer is the second-most common cause of death in the United States after cardiovascular disease, causing more than 500,000 fatalities annually. The most common cancers are breast, prostate, lung, and colorectal. The leading cause of cancer death is lung cancer. Cancer is a group of more than 100 different diseases, characterized by uncontrolled cellular division and **hyperplasia** (abnormal cell growth), local tissue invasion (breaking through boundaries that separate cell types within some organs), and **metastasis** (spreading of cancer cells from the primary site to secondary sites). Cancer cells are also referred to as *tumors* or *neoplasms*. Tumors can be benign or malignant. **Benign** tumors are generally slow growing and resemble normal cells. They are localized and not harmful. **Malignant** tumors often proliferate more rapidly and have an atypical appearance. This atypical appearance is because cancer cells, unlike normal cells, do not continue to mature. Instead, their rapid multiplication causes them to become more and more atypical—a process often called *differentiation*. They invade and destroy surrounding tissues, and they induce the formation of new blood vessels (*angiogenesis*) that act as the tumor's own blood supply to help spread malignant cells to other tissues.

Chemotherapy uses chemical agents to interact with cancer cells to stop or control the growth of the cancer. For example, during World War II, soldiers exposed to nitrogen mustard experienced low white blood cell (WBC) counts. Today, nitrogen mustard is used to treat patients with lymphoid leukemia and lymphomas. However, because chemotherapeutic drugs cannot distinguish between normal cells and cancer cells, both types of cells are affected by chemotherapy. But the killing effect of chemotherapeutic agents has selectivity for cancer cells over normal host cells and thus normal host cells are able to repair themselves and continue to grow.

Chemotherapy, as used for the treatment of cancer, may be termed *primary, palliative, adjuvant,* or *neoadjuvant* agent. For some cancers, chemotherapy alone can destroy all the cancer cells and cure the cancer, which is *primary* treatment. As an **adjuvant** treatment (one that aids or contributes), chemotherapy is given before or after other methods of treatment, such as surgery and radiation, to reduce the risk of recurrence or to prolong survival. **Palliative** treatment, which eases a disease's effects but does not cure, may be used if a cure is not possible to minimize the discomfort caused by cancer or to slow the progression of the disease and prolong the patient's life. Chemotherapy may also be given in the *neoadjuvant* or preoperative setting. The goal in this setting is to make other treatments more effective by reducing tissue damage, decreasing tumor size, or destroying micrometastases.

Neoplasms

Tumors arise from any of the four basic tissue types: epithelial, connective (blood, bone, and cartilage), muscle, and nerve. Benign tumors are named by adding the suffix *-oma* to the name of the cell type. For example, *adenomas* are benign growths of glandular origin. On the other hand, *carcinomas* are malignant growths arising from epithelial cells. An **adenocarcinoma** is a malignant tumor arising from glandular origin. Malignant growths of muscle or connective tissue are called **sarcomas**. Another term used frequently in the description of malignancy is *carcinoma in situ*. In this instance, the cancer is limited to the epithelial cells where it began. Because cancers are most curable with surgery or radiation before they have metastasized, early detection and treatment is very important. In addition, small tumors are more responsive to chemotherapy than are large tumors. Early diagnosis is difficult for many cancers because they do not produce clinical signs or symptoms until they have become large or have metastasized.

Tumors are constantly shedding neoplastic cells into the systemic circulation or surrounding lymphatic nodules. Cells of benign tumors resemble the cells from which they developed. These masses seldom metastasize, and after they are removed, they rarely recur. In contrast, malignant tumors invade and destroy the surrounding tissues. Malignant tumors tend to metastasize, so recurrences are common after the removal or destruction of the primary tumor.

ONCOGENES

Recent explorations into the causes of cancer have centered on the role of genes that cause cancer. There are two major classes of genes involved in carcinogenesis: *oncogenes* and *tumor suppressor*. **Oncogenes** develop from normal genes, termed *protooncogenes*. Protooncogenes are present in all cells and are essential regulators of normal cellular functions, including the cell cycle. Genetic alteration of the protooncogenes may activate the oncogenes. These genetic alterations may be caused by such **carcinogenic** (cancer-causing) agents as radiation, chemicals, or viruses. **Tumor suppressor genes** are another category of genes involved in carcinogenesis. The normal function of these genes is to regulate and inhibit inappropriate cellular growth and proliferation. Gene loss or mutation can result in the loss of control over normal cell growth.

THE CELL CYCLE AND MOLECULAR BIOLOGY

The ability of chemotherapy to kill cancer cells depends on its ability to stop cell division. Usually, cancer drugs work by damaging the ribonucleic acid

(RNA) or deoxyribonucleic acid (DNA) that tells the cell how to copy itself for division. If the cancer cells are unable to divide, they die. The faster cancer cells divide, the more likely it is that chemotherapy will kill the cells, causing the tumor to shrink. Both cancer cells and normal cells reproduce themselves in a series of steps known as the *cell cycle.* There are usually four steps after the resting (G_0) stage:

✳ G_0: The resting or dormant stage when cells have not started to divide. Cells spend much of their lives in this phase. Depending on their type, different cells can last just a few hours or a few years. When cells receive a signal to reproduce, they move into the G_1 phase (Figure 16-1 ■).

✳ G_1: The first gap phase. The cell starts making proteins to prepare for division. This phase lasts about 18 to 30 hours.

✳ S: DNA synthesis occurs. The chromosomes containing the genetic code are copied so both of the new cells formed have the right amount of DNA. This phase lasts about 18 to 20 hours.

✳ G_2: The second gap phase. This occurs just before the cell starts splitting into two cells. It lasts from 2 to 10 hours.

✳ M: **Mitosis** (when one cell splits into two new cells) occurs. This lasts only 30 to 60 minutes.

Most human cells exist in the G_0 phase, and most cancer cells in the G_0 stage are not sensitive to the effects of chemotherapy. Not all cancer cells proliferate faster than normal cells. Many anticancer drugs target rapidly proliferating cells, and these agents may act at selective or multiple sites of the cell cycle. Agents with major activity in a particular phase of the cell cycle are known as *cell cycle phase–specific agents.* Many antineoplastic agents interfere with the

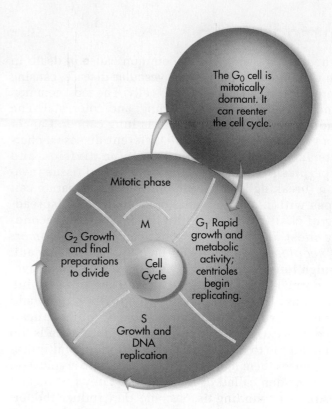

Figure 16-1 ■ The four steps of the cell cycle.

cellular synthesis of DNA, RNA, and proteins. The genetic information is encoded in DNA by the precise sequencing of basic structural subunits of DNA, known as **nucleotides**. The goal of chemotherapy is to selectively destroy tumor cells, which can be achieved by targeting specific growth characteristics of most tumors. Agents used in cancer chemotherapy are commonly categorized by their mechanism of action or by their origin.

Focus Point

The Seven Warning Signs of Cancer

1. Change in bowel or bladder habits
2. A sore that does not heal
3. Unusual bleeding or discharge
4. Thickening or lump in breast or elsewhere
5. Indigestion or difficulty swallowing
6. Obvious change in a wart or mole
7. Nagging cough or hoarseness

Focus on Pediatrics

Warning Signs of Cancer in Children

1. Unexplained or persistent lump
2. Unexplained or persistent limping
3. Unexplained normocytic anemia
4. Unexplained thrombocytopenic bruising
5. Unexplained weight loss
6. Abdominal mass
7. Unexplained persistent headache or vomiting on awakening

✳ Apply Your Knowledge 16.1

The following questions focus on what you have just learned about various cancer cells and molecular biology.

CRITICAL THINKING

1. What are oncogenes?
2. What are the four steps of the cell cycle? Explain them.
3. What are the warning signs of cancer in children?
4. Compare carcinoma with sarcomas.
5. In what stage of the cell cycle does DNA synthesis occur?
6. What is mitosis?

Cancer Therapy

Five primary methods are used in the approach to cancer treatment: surgery, radiation therapy, chemotherapy, immunotherapy, and hormonal therapy. Surgery remains the treatment of choice for many solid tumors. Radiation treatment was first used for cancer treatment in the late 1800s. Although very effective for treating many types of cancer, surgery and radiation are local treatments. Systemic diseases, such as leukemia, cannot be treated this way. Chemotherapy and hormonal therapy access the systemic circulation. Immunotherapy uses the stimulation of the host's immune system to fight against the cancer. The response to chemotherapy may be described as *cure*, *complete response*, **partial response**, **stable disease**, or *progression of disease*. A *cure* implies that the patient is entirely free of disease and has the same life expectancy as a cancer-free individual. *Complete response* means complete disappearance of all cancer and no evidence of new disease for at least 1 month after treatment. A *partial response* is defined as a 50% or greater decrease in the tumor size or other objective disease markers and no evidence of any new disease for at least 1 month. A patient whose tumor size neither grows nor shrinks significantly has *stable disease*.

Depending on the type of cancer and the drug used, chemotherapy agents may be administered orally, intramuscularly (IM), subcutaneously, or intravenously (IV). IV administration is the most common method of administration. Oral chemotherapy is becoming more popular than ever because of its ease of use. The most common antineoplastic agents are listed in Table 16-1 ■.

Table 16-1 ■ Common Agents Used in the Treatment of Cancer

GENERIC NAME	TRADE NAME	COMMON DOSAGE RANGE	ROUTE OF ADMINISTRATION
Alkylating Agents			
chlorambucil (nitrogen mustard)	Leukeran	0.1–0.2 mg/kg/d	PO
cyclophosphamide	Cytoxan	1–5 mg/kg/d	PO
		10–15 mg/kg q7–10d or 3–5 mg/kg twice weekly	IV
ifosfamide	Ifex	1.2 g/m^2/d for 5 d	IV
mechlorethamine (nitrogen mustard)	Mustargen	0.4 mg/kg in 1–4 divided doses	IV, intracavity
melphalan	Alkeran	2–10 mg/d (0–15 mg/kg/d) for 7 d	PO
Ethyleneimines			
altretamine	Hexalen	260 mg/m^2/d for 14 or 21 d in a 28-d cycle	PO
thiotepa	Immunex	0.3–0.4 mg/kg	IV
		0.6–0.8 mg/kg	Intravesicular directly into the bladder
Alkyl Sulfonate			
busulfan	Busulfex	4–8 mg/d	PO
		0.8 mg/kg q6h for 4 d	IV
Miscellaneous			
carboplatin	Paraplatin	On day 1 every 4 weeks	IV infusion
cisplatin	Platinol-AQ	20–100 mg/m^2/d (schedule depends on type of cancer; up to 360 mg/m^2)	IV
procarbazine	Matulane	2–4 mg/kg/d for 1 wk and then 4–6 mg/kg/d until WBCs are less than 4,000/mm^3	PO
Antimetabolites			
capecitabine	Xeloda	2,500 mg/m^2/d in two divided doses for 2 wk	PO
fluorouracil	5-FU, Efudex, Adrucil	6–2 mg/kg/d	IV
mercaptopurine	6-MP, Purinethol	1.5–2.5 mg/kg/d	PO
methotrexate	Rheumatrex, Folex, Trexall	10–30 mg/kg/d for 4–8 d with 7–10-d rest interval	PO
		10–30 mg	IM
		20–500 mg/m^2	IV

GENERIC NAME	TRADE NAME	COMMON DOSAGE RANGE	ROUTE OF ADMINISTRATION
Mitotic Inhibitors (Plant Alkaloids)			
etoposide	VePesid, Toposar, VP-16	35–100 mg/m^2/d	PO, IV
teniposide	Vumon	165 mg/m^2 in combination twice weekly for 4.5 wk	IV
vinblastine	Velban	3.7–11.1 mg/m^2	IV
vincristine	Oncovin, Vincasar PFS	1.4 mg/m^2	IV
vinorelbine	Navelbine	15–30 mg/m^2	IV
Antitumor Antibiotics			
bleomycin	Blenoxane	0.25–0.50 units/kg/d	IM, IV, subcutaneously
daunorubicin	Cerubidine	30–60 mg/m^2/d	IV
doxorubicin	Adriamycin	20–75 mg/m^2	IV
epirubicin	Ellence	100–120 mg/m^2 infused over 3–5 min on day 1 of a 3–4 wk cycle or 50–60 mg/m^2 on day 1 and day 8 of a 3–4 wk cycle	IV
idarubicin	Idamycin	12 mg/m^2/d for 3 d	IV
mitomycin C	Mutamycin	10–20 mg/m^2	IV
plicamycin	Mithracin	20–30 mcg/kg day for 8–10 d	IV
valrubicin	Valstar	800 mg in 75 mL of solution once a week for 6 wk	Instilled into the urinary bladder
Hormonal Therapy			
Corticosteroids			
dexamethasone	Provera	0.25–4 mg bid to qid	PO
	Depo-Provera	8–6 mg every 1–3 wk	IM
prednisone	Deltasone	5–60 mg/d in single or divided doses	PO
Estrogens			
estramustine	Emcyt	10–16 mg/kg/d in 3–4 divided doses for up to 3 y	PO
tamoxifen	Nolvadex	10–20 mg 1–2 times/d	PO
Progestins			
megestrol	Megace	40–320 mg/d in divided doses	PO

(*continued*)

Table 16-1 ■ **Common Agents Used in the Treatment of Cancer** (*continued*)

GENERIC NAME	TRADE NAME	COMMON DOSAGE RANGE	ROUTE OF ADMINISTRATION
Gonadotropins			
goserelin	Zoladex	3.6 mg once every 4 wk or 10.8 mg depot every 3 mo	Subcutaneous implants
leuprolide	Lupron,	1 mg/d	Subcutaneous
	Eligard	7.5 mg monthly as depot injection	IM
Antiandrogens			
bicalutamide	Casodex	50 mg/d	PO
flutamide	Eulexin	250 mg three times/d at 8-h intervals	PO
nilutamide	Nilandron	300 mg/d for 3 d	PO

bid, twice a day; IV, intravenous; PO, oral; qid, four times a day; WBC, white blood cell.

Focus Point

Bone Marrow Depression

Depression of bone marrow is usually the most serious limiting toxicity of cancer chemotherapy.

Focus On

Alkylating Agents

Alkylating agents cause replacement of hydrogen by an alkyl group, specifically one that inhibits cell division and growth. There are five major types of alkylating agents:

1. Nitrogen mustards
2. Ethyleneimines
3. Alkyl sulfonates
4. Nitrosoureas
5. Temozolomide

Acquired resistance to alkylating agents is a common event, but resistance of a cancer to one alkylating agent does not always imply cross-resistance to others.

How do they work?

Alkylating agents act directly on DNA, causing cross-linking of DNA strands, abnormal base pairing, or DNA strand breaks, thus preventing the cells from dividing. They are cell cycle phase–nonspecific but are most active in the resting phase.

How are they used?

Alkylating agents are generally of greatest value in treating slow-growing cancers. They are not as effective on rapidly growing cells.

What are the adverse effects?

This class has a dose-limiting toxicity to bone marrow and intestinal mucosa. Alkylating agents cause oral mucosa ulceration and intestinal denudations. All alkylating agents can cause instances of pulmonary fibrosis and venoocclusive disease in the liver; renal failure; or central neurotoxicity with seizures, coma, and, at times, death. Most alkylating agents cause **alopecia** (hair loss). Central nervous system toxicity is indicated by nausea and vomiting. Ifosfamide (Ifex) is the most neurotoxic of this class, producing altered mental status, coma, generalized seizures, and paralysis. All alkylating agents have toxic effects on the reproductive system.

What are the contraindications and interactions?

Alkylating agents are contraindicated during pregnancy, especially during the first trimester, because they are **teratogenic** (able to cause birth defects in fetuses). Alkylating agents may interact with antidepressants; other anticancer medications; warfarin (Coumadin); and such prescription and nonprescription medications as certain vaccines, aspirin, and vitamins.

What are the most important points patients should know?

Teach patients about the manifestation of bone marrow depression. Advise patients to avoid contact with people who have colds or other infections during susceptible times (for example, after a course of therapy). Warn patients that hair loss may occur from the head, eyelashes, nose, and pubic area, but reassure them that their hair will grow back after the course of therapy is complete.

Focus Point

Tyramine and Procarbazine

Procarbazine (Matulane) is available as a 50-mg capsule. It can cause an acute disulfiram-like reaction (flushing, headache, acute vomiting, and chest or abdominal pain) with alcohol. Avoid tyramine-containing foods (for example, aged cheese, chocolate, pickles, aged meat, wine), which can cause a life-threatening elevation in blood pressure.

Focus On

Antimetabolites

Antimetabolites prevent cancer cell growth by affecting DNA production. They are only effective against cells that are actively participating in cell metabolism. The classes of antimetabolites include:

1. Purine antagonists: mercaptopurine
2. Adenosine antagonists: fludarabine
3. Pyrimidine antagonists: fluorouracil
4. Folic acid antagonists: methotrexate

How do they work?

Antimetabolites replace natural substances as building blocks in DNA molecules, altering the function of enzymes required for cell metabolism and protein synthesis. They are cell cycle phase–specific and are most effective during the S-phase of cell division.

How are they used?

Mercaptopurine (Purinethol) is useful in the maintenance therapy of children with acute and chronic myelocytic leukemia. Fludarabine (Fludara) is used in the treatment of chronic lymphocytic leukemia and non-Hodgkin's lymphoma. Capecitabine (Xeloda) is used for metastatic breast and colorectal cancers. It is a *prodrug* (a modified, pharmacologically inactive form of a pharmacologic agent) of fluorouracil (Adrucil) and undergoes hydrolysis in the liver to form the active drug. Fluorouracil is prescribed for the treatment of *keratoses* (overgrowths of horny skin tissue) and basal cell carcinomas (skin cancer). Methotrexate (Trexall) is used for acute lymphoblastic leukemia, meningeal leukemia, and head and neck cancers (and for such noncancerous disorders as rheumatoid arthritis and psoriasis).

What are the adverse effects?

The adverse effects of mercaptopurine include anorexia, nausea, vomiting, hepatotoxicity, bone marrow depression, and hyperuricemia. Fludarabine may cause headache, hearing loss, sleep disorders, and depression. It may also cause bone marrow toxicity, pneumonia, dyspnea (difficulty breathing), epistaxis (nosebleed), and edema. Fluorouracil causes marked myelosuppression. It can also result in gastrointestinal (GI) disturbances, alopecia, dermatitis, and nail changes.

(Continued)

Focus On (Continued)

Methotrexate commonly causes skin rashes, hyperpigmentation, photosensitivity, hyperuricemia, inflammation of the tongue, and alopecia. Serious adverse effects include severe leukopenia, bone marrow aplasia, and thrombocytopenia.

What are the contraindications and interactions?

Mercaptopurine is contraindicated in patients with a history of resistance to this agent. It must be avoided in the first trimester of pregnancy, in women who are lactating, and in patients who have acute infectious diseases. Fluorouracil, mercaptopurine, and methotrexate are contraindicated in patients with severe bone marrow depression and renal dysfunction. Mercaptopurine may interact with allopurinol (Zyloprim); warfarin (Coumadin); and certain drugs used to treat ulcerative colitis, such as mesalamine (Asacol), olsalazine (Dipentum), and sulfasalazine (Azulfidine). Patients should be instructed not to start or stop any prescription or nonprescription medications while taking this drug and to tell their health-care providers about all medications they are currently taking before taking mercaptopurine.

What are the most important points patients should know?

Advise patients that antimetabolites may cause bone marrow suppression and damage to the GI lining, such as stomatitis (a group of diseases affecting the mucous membranes of the mouth) and ulceration.

Focus on Natural Products

Green Tea as an Antioxidant

Green tea has a reputation as a healthful drink, with studies suggesting it may reduce the incidence of a variety of cancers, including cancers of the colon, pancreas, and stomach. Green tea contains high levels of polyphenols, which exhibit antioxidant and chemopreventive properties. However, green tea is not a proven cure for cancer. As often happens with natural supplements that are supported primarily by observational trials, results of these studies are inconsistent. Also, green tea should not be given to infants or young children.

Focus On

Mitotic Inhibitors (Plant Alkaloids)

Plant alkaloids are typically physiologically active organic bases containing nitrogen (and usually oxygen) that occur in seed plants. They are called *mitotic inhibitors* because they prevent cell division (or *meiosis*). The primary plant alkaloids are vincristine (Oncovin) and vinblastine (Velban). Examples of plant alkaloids are listed in Table 16-1.

How do they work?

Mitotic inhibitors act throughout the cell cycle, and some of these agents are more effective during the S- and M-phases of the cell cycle. They inhibit DNA and RNA synthesis.

How are they used?

Mitotic inhibitors are used to treat cancer of the breast, bladder, ovaries, and lungs as well as leukemias, lymphomas, and testicular cancer.

What are the adverse effects?

These agents may cause nausea, vomiting, diarrhea, alopecia, dizziness, weakness, headache, depression, and stomatitis. The adverse effects of mitotic inhibitors may also cause anemia and hyperpigmentation of the nails, tongue, or oral mucosa.

What are the contraindications and interactions?

Mitotic inhibitors are contraindicated in severe cardiac disease, hypocalcemia, bleeding disorders, myelosuppression, and pregnancy. Some of these drugs, such as plicamycin (Mithracin), must be used cautiously in patients with hepatic or renal impairment. Mitomycin (Mutamycin) may cause acute shortness of breath and severe bronchospasm if it is used with mitotic inhibitors. These agents may decrease phenytoin (Dilantin) levels.

Erythromycin (Eryc) and itraconazole (Sporanox) may increase vinblastine toxicity.

What are the important points patients should know?

Be sure patients are aware that mitotic inhibitors may produce serious toxicity with bone marrow depression and GI damage. Advise them that if they have diarrhea to avoid foods that are likely to cause GI irritation, such as coffee, spicy foods, fruits, and raw vegetables.

Focus on Geriatrics

Toxicity of Antineoplastic Drugs in Elderly Patients

Older adults—many of whom may have such chronic diseases as cardiovascular disease or kidney impairment—are at higher risk for adverse effects when they are being treated with antineoplastic drugs. As a result, lower dosages of antineoplastics should be administered to these patients. Creatinine clearance is used to monitor renal function in elderly patients.

Focus On

Hormonal Therapy

Hormonal agents are frequently prescribed in antineoplastic therapy. These agents may selectively suppress the growth of certain tissues of the body without causing a cytotoxic action. The sex hormones, such as estrogens, progestins, and androgens, are generally used to change the hormonal environment of tissues dependent on these agents for their growth. For example, the administration of antiandrogens or estrogens is beneficial in the treatment of prostatic cancer. On the other hand, these hormones can be useful in treating breast or endometrial cancers.

How do they work?

Hormonal agents are a class of heterogeneous compounds that have various effects on cells. These agents block either hormone production or hormone action. Their action on malignant cells is highly selective. Steroids inhibit migration of WBCs and inhibit the production of products of the arachidonic acid cascade. Estrogen works by promoting the release of calcitonin and by enhancing the availability of vitamin D_3 to increase bone formation in postmenopausal patients with breast cancer.

Progestins inhibit secretion of pituitary gonadotropins by positive feedback. Antiestrogens bind to estrogen receptors, which prevents estrogen from binding to these receptors. Antiandrogens act by blocking the synthesis of endogenous testosterone.

How are they used?

Hormones and their antagonists have various uses in the treatment of malignant tumors. Steroids are especially useful in treating acute lymphocytic leukemia. They are also used in conjunction with radiation therapy to reduce radiation edema. Sex hormones are used in carcinomas of the reproductive tract; for example, estrogen may be given to patients with testicular cancer or to patients with certain carcinomas of the breast.

What are the adverse effects?

GI disturbances are common adverse effects associated with these drugs. Impaired fertility may result from treatment with sex hormone antagonists. In women, menstrual irregularities may develop depending on premenopausal or menopausal stages of life.

(Continued)

Focus On (Continued)

What are the contraindications and interactions?

Most hormones are contraindicated during pregnancy because they are harmful to fetuses. These drugs should be used during pregnancy only in circumstances in which the benefits of treatment far outweigh the risk of harm to the fetus. Interactions with hormonal therapies occur with tamoxifen (Nolvadex), alcohol, St. John's wort, zinc, magnesium, vitamin B, and thyroid supplements.

What are the important points patients should know?

Warn patients that hormonal agents are contraindicated during pregnancy and that menstrual irregularities are common. If appropriate, advise female patients to use strict contraception and to avoid pregnancy for 3 to 4 months after completing the course. Some sources advise that men and women should avoid conceiving a child for about 2 years after treatment.

Focus Point

Possibility of Infertility

It is important to instruct patients that infertility, which may occur with antineoplastic agents, may not be reversible.

Focus On

Antitumor Antibiotics

Antitumor antibiotics are made from natural products produced by species of the soil fungus *Streptomyces*. They are very effective in the treatment of certain tumors. The classifications of these agents are listed in Table 16-1.

How do they work?

The majority of antitumor antibiotics inhibit DNA and RNA synthesis, causing cell death.

How are they used?

Antitumor antibiotics are used only to treat cancer and are not used to treat infections. The effects of each of the antitumor antibiotics are as follows:

✳ Doxorubicin (Adriamycin) is used in the treatment of breast, ovarian, and bone cancers. It is also used in the therapy for acute lymphoblastic and myeloblastic leukemias. Doxorubicin is generally used in combination with surgery, radiation, and immunotherapy.

✳ Daunorubicin (Cerubidine) is the first-line treatment for advanced HIV-associated Kaposi's sarcoma. It is also used for testicular cancer, Wilms's tumor, and choriocarcinoma.

✳ Idarubicin (Idamycin) can be used for treating acute monocytic leukemia and solid tumors.

✳ Plicamycin (Mithracin) is used to treat hypercalcemia associated with advanced neoplasms and testicular cancer.

✳ Bleomycin (Blenoxane) is used in squamous cell carcinomas (skin cancer) of the head, neck, penis, and cervix. It is also used for the treatment of lymphomas and testicular carcinoma.

✳ Mitomycin (Mutamycin) is used in combination with other chemotherapeutic agents in palliative and adjunctive treatment of breast, stomach, and pancreatic cancers.

What are the adverse effects?

Bone marrow suppression is a major adverse effect of antitumor antibiotics. Stomatitis, GI upset, and alopecia can occur during treatment but cease when treatment is discontinued. Bleomycin is less toxic to bone marrow but tends to cause hyperpigmentation, redness, and sometimes ulceration of the skin. Pulmonary fibrosis can occur during therapy. Mitomycin may induce serious renal impairment.

What are the contraindications and interactions?

Antitumor antibiotics are contraindicated in patients with known hypersensitivity to these agents. Some antitumor antibiotics have toxic effects on the heart, kidneys, and liver. Therefore, they are contraindicated in patients with diseases of these organs. Plasma digoxin (Lanoxin) levels may decrease when administered with bleomycin. When bleomycin is used with cisplatin (Platinol), there is an increased risk of bleomycin toxicity. Mitomycin and plicamycin may have an additive bone marrow depressant effect when used with other antineoplastic agents. There is an increased risk of bleeding when plicamycin is administered with aspirin, heparin (Hep-Lock), warfarin (Coumadin), or nonsteroidal anti-inflammatory drugs.

What are the important points patients should know?

Advise patients that bone marrow suppression is a major adverse effect of these drugs. Because cardiac toxicity is observed with antitumor antibiotics, instruct patients to report to their physicians if they experience cardiac problems.

✳ Apply Your Knowledge 16.2

The following questions focus on what you have just learned about various cancer therapies.

CRITICAL THINKING

1. What are the five primary methods used to treat cancer?
2. What is the most common method of administration of chemotherapy agents for the treatment of cancer?
3. What are the trade names of nitrogen mustard, melphalan, busulfan, and bleomycin?
4. What is the most serious toxicity of cancer chemotherapy?
5. What are the five major types of alkylating agents?
6. What are four examples of antimetabolites?
7. Why does green tea reduce the incidence of colon, pancreas, and stomach cancers?
8. What are the mechanisms of action of antitumor antibiotics?

Biologic Response Modifiers

Biologic response modifiers include agents that affect the patient's biologic response to a neoplasm in a beneficial way. Included in this class are agents that act indirectly to mediate antitumor effects or directly on the tumor cells. Recombinant DNA technology has greatly facilitated the identification and production of a number of human proteins, with potent effects on the function and growth of normal and neoplastic cells. Interferons, interleukin-2, tumor necrosis factor, and monoclonal antibodies are types of human proteins.

An example of how the biologic response modifiers are produced is that of **monoclonal antibodies**. These are produced by fusing a single immune cell to tumor cells that are grown in cultures, known as **hybridomas**. Large quantities of these identical antibody cells are produced (rather like clones)—all with the same specific antigen as their target. The advantage of monoclonal antibodies is they can be used to target and then purify the *specific* protein that induced their formation. Interferons are another type of biologic response modifiers that are discussed in detail in this chapter.

Focus On

Interferons

Interferons are a group of blood proteins that have antiviral effects. The genes that produce some of the interferons have been isolated, and those interferons are now commercially produced by means of genetic engineering. Interferons are naturally produced in response to viral infections or other biological inducers, such as some tumors.

There are three types of interferons: alpha (2a and 2b), beta, and gamma.

* Alfa (called alfa when referring to drugs)—produced by WBCs
* Beta—produced by connective tissue cells
* Gamma—produced by T lymphocytes

(Continued)

Focus On (Continued)

Only interferon alfa-2b (Intron A) is effectively used for some cancers. Thus, only alfa-2b will be discussed here.

How does it work?

Interferon alfa-2b (Intron A) is a natural product induced virally in peripheral WBCs. Interferon alfa-2b is obtained by the recombinant DNA technology of *Escherichia coli*, bearing an interferon alfa-2b gene from human leukocytes.

How is it used?

Interferon alfa-2b is a chemotherapy agent that has been used for years to treat kidney cancers, lymphoma, and melanoma. It is given IV or IM with the method and schedule of administration determined by the actual cancer type and the extent of its growth. It is usually administered daily for a specific period of days.

What are the adverse effects?

Patients receiving high IV doses of this agent are closely monitored in a hospital for adverse effects, which may include nausea; vomiting; weight gain; fluid retention; and damage to the liver, lungs, nerves, or kidneys.

What are the contraindications and interactions?

Contraindications include hypersensitivity to interferon alfa-2b or to any components of this product. Safe use during pregnancy, lactation, or in children younger than 18 years is not established.

Interferon alfa-2b should be used cautiously in severe, pre-existing cardiac, renal, or hepatic disease; pulmonary disease; and diabetes mellitus and in those prone to ketoacidosis. This agent may increase theophylline (Elixophyllin) levels, and zidovudine (Retrovir) may increase hematologic toxicity.

What are the important points patients should know?

Teach patients techniques for reconstituting and administrating these drugs. Warn them not to change brands of interferon without first consulting their physicians. Advise patients about adverse effects and when to notify their physicians about those that cause significant discomfort. Advise women not to breast-feed while taking these drugs without consulting their physicians.

Focus Point

Interferon Administration Changes

All changes in interferon administration must be directed by a physician. Patients should never change the times or doses specified for taking interferons.

✳ Apply Your Knowledge 16.3

The following questions focus on what you have just learned about biologic response modifiers.

CRITICAL THINKING

1. What are interferons?
2. What is interleukin-2?
3. What is tumor necrosis factor?
4. What are monoclonal antibodies?
5. What is the advantage of monoclonal antibodies?

PRACTICAL SCENARIO 1

A 68-year-old man has undergone adjuvant chemotherapy for completely resected colon cancer that involved several pericolonic lymph nodes at the time of his surgical resection. After a few days of experiencing diarrhea, he calls his physician. He tells his physician that he has experienced approximately five to six loose, watery stools per day over the past few days. He is mildly lightheaded when walking around.

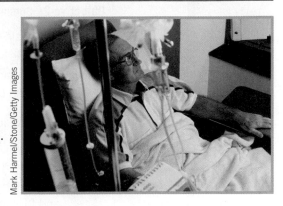
Mark Harmel/Stone/Getty Images

Critical Thinking Questions

1. What is the most likely cause of this patient's ongoing diarrhea?
2. What are the consequences of ongoing diarrhea, and why do you think the physician might instruct this patient to report to the clinic or emergency room immediately?
3. What advice on diet might you offer this patient after he has been seen by his physician?

PRACTICAL SCENARIO 2

A 38-year-old woman complained of pain in the left iliac region of her pelvis, which worsened over several months. She went to her physician, and after a laparoscopy and biopsy, it was discovered she had ovarian cancer.

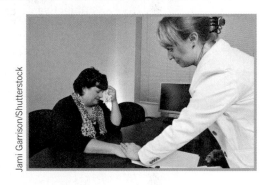
Jami Garrison/Shutterstock

Critical Thinking Questions

1. If the cancer has not metastasized, what would be the common treatments after surgical removal of the ovary?
2. If the cancer has metastasized to other sites, what would be the most appropriate treatments?

Chapter Capsule

This section repeats the objectives from the beginning of the chapter and then provides a summary of the most important concepts for the objective. Use this section as a quick review and to check your knowledge.

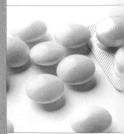

Objective 1: List the seven warning signs of cancer.

- Changes in bowel or bladder habits
- A sore that does not heal
- Unusual bleeding or discharge
- Thickening or lump in breast or elsewhere
- Indigestion or difficulty swallowing
- Obvious change in a wart or mole
- Nagging cough or hoarseness

Objective 2: Summarize the basic cell cycle and its importance in the use of antineoplastic agents.

- The basic cell cycle—G_0 (resting or dormant stage), G_1 (the first gap phase), S (DNA synthesis occurs), G_2 (the second gap phase), and M (mitosis occurs)
- Some antineoplastic agents target cancer cells in various stages of the cell cycle, which, in part, determines how and when they are used

Objective 3: List commonly used antineoplastic agents in each class.

- Alkylating agents—nitrogen mustards, ethyleneimines, alkyl sulfonates, nitrosoureas, and triazenes
- Antimetabolites—purine antagonists, adenosine antagonists, pyrimidine antagonists, and folic acid antagonists
- Mitotic inhibitors (plant alkaloids)—vincristine and vinblastine
- Hormonal therapy—estrogens, progestins, and androgens
- Antitumor antibiotics—doxorubicin, daunorubicin, idarubicin, plicamycin, bleomycin, and mitomycin
- Biologic response modifiers—interferons, interleukin-2, tumor necrosis factor, and monoclonal antibodies

Objective 4: Explain the mechanism of action of each class of antineoplastic agents.

- Alkylating agents—cell cycle phase–nonspecific; most active in resting phase; act directly on DNA, causing cross-linking of DNA strands, abnormal base pairing, or DNA strand breaks, thus preventing the cell from dividing
- Antimetabolites—cell cycle phase–specific; most effective during S-phase; replace natural substances as building blocks in DNA molecules, altering the function of enzymes required for cell metabolism and protein synthesis
- Mitotic inhibitors—act throughout cell cycle; some are most effective during S- and M-phases; inhibit DNA and RNA synthesis
- Hormonal agents—highly selective; either block hormone production or block hormone action
- Antitumor antibiotics—most inhibit DNA and RNA synthesis, causing cell death
- Biologic response modifiers—affect biologic responses to a neoplasm in beneficial ways—sometimes acting indirectly to mediate antitumor effects or directly on the tumor cells

Objective 5: Discuss how steroids, estrogen, progestins, antiestrogens, and antiandrogens work in the treatment of cancer.

- Steroids—inhibit migration of WBCs and inhibit production of products of the arachidonic acid cascade
- Estrogens—promote the release of calcitonin and enhance the availability of vitamin D3 to increase bone formation in postmenopausal patients with breast cancer
- Progestins—inhibit secretion of pituitary gonadotropins by positive feedback
- Antiestrogens—bind to estrogen receptors, preventing estrogen from binding to these receptors
- Antiandrogens—block the synthesis of endogenous testosterone

Objective 6: Explain how biologic response modifiers are created and how they work.

- Human proteins modified by recombinant DNA technology to produce agents with potent effects on the function and growth of normal and neoplastic cells
- Examples—interferon, interleukin-2, tumor necrosis factor, and monoclonal antibodies

Objective 7: Describe the advantages of using monoclonal antibodies in the treatment of cancer.

■ Monoclonal antibodies—can be used to specifically track down and purify the specific protein that induced their formation

Objective 8: Identify the common side effects of chemotherapy treatment.

■ Alkylating agents—oral mucosal ulceration and intestinal denudations, pulmonary fibrosis and venoocclusive disease in the liver, renal failure, or central neurotoxicity with seizures, coma, and at times, death; most of these agents cause hair loss; some cause nausea and vomiting; ifosfamide is the most neurotoxic of this class, producing altered mental status, coma, generalized seizures, and paralysis. All these agents have toxic effects on the reproductive system.

■ Antimetabolites—nausea, vomiting, hepatotoxicity, bone marrow depression, headache, hearing loss, sleep disorders, depression, myelosuppression, GI disturbances, hair loss, dermatitis, nail changes, skin rashes, hyperpigmentation, photosensitivity, hyperuricemia, and inflammation of the tongue. Methotrexate may cause serious adverse effects, including severe leukopenia, bone marrow aplasia, and thrombocytopenia.

■ Mitotic inhibitors (plant alkaloids)—nausea; vomiting; diarrhea; hair loss; dizziness; weakness; headache; depression; stomatitis; anemia; and hyperpigmentation of the nails, tongue, and oral mucosa

■ Hormonal therapy—GI disturbances, possible impaired fertility, menstrual irregularities

■ Antitumor antibiotics—bone marrow suppression, stomatitis, GI upset, hair loss, hyperpigmentation, skin ulceration, pulmonary fibrosis, serious renal impairment

■ Biologic response modifiers—nausea; vomiting; weight gain; fluid retention; and damage to the liver, lungs, nerves, or kidneys

Internet Sites of Interest

■ Health-care workers who are exposed to antineoplastic agents when working with patients are at risk for toxicity. See the Centers for Disease Control and Prevention (CDC) publication about occupational hazards at **http://www.cdc.gov/niosh/docs/2004-102**.

■ The Virtual Library of Biochemistry, Molecular Biology, and Cell Biology provides information on the cell cycle. Click on the Cell Cycle link at **http://www.biochemweb.org**. Many other resources are available from this website.

■ Hormone therapy for treatment of reproductive cancers is discussed on the Mayo Clinic website at: **http://www.mayoclinic.com**. Search for "reproductive cancer."

■ The American Cancer Society has a wealth of information for patients and health-care providers on its website at **http://www.cancer.org**.

myhealthprofessionskit

Go to www.myhealthprofessionskit.com to access the Companion Website created for this textbook. Simply select "Basic Health Science" from the choice of disciplines. Find this book and then log in using your username and password to access interactive learning games, assessment questions, animations, and more.

Checkpoint Review 3

Select the best answer for the following questions.

1. Vitamin requirements are measured by which of the following units?
   a. Milligrams
   b. Centigrams
   c. Micrograms
   d. a and c

2. Vitamin B_1 is also called:
   a. Riboflavin
   b. Cobalamin
   c. Thiamine
   d. Retinol

3. Which of the following is the newest COX-2 inhibitor for the treatment of osteoarthritis?
   a. Celecoxib (Celebrex)
   b. Meloxicam (Mobic)
   c. Oxycodone (Percolone)
   d. Fentanyl (Duragesic)

4. Which of the following vaccines is used for the prevention of viral infections?
   a. Q fever
   b. Pertussis
   c. Yellow fever
   d. Plague

5. Which of the following minerals acts in bone formation, impulse conduction, myocardial contractions, and the blood-clotting process?
   a. Sodium
   b. Phosphorus
   c. Iodine
   d. Calcium

6. Which of the following is the trade name of naloxone?
   a. Demerol
   b. Talwin
   c. Narcan
   d. Stadol

7. Zinc is a very important trace element for which of the following conditions?
   a. During hemoglobin synthesis and energy production
   b. During periods of rapid tissue growth
   c. Gaining too much weight
   d. Kidney failure

8. Which of the following vitamins is an antioxidant?
   a. Tocopherol (vitamin E)
   b. Cholecalciferol (vitamin D)
   c. Phylloquinone (vitamin K)
   d. Cobalamin (vitamin B_{12})

9. Patients should be instructed to drink several full glasses of water when taking which of the following antimicrobial drugs?
   a. Penicillins
   b. Sulfonamides
   c. Fluoroquinolones
   d. Aminoglycosides

10. Acetaminophen should be avoided in which of the following patients?
    a. Those taking antacids
    b. Those drinking milk
    c. Those drinking alcohol
    d. Those taking antibiotics

11. The sulfonamides block the biosynthetic pathway of which of the following?
    a. Folic acid
    b. Bacterial proteins
    c. Bacterial nucleic acid
    d. Bacterial lipids

12. The presence of food in the GI tract reduces is the absorption of many anti-infective agents including which of the following:
    a. Penicillin V
    b. Doxycycline
    c. Minocycline
    d. All of the above

13. Which of the following foods contains very high amounts of tyramine, which may interact with MAO inhibitors and cause hypertensive crises?
    a. Bananas
    b. Cottage cheese
    c. Red meat
    d. Red apples

14. Ethanol impairs absorption of which of the following vitamins?
    a. Thiamine (vitamin B_1)
    b. Cobalamin (vitamin B_{12})
    c. Ascorbic acid (vitamin C)
    d. Tocopherol (vitamin E)

15. Black "hairy" tongue (temporary overgrowth of harmless bacteria or yeast in the mouth) is a side effect of oral administration of which of the following antibacterials?

a. Tetracycline
b. Erythromycin
c. Penicillin
d. Streptomycin

16. Opioid receptors in the brain stem are responsible for the respiratory depressant effects produced by which of the following?

a. Nonopioid analgesics
b. Nonopioid antagonists
c. Opioid antagonists
d. Opioid analgesics

17. Fluoride's main function in human nutrition is to prevent:

a. Retarded physical growth
b. Formation of kidney stones
c. Dental caries
d. Wilson's disease

18. Which of the following is the major adverse effect of aminoglycosides?

a. Hepatotoxicity
b. Nephrotoxicity
c. Neurotoxicity
d. GI toxicity

19. Most of the currently used opioid analgesics act primarily at which of the following receptors?

a. Mu   b. Delta   c. Kappa   d. Gamma

20. Which of the following is the major adverse effect of meperidine?

a. Hypertensive crisis
b. Agitation
c. Hallucinations
d. Respiratory depression

21. Essential fatty acids are required for the formation of:

a. Prostaglandins
b. Insulin
c. Vitamin K
d. Enzymes

22. Aspirin appears to impede clotting by blocking which of the following?

a. Opioid receptors
b. Calcium channels
c. Prostaglandin formation
d. All of the above

23. Which of the following antibiotics may impair bone growth and discolor the teeth in children?

a. Macrolides
b. Aminoglycosides
c. Sulfonamides
d. Tetracyclines

24. Talwin is the trade name of:

a. Meperidine
b. Pentazocine
c. Fentanyl
d. Naloxone

25. Patients should notify their physicians if blood appears in their stools, vomitus, or urine if they are taking:

a. Indomethacin
b. Antacids
c. Acetaminophen
d. Benzodiazepines

26. All the following infections may be transmitted by mosquitoes except:

a. West Nile virus
b. Malaria
c. Rabies
d. Encephalitis

27. Which of the following antibiotics is in the class of macrolides?

a. Erythromycin
b. Ciprofloxacin
c. Doxycycline
d. Rifampin

28. Which of the following is the most common adverse effect of vaccinations?

a. Convulsions
b. Liver impairment
c. Malaise
d. Allergic reaction

29. A booster dose of adult diphtheria and tetanus toxoid is recommended every:

a. 2 years
b. 5 years
c. 10 years
d. Not required

30. Ganciclovir is used for the prophylaxis and systemic treatment of which of the following infections?

a. Respiratory syncytial virus
b. Hepatitis C virus
c. Advanced HIV
d. Cytomegalovirus

31. Which of the following was the leading cause of invasive bacterial disease (meningitis) among children until pediatric immunization was introduced in 1988?
    a. Measles
    b. Polio
    c. *Haemophilus influenzae* type b
    d. Varicella

32. Which of the following is the trade name for doxycycline?
    a. Minocin
    b. Vibramycin
    c. Terramycin
    d. Aureomycin

33. Which of the following vaccines may be given at birth?
    a. Varicella (chicken pox)
    b. Rubella (German measles)
    c. Hepatitis B
    d. Influenza

34. Which of the following agents may cause a reddish-orange discoloration of body fluids, including tears, urine, and saliva?
    a. Isoniazid
    b. Chloramphenicol
    c. Spectinomycin
    d. Rifampin

35. Amantadine is used to prevent or treat symptoms of:
    a. Mumps
    b. Influenza A
    c. Hepatitis A
    d. Hepatitis C

36. Which of the following vaccines is recommended every year for those at a high risk for complications?
    a. Influenza
    b. Meningococcal
    c. Typhoid
    d. Cholera

37. Meningococcal polysaccharide vaccine must be administered via which of the following routes?
    a. Subcutaneously
    b. Intramuscularly
    c. Intravenously
    d. Inhalation

38. The second-most common cause of death in the United States is:
    a. Cardiovascular disease
    b. Car accidents
    c. Cancer
    d. Infectious diseases

39. The ability of chemotherapy to kill cancer cells depends on which of the following factors?
    a. Its ability to destroy specific tissues
    b. Its ability to stop cell division
    c. Its ability to cause necrosis of tissues
    d. All of the above

40. Which of the following vaccines is recommended only in extremely high-risk individuals in whom other controls are impractical?
    a. Q fever
    b. Rabies
    c. Tuberculosis
    d. Typhoid

41. DNA synthesis occurs in which of the following phases of the cell cycle?
    a. G_0 b. G_1 c. S   d. M

42. Chemotherapy agents may be administered by which of the following routes?
    a. Intramuscularly
    b. Orally
    c. Subcutaneously
    d. All of the above

43. Which of the following vaccines is recommended between 12 and 15 months of age?
    a. Hepatitis B
    b. *Haemophilus influenzae* b
    c. Diphtheria, tetanus, pertussis
    d. Measles, mumps, rubella

44. Which of the following is an example of antimetabolites?
    a. Nitrogen mustards
    b. Ethyleneimines
    c. Adriamycin
    d. Fluorouracil

45. Which of the following antitumor antibiotics is the first-line treatment for advanced HIV-associated Kaposi's sarcoma?
    a. Doxorubicin (Adriamycin)
    b. Daunorubicin (Cerubidine)
    c. Idarubicin (Idamycin)
    d. Plicamycin (Mithracin)

46. Interferons are a group of blood proteins that have which of the following effects?
    a. Antiviral
    b. Antiprotozoal
    c. Antibiotic
    d. None of the above

47. Acyclovir is used to treat all the following except:
    a. Chicken pox
    b. Hepatitis B
    c. Herpes zoster (shingles)
    d. Herpes simplex encephalitis

48. Which of the following is the major adverse effect of didanosine (antiviral drug)?
    a. Hepatitis and heart failure
    b. Peripheral neuropathies and pancreatitis
    c. Nephritis and pulmonary edema
    d. Ototoxicity and glaucoma

For questions 49–53, match the lettered drug to the numbered description.

DESCRIPTION

_____ 49. Used for the relief of nonproductive cough and for moderate to severe pain

_____ 50. Related to its inhibition of prostaglandin

_____ 51. Used for the treatment of osteoarthritis and rheumatoid arthritis in adults

_____ 52. Has caused liver damage in patients who consume three or more alcoholic drinks per day

_____ 53. Used for narcotic overdose

TERM

a. celecoxib
b. naloxone
c. acetaminophen
d. ibuprofen
e. hydrocodone

For questions 54–58, match the lettered term to the numbered description.

DESCRIPTION

_____ 54. A fungal is also called this

_____ 55. A common opportunistic infection (candidiasis) is also known as this

_____ 56. Caused by *Plasmodium vivax*

_____ 57. Responsible for causing dysentery

_____ 58. Caused by the flagellated protozoan lamblia

TERM

a. *Entamoeba histolytica*
b. Giardiasis
c. Moniliasis
d. Malaria
e. Mycosis

Select terms from your reading to fill in the blanks.

59. _____ is prescribed for asymptomatic and symptomatic trichomoniasis in females and males.

60. Iodoquinol is an anti-infective, antiamebicide, and _____ agent.

61. Substances produced by microorganisms that, in low concentrations, are able to inhibit or kill other microorganisms are called _____.

62. The most common sources of natural antibiotics are molds and _____.

63. Systemic antibacterial agents that are able to kill microbes are called _____.

64. Today, sulfamethoxazole is the most commonly used sulfonamide and is usually combined with trimethoprim and abbreviated _____.

65. The cephalosporins are a group of antibiotics closely related to the _____.

66. First-generation cephalosporins have their highest activity against _____ bacteria.

67. The serious adverse effects of aminoglycosides include ototoxicity and _____.

68. Macronutrients are needed by the body in relatively _____ _____ and constitute the bulk of the diet.

69. The daily requirement for carbohydrates is _____% to _____% of one's total caloric intake.

70. Deficiency of thiamine (vitamin B_1) leads to a disease called _____.

71. Pyridoxine (vitamin B_6) is prescribed to treat _____ during pregnancy.

72. _____ is the ability to resist infection and disease through the activation of specific defenses.

73. Active immunity is a form of acquired immunity that develops in an individual in response to an _____.

74. Immune globulin is produced by _____.

75. The treatment of patients with diphtheria requires a specific _____.

Unit 4

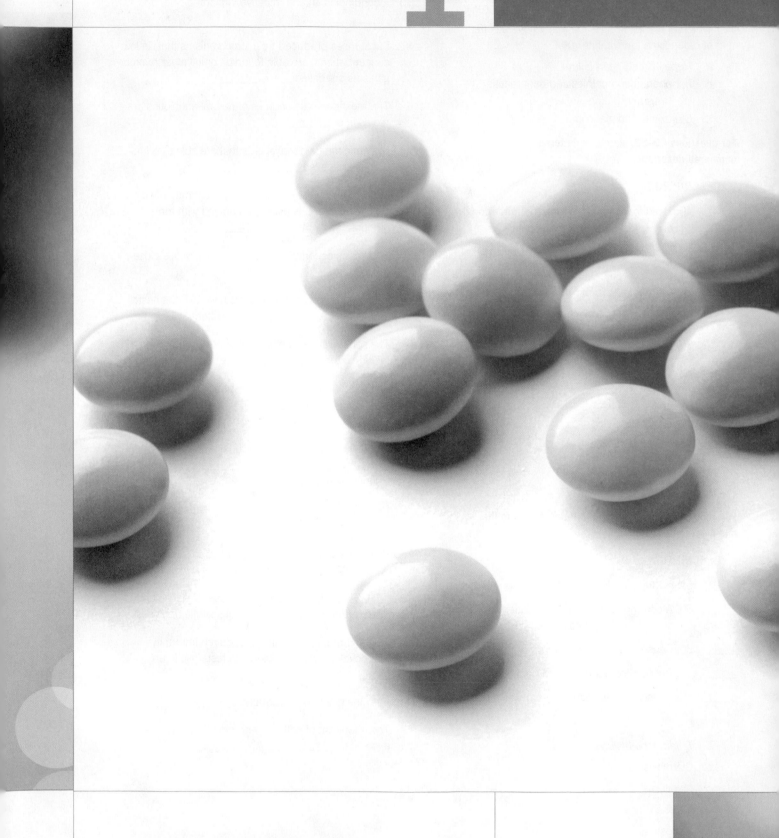

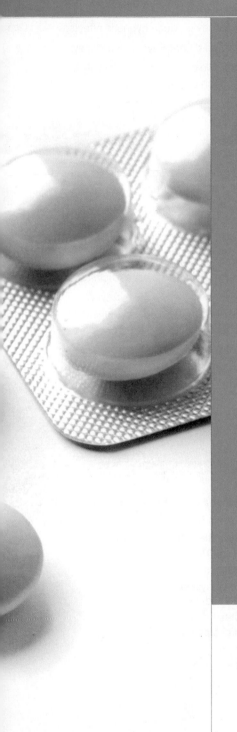

DRUG EFFECTS ON SPECIFIC SYSTEMS

" The nervous and endocrine systems involve high-level integration in the brain and have the ability to influence processes in distant regions of the body and to extensively use negative feedback. "

Chapter 17

Drugs Used to Treat Central Nervous System Conditions

Chapter Objectives

After completing this chapter, you should be able to:

1. Describe the four major parts of the brain.

2. Name three benzodiazepine hypnotic drugs and explain the mechanism by which they produce hypnotic effects.

3. List three different types of epilepsy.

4. Name two drugs used specifically to treat each type of epilepsy.

5. Describe the mechanisms of action of drugs that increase dopamine or decrease acetylcholine levels in the basal ganglia.

6. Describe five adverse effects associated with antianxiety drugs.

7. Describe the common adverse effects and the specific neurologic conditions caused by antipsychotic drugs.

8. Explain the use of lithium in mania and the adverse effects associated with its use.

9. Describe the main adverse effects of antipsychotic drugs.

10. Identify three of the most common types of drugs used to treat patients with depression.

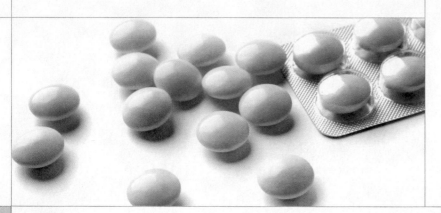

Key Terms

Introduction

Thinking, remembering, feeling, moving, and being aware of the world require activity from the nervous system. The human brain has about 100 billion **neurons** (or nerve cells) that help to coordinate all other body functions to maintain homeostasis and to enable the body to respond to changing conditions. The neurons release chemical substances called neurotransmitters that allow communication from one nerve cell to another. The most common neurotransmitters are acetylcholine, norepinephrine, dopamine, serotonin, gamma-aminobutyric acid (GABA), and glutamate. Some mental disorders or conditions are associated with abnormal changes in the activity or amount of a specific neurotransmitter.

The Nervous System

The organs of the nervous system can be divided into two groups. One group, consisting of the brain and spinal cord, forms the **central nervous system** (CNS). The other group, composed of the nerves (peripheral nerves) that connect the central nervous system to other body parts, is called the **peripheral nervous system** (PNS). Together, these systems provide three general functions: sensory, integrative, and motor (see Figure 17-1 ■).

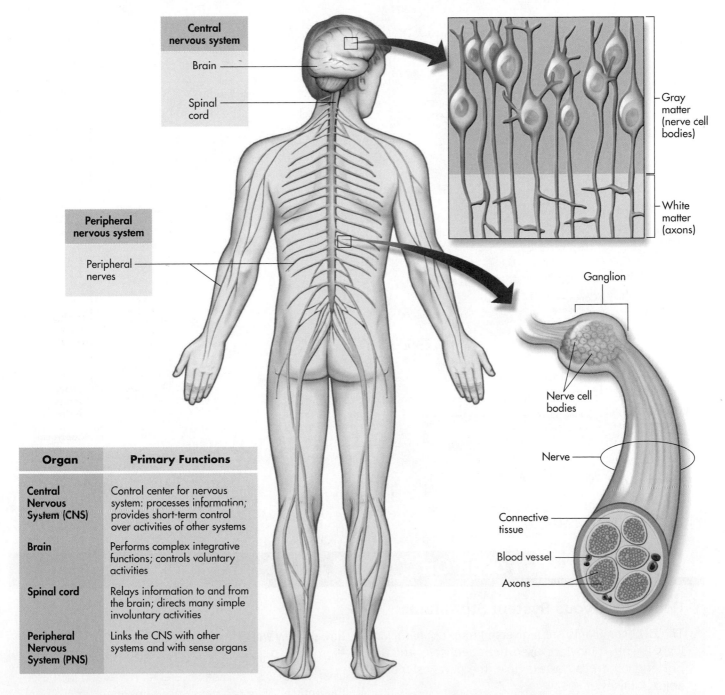

Organ	Primary Functions
Central Nervous System (CNS)	Control center for nervous system: processes information; provides short-term control over activities of other systems
Brain	Performs complex integrative functions; controls voluntary activities
Spinal cord	Relays information to and from the brain; directs many simple involuntary activities
Peripheral Nervous System (PNS)	Links the CNS with other systems and with sense organs

Figure 17-1 ■ The central nervous system (CNS) includes the brain and spinal cord. The peripheral nervous system includes the nerves throughout the body that exit from the spinal cord.

The brain can be divided into four major portions—the cerebrum, diencephalon, brain stem, and cerebellum. The **cerebrum** (the largest part of the brain) includes nerve centers associated with sensory and motor functions and provides higher mental functions, including memory and reasoning. The cerebrum is composed of an outer cerebral cortex and inner cerebral medulla. In the medulla, there is a group of cell bodies (gray matter) known as the **basal ganglia**. The basal ganglia are involved in the regulation of motor activity. Degeneration of certain neurons within the basal ganglia is responsible for Parkinson's disease. The *diencephalon* also processes sensory information. Nerve pathways in the brain stem connect various parts of the nervous system and regulate certain visceral activities. The cerebellum includes centers that coordinate voluntary muscular movements.

The spinal cord is a slender nerve column that passes downward from the brain into the vertebral canal, continuing on to the peripheral organs and skeletal muscle, carrying motor impulses. Nerve axons travel from the peripheral parts of the body, such as the skin, muscles, and visceral organs, to the brain, carrying sensory information (see Figure 17-2 ■).

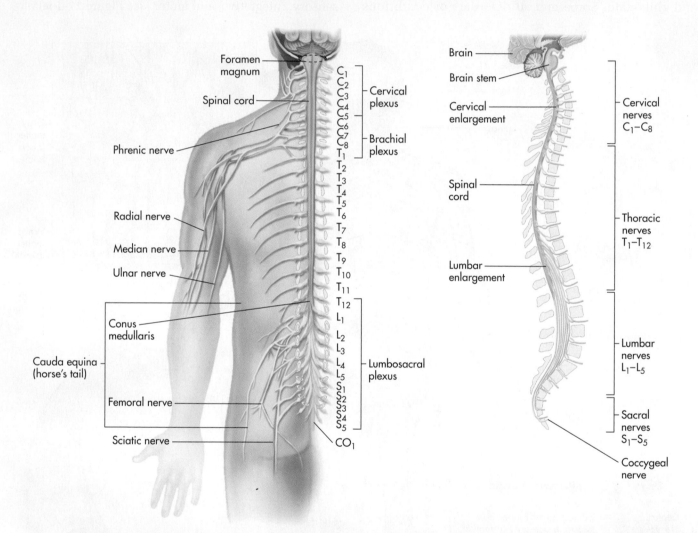

Figure 17-2 ■ The spinal cord.

Focus On

Central Nervous System Stimulants

The CNS stimulants are a diverse group of pharmacologic agents. Many are used therapeutically and are prescription drugs (for example, the psychostimulant amphetamines).

How do they work?

The exact mechanism of action of CNS stimulants is not clear, but they stimulate the cerebral cortex and increase the activity of norepinephrine, dopamine, and other catecholamines at CNS **synapses** (the point of contact between nerve cells with each other or other types of cells). This increased activity can lead to many effects, including euphoria, reduced appetite, insomnia, and wakefulness.

How are they used?

The indirect-acting sympathomimetics (for example, methylphenidate [Ritalin] and the amphetamines) are more potent CNS stimulants than caffeine but have limited therapeutic use. They are used in the treatment of attention deficit hyperactivity disorder (ADHD), narcolepsy, and obesity. However, because these CNS stimulants convey a sense of self-confidence, well-being, and euphoria, they are highly addictive. Some of these agents are widely abused (such as amphetamines and especially methamphetamine).

What are the adverse effects?

The most common adverse effects include headache, palpitations, cardiac dysrhythmias, hypertension, nervousness, and nausea.

What are the contraindications and interactions?

CNS stimulants are contraindicated in persons who are hypersensitive to sympathomimetic amines; have a history of drug abuse; are severely agitated; have hyperthyroidism, diabetes mellitus, moderate to severe hypertension, advanced arteriosclerosis, angina pectoris, or other cardiovascular disorders; or have glaucoma. Safety during pregnancy and lactation is not established. These agents should be used cautiously in those with mild hypertension. Acetazolamide (Diamox) and sodium bicarbonate decrease amphetamine elimination; ammonium chloride and ascorbic acid (Ascorbicap) increase amphetamine elimination.

What are the important points patients should know?

Advise patients that when taking CNS stimulants for a prolonged period, withdrawal symptoms could occur. A gradual decrease is essential to prevent withdrawal effects.

Focus on Pediatrics

The Need for Counseling in Attention Deficit Hyperactivity Disorder

Families of children with ADHD should be encouraged to seek counseling for support and reassurance. Drug treatment alone is an insufficient form of therapy.

Anxiety and Insomnia

Anxiety is a very common disorder. In many cases, anxiety is self-limiting, and recourse to medications is not necessary. Occasionally, however, anxiety is so stressful and mentally painful that drug therapy is required. Anxiety and stress are part of everyday life, and it is important that education programs include life skills that help people develop coping mechanisms. Furthermore, anxiety may be accompanied by mild reactive or even endogenous depression.

Sleep and its importance for normal living is a process that is still little understood. Sleep disturbances are extremely common, and if continuous, they have the potential to seriously disrupt normal day-to-day living. Many people with sleep disorders want to turn to drugs to solve their problem.

Sedatives and Hypnotics

A sedative diminishes the activity of the CNS. This effect on the CNS can, in many circumstances, relieve anxiety, which is why sedatives are often referred to as *anxiolytics. Hypnotic* is the term used to describe a substance that induces sleep. Many of the drugs in these categories are addictive if taken regularly for even short periods. In some cases, addiction has been known to occur in about 10 days. Thus, the use of these drugs is controversial. If prescribed, they should be taken for only limited periods (no more than 7 days under normal circumstances).

The use of hypnotics in the treatment of short-term insomnia is often beneficial in cases in which the insomnia can be predicted. There are least two stages of sleep: the first called *rapid eye movement (REM)*, which is the dreaming stage, and the second is *non-REM* stage. It seems that many hypnotics upset the REM stage of sleep.

The difference between most hypnotics and anxiolytics is the dosage, not the drug. Therefore, the drugs are dealt with according to their chemical classification and not their therapeutic classification except when there is no overlap.

Focus Point

Sleep with Hypnotics

It is important to remember that no currently available hypnotics induce what could be termed "natural sleep."

Focus On

Benzodiazepines

Benzodiazepines may be used as sedatives or hypnotics. However, it is wise to attempt treatment options with less addictive potential before using a benzodiazepine for this purpose. Table 17-1 ■ shows some of the most commonly prescribed benzodiazepines.

How do they work?

The mechanism of action of benzodiazepines on the CNS appears to be closely related to their ability to increase the action of the neurotransmitter GABA.

How are they used?

Indications for the use of benzodiazepines include generalized anxiety disorders, panic disorders, insomnia, myoclonic and **absence seizures** (brief seizures characterized by arrest of activity and occasional muscle contractions and relaxations), status epilepticus, and muscle relaxation. In **seizures** (abnormal electrical activity in the brain), injectable forms of diazepam (Valium) and lorazepam (Ativan) are commonly used initially to stop the repetitive seizure activity and then long-acting drugs, such as phenytoin (Dilantin), are given to prevent the recurrence of seizures.

What are the adverse effects?

The adverse effects of the benzodiazepines include drowsiness, **ataxia** (an inability to coordinate muscle activity), impaired judgment, rebound insomnia, and the development of tolerance. Overdosage may result in CNS and respiratory depression as well as hypotension and coma. Gradual withdrawal of these drugs is recommended. Sudden withdrawal of benzodiazepines may cause such serious problems as seizures, severe anxiety, sensory disturbances, schizophrenia, and suicidal thoughts.

What are the contraindications and interactions?

If taken during pregnancy, benzodiazepines are likely to cause fetal abnormalities, and flurazepam (Dalmane) is entirely contraindicated during pregnancy. Benzodiazepines are also contraindicated in individuals with severe liver and kidney disorders and in children who are hyperactive.

Benzodiazepines increase CNS depression with alcohol and omeprazole (Prilosec). They also increase pharmacologic effects if combined with cimetidine (Tagamet), disulfiram (Antabuse), or hormonal contraceptives. The effects of benzodiazepines decrease with theophylline (Bronkodyl) and ranitidine (Zantac).

What are the important points patients should know?

Instruct patients about methods, such as relaxation, they can use to decrease anxiety. Advise patients not to stop the medication abruptly after prolonged use because withdrawal symptoms may occur. Warn patients not to drink alcohol or take other CNS depressants while taking hypnotics or anxiolytics.

Instruct patients about methods to assist with sleep, such as avoiding coffee, heavy meals, and excessive stimuli close to bedtime. Caution them against driving or operating machinery because dizziness or drowsiness might occur.

Table 17-1 ■ Commonly Used Benzodiazepines

GENERIC NAME	TRADE NAME	AVERAGE ADULT DOSAGE	ROUTE OF ADMINISTRATION
alprazolam	Xanax	0.25–0.5 mg tid up to 4 mg/d in divided doses	PO
chlordiazepoxide	Librium	5–25 mg tid–qid	PO
		25–100 mg; then 25–50 mg tid–qid PRN	IM, IV
clorazepate	Tranxene	7.5–60 mg in divided doses tid	PO
diazepam	Valium	2–10 mg bid–qid	PO
		2–20 mg; may be repeated in 1–4 h PRN	IM, IV
		0.2 mg/kg only once q5d	Rectal
estazolam	ProSom	1–2 mg at bedtime	PO
flurazepam	Dalmane	30 mg at bedtime; 15 mg may suffice	PO
halazepam	Paxipam	20–40 mg tid–qid	PO
lorazepam	Ativan	1–10 mg/d in divided doses, with largest dose at bedtime	PO
		0.05–4 mg/kg	IM
		0.004 mg/kg but no greater than 2 mg/kg total	IV
midazolam	Versed	0.07–0.08 mg/kg 30–60 min before procedure	IM
		1–1.5 mg; may repeat in 2 min PRN	IV
oxazepam	Serax	10–30 mg tid–qid	PO
quazepam	Doral	7.5–15 mg until desired response is seen	PO
temazepam	Restoril	15–30 mg at bedtime	PO
triazolam	Halcion	0.125–0.5 mg at bedtime	PO

IM, intramuscular; IV, intravenous; PO, oral; PRN, as needed; qid, four times a day; tid, three times a day.

Focus Point

Oral Contraceptives and Benzodiazepines

Women who are taking benzodiazepines should not use oral contraceptives because the drug combination may cause increased sedative effects, and high levels of the benzodiazepine may accumulate in the blood plasma.

Focus on Geriatrics

Diazepam

Elderly patients usually require lower dosages of diazepam to decrease ataxia and avoid oversedation. Apnea and cardiac arrest may occur when diazepam is given to elderly patients, very ill people, and individuals with limited pulmonary reserve.

Focus On

Barbiturates

Barbiturates are classified as CNS agents, anticonvulsants, and sedative–hypnotic drugs.

How do they work?

The sedative and hypnotic effects of barbiturates, such as phenobarbital (Luminal), appear to be primarily attributable to interference with impulse transmission of the cerebral cortex by the inhibition of the reticular activating system (a part of the brain that appears to control sleep and wakefulness). CNS depression may range from mild sedation to coma depending on the dosage, route of administration, degree of nervous system excitability, and drug tolerance. Initially, barbiturates suppress REM sleep, but with chronic therapy, REM sleep returns to normal. In seizure disorders, phenobarbital limits the spread of seizure activity by increasing the threshold for motor cortex stimuli. Barbiturates are habit forming.

How are they used?

Barbiturates are primarily used to treat insomnia, although they are also used for partial **epilepsy** (brain dysfunction that is caused by excessive discharge of neurons) and tonic–clonic seizures.

What are the adverse effects?

The most common adverse effect associated with barbiturates is sedation, which can range from mild sleepiness or drowsiness to somnolence. The barbiturate phenobarbital may also cause nausea, vomiting, constipation or diarrhea, bradycardia, skin rash, fever, and headache. The toxic effects of barbiturates include respiratory depression, circulatory shock, and renal or hepatic damage.

What are the contraindications and interactions?

Barbiturates are contraindicated in anyone with a familial history of **porphyria** (a genetic disorder caused by deficiency of enzymes of the heme biosynthetic pathway) and in cases of severe respiratory or kidney disease. They should be avoided in patients with a history of previous addiction to sedative–hypnotics or uncontrolled pain and in women who are pregnant or lactating. Alcohol may interact with barbiturates because of these agents' similar CNS depressant qualities. The barbiturate phenobarbital may decrease absorption and increase metabolism of oral anticoagulants and may also increase metabolism of corticosteroids and oral contraceptives.

What are the important points patients should know?

Instruct patients about methods, such as relaxation, they can use to decrease anxiety. Advise patients not to stop the medication abruptly after prolonged use because withdrawal symptoms may occur. Warn patients not to drink alcohol or take other CNS depressants while taking hypnotics or anxiolytics.

Instruct patients about methods to assist with sleep, such as avoiding coffee, heavy meals, and excessive stimuli close to bedtime. Caution them against driving and operating machinery because dizziness or drowsiness might occur.

✱ Apply Your Knowledge 17.1

The following questions focus on what you have just learned about the nervous system, CNS stimulants, and sedatives and hypnotics.

CRITICAL THINKING

1. What are the four major portions of the brain?
2. What disorders will be the result of degeneration of the basal ganglia?
3. What are the two major functions of the brain?
4. What is the mechanism of action of CNS stimulants?
5. What are the differences between sedatives and hypnotics?
6. What are the significant adverse effects of overdosage of benzodiazepines?
7. What are the trade names of oxazepam, midazolam, diazepam, and alprazolam?
8. What are the contraindications of barbiturates?

CHAPTER SEVENTEEN Drugs Used to Treat Central Nervous System Conditions ✳ **289**

Epilepsy

The terms **convulsion** (violent spasms) and *seizure* are often used interchangeably and basically have the same meaning. A seizure is a periodic attack of disturbed cerebral function. A seizure may also be defined as an abnormal disturbance in the electrical activity in one or more areas of the brain.

Seizures may be classified as generalized **tonic–clonic** (contraction–relaxation) seizures (previously termed *grand mal*); generalized absence seizures (previously called *petit mal*); generalized myoclonic seizures; and partial seizures. Status epilepticus is an emergency condition that may result in brain injury or death if not treated immediately.

Epilepsy is a permanent, recurrent seizure disorder. Examples of the known causes of epilepsy include brain injury at birth, head injuries, and inborn errors of metabolism. In some patients, the cause of epilepsy is never determined.

Antiseizure Drugs (Anticonvulsants)

The categorizations of antiseizure drugs that follow are based on chemical structure and mechanism of action. Chemical groupings include the hydantoins, succinimides, benzodiazepines, and barbiturates.

In addition, several miscellaneous drugs are used as anticonvulsants, such as carbamazepine (Tegretol), valproic acid or valproate (Depakote), primidone (Mysoline), gabapentin (Neurontin), and lamotrigine (Lamictal). All can depress abnormal neural discharges in the CNS, resulting in an inhibition of seizure activity. Drugs that control generalized tonic–clonic seizures are not effective for absence seizures. If both conditions are present, then combined drug therapy is required. Table 17-2 ■ lists the most commonly used antiseizure medications.

Table 17-2 ■ **Most Commonly Prescribed Antiseizure Drugs**

GENERIC NAME	TRADE NAME	AVERAGE ADULT DOSAGE	ROUTE OF ADMINISTRATION
Hydantoins			
fosphenytoin	Cerebyx	Individualized	IM, IV
phenytoin	Dilantin	50–200 mg bid–tid	PO
Succinimides			
ethosuximide	Zarontin	500 mg/d	PO
methsuximide	Celontin	300–1,200 mg/d	PO
phensuximide	Milontin	1–3 g/d in divided doses	PO
Benzodiazepines			
diazepam	Valium	5–10 mg; repeat if needed at 10- to 15-min intervals to 30 mg and then repeat if needed q2–4h	IM, IV
lorazepam	Ativan	4 mg injected slowly at 2 mg/min; may repeat once after 10 min	IV
Barbiturates			
mephobarbital	Mebaral	400–600 mg/d in divided doses	PO
phenobarbital	Barbital	Anticonvulsant: 100–300 mg/d	PO
		Anticonvulsant: 200–600 mg up to 20 mg/kg	IM, IV
		Status epilepticus: 15–18 mg/kg in single or divided doses (maximum, 20 mg/kg)	IV

(continued)

Table 17-2 ■ **Most Commonly Prescribed Antiseizure Drugs** (*continued*)

GENERIC NAME	TRADE NAME	AVERAGE ADULT DOSAGE	ROUTE OF ADMINISTRATION
Miscellaneous Antiseizure Drugs			
carbamazepine	Tegretol	100–400 mg tid	PO
gabapentin	Neurontin	100–800 mg tid–qid	PO
lamotrigine	Lamictal	500 mg bid (maintenance) Starting dosage depends on patient weight and other variables	PO
levetiracetam	Keppra	500 mg bid	PO
pregabalin	Lyrica	100 mg tid based on creatinine clearance	PO
primidone	Mysoline	250 mg–2 g in divided doses	PO
topiramate	Topamax	200–400 mg/day in two divided doses	PO
valproate	Depakote	125–250 mg tid–qid	PO
valproic acid	Depakene	100–200 mg bid–tid	PO

bid, twice a day; IM, intramuscular; IV, intravenous; PO, oral; tid, three times a day.

Focus on Natural Products

Drug Interactions with Kava

The dried, crushed roots and rhizome of the kava plant, an Australasian shrubby pepper found in abundance on the islands of the South Pacific, are often used as an antiepileptic and dietary supplement to reduce stress and anxiety. Kava is available in many different oral forms, such as teas, cold drink powders, and paste. It should not be used in patients who have Parkinson's disease, and concurrent use with carbidopa and levodopa is contraindicated. Antipsychotics taken with kava may result in neuroleptic movement disorders. Barbiturates, benzodiazepines, and CNS depressants in general may cause increased sedation when taken with kava.

Focus On

Phenytoin

The most commonly used and recognizable drug in this group is phenytoin (Dilantin), which was first synthesized in 1908. It is the sole clinical representative of the hydantoins in use as an antiseizure drug.

How does it work?

Phenytoin is a hydantoin derivative chemically related to phenobarbital (Luminal). The precise mechanism of anticonvulsant action is not known, but use of this drug is accompanied by reduced voltage, frequency, and spread of electrical discharges within the motor cortex.

How is it used?

Phenytoin is approved by the U.S. Food and Drug Administration (FDA) for partial seizures with complex symptomatology and tonic–clonic seizures, psychomotor, and nonepileptic seizures, such as those caused by head trauma. It is also used to prevent or treat seizures occurring during or after neurosurgery. Phenytoin is prescribed as an antiarrhythmic agent, especially in the treatment of digitalis-induced arrhythmias.

What are the adverse effects?

Phenytoin may cause blurred vision, dizziness, drowsiness, fatigue, thrombocytopenia, and aplastic anemias. Patients should be advised to use caution when driving or operating machinery and performing tasks that require mental alertness. Serum levels above the optimal range may produce confusion, delirium, or psychosis. Dose adjustments may be necessary in patients with renal disease. Chronic use may cause gingival hyperplasia.

What are the contraindications and interactions?

Phenytoin is contraindicated in patients who are hypersensitive to the drug. It must be avoided in patients with seizures caused by hypoglycemia, sinus bradycardia, and complete or incomplete heart block and in pregnant and lactating patients.

There are numerous drug–drug interactions with phenytoin, including antacids, antidiabetic agents, **antipsychotics** (*neuroleptic* drugs that can improve thought disorders), anxiolytics, barbiturates, calcium channel blockers, cardiac glycosides, corticosteroids, estrogens, neuromuscular-blocking agents, opiate agonists, oral contraceptives, progestins, salicylates, sulfonamides, thyroid hormones, tricyclic antidepressants (TCAs), vinca alkaloids, and vitamin D analogues. Phenytoin should be used cautiously in patients with impaired liver or kidney function, alcoholism, blood disorders, and hypotension.

What are the important points patients should know?

Advise patients taking phenytoin that their urine might become discolored to a pink or red-brown color. This discoloration is harmless. For patients with diabetes who are taking phenytoin, advise them that their blood glucose level should be checked more closely because phenytoin can inhibit insulin release. Also, advise patients about the importance of oral hygiene and regular dental checkups to prevent gingivitis and gingival hyperplasia.

Focus on Geriatrics

Phenytoin

Phenytoin should be used cautiously and at lower doses in elderly patients to avoid toxicity.

Focus On

Valproic Acid

Valproic acid (Depakote) is used to treat patients with simple and complex absence seizures. It has been used for other generalized seizures, including primary generalized tonic–clonic, atypical absence, myoclonic, and atonic seizures.

How does it work?

The mechanism of action of valproic acid is unknown. It may be related to the increased bioavailability of the inhibitor neurotransmitter GABA to brain neurons.

How is it used?

Valproic acid is used alone or with other anticonvulsants in the management of absence and mixed seizures and mania and in migraine headache prophylaxis. It is the drug of choice for symptomatic and idiopathic generalized seizures, juvenile myoclonic epilepsy, and childhood absence seizures.

What are the adverse effects?

Adverse effects of valproic acid include nausea, vomiting, hypersalivation, abdominal cramps, liver failure, and cases of life-threatening pancreatitis. Sedation and drowsiness are the most frequently reported adverse effects. There are considerable hematologic effects, and because valproic acid inhibits the secondary phase of platelet aggregation, it may prolong bleeding time.

What are the contraindications and interactions?

Safe use of valproic acid during pregnancy has not been established. Patients taking valproic acid may develop clotting abnormalities. Additive CNS depression may

(*Continued*)

Focus On (Continued)

occur when valproic acid is administered with other CNS depressants. Valproic acid may potentiate the effects of monoamine oxidase inhibitors (MAOIs) and other antidepressant drugs. This drug may alter some laboratory tests, such as thyroid function and urinary ketones. Alcohol and other CNS depressants potentiate its depressant effects. Haloperidol (Haldol), loxapine (Loxitane), maprotiline (Maprotiline HCl), phenothiazines, and TCAs can increase CNS depression or lower seizure thresholds. Aspirin and warfarin (Coumadin) increase the risk of spontaneous bleeding and decrease clotting.

Cimetidine (Tagamet) may increase valproic acid levels and toxicity.

What are the important points patients should know?

Valproic acid may irritate the mouth, throat, and stomach, so if patients are taking the capsule form, instruct them to swallow the capsules whole and not chew, crush, or break them. The syrup form of valproic acid may be added to foods or liquids for a better taste. It is advisable to take valproic acid with meals or snacks to reduce stomach upset.

Ethosuximide

Succinimides are anticonvulsant agents. There is only one member of this group still used in clinical practice: ethosuximide (Zarontin). Ethosuximide is the drug of choice for control of uncomplicated absence seizures. It is generally considered to be the safest of the succinimide drugs. The FDA approved ethosuximide in 1960 as a succinimide-derived anticonvulsant.

How does it work?

Ethosuximide acts to stabilize neuronal excitability, thereby raising the threshold of uncontrolled cerebral discharges (especially within the motor cortex). It does this by delaying the entry of calcium into neuron cells by blocking calcium channels. It suppresses the electroencephalogram pattern associated with lapses of consciousness in absence seizures. Its actual mechanism of action is not understood, but it may act to inhibit neuronal systems.

How is it used?

Ethosuximide is used to manage absence seizures in adults and children older than 6 years of age, myoclonic seizures, and akinetic epilepsy. This agent may be administered with other anticonvulsants when other forms of epilepsy coexist with absence seizures. It is the drug of choice for absence seizures during pregnancy because it is much less teratogenic than other drugs in this category.

What are the adverse effects?

Common adverse effects of ethosuximide include drowsiness, hiccups, ataxia, dizziness, headache, euphoria, restlessness, anxiety, blurred vision, and aggressiveness. Pancytopenia (abnormal reduction in red and white blood cells and platelets), nausea, vomiting, anorexia, abdominal pain, weight loss, diarrhea, and gingival hyperplasia are also seen. Vaginal bleeding, agranulocytosis (depression of granulocyte-producing bone marrow), aplastic anemia, alopecia (hair loss), and muscle weakness have been associated with ethosuximide therapy. Abnormal liver and kidney function test results are sometimes seen.

What are the contraindications and interactions?

Contraindications include hypersensitivity to succinimides and severe liver or kidney disease. Safety during pregnancy, lactation, and in children younger than 3 years has not been established. Ethosuximide decreases the serum levels of primidone (Mysoline). Carbamazepine (Tegretol) decreases ethosuximide levels, and isoniazid (Nydrazid, Laniazid) significantly increases ethosuximide levels.

What are the important points patients should know?

Advise patients about the possibility of blood disorders, and instruct them to report any signs of a sore throat, fever, or bruising of unknown cause to their physician. Warn them against driving or working with heavy machinery because of the adverse effects of succinimides.

Carbamazepine

Carbamazepine (Tegretol) is an oral anticonvulsant drug similar to TCAs. It is used to treat partial seizures—simple and complex—and for tonic–clonic seizures. It is the drug of choice in symptomatic partial seizures. This drug is preferred over phenobarbital because it has fewer adverse effects on behavior and alertness. Carbamazepine is also the drug of choice for the treatment of neuralgias, particularly trigeminal neuralgia (intense pain in the lips, eyes, nose, scalp, forehead, and upper or lower jaw).

How does it work?

Carbamazepine promotes sodium **efflux** (the process of flowing out) across the nerve membranes. As a consequence, carbamazepine reduces neuronal excitability, especially repeated firing of the same neuron. Unlike phenytoin, carbamazepine leaves the motor cortex relatively unaffected.

How is it used?

FDA-approved uses are for partial seizures, tonic–clonic seizures, and trigeminal neuralgia. However, this drug is often used to treat many other disorders, such as depression and bipolar disorder.

What are the adverse effects?

Severe cardiovascular disturbances, blood disorders, altered urination, and liver or kidney dysfunctions are adverse effects of carbamazepine in addition to those generally associated with antiseizure drugs. Elderly patients may be more susceptible to confusion or agitation. Carbamazepine commonly causes blurred vision, dizziness, drowsiness, and fatigue.

What are the contraindications and interactions?

Absolute contraindications for use of carbamazepine are hypersensitivity and cardiac or liver impairment. It should be used with extreme caution in pregnant women because it crosses the placenta and has been implicated in a number of fetal abnormalities.

Drug interactions occur with antineoplastic agents, antiretroviral protease inhibitors, barbiturates, calcium channel blockers, corticosteroids, MAOIs, neuromuscular blockers, opiate agonists, oral contraceptives, progestins, estrogens, halogenated anesthetics, thyroid hormones, and TCAs.

What are the important points patients should know?

Inform patients about the possibility of blood disorders. Advise them to report any signs of a sore throat, mucosal ulceration, petechiae (minute hemorrhagic spots in the skin), or bruising of unknown cause.

✳ Apply Your Knowledge 17.2

The following questions focus on what you have just learned about antiseizure medications.

CRITICAL THINKING

1. What are the classifications of seizures?
2. What are the causes of epilepsy?
3. What are the most commonly prescribed antiseizure drugs?
4. What are the trade names of ethosuximide, phenytoin, valproic acid, and carbamazepine?
5. What are the indications of phenytoin?
6. What are the indications of valproic acid?
7. What is the drug of choice for the control of uncomplicated absence seizures?
8. What are the indications of carbamazepine?

Parkinson's Disease

Parkinson's disease was first described by English physician James Parkinson in 1817. It is a disease that principally occurs in elderly individuals, but it can also develop in middle-aged people. Parkinson's disease is a nervous system disorder characterized by movement abnormalities, such as tremors of the extremities and head, and great difficulty in the coordination of fine muscle movement. The other salient feature is *hypokinesia*, an inability or slowness in initiating movements. Other signs and symptoms include a shuffling gait and skeletal muscle rigidity. Often, the affected person breaks into a run to stop from falling.

The incidence of Parkinson's disease is about 1% in people older than 60 years, so it is not an uncommon disease. Its cause is unknown, but a considerable amount is known about the CNS defect that leads to the illness.

This defect is in the basal ganglia portion of the midbrain known as the **substantia nigra** (a large cell mass involved in metabolic disturbances associated with Parkinson's disease). This part of the brain is important in the initiation and control of muscular movement.

Skeletal muscle movements are initiated in the motor cortex of the brain and pass through the basal ganglia and thalamus to the spinal cord along the corticospinal tract.

In the pathways of the substantia nigra, there is a balance between dopamine and acetylcholine in normal individuals. In patients with Parkinson's disease, a lack of dopaminergic activity leads to an imbalance between these neurotransmitters (Figure 17-3 ■).

Parkinsonism is a term that refers to the symptoms produced by certain drugs, poisons, and traumatic lesions in the basal ganglia. When the cause is known, the disease is termed *secondary parkinsonism*, as opposed to *primary parkinsonism*. Secondary parkinsonism is sometimes only temporary if the symptoms are caused by drugs. Secondary parkinsonism is not the same as Parkinson's disease.

There is no cure for Parkinson's disease. Drugs have been developed that can help patients manage many of the symptoms, but they do not stop the progression of the disease. However, patients with Parkinson's disease frequently experience dramatic swings in mobility and mood (known as being "on" or "off"), which may depend on the severity of the disease or the timing of the medication doses.

Because surgical treatment is still experimental, the usual way to treat people with this condition is to try to rebalance dopamine and acetylcholine by using drugs. Two methods are used to correct the condition: Decrease the muscarinic activity (by using antimuscarinic drugs) or increase the dopaminergic activity (by increasing dopamine levels, blocking its breakdown, or mimicking its action).

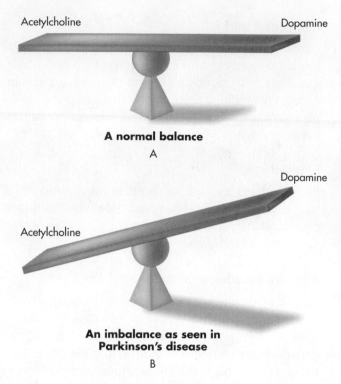

Figure 17-3 ■ Normal (**A**) and abnormal (**B**) balance between dopamine and acetylcholine.

Focus On

Anticholinergic Drugs (Muscarinic Antagonists)

The most commonly used agents in this class are benztropine (Cogentin) and trihexyphenidyl (Trihexy). Amantadine (Symmetrel) is sometimes useful for tremor or for making levodopa work better, but exactly how it works is not clear. It may also dramatically reduce dyskinesia (difficulty in making voluntary movements) in some patients.

How do they work?

Anticholinergic agents work by inhibiting the muscarine receptors in the basal ganglia, lessening the imbalance between the extrapyramidal and pyramidal pathways by blocking the effect of acetylcholine. Table 17-3 ■ lists anticholinergic drugs used for Parkinson's disease.

How are they used?

Only centrally acting anticholinergic drugs are effective for Parkinson's disease. These medications can also be prescribed in combination with other antiparkinsonian drugs.

What are the adverse effects?

CNS adverse effects include anxiety, which is experienced by 30% to 50% of all patients, and, more seriously, agitation or confusion. The anticholinergic effects include dry mouth and decreased sweating and heat release. Other serious adverse reactions include urticaria, urine retention, paresthesias, and sinus tachycardia.

What are the contraindications and interactions?

The safe use of anticholinergic agents in pregnant patients has not been established. They should not be given with other antimuscarinics because additive effects may occur.

What are the important points patients should know?

Instruct patients to avoid alcohol consumption because this combination may intensify the CNS depressant effects. Advise patients that constipation can occur and urge them to consume a high-fiber diet. Because drowsiness is a common effect of these drugs, advise patients to avoid driving a car or operating heavy machinery.

Table 17-3 ■ Anticholinergic Drugs Used for Parkinson's Disease

GENERIC NAME	TRADE NAME	AVERAGE ADULT DOSAGE	ROUTE OF ADMINISTRATION
benztropine	Cogentin	0.5–1 mg/d; gradually increase as needed up to 6 mg/d	PO
biperiden	Akineton	2 mg 1–4 times/d	PO
diphenhydramine	Benadryl	25–50 mg tid–qid	PO
procyclidine	Kemadrin	2.5–5 mg tid	PO
trihexyphenidyl	Artane	1 mg on day 1; 2 mg on day 2; then increase by 2 mg every 3–5 d, up to 6–10 mg/d	PO

PO, oral; qid, four times a day; tid, three times a day.

Focus On

Dopaminergic Drugs

The first drug approved specifically for Parkinson's disease (in 1970)—and still the most commonly administered therapy—is levodopa (Larodopa). In most patients, it significantly improves mobility and allows them to function relatively normally. A number of chemicals, such as carbidopa (a drug that prevents peripheral metabolism of levodopa and is marketed as Lodosyn), are able to prolong the effects of levodopa and help reduce its side effects. The combination drug carbidopa–levodopa is marketed in the United States as Sinemet. Dopaminergic agents used for Parkinson's disease are listed in Table 17-4 ■.

How do they work?

Dopaminergic agents, such as levodopa, are metabolic precursors of dopamine, a catecholamine neurotransmitter. Unlike dopamine, levodopa readily crosses the blood–brain barrier. Its precise mechanism of action is unknown.

How are they used?

The dopaminergic agent levodopa is used in idiopathic Parkinson's disease, postencephalitic and arteriosclerotic parkinsonism, and parkinsonism symptoms associated with manganese and carbon monoxide poisoning.

What are the adverse effects?

The debilitating side effects of dopaminergic agents include dyskinesia, hallucinations, and mental confusion. A major long-term complication is loss of efficacy after about 5 years of therapy. Abrupt discontinuation should be avoided because some patients experience a complex called *neuroleptic malignant syndrome (NMS)*, especially if they are also taking **neuroleptic** agents (psychotropic drugs used to treat psychosis). Manifestations of NMS include tachycardia, muscular rigidity, fever, mental status changes, diaphoresis, tachypnea, and increases in serum creatinine levels.

What are the contraindications and interactions?

Dopaminergic agents should be administered with extreme caution to patients who have cardiac disease. Other drugs work differently. The so-called *dopamine agonists*, such as bromocriptine (Parlodel), ropinirole (Requip), pergolide (Permax), and pramipexole (Mirapex), work directly on the target cells of the substantia nigra in a way that imitates dopamine. Dopamine agonists are often used in combination with levodopa.

Unfortunately, all drugs used to treat Parkinson's disease may have side effects. Although some people never experience such side effects, others are very sensitive to the medications and may be unable to tolerate them. Most commonly, the side effects of antiparkinsonian drugs are mental confusion, hallucinations, and dyskinesia. Because effective treatment of Parkinson's disease is often a matter

(Continued)

Focus On (Continued)

of balancing beneficial effects of drugs against their side effects, many people prefer to see experienced specialists.

What are the important points patients should know?

Instruct patients to take dopaminergic agents with food to avoid gastrointestinal irritation. Levodopa may discolor urine and perspiration. Advise patients to avoid foods rich in vitamin B_6 (such as beans and cereals) and alcohol. Bromocriptine can cause postural hypotension, so advise patients to rise slowly from a lying position. Also, instruct patients to regularly visit their dentists to prevent dental problems caused by the inhibition of salivation. Dopaminergic agents should never be stopped abruptly because of a possible rebound of parkinsonism.

Table 17-4 ■ Dopaminergic Drugs Used for Parkinson's Disease

GENERIC NAME	TRADE NAME	AVERAGE ADULT DOSAGE	ROUTE OF ADMINISTRATION
amantadine	Symmetrel	100 mg bid	PO
bromocriptine	Parlodel	1.25– 2.5 mg/d up to 100 mg/d in divided doses	PO
carbidopa–levodopa	Sinemet	1 tablet containing 10 mg carbidopa/100 mg levodopa or 25 mg carbidopa/100 mg levodopa tid; increased by 1 tablet every day or every other day, up to 6 tablets/d	PO
levodopa	L-Dopa, Larodopa	500 mg–1 g/d	PO
pergolide	Permax	Start with 0.5 mg/d for 2 d; then increase by 0.1 or 0.15 mg/d q3d for 12 d; and then increase by 0.25 mg every third day until reaching the desired effect	PO
pramipexole	Mirapex	Start with 0.125 mg tid for 1 wk; double this dose for the next week; continue to increase by 0.25 mg/dose tid q1wk to the desired dose of 1.5 mg tid	PO
ropinirole	Requip	Start with 0.25 mg tid; increase q1wk by 0.25 mg/dose to the target dose of 1 mg tid	PO
tolcapone	Tasmar	100 mg tid (maximum, 600 mg/d)	PO

bid, twice a day; PO, oral; tid, three times a day.

✳ Apply Your Knowledge 17.3

The following questions focus on you what have just learned about Parkinson's disease and antiparkinsonian drugs.

CRITICAL THINKING

1. What are the major signs and symptoms of Parkinson's disease?
2. What is the role of the substantia nigra involved with Parkinson's disease?
3. What is the relationship between dopamine and acetylcholine?
4. What is the difference between Parkinson's disease and parkinsonism?
5. What is the mechanism of action of levodopa?
6. What is the result of abrupt discontinuation of dopaminergic agents?
7. What is the mechanism of action of anticholinergic drugs?
8. What are the trade names of benztropine, procyclidine, levodopa, amantadine, and bromocriptine?

Schizophrenia

Schizophrenia is one of the most common psychotic disorders. Almost 1.6% of the population (about 2 million people in the United States), across all cultural groups, are affected by this disorder during their lifetimes. It occurs more commonly in urban populations and in lower socioeconomic groups. The cause of schizophrenia is unknown.

Manifestations of schizophrenia include either positive or negative symptoms. Positive symptoms tend to be exaggerations of normal functioning. For example, a distortion of perceptions may manifest as hallucinations (hearing or seeing things that are not real) and as distortions of thought processes, which may manifest as delusions. Negative symptoms include terseness in speech, social withdrawal, anhedonia (the inability to experience pleasure), and apathy. Symptoms usually manifest during the early years of adulthood. The illness is chronic, and fewer than 20% of patients recover fully from a single episode of psychosis.

PSYCHOACTIVE DRUGS

The past 3 decades of research in the neurosciences have dramatically increased our understanding of the neurobehavioral aspects of mental illness. The 1990s were referred to as the *decade of the brain*, and the more recent discovery of the human genome was accomplished in 2000. Historically, the advent of the first psychotropic medications in the 1950s significantly changed the treatment of people with mentally illnesses.

More than 1,500 compounds, classified as *psychoactive* or *psychotropic* drugs, have been described. Approximately 20% of all prescriptions written in the United States are for medications intended to alter mental processes and behavior. Those agents used in the treatment of people with psychotic illnesses and depressant disorders are the focus of this chapter. One of the major uses of antipsychotic drugs is the treatment of people with schizophrenia.

Focus On

Antipsychotic Drugs

The terms *antipsychotic* and *neuroleptic* are used interchangeably to denote a group of drugs that have been used mainly for treating schizophrenia but are also effective in some other psychoses and agitated states. A new type of antipsychotic medication became available with the introduction of clozapine (Clozaril) in 1990. After its success, other medications with similar clinical profiles were developed. These *atypical* antipsychotic agents are effective against the positive and the negative symptoms of schizophrenia. Although the atypical agents are more expensive than the typical drugs, recent evaluations of the total costs of treatment show that atypical drugs are economically superior. This is because the increased efficacy and higher rate of compliance result in fewer hospital admissions and other emergency interventions.

(Continued)

Focus On (Continued)

Typical antipsychotics are available in several different groups. Structurally, they can be divided into phenothiazines, thioxanthenes, butyrophenones, dihydroindolone derivatives, and dibenzodiazepines. Common typical and atypical antipsychotic drugs are listed in Table 17-5 ■.

How do they work?

The mechanism of action of the antipsychotic agents is complex, and many details remain to be established. However, the evaluation of properties shared by effective antipsychotic agents provides clues to their mechanism of action. All the typical antipsychotic agents block postsynaptic dopaminergic receptors and act as competitive antagonists of dopamine centrally and peripherally.

How are they used?

Antipsychotic drugs are effective mainly against the positive symptoms of schizophrenia. In addition to their use in treating schizophrenia, several of these drugs are also effective antiemetic and antinausea agents.

What are the adverse effects?

The main adverse effects of antipsychotic drugs include sedation, dry mouth, sexual dysfunction, **akathisia** (difficulty in initiating muscle movement), **bradykinesia** (extremely slow movement), rigidity, and sometimes **tardive dyskinesia** (slowed ability to make voluntary movements).

What are the contraindications and interactions?

Many of the contraindications to the use of these drugs are similar. They are contraindicated in comatose patients who have received large amounts of CNS depressant drugs (such as alcohol and barbiturates).

What are the important points patients should know?

Advise family members of psychiatric outpatients about the adverse effects of drug therapy and any adverse reactions that may occur because they will be responsible for administering antipsychotic drugs to the patient. They should suggest that the patient use hard candy or ice chips for a dry mouth. Advise the patient not to drive a car or operate machinery until a maintenance dose has been established. Instruct patients who are taking phenothiazines, such as chlorpromazine (Thorazine), that their urine may turn pink or red-brown and that this discoloration is not harmful.

Table 17-5 ■ Common Typical and Atypical Antipsychotic Drugs

GENERIC NAME	TRADE NAME	AVERAGE ADULT DOSAGE	ROUTE OF ADMINISTRATION
Typical			
chlorpromazine	Thorazine	25–100 mg tid–qid up to 1,000 mg/d	PO
		25–50 mg up to 600 mg q4–6h; switch to oral dosage as soon as possible	IM
fluphenazine	Permitil, Prolixin	0.5–10 mg/d in divided doses q6–8h; usual daily dose is less than 3 mg	PO
		2.5–10 mg/d (range: 2.5–10 mg) q6–8h	IM
haloperidol	Haldol	Initial dosage range: 0.5–5 mg bid–tid	PO
		2–5 mg (up to 10–30 mg) q60 min or q4–8h PRN; switch to oral dose as soon as possible	IM
lithium	Eskalith, Lithobid	600 mg tid or 900 mg slow-release form bid to produce effective serum levels of 1–1.5 mEq/L	PO

GENERIC NAME	TRADE NAME	AVERAGE ADULT DOSAGE	ROUTE OF ADMINISTRATION
loxapine	Loxitane	Initially, 10 mg bid, rapidly increased to 60–100 mg/d in 2–4 divided doses	IM
		12.5–50 mg q4–6h; when controlled, change to oral dose	IM
mesoridazine	Serentil	Initially, 50 mg tid, up to 400 mg/d	PO
		25 mg; may repeat in 30–60 min	IM
molindone	Moban	50–75 mg/d in three or four divided doses; may be increased to 100 mg/d in 3–4 d	PO
perphenazine	Trilafon	4–16 mg bid–qid; reduce as soon as possible; avoid dosages greater than 64 mg/d	PO
		Initially 5–10 mg q6h, not exceeding 30 mg/d	IM
		Dilute to 0.5 mg per mL; give no more than 1 mg per injection at no less than 1- to 2-min intervals; do not exceed 5-mg total dose	IV
prochlorperazine	Compazine	Initially 5–10 mg tid–qid; gradually increase q2–3 d up to 50–150 mg/d	PO
		10–20 mg q2–4h; switch to oral therapy as soon as possible	IM
		2.5–10 mg q6–8h (maximum: 40 mg/d)	IV
		25 mg bid up to 40 mg/d	Rectal
promazine	Sparine	10–200 mg q4–6h up to 1,000 mg/d	PO/IM
thioridazine	Mellaril	50–100 mg tid; may increase up to 800 mg/d	PO
trifluoperazine	Stelazine	1–2 mg bid; may increase up to 20 mg/d in hospitalized patients	PO
		1–2 mg q4–6h (maximum, 10 mg/d)	IM
Atypical			
aripiprazole	Abilify	10–15 mg/d	PO
clozapine	Clozaril	25 mg/d in 1–2 doses; gradually increase by 25–50 mg/d, up to 300–450 mg/d, by end of week 2	PO
olanzapine	Zyprexa	5–10 mg/d; increase by 5 mg/d at 1-wk intervals	PO
quetiapine	Seroquel	25 mg bid; increase by 25–50 mg bid, up to 800 mg/d	PO
risperidone	Risperdal	2 mg/d (maximum dosage: 4–8 mg/d)	PO
ziprasidone	Geodon	40 mg/d	IM, PO

bid, twice a day; IM, intramuscular; PO, oral; PRN, as needed; qid, four times a day; tid, three times a day.

Focus On

Lithium Carbonate

Lithium carbonate (Eskalith) can control symptoms in the manic and depressive phases of psychotic disorders and is also used to treat bipolar disorder.

How does it work?

Lithium's exact mechanism of action is unclear. Therefore, therapeutic levels of lithium must be considered individually. Therapeutic effects usually take 1 to 2 weeks to be observed.

How is it used?

Lithium is used in the control and the prophylaxis of acute mania and the acute manic phase of mixed bipolar disorder.

What are the adverse effects?

Common adverse effects of lithium include nausea and tremors, which subside with continued treatment. Overdose may cause vomiting, diarrhea, dizziness, headache, drowsiness, tinnitus, loss of equilibrium, disorientation, and short-term memory loss. Toxic levels may cause kidney and heart damage. Therefore, serum concentration levels should be monitored on a regular basis.

What are the contraindications and interactions?

Lithium should be avoided in pregnant women or patients with thyroid disorders. Carbamazepine (Tegretol), haloperidol (Haldol), and phenothiazines increase the risk of neurotoxicity when they are used with lithium.

What are the important points patients should know?

Advise patients to drink plenty of fluids—at least 2 to 3 liters per day, during the stabilization period and at least 1 to 1-1/2 liters per day during ongoing therapy. Alert them that urine output will be increased and diluted and that they may have persistent thirst. Dose reduction may be indicated. Instruct patients to contact their physicians if diarrhea or fever develops. Warn patients to avoid hot environments and excessive use of caffeinated beverages. Warn patients against driving and engaging in other potentially hazardous activities until the response to the drug is known.

Focus Point

Lithium, Contraception, and Pregnancy

Women who are taking lithium should use effective contraceptive measures. If therapy must be continued during pregnancy, serum lithium levels should be closely monitored to prevent toxicity.

✻ Apply Your Knowledge 17.4

The following questions focus on what you have just learned about psychoactive drugs.

CRITICAL THINKING

1. What are the manifestations of schizophrenia?
2. What are the effects of atypical antipsychotic agents?
3. What are the differences between atypical and typical antipsychotic agents?
4. What are the indications of lithium?
5. What are the contraindications of lithium?
6. What are the trade names of haloperidol, lithium, mesoridazine, olanzapine, and clozapine?

Depression

Major depression is one of the most common psychiatric disorders in the United States. About 5% to 6% of the population is depressed. Depression may be "reactive" (in response to a stimulus such as the loss of a loved one) or "endogenous" (a chemical disorder in the brain). The majority of antidepressant medications are used chiefly in the management of endogenous depression. Symptoms of depression include feelings of doom, a lack of self-worth, an inability to sense pleasure, loss of energy, an inability to concentrate, changes in sleep habits, and thoughts of suicide.

ANTIDEPRESSANTS

Antidepressants are classified into several groups on the basis of their chemical structures and antidepressant action in the brain. The most commonly used drugs are listed in Table 17-6 ■ and include TCAs, MAOIs, and selective serotonin reuptake inhibitors (SSRIs). Another class that is used less commonly is the selective serotonin–norepinephrine reuptake inhibitors (SSNRIs), also known as the serotonin–norepinephrine reuptake inhibitors (SNRIs). These include venlafaxine (Effexor), duloxetine (Cymbalta), and several other less commonly used medications.

Table 17-6 ■ Classifications of Antidepressants

GENERIC NAME	TRADE NAME	AVERAGE ADULT DOSAGE	ROUTE OF ADMINISTRATION
Tricyclic Antidepressants			
amitriptyline	Elavil	Up to 300 mg/d in divided doses	PO
amoxapine	Asendin	Start at 50 mg bid–tid; may increase on day 3 to 100 mg tid	PO
clomipramine	Anafranil	50–150 mg/d in single or divided doses	PO
desipramine	Norpramin	100–300 mg/d	PO
doxepin	Sinequan	25–30 mg/d in divided doses	PO
imipramine	Tofranil	75–300 mg/d in divided doses	PO
nortriptyline	Aventyl, Pamelor	25 mg tid–qid	PO
protriptyline	Vivactil	15–40 mg/d in 3–4 divided doses (maximum: 60 mg/d)	PO
trimipramine	Surmontil	100–300 mg/d in divided doses	PO
Monoamine Oxidase Inhibitors			
phenelzine	Nardil	15 mg tid rapidly increased to at least 60 mg/d; may need up to 90 mg/d	PO
tranylcypromine	Parnate	30–60 mg/d in divided doses at 3-wk interval	PO
Selective Serotonin Reuptake Inhibitors			
citalopram	Celexa	20–40 mg/d	PO
escitalopram	Lexapro	10 mg/d; may increase to 20 mg after 1 wk	PO
fluoxetine	Prozac, Prozac weekly, Sarafem	20 mg/d in the morning; may increase by 40–80 mg/d in divided doses; weekly dose: 1 capsule/wk	PO
fluvoxamine	Luvox	50–300 mg/d in divided doses	PO
paroxetine	Paxil	20–50 mg/d	PO
sertraline	Zoloft	50–200 mg/d	PO

bid twice a day; PO, oral; qid, four times a day; tid, three times a day.

Focus On

Tricyclic Antidepressants

Historically, drugs from this group have been the first choice in the treatment of depression and include imipramine (Tofranil), amitriptyline (Elavil), doxepin (Sinequan), and related drugs.

How do they work?

TCAs increase the effect of norepinephrine and serotonin in the CNS by blocking their reuptake by the neurons.

How are they used?

TCAs are used for endogenous depression and occasionally for reactive depression.

What are the adverse effects?

Adverse effects derive from the fact that TCAs have secondary actions, including antimuscarinic, antihistamine, and antiadrenergic activity. The first action accounts for dry mouth, blurred vision, constipation, urine retention, and tachycardia. Mental confusion and sedation arise from a central antihistamine action, and postural hypotension can occur as a result of an antiadrenergic effect.

When used together with antihypertensive agents, orthostatic hypotension may increase. Norepinephrine and other sympathomimetics may increase cardiac toxicity when they are used with TCAs.

What are the contraindications and interactions?

TCAs are contraindicated in patients who are hypersensitive to these drugs. They must be avoided in patients during the acute recovery period after a heart attack and in patients with severe renal or hepatic impairment. MAOIs may precipitate hyperpyrexic crisis, tachycardia, or seizures as a result of drug interaction with TCAs.

What are the important points patients should know?

Warn patients against stopping TCAs abruptly. Advise patients to take these drugs at bedtime to promote a normal sleep pattern. Instruct patients to report having severe postural hypotension to their physicians and explain that the drug's effectiveness begins after about 2 weeks of use. Antidepressant treatment needs to continue even after recovery because of the potential for a relapse.

Focus on Geriatrics

Effect of Tricyclic Antidepressants on the Prostate Gland

Elderly men with enlarged prostate glands are at higher risk for urine retention when taking TCAs.

Focus Point

Tricyclic Antidepressants and Other Medications

Patients taking TCAs should not take any medications, including over-the-counter (OTC) medications, without notifying their physicians.

Focus on Natural Products

Drug Interactions with St. John's Wort

St. John's wort is a flower grown throughout the world and is used to treat patients with mild to moderate depression and anxiety. It is administered orally for this purpose. St. John's wort should not be used during pregnancy and lactation. Interactions with St. John's wort occur with TCAs, MAOIs, SSRIs, alcohol, and foods that are high in tyramine or catecholamines. The major problem in using St. John's wort for depression and anxiety is that this herbal supplement may take 4 to 6 weeks to become effective. It may also cause increased photosensitivity.

Focus On

Selective Serotonin Reuptake Inhibitors

SSRIs are relatively newer antidepressants that have had a tremendous impact on prescribing patterns. They are now considered the first-line drugs in the treatment of patients with major depression.

How do they work?

SSRIs primarily block the effect of serotonin reuptake. Clinical studies have found that, generally, SSRIs have comparable efficacy to TCAs. However, TCAs have been found to be more effective in the treatment of patients with severe depression.

How are they used?

SSRIs are commonly used for depression, geriatric depression, obsessive-compulsive disorder, bulimia nervosa, and premenstrual dysphoric disorder.

What are the adverse effects?

In general, the adverse effects of SSRIs are relatively mild, of shorter duration than those of TCAs, and diminish as treatment continues. Cardiac toxicity and the risk of death after overdose are less likely than with TCAs.

Common adverse effects include headache, nausea, vomiting, tremor, insomnia, dizziness, and diarrhea.

What are the contraindications and interactions?

SSRIs must be avoided in patients who are hypersensitive to them. SSRIs should not be used concurrently with MAOIs or thioridazine (Mellaril). These drugs should not be used during pregnancy or in children younger than 7 years. SSRIs should be used with caution in patients with hepatic or renal impairment, renal failure, lactation, cardiac disease, or diabetes mellitus.

What are the important points patients should know?

Advise patients to report withdrawal symptoms, including abdominal pain, diarrhea, nausea, headache, sweating, and insomnia. Tell patients to take great care when driving and operating machinery while on antidepressant therapy, especially during the initial stages of treatment. Instruct patients to take SSRIs in the morning to minimize the incidence of insomnia and to avoid alcohol because of the additive CNS depressant effects.

Focus on Geriatrics

Taking SSRIs

All SSRIs should be administered with food. Patients—particularly older adults and nutritionally compromised patients—should be weighed weekly to monitor weight loss.

Focus On

Monoamine Oxidase Inhibitors

The therapeutic response rate with all antidepressants is similar, and the selection of the proper agent depends on the side effects the patient experiences from the drugs. MAOIs are second- or third-line antidepressants because of the numerous interactions with prescription and OTC medications as well as with certain foods and beverages.

How do they work?

MAOIs are thought to act by preventing the natural breakdown of neurotransmitters, but their precise mode of action is not known. It is also thought that MAOIs are able to inhibit hepatic microsomal drug-metabolizing enzymes; thus, they may intensify and prolong the effects of many drugs.

How are they used?

Until the availability of SSRIs, MAOIs were the most effective antidepressants available. These agents are used to manage endogenous depression, the depressive phase of manic-depressive (bipolar) psychosis, and severe exogenous (reactive) depression that is not responsive to more commonly used therapies.

What are the adverse effects?

Common adverse reactions of MAOIs are less serious than those observed during TCA therapy but consist of antimuscarinic and antiadrenergic effects. Orthostatic hypotension is a common adverse effect of MAOIs. Nausea, constipation, dry mouth, diarrhea, dizziness, vertigo, and headache are also seen. A serious hypertensive crisis may occur if a patient taking MAOIs eats a food containing tyramine (an amino acid present in some foods).

What are the contraindications and interactions?

MAOIs are contraindicated in those with epilepsy, liver disease, and serious cardiovascular disease. These drugs are also contraindicated in patients with known hypersensitivity to them.

What are the most important points patients should know?

Instruct patients to avoid foods that contain tyramine and provide a list of these foods, which includes cheese, sour cream, yogurt, chicken liver, beef, coffee, tea, caffeinated sodas, chocolate, pickled herring, soy sauce, yeast extracts, and fruits and vegetables (dried beans, fava beans, figs, raisins, avocados, bananas, and raspberries). Inform patients that the drug's effectiveness occurs after about 2 weeks of therapy.

Focus Point

Diet and Monoamine Oxidase Inhibitors

Patients taking MAOIs must avoid foods containing tyramine to avoid severe hypertension, heart attack, adverse reactions, and death.

✳ Apply Your Knowledge 17.5

The following questions focus on what you have just learned about TCAs, SSRIs, and MAOIs.

CRITICAL THINKING

1. What is endogenous depression?
2. What are the classifications of antidepressants?
3. Which class of antidepressants are relatively newer drugs?
4. Which class of antidepressants was most effective before the availability of selective serotonin reuptake inhibitors?
5. What are the trade names of clomipramine, doxepin, phenelzine, citalopram, and paroxetine?

PRACTICAL SCENARIO 1

The father of an 18-year-old teenager calls the physician's office, stating that his son, who has been diagnosed with schizophrenia, has become increasingly withdrawn and does not seem interested in doing anything at all. He says his son is taking the antipsychotic clozapine (Clozaril), and he believes his son's condition should be better. His father states he is worried because his son also seems to have strange movements—he seems to move very slowly.

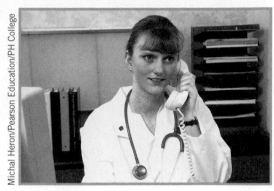

Michal Heron/Pearson Education/PH College

Critical Thinking Questions

1. As the medical assistant who takes the phone call, what might you say to alleviate some of the father's anxiety as you take down the details to relay to the physician?
2. What questions would you ask the father about his son's personality, mood, and physical changes?
3. What teaching points might you offer the father during the phone call?

PRACTICAL SCENARIO 2

A 45-year-old woman has had major depression. Recently, she attempted suicide. Her family history includes a sister who also had depression and committed suicide 3 years earlier.

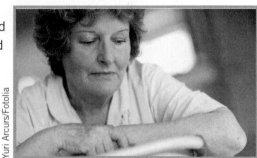

Yuri Arcurs/Fotolia

Critical Thinking Questions

1. In your opinion, what would be the best of the popular medications for this patient to treat her depression?
2. If she takes an MAOI, what precautions should she take concerning foods to avoid drug–food interactions?

Chapter Capsule

This section repeats the objectives from the beginning of the chapter and then provides a summary of the most important concepts for that objective. Use this section as a quick review and to check your knowledge.

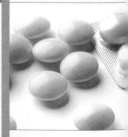

Objective 1: Describe the four major parts of the brain.

- Cerebrum—the largest part, which includes nerve centers associated with sensory and motor functions and provides higher mental functions, including memory and reasoning; composed of an outer cerebral cortex and inner cerebral medulla
- Diencephalon—also processes sensory information
- Brain stem—contains nerve pathways that connect various parts of the nervous system and regulate certain visceral activities
- Cerebellum—includes centers that coordinate voluntary muscular movements

Objective 2: Name three benzodiazepine hypnotic drugs and explain the mechanism by which they produce hypnotic effects.

- Diazepam—appears to act at the limbic and subcortical levels of the CNS
- Lorazepam—effects are mediated by GABA; it acts on the thalamic, hypothalamic, and limbic levels of the CNS
- Phenytoin—precise mechanism is not known, but it appears to reduce the voltage, frequency, and spread of electrical discharges within the motor cortex

Objective 3: List three different types of epilepsy.

- Generalized tonic–clonic seizures
- Generalized absence seizures
- Partial seizures

Objective 4: Name two drugs used specifically to treat each type of epilepsy.

- Phenytoin, carbamazepine—generalized tonic–clonic seizures
- Valproic acid, ethosuximide—generalized absence seizures
- Phenytoin, carbamazepine—partial seizures

Objective 5: Describe the mechanisms of action of drugs that increase dopamine or decrease acetylcholine levels in the basal ganglia.

- Anticholinergic agents—work by inhibiting the muscarine receptors in the basal ganglia, lessening the imbalance between the extrapyramidal and pyramidal pathways by blocking the effect of acetylcholine
- Dopaminergic drugs (such as levodopa)—the exact mechanism of action is unknown

Objective 6: Describe five adverse effects associated with antianxiety drugs.

- Drowsiness
- Nausea
- Bradycardia
- Skin rash
- Fever

Note: There are more adverse effects, but these five are the most common.

Objective 7: Describe the common adverse effects and the specific neurologic conditions caused by antipsychotic drugs.

- Common adverse effects—nausea, vomiting, diarrhea, dizziness, headache, drowsiness, tinnitus, disorientation, and short-term memory loss
- Neurological conditions—tremors, loss of equilibrium, and neurotoxicity (when combined with carbamazepine, haloperidol, and phenothiazines)

Objective 8: Explain the use of lithium in mania and the adverse effects associated with its use.

- Lithium—controls symptoms in the manic and depressive phases of psychotic disorders; used for the control and prophylaxis of acute mania and the acute manic phase of mixed bipolar disorder

- Adverse effects—nausea, tremors (which subside with continued treatment), vomiting, diarrhea, dizziness, headache, drowsiness, tinnitus, loss of equilibrium, and short-term memory loss; at toxic levels, kidney and heart damage

Objective 9: Describe the main adverse effects of antipsychotic drugs.

- Sedation, dry mouth, sexual dysfunction, akathisia, bradykinesia, and rigidity; sometimes, tardive dyskinesia

Objective 10: Identify three of the most common types of drugs used to treat patients with depression.

- The most common types of drugs used to treat depression include the tricyclic antidepressants, monoamine oxidase inhibitors, and selective serotonin reuptake inhibitors.

 ## Internet Sites of Interest

- Find a concise description of sedative–hypnotic agents on the Psychology Today website at **http://www.psychologytoday.com**. Search for "sedative."

- The National Institute of Neurological Disorders and Stroke contains a comprehensive site for information on epilepsy, including support organizations and fact sheets for patients and caregivers, at **http://www.ninds.nih.gov/disorders/epilepsy**.

- For an overview of anticonvulsant medications, click "Neuro Med" and then look for "anticonvulsant" on Neuroland's website at **http://neuroland.com**.

- In-depth information on a variety of topics related to schizophrenia, including symptoms and diagnosis, drug therapy, support groups, and frequently asked questions, can be found at **http://www.schizophrenia.com**.

- Information about bipolar disorder and medications used to treat it can be found at **http://www.pendulum.org**.

- The National Institute of Mental Health discusses the latest treatments for schizophrenia, depression, and other psychiatric disorders at **http://www.nimh.nih.gov**.

Chapter 18

Drugs Used to Treat Autonomic Nervous System Conditions

Chapter Objectives

After completing this chapter, you should be able to:

1. List the two divisions of the nervous system and their subdivisions.
2. Explain the basic functional unit cell of the nervous system.
3. Define the terms *cholinergic* and *adrenergic*.
4. Describe the fight-or-flight response.
5. List the two main adrenergic receptors and what they respond to.
6. Explain the actions of adrenergic agonists.
7. Explain the actions of receptor agonists.
8. Define *adrenergic antagonists*.
9. List the two types of cholinergic receptors.
10. Discuss parasympathomimetics (also called *cholinergic agonists*).

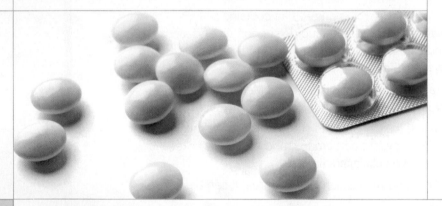

Key Terms

adrenergic (add-ruh-NUR-jik) (page 310)

alpha-adrenergic receptors (AL-fuh add-ruh-NUR-jik ree-SEP-ters) (page 312)

anticholinergics (an-tee-kol-in-UR-jiks) (page 322)

beta-adrenergic receptors (BAY-tuh add-ruh-NUR-jik) (page 312)

catecholamines (kah-teh-KOH-luh-meenz) (page 312)

cholinergic (kol-in-UR-jik) (page 309)

cholinergic blockers (page 322)

fight-or-flight response (page 312)

muscarinic receptors (MUS-kah-RIN-ik) (page 322)

nicotinic receptors (NIK-oh-TIN-ik) (page 322)

parasympathetic nervous system (pair-ah-SIM-pah-THET-ik) (page 309)

parasympatholytics (pair-ah-SIM-pa-tho-LIH-tiks) (page 322)

peripheral nervous system (per-IF-urr-ul) (page 309)

sympathetic nervous system (SIM-pah-THET-ik) (page 309)

sympathomimetics (sim-pah-tho-MI-met-iks) (page 315)

Introduction

The two major systems controlling bodily functions are the nervous system and the endocrine system. These systems involve high-level integration in the brain and have the ability to influence processes in distant regions of the body as well as to extensively use negative feedback. Both use chemicals to transmit information. In the endocrine system, these chemicals (hormones) are released into the blood circulation and travel to interact with receptors in target tissue. In the nervous system, these chemicals (transmitters) are released from nerve terminals in the synaptic cleft (axons) and interact with receptors on neurons or effectors.

These two systems work closely with each other to control all the body's functions. They are the most complicated and difficult parts of the anatomy and physiology of the body. For this reason, neuropharmacology is a challenging subject for allied health-care students.

Anatomy of the Autonomic Nervous System

The nervous system is divided into two main parts: the central nervous system (CNS), which comprises the brain and spinal cord, and the **peripheral nervous system** (PNS), that part of the nervous system that is outside the brain and spinal cord (Figure 18-1 ■). The autonomic nervous system (ANS) is a division of the PNS, which can itself be divided into two sections: motor and sensory neurons. In turn, motor neurons can be divided into two divisions that generally possess opposing functions: the **sympathetic nervous system** (which accelerates heart rate, constricts blood vessels, and raises blood pressure) and the **parasympathetic nervous system** (which slows the heart rate, increases intestinal and glandular activity, and relaxes muscles). This division is an anatomical division rather than a strict neurotransmitter division. Each division uses two efferent neurons to carry neural signals to effector tissues with the specific receptors.

The neuron is the basic functional unit cell of the nervous system. Therefore, these cells must communicate with each other and the other tissues of the body. The communication sites of neurons are called synapses, which are actually junctions that nerve impulses pass across. The nerve starting the original impulse is known as the *presynaptic nerve*. The nerve that originates after the synapse is called *postsynaptic nerve.*

The space between each synapse (called the *synaptic* cleft) is bridged by chemicals called *neurotransmitters*. The two primary neurotransmitters in the ANS are acetylcholine (ACh) and norepinephrine (NE), although many different types of neurotransmitters exist throughout the nervous system. Many drugs act as neurotransmitters. Drugs can also be used to block or enhance the activity of these neurotransmitters (Figure 18-2 ■).

Sympathetic Nervous System

A *ganglion* is an aggregation of nerve cell fibers. Sympathetic preganglionic fibers exit the CNS through the thoracic and lumbar spinal nerves. Sympathetic preganglionic fibers terminate in ganglia located in the two paravertebral chains that lie on either side of the spinal cord. Thus, sympathetic preganglionic fibers are short and can activate diffuse numbers of postganglionic neurons. ACh is the neurotransmitter released by the preganglionic sympathetic neuron. Postganglionic sympathetic neurons project long fibers to innervate the sympathetic target tissue. The major neurotransmitter released by the postganglionic neuron is NE. However, in sweat glands, the postganglionic neuron releases ACh. Dopamine serves as the postganglionic neurotransmitter in renal smooth muscle. The adrenal medulla also receives sympathetic preganglionic fibers that release ACh and bind to nicotinic receptors. This results in the release of epinephrine and NE into the blood circulation, where they act as hormones at adrenergic receptors throughout the body (Figure 18-3 ■).

Parasympathetic Nervous System

Parasympathetic preganglionic fibers exit the CNS through the cranial nerves and the sacral spinal roots and then travel to innervated tissues. Most preganglionic parasympathetic fibers terminate on ganglion cells. Innervation (neural or electrical arousal) of the target tissue is far less divergent than in the sympathetic nervous system. Just as in the sympathetic division, parasympathetic preganglionic neurons release ACh at the ganglia. The parasympathetic postganglionic neurons also release ACh, which binds to the target tissue.

Neurotransmitters of the Autonomic Nervous System

Neurons in the ANS can be classified into two groups based on the neurotransmitter they release. Neurons that release ACh are termed **cholinergic**. Cholinergic neurons include:

✳ Preganglionic neurons in the sympathetic and parasympathetic nervous systems

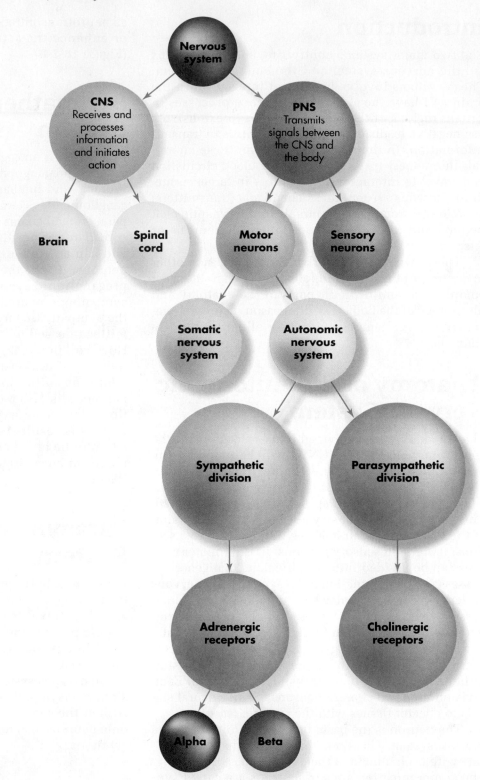

Figure 18-1 ■
Divisions of the nervous system.

✳ Parasympathetic postganglionic neurons
✳ Somatic transmission at the neuromuscular junction
✳ Sympathetic postganglionic fibers that innervate sweat glands

Accordingly, receptors to which ACh binds are also termed *cholinergic*. There are more specific designations for cholinergic receptor–based selectivity for agonist/antagonist binding and anatomical location. Neurons that release NE, epinephrine, or dopamine are termed **adrenergic**. Similarly, receptors to which these adrenergic agonists bind are also termed *adrenergic*. Besides acting as direct agonists or antagonists at cholinergic and adrenergic receptors, drugs can affect the synthesis, storage, release, and termination of neurotransmitters in the ANS.

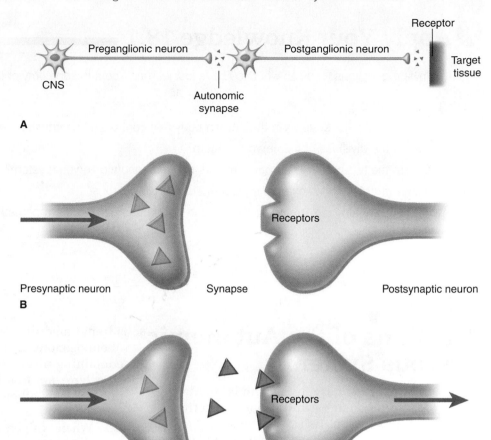

Figure 18-2 ■

In the autonomic pathway (**A**), nerve impulses (**B**; shown as arrows) travel along a presynaptic neuron to reach the junction between two neurons called the *synapses*. Chemicals called neurotransmitters (shown as triangles) must cross the synapses to carry the nerve impulse to the postsynaptic neuron. When the neurotransmitters cross the synapses, they reach a receptor (**C**). Many drugs act as neurotransmitters or they act by blocking the neurotransmitters from reaching a receptor or enhancing the activity of neurotransmitters so that more of them reach the receptor.

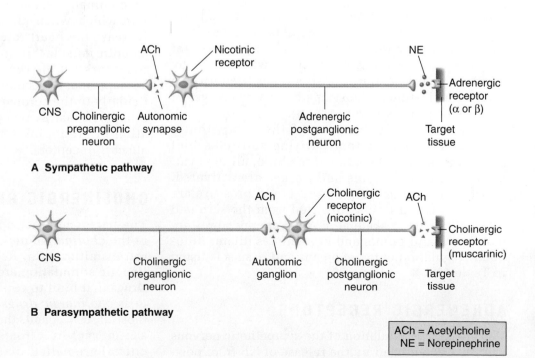

Figure 18-3 ■

Receptors in the autonomic nervous system. **A:** Sympathetic pathways (acetylcholine [ACh] and norepinephrine [NE]).
B: Parasympathetic pathway (ACh).

ACh = Acetylcholine
NE = Norepinephrine

✺ Apply Your Knowledge 18.1

The following questions focus on what you have just learned about the anatomy of the ANS.

CRITICAL THINKING

1. What are two major systems in the human body that control and coordinate the other systems?
2. What are the divisions of the nervous system?
3. What are the two primary neurotransmitters in the autonomic nervous system?
4. What are the definitions of adrenergic and cholinergic neurons?
5. What neurotransmitters are released from the parasympathetic and sympathetic postganglionic neurons?

Functions of the Autonomic Nervous System

The parasympathetic nervous system is required for life; it maintains such essential body functions as digestion and excretion. Its actions generally oppose those of the sympathetic system. At times of "rest and digest," the parasympathetic nervous system dominates the sympathetic nervous system. Rather than discharging as a complete system, the parasympathetic nervous system operates in discrete units based on the specific needs of the body. Discharging as a complete system would produce massive, undesirable symptoms (such as in organophosphate poisoning).

The sympathetic nervous system adjusts body functions in response to such stressors as trauma, fear, hypoglycemia, cold, or exercise. The **fight-or-flight response** (the reaction in the body when faced by a sudden threat or source of stress) has been used to describe activation of the sympathetic nervous system during emergencies (Figure 18-4 ■).

Remember that because of the sympathetic nervous system's anatomic wiring and release of epinephrine from the adrenal medulla, all the sympathetic effector organs and tissues are activated. Heart rate, cardiac output, and blood pressure are increased; blood flow is diverted from the skin and internal organs to skeletal muscle; energy stores are mobilized; and pupils and bronchioles dilate. Autonomic regulation of target organs and tissues is listed in Table 18-1 ■.

ADRENERGIC RECEPTORS

The effects of stimulation of the sympathetic nervous system are mediated by the release of NE from postganglionic nerve terminals and epinephrine from the adrenal medulla. NE and epinephrine are two types of endogenous **catecholamines** (chemical compounds containing nitrogen that are derived from the amino acid *tyrosine*) that bind to adrenergic receptors and produce sympathetic effects.

The two main adrenergic receptors are alpha and beta. Whereas alpha-adrenergic receptors are divided into α_1 and α_2, beta-adrenergic receptors are divided into β_1 and β_2. **Alpha-adrenergic receptors** (parts of cells that respond to adrenaline) are found in vascular smooth muscle and, when stimulated by NE or epinephrine, cause vasoconstriction.

Beta-adrenergic receptors (receptors that respond to NE or epinephrine) are found on smooth and cardiac muscle membranes. In the heart, the predominant beta-adrenergic receptors are β_1 receptors, which, when stimulated by NE and epinephrine, increase the heart rate and force of contraction. In smooth muscle, the predominant beta-adrenergic receptors are β_2 receptors. When stimulated by epinephrine, β_2 receptors produce vasodilation, particularly in the coronary arteries and skeletal muscle blood vessels. β_2 receptors can produce the relaxation of bronchiolar smooth muscle. NE does not affect β_2 receptors.

CHOLINERGIC RECEPTORS

The parasympathetic nervous system, also known as the *cholinergic nervous system*, releases the neurotransmitter ACh. Receptors that respond to cholinergic stimulation are called *cholinergic receptors*. Drugs that bind to cholinergic receptors are referred to as *cholinergic drugs* and exhibit effects similar to those of ACh. Agents that bind to cholinergic receptors and prevent ACh from acting on its receptors (antagonism) are called *cholinergic-blocking drugs* (see Figure 18-3).

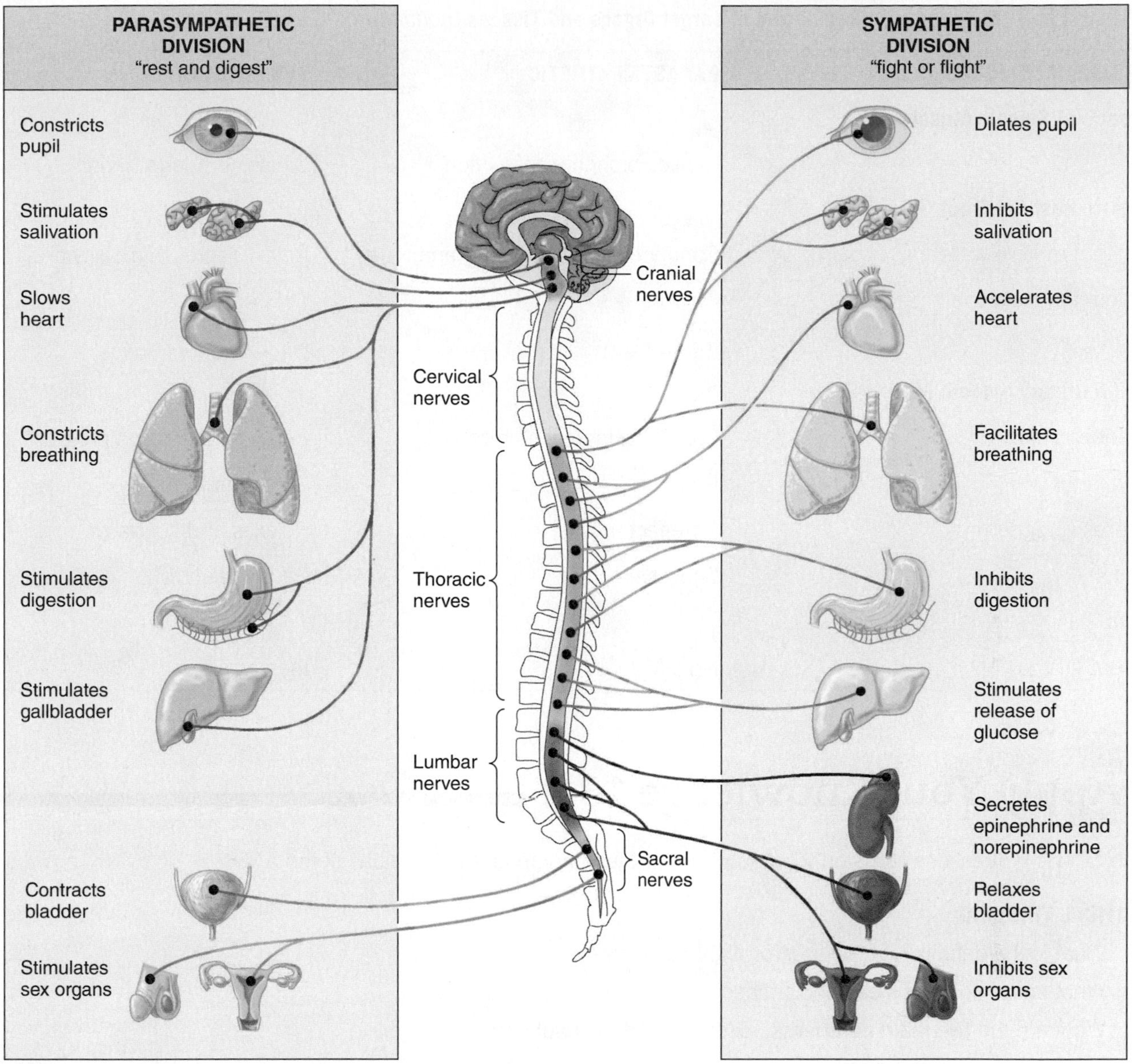

Figure 18-4 ■
"Rest and digest" effects of the parasympathetic nervous system; "fight-or-flight" effects of the sympathetic nervous system.

Table 18-1 ■ Autonomic Regulation of Target Organs and Tissues

ORGANS OR TISSUES	PARASYMPATHETIC	SYMPATHETIC
Eyes		
Pupillary response	Causes constriction (miosis)	Causes dilation (mydriasis)
Heart		
	Decreases heart rate	Increases heart rate
	No effect	Increases arrhythmias
Blood Vessels		
Skin	No effect	Causes vasoconstriction
Skeletal muscle vessels	No effect	Relax; cause vasodilation

(continued)

Table 18-1 ■ Autonomic Regulation of Target Organs and Tissues (*continued*)

ORGANS OR TISSUES	PARASYMPATHETIC	SYMPATHETIC
Bronchial Smooth Muscle		
	Causes bronchoconstriction	Causes bronchodilation
Gastrointestinal Tract		
Smooth muscle walls	Contract; increase motility and tone	Relax; decrease motility and tone
Smooth muscle sphincter	Relaxes	Contracts
Secretion	Increases	No effect
Genitourinary Smooth Muscle		
Bladder wall	Contracts; increase pressure	Relaxes; decreases pressure
Sphincter	Relaxes	Contracts
Uterus (pregnant)	No effect	Relaxes and contracts
Penis	Causes erection	Causes ejaculation
Skin		
Sweat glands	No effect	Increases

✳ Apply Your Knowledge 18.2

The following questions focus on what you have just learned about the functions of the ANS.

CRITICAL THINKING

1. What is the definition of the fight-or-flight response?
2. What are endogenous catecholamines?
3. What are the two main adrenergic receptors and their subdivisions?
4. What is the "rest and digest" response?
5. What is the effect of the sympathetic nervous system on the eyes, heart, and bronchial smooth muscle?
6. What is the effect of the parasympathetic nervous system on the bladder wall, penis, bronchial smooth muscle, and uterus (in pregnant women)?
7. What are cholinergic receptors?
8. What is another name of the parasympathetic nervous system?

Focus on Geriatrics

Effects of Stress in Elderly Patients

Elderly people experience many losses and changes in their lives. These changes may be incremental and, over time, become stressful and possibly overwhelming. Stress can have physical, emotional, intellectual, social, and spiritual consequences. Usually, the effects are mixed because stress affects every person uniquely.

Drug Effects on the Autonomic Nervous System

Autonomic drugs are categorized based on which receptors can be stimulated or blocked.

1. **Sympathomimetics** (or adrenergic agonists) produce symptoms of the fight-or-flight response and stimulate the sympathetic nervous system.

2. Parasympathomimetics (or cholinergic agonists) produce symptoms of the rest-and-relaxation response and stimulate the parasympathetic nervous system.

3. Adrenergic blockers produce actions opposite to sympathomimetics and inhibit the sympathetic nervous system.

4. Anticholinergics (or cholinergic blockers) produce actions opposite to parasympathomimetics and inhibit the parasympathetic nervous system.

Focus on Natural Products

Essential Fatty Acids

Essential fatty acids, which cannot be manufactured by the body, are most commonly found in poly-unsaturated vegetable oils. Both omega-3 and omega-6 fatty acids are converted in the body into powerful hormone-like substances (prostaglandins) that affect almost every biologic function, including the regulation of smooth muscle and autonomic reflexes. Omega-6 fatty acids are present in food sources, and it is important to balance their intake with omega-3 fatty acids, which are found in fish and flaxseed oil. Adding 1 Tbsp of flaxseed oil to your daily diet is beneficial.

ADRENERGIC AGONISTS OR SYMPATHOMIMETIC DRUGS

The adrenergic agonists are categorized as catecholamines and noncatecholamines. The catecholamines include NE, which is released at the nerve terminals; epinephrine, from the adrenal medulla; and dopamine, from sites in the brain, kidneys, and gastrointestinal (GI) tract. These types of drugs can be made synthetically to produce the same effects as those of the naturally secreted neurotransmitters. The noncatecholamines have somewhat similar actions to the catecholamines but are more selective of receptor sites, are not quite as fast acting, and have a longer duration. The medications of the adrenergic agonist class mimic the sympathetic nervous system and are also called *sympathomimetics* or *adrenergic agonists*. Classifications of sympathomimetic drugs are listed in Table 18-2 ■.

Table 18-2 ■ Classifications of Sympathomimetic Drugs

GENERIC NAME	TRADE NAME	PRIMARY USE
Catecholamines		
dopamine	Intropin (α_1 and β_1)	Shock
epinephrine	Adrenalin, Primatene (α and β)	Asthma, cardiac arrest
isoproterenol	Isuprel (β_1 and β_2)	Asthma, dysrhythmias, heart failure
norepinephrine	Levarterenol, Levophed (α and β)	Shock
Alpha$_1$ Agonists		
methoxamine	Vasoxyl	Maintains blood pressure during anesthesia
midodrine	Pro Amatine	Orthostatic hypotension
oxymetazoline	Afrin	Nasal congestion
phenylephrine	Neo-Synephrine	Nasal congestion
xylometazoline	Otrivin	Nasal congestion

(continued)

Table 18-2 ■ Classifications of Sympathomimetic Drugs (*continued*)

GENERIC NAME	TRADE NAME	PRIMARY USE
Alpha$_2$ Agonists		
apraclonidine	Iopidine	Operative eye pressure, glaucoma
clonidine	Catapres (in the CNS)	Hypertension
guanabenz	Wytensin	Hypertension
guanfacine	Tenex	Hypertension
methyldopa	AdoMet (in the CNS)	Hypertension
Beta$_1$ Agonists		
dobutamine	Dobutrex	Cardiac stimulant
Beta$_2$ Agonists		
albuterol	Ventolin	Asthma
metaproterenol	Alupent	Asthma
ritodrine	Yutopar	Slows uterine contractions
salmeterol	Serevent	Decongestant
terbutaline	Brethine	Asthma
Miscellaneous Adrenergic Agonists		
amphetamine*	Generic	Narcolepsy, ADD, obesity
ephedrine	Generic	Allergies, asthma, narcolepsy
methylphenidate*	Ritalin	ADHD, obesity
pemoline	Cylert	ADHD
pseudoephedrine	Sudafed (α and β)	Rhinitis, coryza, sinusitis

*Discussed in Chapter 17 as central nervous system (CNS) stimulants. These agents are primarily used for their CNS effects and are not used for the same indications as pseudoephedrine and other similar agents. Ephedrine has strictly controlled uses within the United States.

ADD, attention deficit disorder; ADHD, Attention deficit hyperactivity disorder.

As previously discussed, there are two principal types of adrenoreceptors: alpha (α) and beta (β). These receptors have been further subdivided into the main subtypes of α_1, α_2, β_1, and β_2.

The activation of alpha and beta receptors through the administration of adrenergic agonists produces effects consistent with sympathetic (fight-or-flight) stimulation.

Focus On

Alpha$_1$-Receptor Agonists

Alpha$_1$ receptors are located on blood vessels and influence blood pressure and blood flow into the tissues (called *tissue perfusion*). Resistance to blood flow is determined by the diameter of the vessels. Alpha$_1$ receptors are also found on the muscles of the iris; on smooth muscle of the GI tract and male and female reproductive tracts; and in liver cells, sweat glands, and sphincters of the urinary bladder.

How do they work?

The stimulation of α_1 receptors causes vasoconstriction of blood vessels, dilation of the pupils (mydriasis), decreased GI motility, contraction of the external sphincter of the bladder, decreased bile secretion, and stimulation of sweat glands.

How are they used?

Alpha$_1$-receptor agonists are used to treat hypotension, nasal congestion, and subconjunctival hemorrhage (red eye).

What are the adverse effects?

The common adverse effects of α_1-receptor agonists are hypertension, blurred vision, constipation, urine retention, gooseflesh, and sweating.

What are the contraindications and interactions?

Alpha$_1$-receptor agonists are contraindicated for severe coronary or cardiovascular disease; glaucoma; hypovolemia (within 2 weeks of taking monoamine oxidase inhibitors [MAOIs]); acute kidney disease; urine retention; pheochromocytoma (adrenal tumor); thyrotoxicosis (hyperthyroidism or Graves's disease); sensitivity to adrenergic substances; supine hypertension (that is, when lying down); ventricular tachycardia; and for pregnant, lactating, and very young patients. Drug interactions occur with digoxin, doxazosin, ephedrine, guanethidine, halothane, methyldopa, oxytocin, phentolamine, phenothiazines, phenylpropanolamine, prazosin, pseudoephedrine, reserpine, alpha blockers, beta blockers, atropine, MAOIs, terazosin, tricyclic antidepressants (TCAs), vasopressin, and ergot alkaloids.

What are the important points patients should know?

Instruct patients taking α_1-receptor agonists to inform their health-care providers if they have high blood pressure, thyroid disease, an enlarged prostate, glaucoma, or are breastfeeding. Also, instruct patients to inform their doctors of other prescriptions they are taking, such as antihypertensive medicines, thyroid medications, other decongestants, and TCAs. Caution them against taking more than the prescribed dosage or of combining these medications with over-the-counter (OTC) drugs without consulting their health-care providers.

Alpha$_2$-Receptor Agonists

Alpha$_2$ receptors are believed to be located on the presynaptic neurons, and they seem to function as controllers of neurotransmitter release by the presynaptic neurons. They are often used in reducing blood pressure.

How do they work?

These agonists stimulate alpha$_2$ adrenergic receptors in the CNS to inhibit sympathetic vasomotor centers. They reduce plasma concentrations of NE, decrease systolic blood pressure and heart rate, and inhibit renin release from the kidneys.

How are they used?

These agonists are used to treat hypertension—either alone or with diuretic or other hypertensive agents. They are also used epidurally as adjunct therapy for severe pain.

What are the adverse effects?

Adverse effects of these agonists include hypotension, peripheral edema, dry mouth or eyes, constipation, drowsiness, dizziness, rash, pruritus, impotence, nausea and vomiting, hepatitis, hallucinations, depression, and recurrent herpes simplex.

What are the contraindications and interactions?

These agonists are contraindicated in pediatric, pregnant, and lactating patients; hypertension that is associated with toxemia of pregnancy; polyarteritis nodosa (swollen or damaged arteries); scleroderma (skin hardening); hepatitis; cirrhosis; pheochromocytoma; and blood dyscrasias. Interactions include alcohol and other CNS depressants, amphetamines, TCAs, ephedrine, haloperidol, levodopa, lithium, MAOIs, methotrimeprazine, opiate analgesics, phenothiazines, phenoxybenzamine, digoxin, calcium channel blockers, or beta blockers.

What are the important points patients should know?

Instruct patients with hypertension that excessive sodium leads to fluid retention and to avoid foods that are high in sodium, including canned, frozen, or dehydrated soup; processed cheese; salted biscuits; potato chips; and pretzels.

(Continued)

Focus On (Continued)

. . . .

Beta$_1$-Receptor Agonists

Beta$_1$ receptors are located on the myocardium, adipocytes (fat cells), sphincters and smooth muscle of the GI tract, and renal arterioles.

How do they work?

Beta$_1$-receptor agonists increase the rate and force of contraction of the heart, increase lipolysis in adipose tissue, decrease digestion and GI motility, and increase glomerular filtration.

How are they used?

Beta$_1$-receptor agonists are used to treat circulatory shock, hypotension, and cardiac arrest. Two important drugs represent this group: dobutamine (Dobutrex), a selective β_1-receptor agonist, and isoproterenol (Isuprel), a nonselective β_1-receptor agonist.

What are the adverse effects?

The common adverse effects of β_1-receptor agonists include hypertension, tachycardia, and constipation.

What are the contraindications and interactions?

Beta$_1$-receptor agonists are contraindicated in patients with a history of hypersensitivity to other sympathomimetic amines (nitrogen compounds); in those with ventricular tachycardia; in pediatric, pregnant, or lactating patients; or after an acute myocardial infarction (MI). Interactions can occur with general anesthetics (especially cyclopropane and halothane), such beta-adrenergic blocking agents as metoprolol and propranolol, MAOIs, and TCAs.

What are the important points patients should know?

Alert patients that sputum and saliva may turn pink after the inhalation of isoproterenol. Warn patients not to breastfeed when taking these agents. Patients should not increase, decrease, or omit doses or change intervals between doses. Advise patients to immediately report anginal pain to their health-care providers.

. . . .

Beta$_2$-Receptor Agonists

These adrenoreceptors are distributed on the smooth muscle of the bronchioles; in skeletal muscle; in blood vessels supplying the brain, heart, kidneys, and skeletal muscle; in the uterus; and in liver cells.

How do they work?

Stimulation of β_2 receptors results in bronchodilation; increased skeletal muscle excitability; vasodilation of blood vessels to the brain, heart, kidneys, and skeletal muscle; and relaxation of the uterus in pregnancy.

How are they used?

Beta$_2$-receptor agonists are used in patients with chronic obstructive airway disease, circulatory shock, premature labor, and peripheral vascular disease.

What are the adverse effects?

The common adverse effects of β_2-receptor agonists include muscle tremor (in the hands), increased muscle tension, and feelings of warmth. These agents also cause hyperglycemia (increased blood glucose).

What are the contraindications and interactions?

Beta$_2$-receptor agonists are contraindicated in pediatric, pregnant, or lactating patients; in those who are sensitive to other sympathomimetic agents; and in patients with cardiac arrhythmias associated with tachycardia or digitalis intoxication, hyperthyroidism, preeclampsia (hypertension during pregnancy), eclampsia (coma and convulsions related to pregnancy), intrauterine infection, hypertension, diabetes mellitus, hypovolemia (decrease in volume of circulating blood), thyrotoxicosis, asthma that is treated with beta-mimetics, hypersensitivity, coronary artery disease (within 14 days of MAOI therapy), and angle-closure glaucoma. Interactions can occur with beta-adrenergic blockers, corticosteroids, epinephrine, other sympathomimetic bronchodilators, MAOIs, and TCAs.

What are the important points patients should know?

Instruct patients about using the inhaler correctly and have them demonstrate the technique for you. Warn patients not to change the dose or frequency of doses. Patients should know that these drugs may cause dizziness (albuterol) or tremor (metaproterenol), so advise them to change positions slowly. They should not take other OTC drugs or breastfeed without first consulting their health-care providers. Advise patients to report if the drug fails to reduce symptoms.

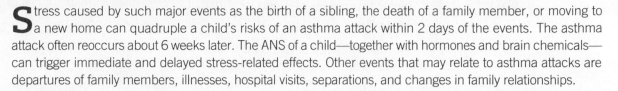

Focus on Pediatrics

Stress and Childhood Asthma

Stress caused by such major events as the birth of a sibling, the death of a family member, or moving to a new home can quadruple a child's risks of an asthma attack within 2 days of the events. The asthma attack often reoccurs about 6 weeks later. The ANS of a child—together with hormones and brain chemicals—can trigger immediate and delayed stress-related effects. Other events that may relate to asthma attacks are departures of family members, illnesses, hospital visits, separations, and changes in family relationships.

ADRENERGIC ANTAGONISTS OR SYMPATHOLYTICS

Similar to sympathomimetic agents, sympatholytics can act either directly or indirectly. Direct-acting sympatholytics are antagonists that have an affinity for a receptor but block the normal response. Adrenergic antagonists can show specificity for one receptor or subtype. Indirect-acting agents block adrenergic nerve transmission—usually by inhibiting the release of neurotransmitters or depleting the stores of transmitters. Table 18-3 ■ lists the common adrenergic antagonists.

Table 18-3 ■ Adrenergic Antagonists

GENERIC NAME	TRADE NAME	AVERAGE ADULT DOSE	ROUTE OF ADMINISTRATION	PRIMARY USE
Alpha-Receptor Antagonists				
doxazosin	Cardura	Start 1 mg at bedtime and titrate up to max of 16 mg/d in one or two divided doses	PO	Hypertension
phenoxybenzamine	Dibenzyline	5–10 mg bid; may increase by 10 mg/d at 4-d intervals to desired response	PO	Pheochromocytoma
phentolamine	Regitine	2–5 mg as needed	IV, IM	Hypertensive episode during surgery
prazosin	Minipress	Start 1 mg at bedtime and then 1 mg bid or tid; may increase to 20 mg/d in divided doses	PO	Hypertension
terazosin	Hytrin	Start 1 mg at bedtime and then 1–5 mg/d (maximum: 20 mg/d)	PO	Hypertension, urinary obstruction
Beta-Receptor Antagonists (Nonselective)				
labetalol	Normodyne	100 mg bid (maximum: 2,400 mg/d)	PO	Hypertension
		20 mg slowly (maximum: 300 mg total dose)	IV	Hypertension
nadolol	Corgard	40 mg/d (maximum: 320 mg/d in one or two divided doses)	PO	Hypertension, angina

(continued)

Table 18-3 ■ Adrenergic Antagonists (*continued*)

GENERIC NAME	TRADE NAME	AVERAGE ADULT DOSE	ROUTE OF ADMINISTRATION	PRIMARY USE
pindolol	Visken	5 mg bid (maximum: 60 mg/d in two or three divided doses)	PO	Hypertension
		15–40 mg/d in three or four divided doses	PO	Angina pectoris
propranolol	Inderal	10–40 mg bid (maximum: 480 mg/d)	PO	Hypertension, angina, acute MI, and dysrhythmias
timolol	Betimol	10–45 mg in bid–tid/d (maximum: 60 mg/d in two divided doses)	PO	Hypertension, angina
Beta-Receptor Antagonists (Selective)				
acebutolol	Sectral	200–800 mg/d in one or two divided doses (maximum: 1200 mg/d)	PO	Hypertension, dysrhythmias
atenolol	Tenormin	25–50 mg/d (maximum: 100 mg/d)	PO	Hypertension, angina pectoris
		5 mg q5min in two doses	IV	MI
esmolol	Brevibloc	25–50 mg/d (maximum: 100 mg/d)	IV	Supraventricular tachydysrhythmias
metoprolol	Lopressor	50–100 mg/d in one or two divided doses (maximum: 450 mg/d)	IV	Hypertension
		100 mg/d in two divided doses (maximum: 400 mg/d)	PO	Angina pectoris
		5 mg q2min for three doses and then PO therapy	PO	MI
		50 mg q6h for 48 h and then 100 mg bid	PO	MI

bid, bid twice a day; IM, intramuscular; MI, myocardial infarction; IV, intravenous; PO, oral; tid, three times a day.

Focus On

Alpha-Receptor Antagonists

Alpha-receptor antagonists can work in a reversible or an irreversible manner. Some are nonselective and antagonize α_1 and α_2 receptors. Others are highly selective for α_1 receptors. All antagonize the effects of endogenous catecholamines.

How do they work?

These antagonists selectively inhibit the actions of alpha adrenoreceptors, producing vasodilation in arterioles and veins, with the result that peripheral vascular resistance and blood pressure are reduced.

How are they used?

Applications for alpha-receptor antagonists include control of hypertension and treatment of patients with peripheral vascular disease, adrenal medulla tumor (pheochromocytoma), and urinary retention.

What are the adverse effects?

The common adverse effects of alpha-receptor antagonists include nasal congestion and stuffiness, postural hypotension (which occurs on sitting or standing), inhibition of ejaculation, and lack of energy.

What are the contraindications and interactions?

A contraindication for the use of alpha-receptor antagonists is known hypersensitivity to any of these drugs. Interactions can occur with diuretics, ephedrine, epinephrine, methoxamine, NE, other hypotensive agents, nonsteroidal anti-inflammatory drugs, and phenylephrine.

What are the important points patients should know?

Because these drugs may cause dizziness, advise patients to change positions slowly. Patients should avoid driving for at least 12 hours after taking the first dose to determine side effects. Patients should not breastfeed while taking these drugs or take OTC drugs for coughs, colds, or allergies without discussing it with their health-care providers.

Beta-Receptor Antagonists

Beta$_2$ antagonists work against the effects of catecholamines at beta adrenoreceptors. Beta-blocking drugs reduce receptor occupancy by beta agonists. Most of these agents are pure antagonists and occupy beta receptors, causing no activation of the receptors.

How do they work?

Beta blockade by these antagonists results in vasodilation, decreased peripheral resistance, and orthostatic hypotension. These agents work primarily on cardiac muscle, competitively blocking beta-adrenergic receptors within the heart.

How are they used?

These agents are used in the management of hypertension—sometimes with a thiazide diuretic—for patients who have failed to respond to diet, exercise, and weight reduction. They are also used to treat cardiac arrhythmias, MI, tachyarrhythmias, hypertrophic subaortic stenosis (thickening of the ventricular septum or wall), angina pectoris, pheochromocytoma, and hereditary essential tremor.

What are the adverse effects?

Common adverse effects of beta-receptor antagonists are dizziness, lethargy, insomnia, and diarrhea.

What are the contraindications and interactions?

Beta-blockers are contraindicated in patients with known hypersensitivity, heart block, severe heart failure, cardiogenic shock, and other severe circulatory disorders. These agents should be avoided in patients with a history of asthma or chronic obstructive airway disease unless no alternative is available. Interactions can occur with phenothiazines, beta-adrenergic agonists, atropine, TCAs, diuretics and other hypotensive agents, tubocurarine, cimetidine, and antacids.

What are the important points patients should know?

Teach patients to take their heart rate and blood pressure and to report a decrease in either. Because these drugs may cause dizziness, advise patients to change positions slowly. Patients should avoid driving for at least 12 hours after taking the first dose to determine side effects. Patients should not breastfeed while taking these drugs or take OTC drugs for coughs, colds, or allergies without discussing it with their health-care providers. Warn patients not to discontinue these drugs suddenly. Advise patients to check with their health-care providers before taking OTC medications.

(Continued)

Focus On (*Continued*)

. . . .

Parasympathomimetics or Cholinergic Agonists

Cholinergic agonists (also called *parasympathomimetics* or *cholinomimetics*) stimulate the parasympathetic nervous system because they mimic the parasympathetic neurotransmitter ACh. This neurotransmitter is located at the ganglions and the parasympathetic terminal nerve endings. It stimulates the receptors in tissues, organs, and glands. There are two types of cholinergic receptors: (1) **muscarinic receptors** (which innervate smooth muscle and slow the heart rate) and (2) **nicotinic receptors** (which affect the skeletal muscles). Many cholinergic drugs are nonselective and can therefore affect the muscarinic and the nicotinic receptors. However, selective cholinergic drugs for the muscarinic receptors do not affect the nicotinic receptors.

How do they work?

The rapid destruction of systemically administered ACh by cholinesterases makes the endogenous (self-produced) neurotransmitter of limited clinical value. Clinically useful cholinomimetic drugs are either cholinergic agonists that are resistant to the hydrolytic (water-eliminating) action of cholinesterases or agents that inhibit cholinesterases. Based on their mechanisms of action, cholinomimetic drugs may be classified as direct-acting agents (agonists) or indirect-acting agents (anticholinesterases).

How are they used?

Pilocarpine (Isopto-Carpine) is a direct-acting cholinergic drug that is used most commonly in ophthalmology to reduce elevated intraocular pressure in patients with glaucoma and induce miosis. Specific muscarinic agonist drugs that are nonspecific may be used in the treatment of constipation that is caused by a lack of muscle tone (called *atonic*), congenital megacolon, and postoperative and postpartum intestinal ileus (that is, an obstructed bowel). Bethanechol (Urecholine) has been used to increase the tone of the lower esophageal sphincter in the treatment of patients with reflux esophagitis. In the genitourinary tract, muscarinic agonists are useful in the treatment of those with postoperative and postpartum nonobstructive urine retention and neurogenic urinary bladder with retention. The primary use of the drug in the cardiovascular field is in the diagnosis of atrial tachycardia. In pulmonary practice, the hypersensitivity of patients with asthma to bronchiolar constriction induced by cholinomimetics makes methacholine useful in the diagnosis of asthma. Muscarinic agonists are also known to increase secretion of the salivary and lacrimal glands. They are used to treat symptoms of dry mouth caused by radiotherapy for cancer of the head and neck. The most common cholinomimetic drugs are summarized in Table 18-4 ■.

What are the adverse effects?

Adverse effects produced by the cholinomimetics can be predicted based on the pharmacodynamic activity of the drugs. Thus, undesirable effects may include flushing, sweating, abdominal cramps, difficulty in visual accommodation, headache, and convulsions at high doses. Specific GI adverse effects include nausea, vomiting, diarrhea, and abdominal pain. Other adverse effects are bronchospasm, excessive salivation, and urinary frequency.

What are the contraindications and interactions?

Muscarinic drugs are contraindicated in the presence of atrioventricular arrhythmias, coronary insufficiency, hyperthyroidism, asthma, and peptic ulcer. Interactions can occur with ambenonium, neostigmine, and other cholinesterase inhibitors; mecamylamine; procainamide; quinidine; atropine; epinephrine; beta-adrenergic agonists; and parasympathomimetic drugs.

What are the important points patients should know?

Advise patients to inform their health-care providers of any other drugs they are taking. Because these drugs may cause dizziness, caution patients to change positions slowly. Warn patients not to breastfeed without a health-care provider's approval. Explain to patients that they may experience increased sweating and urinary frequency.

Cholinergic Blockers

Drugs that inhibit the actions of ACh by occupying the ACh receptors are called *cholinergic antagonists* or **cholinergic blockers** (also called **anticholinergics** or **parasympatholytics**). The major body tissues and organs affected by the cholinergic-blocking agents include the heart, respiratory tract, urinary bladder, eyes, GI tract, and sweat glands.

Table 18-4 ■ Cholinergic Agents

GENERIC NAME	TRADE NAME	AVERAGE ADULT DOSE	ROUTE OF ADMINISTRATION	PRIMARY USE
Direct-Acting Cholinergic Agonists				
bethanechol	Duvoid	10–50 mg qid (maximum: 120 mg/d)	Subcutaneously	Nonobstructive urine retention
	Urabeth	2.5–5 mg; repeat at 15–30 min intervals PRN	PO	
carbachol	Miostat	1–2 drops q4–8h; 0.5 mL injected	Intraocular; topical	Glaucoma
cevimeline	Evoxac	30 mg tid	PO	Dry mouth from Sjögren's syndrome
pilocarpine	Pilocar	1–2 gtt in eye 1–6 times/d	Ocular	Glaucoma
Indirect-Acting Cholinergic Agonists				
ambenonium	Mytelase	5–75 mg qid	PO	Myasthenia gravis
edrophonium	Enlon, Tensilon	2 mg injected over 15–30 sec; if no reaction, inject 8 mg after 45 sec	IV	Diagnosis of myasthenia gravis
neostigmine	Prostigmin	15–375 mg/d in three to six divided doses	PO	Myasthenia gravis, urine retention
pyridostigmine	Mestinon	60 mg–1.5 g/d 180–540 mg one or two times/d by sustained release	PO	Myasthenia gravis
tacrine	Cognex	10–40 mg/d (maximum: 160 mg/d)	PO	Alzheimer's disease

PO, oral; PRN, as needed; qid, four times a day; tid, three times a day.

Focus On

Atropine

Atropine (Atropair, AtroPen) is a classic anticholinergic or muscarinic antagonist drug. Atropine was first derived from the belladonna plant. Scopolamine was the second belladonna alkaloid produced. Atropine and scopolamine act on the muscarinic receptor, but they have little effect on the nicotinic receptor.

How does it work?

Atropine acts by selectively blocking all muscarinic responses to ACh—whether excitatory or inhibitory. Selective depression of the CNS relieves the rigidity and tremor of Parkinson's syndrome.

How is it used?

Atropine is used adjunctively to treat the symptoms of GI disorders; to treat ophthalmic disorders, various cardiac conditions, bronchial conditions, chronic obstructive airway disease, and upper respiratory infections; and to counteract mushroom poisoning. It is also used in preoperative situations.

What are the adverse effects?

The common adverse effects of atropine and atropine-like drugs include dry mouth, decreased perspiration,

(Continued)

Focus On (*Continued*)

blurred vision, tachycardia, constipation, and urine retention. Other adverse effects are nausea, headache, dry skin, abdominal distension, hypotension or hypertension, impotence, photophobia, and coma.

What are the contraindications and interactions?

Atropine is contraindicated for patients with hypersensitivity to belladonna alkaloids, with angle-closure glaucoma, parotitis (inflammation of the saliva glands), obstructive uropathy, intestinal atony (muscular weakness), paralytic ileus, GI obstructions, severe ulcerative colitis, toxic megacolon, tachycardia, acute hemorrhage, and myasthenia gravis (muscle weakness brought on by movement) and in pregnant or lactating patients. Interactions include amantadine, antihistamines, TCAs, quinidine, disopyramide, procainamide, levodopa, methotrimeprazine, and phenothiazines.

What are the important points patients should know?

Encourage patients receiving atropine to use frequent mouth rinses, chew gum, or suck on sugarless sourball candy to relieve dry mouth. Meticulous dental hygiene should be encouraged. Caution patients to avoid driving. Warn patients not to breastfeed while taking this drug. Tell patients to report a fast heartbeat or palpitations.

Focus Point

Ecstasy and the Autonomic Nervous System

3,4 methylenedioxymethamphetamine (MDMA) is an illegal drug known as Ecstasy. Other names for MDMA are *Adam, XTC, Doves*, and just *E*. Originally patented as an appetite suppressant, data now show that MDMA may be toxic to the brain. This drug is a serious problem in the United States because of its trendiness among teenagers, who may be unaware of its harmful effects. Studies have shown a 20% to 60% reduction in healthy serotonin cells in the brains of MDMA users, damaging their ability to remember and to learn. Tests on the brains of monkeys showed brain damage that remained visible 7 years after the monkeys were given MDMA.

✱ Apply Your Knowledge 18.3

The following questions focus on what you have just learned about drug effects on the ANS.

CRITICAL THINKING

1. What is the mechanism of action of alpha$_1$-receptor agonists?
2. What are the indications of beta$_1$-receptor agonists?
3. What are the contraindications of beta$_2$-receptor agonists?
4. What is the mechanism of action of beta-receptor antagonists?
5. What are the trade names of propranolol, prazosin, atenolol, metaproterenol, and dopamine?
6. What is the mechanism of action of cholinergic blockers?
7. What are the two types of cholinergic receptors and their effect on the body?
8. What are the trade names of bethanechol, pilocarpine, nadolol, metoprolol, and terbutaline?

PRACTICAL SCENARIO 1

The emergency medical services (EMS) team has brought a 54-year-old female patient to the emergency department where you are working. The EMS personnel state that the patient was found wandering in a nearby park by a jogger who called 911 from her cell phone after the woman screamed obscenities at her and then fell, seriously scraping her arm and face. The woman is bleeding, disoriented, combative, and accusing the EMS team of stealing her purse. Her hands are shaking severely, and she is shouting at the doctors and nurses that she needs a bottle. The woman's clothing is dirty, and you can smell stale body odor and urine.

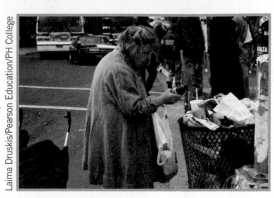

Laima Druskis/Pearson Education/PH College

Critical Thinking Questions

1. Based on your first impressions of this patient's actions and appearance, what do you suspect she is suffering from? (*Hint*: Think about what you learned in Chapters 1 and 9.)
2. What short- and long-term health risks would you suspect this patient faces?
3. Why do you think the patient's hands are shaking, and what do you think causes her confusion and combativeness?
4. What assessments do you think are needed for this patient?

PRACTICAL SCENARIO 2

A 62-year-old woman with a history of glaucoma went to her family physician with symptoms of the common cold. Her physician prescribed medication for her nasal congestion. After two days of use, she noticed that her vision was blurred and she had a severe headache. She was taken to the emergency room of the local hospital.

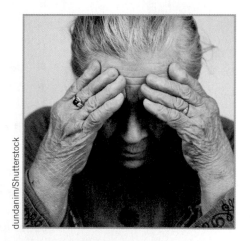

dundanim/Shutterstock

Critical Thinking Questions

1. What is the relationship between nasal decongestants and the woman's history of glaucoma?
2. List the other contraindications of alpha$_1$-receptor agonists.

Chapter Capsule

This section repeats the objectives from the beginning of the chapter and then provides a summary of the most important concepts for that objective. Use this section as a quick review and to check your knowledge.

Objective 1: List the two divisions of the nervous system and their subdivisions.

- Central nervous system (CNS): brain and spinal cord
- Peripheral nervous system (PNS)

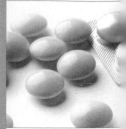

▢ Autonomic nervous system (ANS)

- Motor neurons
  - ◆ Sympathetic nervous system
  - ◆ Parasympathetic nervous system
- Sensory neurons

Objective 2: Explain the basic functional unit cell of the nervous system.

- Neurons—carry nervous system signals throughout body

Objective 3: Define the terms *cholinergic* and *adrenergic*.

- Cholinergic—liberating or activated by the neurotransmitter acetylcholine
- Adrenergic—liberating or activated by norepinephrine, epinephrine, or dopamine

Objective 4: Describe the fight-or-flight response.

- The body's reaction to a sudden threat or source of stress, such as trauma, fear, hypoglycemia, cold, or exercise
- Activates the sympathetic nervous system during emergencies

Objective 5: List the two main adrenergic receptors and what they respond to.

- Alpha receptor—responds to adrenaline
- Beta receptor—responds to norepinephrine and epinephrine

Objective 6: Explain the actions of adrenergic agonists.

- Mimic the sympathetic nervous system
- Produce fight-or-flight symptoms

Objective 7: Explain the actions of receptor agonists.

- Alpha-receptor agonists—influence blood pressure and tissue perfusion
- Beta-receptor agonists—work against catecholamines, reducing receptor occupancy by beta agonists

Objective 8: Define *adrenergic antagonists*.

- Block adrenergic nerve transmission (usually by inhibiting the release of neurotransmitters or depleting the stores of transmitters)

Objective 9: List the two types of cholinergic receptors.

- Muscarinic receptors—innervate smooth muscle and slow the heart rate
- Nicotinic receptors—affect skeletal muscle

Objective 10: Discuss parasympathomimetics (also called *cholinergic agonists*).

- Parasympathomimetics stimulate the parasympathetic nervous system because they mimic the parasympathetic neurotransmitter acetylcholine, which is located at the ganglions and parasympathetic terminal nerve endings.

- There are two types of cholinergic receptors: muscarinic and nicotinic. Many parasympathomimetics are nonselective, but those that are selective affect only one of these types of receptors.

- They are characterized based on their mechanisms of action as either direct-acting agents (agonists) or indirect-acting agents (anticholinesterases).

- The most common direct-acting cholinergic agonists are bethanechol, carbachol, cevimeline, and pilocarpine.

- The most common indirect-acting cholinergic agonists are ambenonium, edrophonium, neostigmine, pyridostigmine, and tacrine.

 Internet Sites of Interest

- Search **http://faculty.washington.edu/chudler/ehceduc.html** for recent research and a great site called Neuroscience for Kids that explains and uses great graphics to illustrate the concepts of neurotransmitters, the autonomic nervous system, and more.

- Go to the American Heart Association's website (**http://www.heart.org/heartorg**) and then search for "autonomic nervous system." You will find information on how the system works in relation to the cardiovascular system. You can also learn how the ANS impacts blood pressure.

- Search for "autonomic nervous system" on MedlinePlus at **http://www.nlm.nih.gov/medlineplus**.

PEARSON
myhealthprofessionskit™

Go to www.myhealthprofessionskit.com to access the Companion Website created for this textbook. Simply select "Basic Health Science" from the choice of disciplines. Find this book and then log in using your username and password to access interactive learning games, assessment questions, animations, and more.

Chapter 19

Anesthetic Agents

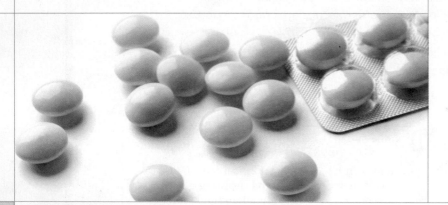

Chapter Objectives

After completing this chapter, you should be able to:

1. Outline the stages of anesthesia.
2. Define the importance of premedications before anesthesia.
3. Explain the action of anesthetics within the central nervous system.
4. List the effects of general anesthetics.
5. Describe the common local anesthetics and their uses.
6. Compare ester and amide local anesthetics
7. List the problems associated with the use of local anesthetics.
8. Explain the indications for spinal anesthesia.
9. Discuss various techniques for local anesthetics.
10. Compare epidural anesthesia with field block anesthesia.

Key Terms

analgesia (an-ul-JEE-zee-ah) (page 329)

anesthesia (an-ess-THEE-zee-ah) (page 329)

anesthetics (an-ess-THET-iks) (page 329)

cryoanesthesia (KRY-o-an-ess-THEE-zee-ah) (page 337)

epidural anesthesia (ep-eh-DUR-al) (page 339)

lipophilic (lie-poh-FIL-lik) (page 332)

preanesthetics (pree-an-ess-THET-ik) (page 330)

regional anesthesia (page 329)

spinal anesthesia (page 339)

subarachnoid (sub-uh-RAK-noyd) (page 339)

volatile liquids (page 332)

Introduction

It was not until the 1840s that surgical anesthesia became possible with the introduction of three agents in quick succession: chloroform, ether, and nitrous oxide. These three agents, when inhaled quickly, led to unconsciousness, and surgical anesthesia was produced. Today, patients having surgery receive medication before, during, and after surgery to achieve specific therapeutic outcomes. Usually, all other medication orders are withheld when a patient goes to surgery.

General **anesthetics** are normally used to produce loss of consciousness before and during surgery. However, for certain minor procedures, an anesthetic may be given in small amounts to relieve anxiety or pain without causing unconsciousness. These are called *local anesthetics*. They numb small areas of tissue where a minor procedure is to be done and are commonly used in dentistry and for minor surgery. **Regional anesthesia** affects a larger (but still limited) part of the body and is often used in obstetrics (labor and delivery). It does not make the person unconscious. Spinal and epidural anesthesia are examples of regional anesthesia.

The ideal anesthetic agent should possess the following characteristics:

* Rapid and pleasant induction and withdrawal from **anesthesia** (loss of sensation, consciousness, or both)
* Skeletal muscle relaxation
* **Analgesia** (pain relief while still conscious)
* High potency
* A wide therapeutic index
* Nonflammability
* Chemical inertness with regard to anesthetic delivery devices

However, in practice, it is common to use a variety of drugs because no single agent meets all these criteria.

Stages of Anesthesia

Before patients reach surgical anesthesia, they go through four stages: analgesia, excitement (delirium), surgical anesthesia, and medullary paralysis.

STAGE 1: **Analgesia** Pain is the first sense to be abolished, and consciousness is still retained. This type of anesthesia is often used in child-birth and in trauma in the form of Entonox, which is a mixture of nitrous oxide and oxygen. The patient inhales the gas until pain recedes but does not inhale enough to reach the unconscious state, thus maintaining some control over the situation. The sense of hearing is often enhanced in this stage.

STAGE 2: **Excitement** This stage may not be a pleasant time of anesthesia. More or less unconscious, the patient may experience shaking and become violent. A sense of extreme fear may be felt, which can produce a phobic response to any suggestion of anesthetics in the future. It is important that the passage from stage 1 to stage 3 be attained as quickly as possible. Sudden death can occur during stage 2, possibly because of vagal nerve inhibition (the vagus nerve extends from the cranium to the abdomen).

STAGE 3: **Surgical anesthesia** This stage is characterized by progressive muscular relaxation. Muscle relaxation is important during many surgical procedures because reflex movements can occur when a scalpel slices through the tissues. This muscular relaxation ends in respiratory paralysis, and unless the patient is on a respirator, death may ensue fairly quickly. These reflexes are abolished with high delivery rates of gaseous anesthetics, but the dividing line between the desired state and respiratory paralysis is narrow. Early anesthetists used various reflexes of the body, such as corneal reflexes and pupillary size, to help them determine when to reduce the amount of anesthetic given to maintain surgical anesthesia but not so much as to return to stage 2. To prevent the danger of respiratory depression, the use of a respirator during surgical procedures is usually obligatory. An endotracheal tube is passed into the trachea, which is connected to the respirator. Unfortunately, the laryngeal reflex (gag reflex) is one of the last reflexes to disappear before stage 4 is reached.

STAGE 4: **Medullary paralysis** This stage begins with respiratory failure and can lead to circulatory collapse. Through careful monitoring, this stage is avoided. If it is reached, it is called an *anesthetic accident*. In the induction of anesthesia with intravenous (IV) anesthetic agents, stages 1 to 3 merge so quickly into one another that they are not apparent.

Focus on Geriatrics

Respiratory Apnea

During the recovery period, the patient must be observed for underventilation by monitoring for respiratory apnea. It is very important to watch elderly patients and those with pre-existing respiratory insufficiency.

Preoperative Medications As Adjuncts to Surgery

Surgical patients are usually given preoperative medications—called **preanesthetics**—45 to 70 minutes before the scheduled surgery. Any delay in administration should be reported promptly to the surgical department.

A combination of preoperative drugs may be ordered to achieve the desired outcomes with minimal side effects. Such outcomes include sedation, reduced anxiety, amnesia to minimize unpleasant surgical memories, increased comfort during preoperative procedures, reduced gastric acidity and volume, increased gastric emptying, decreased nausea and vomiting, and reduced incidence of aspiration by drying oral and respiratory secretions. Table 19-1 ■ lists commonly prescribed preoperative medications.

Table 19-1 ■ Preoperative Medications as Adjuncts to Surgery

GENERIC NAME	TRADE NAME	AVERAGE ADULT DOSAGE	ROUTE OF ADMINISTRATION
Benzodiazepines			
diazepam	Valium	2–10 mg bid–qid or 15–30 mg/d sustained release	PO
		2–10 mg; repeat if needed in 3–4h	IM, IV
lorazepam	Ativan	2–4 mg at least 2 h before surgery	IM
		0.044–2 mg/kg 15–20 min before surgery	IV
midazolam	Versed	Premedicated: 0.15–0.25 mg/kg over 20–30 sec; allow 2 min for effect	IV
		Nonpremedicated: 0.3–0.35 mg/kg over 20–30 sec; allow 2 min for effect	IV
Opioid Analgesics			
meperidine	Demerol	50–150 mg 30–90 min before surgery	IM, subcutaneous
morphine	DepoDur	10–15 mg as single dose 30 min before surgery (maximum: 20 mg)	Epidural
Antacids			
sodium citrate	Bicitra	15–30 mL	PO
H₂-Receptor Antagonists			
cimetidine	Tagamet	300 mg	IM, IV, or PO
famotidine	Pepcid	20 mg	IV
ranitidine	Zantac	50 mg	IM, IV, or PO
Gastric Acid Pump Inhibitors (see Chapter 27 for a complete list)			
lansoprazole	Prevacid	15–60 mg	PO
omeprazole	Prilosec	20–40 mg	PO
Antiemetics			
droperidol	Inapsine	2.5–10 mg 30–60 min before surgery	IM, IV
metoclopramide	Reglan	10 mg administered over 1–2 min	IM, IV
Anticholinergics			
atropine	Atropisol	0.4–0.6 mg	IM, IV
glycopyrrolate	Robinul	0.1–0.3 mg	IM, IV
scopolamine	Hyoscine	0.5–1 mg	IM, IV, subcutaneous

bid, twice a day; IM, intramuscular; IV, intravenous; PO, oral; qid, four times a day.

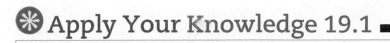

✳ Apply Your Knowledge 19.1

The following questions focus on what you have just learned about the types of anesthesia and the use of preoperative medications as adjuncts to surgery.

CRITICAL THINKING

1. What are the differences between general anesthetics and regional anesthesia?
2. What are the characteristics of anesthetic agents?
3. How many stages of anesthesia exist and which stage is dangerous?
4. Why are preanesthetics used before surgery?
5. Why may a combination of preoperative drugs be ordered?

General Anesthetics

General anesthesia affects the entire body and makes the patient unconscious by depressing the central nervous system (CNS). The unconscious patient is completely unaware of what is going on and does not feel pain from the surgery or procedure. Skeletal muscles relax and reflexes also diminish.

The advantages of general anesthesia include rapid excretion of the anesthetic agent and prompt reversal of its effects when desired. In addition, general anesthesia can be used with all age groups and in any type of surgical procedure.

An ideal anesthetic drug would induce anesthesia smoothly and rapidly while allowing for prompt recovery after its administration is discontinued. The drug would also possess a wide margin of safety and be devoid of adverse effects. No single anesthetic agent is capable of achieving all these desirable effects without some disadvantages when used alone. For this reason, modern anesthesiology practice commonly uses combinations of IV and inhaled drugs, taking advantage of each drug's individual favorable properties while attempting to minimize any potential for adverse reactions.

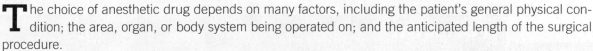

Focus Point

Choosing Appropriate Anesthesia

The choice of anesthetic drug depends on many factors, including the patient's general physical condition; the area, organ, or body system being operated on; and the anticipated length of the surgical procedure.

The anesthetic technique varies depending on the proposed type of diagnostic, therapeutic, or surgical intervention. For minor procedures, conscious sedation is used by using oral or parenteral sedatives in conjunction with local anesthetics. These techniques provide profound analgesia but retain the patient's ability to maintain his or her own airway and to respond to verbal commands. For more extensive surgical procedures, anesthesia frequently includes the use of preoperative benzodiazepines, the induction of anesthesia with IV thiopental or propofol, and the maintenance of anesthesia with a combination of inhaled and IV anesthetic drugs.

Focus on Geriatrics

Adverse Drug Reactions

Older adults are more likely to experience adverse drug reactions than younger adults because, in general, they take more prescription medications. These adverse reactions may be drug–drug interactions, drug–disease interactions (in which a drug may adversely affect a patient with a certain condition), or drug–food interactions.

TYPES OF GENERAL ANESTHETICS

General anesthetics are usually given by inhalation or by IV injection.

Inhalation Anesthetics

Drugs given to induce or maintain general anesthesia are given either as gases or vapors (inhalation anesthetics) or injections (IV anesthetics). Most commonly, these two forms are combined, although it is possible to deliver anesthesia solely by inhalation or injection.

Inhalation anesthetic agents are either **volatile liquids** (easily vaporized) or gases and are usually delivered by using an anesthesia machine. These machines allow mixtures of anesthetic agents with oxygen. Anesthetics and ambient air are delivered to the patient, who is monitored along with the machine's parameters. Liquid anesthetics are vaporized in the machine.

Many compounds have been used for inhalation anesthesia, but only a few are still in widespread use. Today, desflurane (Suprane) and sevoflurane (Ultane) are the most widely used volatile anesthetics. They are often combined with nitrous oxide (Entonox). Older, less popular volatile anesthetics include isoflurane (Forane), halothane (Fluothane, Somnothane), enflurane (Ethrane), and methoxyflurane (Penthrane). The major inhalation anesthetics are listed in Table 19-2 ■.

Table 19-2 ■ General Anesthetics Used by Inhalation

GENERIC NAME	TRADE NAME	PHYSICAL STATE AT ROOM TEMPERATURE
desflurane	Suprane	Volatile liquid
enflurane	Ethrane	Volatile liquid
halothane	Fluothane, Somnothane	Volatile liquid
isoflurane	Forane	Volatile liquid
methoxyflurane	Penthrane	Volatile liquid
nitrous oxide (laughing gas)	Entonox	Gas
sevoflurane	Ultane	Volatile liquid

Focus Point

The Dangers of Malignant Hyperthermia

Malignant hyperthermia is a life-threatening, acute pharmacogenetic disorder that develops during or after anesthesia. This is a disorder that presents itself in some patients undergoing anesthesia and, in some cases, in the postoperative care unit. Hyperthermia is characterized by a rapid increase in body temperature, unexplained tachycardia, unstable blood pressure, muscle rigidity, and cyanosis. The body temperature may increase to above 115°F (46°C).

Focus On

Intravenous Anesthetics

Injectable anesthetics are used for the induction and maintenance of a state of unconsciousness. Anesthetists prefer to use IV injections because they are faster, less painful, and more reliable than intramuscular or subcutaneous injections. Among the most widely used drugs (Table 19-3 ■) are propofol (Diprivan); etomidate (Amidate); such barbiturates as methohexital (Brevital) and thiopental (Pentothal); such benzodiazepines as midazolam (Versed) and diazepam (Valium); and ketamine (Ketalar).

How do they work?

The mechanism of action of most of the IV agents is principally confined to the CNS. A common property of all general anesthetics is that they are all very **lipophilic** (able to dissolve much more easily in lipids than in water). This property is essential because the drug must cross the blood–brain barrier to be effective. Cell membranes are, by nature, lipophilic and hydrophilic depending on the site in the membrane. When the lipophilic anesthetic enters the lipid membrane, the whole membrane is slightly distorted and closes the sodium channels, causing a marginal blockage, which prevents neural conduction (Figure 19-1 ■).

How are they used?

Volatile anesthetics are rarely used as the sole agents for the induction and maintenance of anesthesia. Most commonly, IV and volatile anesthetics are combined in regimens of so-called balanced anesthesia. Of the inhaled anesthetics, nitrous oxide (Entonox), desflurane (Suprane), sevoflurane (Ultane), and isoflurane (Forane) are the most commonly used in the United States.

Use of the more soluble volatile anesthetics has declined during the past decade because more surgical procedures are being performed on an outpatient or short-stay basis. Desflurane (Suprane) and sevoflurane (Ultane) allow a more rapid recovery and produce fewer postoperative adverse effects than halothane (Fluothane, Somnothane) or isoflurane (Forane). Although halothane (Fluothane, Somnothane) is still used in pediatric anesthesia, sevoflurane (Ultane) is rapidly replacing halothane in this setting.

In the past 2 decades, there has been an increasing use of IV drugs in anesthesia—as adjuncts to inhaled anesthetics and in techniques that do not include inhaled anesthetics. IV drugs such as thiopental (Pentothal), etomidate (Amidate), ketamine (Ketalar), and propofol (Diprivan) have faster onsets of anesthetic action than the fastest of the inhaled gaseous agents such as desflurane (Suprane) and sevoflurane (Ultane). Therefore, IV agents are commonly used for induction of anesthesia.

What are the adverse effects?

Because IV (and inhaled) anesthetics affect the CNS, patients may feel drowsy, weak, or tired for as long as a few days after having general anesthesia. Fuzzy thinking, blurred vision, and coordination problems are also possible. For these reasons, anyone who has had general anesthesia should not drive, operate machinery, or perform other activities that could endanger themselves or others for at least 24 hours or longer if necessary.

After general anesthesia, patients may also complain of headache, shivering, muscle pain, mental or mood changes, nausea or vomiting, sore throat, and nightmares.

What are the contraindications and interactions?

IV anesthetics are contraindicated in patients who have received monoamine oxidase inhibitors (MAOIs) within 14 days. Those who are intolerant to benzodiazepines or have hypersensitivity, myasthenia gravis, acute narrow-angle glaucoma, increased intracranial pressure, impaired cerebral circulation, acute alcohol intoxication, intra-arterial injection, a history of paradoxic excitation, status asthmaticus, and acute intermittent or other hepatic porphyrias should not receive general anesthetics. They are contraindicated in shock and coma and during obstetric procedures, labor and delivery, and lactation. They must be used carefully during pregnancy and in children younger than age 12 years. Interactions occur with alcohol and other CNS depressants, MAOIs, anticonvulsants, cimetidine (Tagamet), levodopa (Larodopa), phenytoin (Dilantin), and phenothiazines and in patients who smoke. The general anesthetic propofol (Diprivan) interacts with alfentanil (Alfenta). Midazolam (Versed) and thiopental (Pentothal) interact with the herbal supplements kava-kava and valerian.

What are the important points patients should know?

Because these drugs can interact with medications administered in the perioperative period, ask the patient about the use of over-the-counter medications, including herbal supplements. Instruct the patient in deep breathing and coughing, which reopens the lung alveoli and helps to clear secretions from the lower respiratory tract. Encourage the patient to perform these maneuvers as soon as possible after emergence from deep sedation or general anesthesia.

Table 19-3 ■ General Anesthetics Commonly Given by Injection

GENERIC NAME	TRADE NAMEA	VERAGE ADULT DOSAGE	ROUTE OF ADMINISTRATION
etomidate	Amidate	0.3 mg/kg over 30–60 sec	IV
fentanyl	Sublimaze	Up to 150 mcg/kg PRN	IV
ketaminc	Kelalar	100 mg	IM
methohexital	Brevital sodium	5–12 mL of 1% solution at a rate of 1 mL q5min and then 2–4 mL q4–7 min PRN	IV
midazolam	Versed	Premedicated: 0.15–0.25 mg/kg over 20–30 sec; allow 2 min for effect	
		Nonpremedicated: 0.3–0.35 mg/kg over 20–30 sec; allow 2 min for effect	IV
propofol	Diprivan	2–2.5 mg/kg q10 sec until induction onset	IV
thiopental	Pentothal	Test dose: 25–75 mg and then 50–75 mg at 20–40 sec intervals; additional 50 mg may be given if needed	IV

IM, intramuscular; IV, intravenous; PRN, as needed.

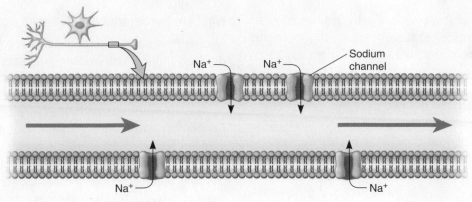

A Normal nerve conduction

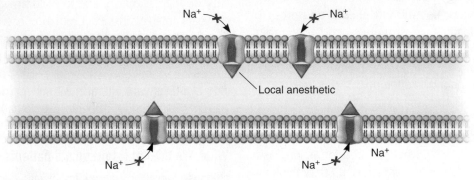

B Local anesthetic blocking sodium channels

Figure 19-1 ■ Mechanism of action of anesthetics: normal nerve conduction (A) and anesthetic blocking sodium channels (B).

Focus on Natural Products

Stopping Herbal Medications Before Surgery

The recent increased use of natural products has been an issue raised by the American Society of Anesthesiologists concerning anesthesia. It is recommended that patients stop taking herbal medications at least 2 to 3 weeks before surgery to decrease the risk of adverse effects resulting from an enhancement or prolongation of anesthetic effects.

Focus Point

Diabetes and Surgery

The stress of surgery in patients with diabetes may increase (rather than decrease) their blood glucose levels. Insulin injections and hypoglycemic medications should be coordinated with the patient, surgeon, and anesthesiologist.

✳ Apply Your Knowledge 19.2

The following questions focus on what you have just learned about general anesthetics.

CRITICAL THINKING

1. What is balanced anesthesia?
2. What are four examples of the inhaled anesthetics (their generic and trade names)?
3. What are the trade names of propofol, midazolam, ketamine, and fentanyl?
4. How long should a patient stop taking herbal medications before surgery to decrease the risk of adverse effects?
5. What is a volatile liquid?
6. What factors affect the anesthetic technique?
7. What are the most widely used volatile anesthetics today?
8. What are the advantages of intravenous injections?

TYPES OF LOCAL ANESTHETICS

Local anesthesia is used to provide regional or topical anesthesia to relieve pain and to provide localized nerve block for surgical procedures without loss of consciousness. Generally, local anesthesia is safer than general anesthesia and allows for more rapid recovery. Local anesthetics are divided into two groups: esters and amides.

Ester-Type Agents

Ester-type local anesthetics have been in use longer than amides. Esters tend to have a rapid onset and short duration of activity (except tetracaine [Pontocaine]). Esters are associated with a higher incidence of allergic reactions because of one of their metabolites: para-amino benzoic acid (PABA). PABA is structurally similar to methylparaben. Ester-type agents include benzocaine, cocaine, procaine, propoxycaine, chloroprocaine, and tetracaine. Because of these possible hypersensitivity reactions, many manufacturers have reformulated some of their products to eliminate methylparaben.

Generally, they are used topically. Procaine 2% (Novocain) is still marketed for use with epinephrine (Adrenalin) but is rarely used. Tetracaine (Pontocaine) is most efficacious as a topical anesthetic but is also 10 times more toxic than procaine. However, amides are often recommended over esters. They are safer and can also be used for topical applications.

Focus On

Amide-Type Agents

The most commonly recognized drug in the class of amides is lidocaine (Xylocaine), which was synthesized in 1943. The amides have several advantages over the esters. Amide local anesthetics do not undergo metabolism to PABA as esters do; therefore, hypersensitivity to amide local anesthetics is rare. Also, they can undergo repeated high-temperature sterilization without losing potency. Most of the local anesthetics in common use today belong to the amide class. These include (in addition to lidocaine) bupivacaine (Marcaine, Sensorcaine); mepivacaine (Carbocaine); etidocaine (Duranest); prilocaine (Citanest); and the most recent, ropivacaine (Naropin).

Lidocaine is supplied in many formulations, including an ointment, a water-soluble jelly, and a 4% solution for topical use; a 5% solution with dextrose for spinal administration; and 0.5%, 1%, 1.5%, and 2% solutions for injection. It is also widely available in a 1% multi dose vial and preprepared with epinephrine (Adrenalin). The most common local anesthetics are summarized in Table 19-4 ■.

How do they work?

Local anesthetics appear to work by inhibiting the movement of sodium through channels in the membrane of a neuron, which in turn inhibits the transmission of nerve impulses. The action of the local anesthetics is dose dependent. The more drug present, the more the inhibition—until a complete block is produced.

(Continued)

Focus On (Continued)

Local anesthetics can also affect sodium channels in other parts of the body, such as the conduction system of the heart. This can lead to an abnormal heartbeat; thus, systemic distribution of local anesthetics is best kept to a minimum.

How are they used?

Local anesthesia is useful in a wide variety of clinical situations. It increases patient comfort and facilitates patient cooperation during procedures. As a diagnostic aid, it helps localize or identify the source of pain. Local anesthesia is warranted for any clinical procedure with a potential for pain, such as incision and drainage of abscesses, laceration repair, biopsy, wart treatment, vasectomy, neonatal circumcision, and dental procedures. Local anesthesia is also used during labor and delivery and for diagnostic procedures, such as gastrointestinal endoscopy. Occasionally, local anesthetics are used to relieve pain associated with pathologic conditions.

What are the adverse effects?

True allergic reactions to local anesthetics are rare and usually involve the ester agents. Allergic reactions are seldom caused by amide anesthetics. There is no cross-reactivity between amide and ester agents.

It is important to keep track of the total anesthetic dose given because toxic effects are dose related. Adverse effects are related to the CNS and, to a lesser degree, the cardiovascular system. Symptoms of toxicity include lightheadedness, dizziness, nystagmus (rhythmical oscillation of the eyeballs), restlessness, disorientation, and psychosis. Slurred speech and tremors often precede seizures. Hypotension, bradycardia, and cardiac arrest may occur.

What are the contraindications and interactions?

Local anesthetics are contraindicated in older adults and debilitated patients and should be used cautiously in children younger than 14 years of age. They should not be used during pregnancy, labor, or lactation. They are contraindicated in patients who are hypersensitive to these agents and who have sepsis, acidosis, heart or spinal block, severe hemorrhage, hypotension and shock, hypertension, cerebrospinal deformities or diseases, blood dyscrasias, supraventricular dysrhythmias, untreated sinus bradycardia, or bowel pathology. They should not be used concurrently with long-term ophthalmic preparations, bupivacaine or chloroprocaine, obstetric paracervical anesthesia, spinal anesthesia, or topical or IV regional anesthesia. Avoid use on infected application or injection sites, on a perforated eardrum or ear discharge, and on large areas. They are contraindicated in patients with a history of malignant hyperthermia and during severe trauma. These drugs interact with the sulfonamides, epinephrine (Adrenalin), MAOIs, antihypertensive agents, isoproterenol (Isuprel), ergonovine (Ergotrate Maleate), tricyclic antidepressants, phenothiazines, other local anesthetics, barbiturates, cimetidine (Tagamet), beta-blockers, quinidine (Quinidex), phenytoin (Dilantin), and procainamide (Procan, Pronestyl).

What are the important points patients should know?

Instruct patients who have received local anesthetics to report such symptoms as lightheadedness, dizziness, disorientation, or slurred speech and to avoid driving and operating heavy machinery.

Table 19-4 ■ Local Anesthetics

GENERIC NAME	TRADE NAME	AVERAGE ADULT DOSAGE	ROUTE OF ADMINISTRATION
Esters			
benzocaine	Americaine, Benzocol, Oracin	Lowest effective dose	Topical
cocaine	None	1%–10% solution (use greater than 4% solution with caution) (maximum: single dose of 1 mg/kg)	Topical
procaine	Novocain	0.25%–0.5% solution	Subcutaneous
tetracaine	Pontocaine	1–2 drops of 0.5% solution diluted with equal volume of 10% dextrose	Topical

GENERIC NAME	TRADE NAME	AVERAGE ADULT DOSAGE	ROUTE OF ADMINISTRATION
Amides			
bupivacaine	Marcaine, Sensorcaine	0.25%–0.75% solution	IM local infiltration, sympathetic block, lumbar epidural, caudal block, peripheral nerve block, retrobulbar block
etidocaine	Duranest	0.5%–1.5% solution (maximum: 300 mg; 400 mg if given with epinephrine)	Percutaneous infiltration, peripheral nerve block (caudal), central neural block
lidocaine	Xylocaine	0.5%–5% solution; solution with glucose (spinal); solution with dextrose (saddle block); jelly, ointment, cream, or solution (topical)	Infiltration, nerve block, epidural, caudal, spinal, saddle block, topical
mepivacaine	Carbocaine	1%–2% solution	Infiltration, nerve block, caudal and lumbar epidurals
ropivacaine	Naropin	5–250 mg (0.5%–1% solution)	Epidural, nerve block

✳ Apply Your Knowledge 19.3

The following questions focus on what you have just learned about local anesthesia.

CRITICAL THINKING

1. What are the main groups of local anesthetics?
2. What are the most common uses of local anesthetics today?
3. Why is it important to keep track of the total amount of anesthetics being administered?
4. What type of local anesthetic has been used for the longest time?
5. What are the trade names of procaine, tetracaine, bupivacaine, lidocaine, and ropivacaine?

SPECIFIC APPLICATIONS

Several local anesthetics can be used with different techniques or specific applications. They include topical anesthesia, infiltration anesthesia, field block anesthesia, nerve block anesthesia, spinal anesthesia, and epidural anesthesia. Techniques for applying local anesthesia are illustrated in Figure 19-2 ■.

Topical Anesthesia

Topical anesthesia involves the placement of a nerve-conduction-blocking agent onto a tissue layer (skin or mucous membrane). This method is used to provide anesthesia on mucous membranes of the urethra, vagina, rectum, and skin. The tissue affected is limited to the area in contact with the topical anesthetic. Topical anesthesia is usually administered by the physician and is achieved with either the use of **cryoanesthesia** or a pharmacologic agent.

Cryoanesthesia involves the reduction of nerve conduction by localized cooling. This may be accomplished with ice or by the use of a cryoanesthesia machine to produce the cooling action. Reduced skin temperature may also be a result of a pharmaceutical agent sprayed onto the skin, such as ethyl chloride. Lidocaine (Xylocaine) and cocaine are examples of topical anesthetic agents. Although the amount of agent applied is limited, the patient must be monitored for toxic reactions.

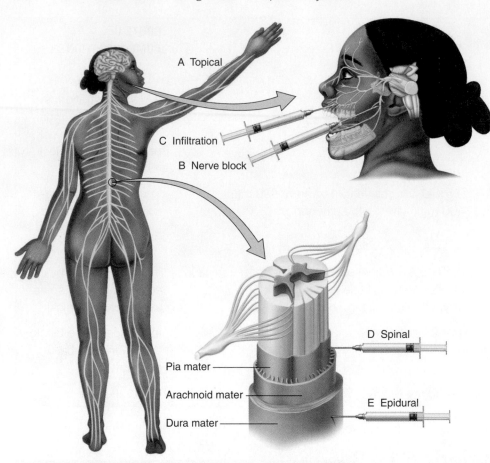

Figure 19-2 ■ Techniques for applying local anesthesia: topical (A), nerve block (B), infiltration (C), spinal (D), and epidural (E).

Focus Point

Contact with Topical Anesthetics

P atients should be advised that when using topical anesthetics for skin conditions, they must not touch their eyes. Also, topical medications should never be applied to areas where there is an open lesion or cut.

Local Infiltration Anesthesia

Local infiltration anesthesia, which works by blocking nerves, is produced by the injection of a local anesthetic solution directly into an area that is painful or about to be operated on. Local infiltration is probably the most common route used to administer local anesthetics and is the simplest form of regional anesthesia. Local infiltration is used primarily for minor surgical procedures, such as the removal of superficial skin lesions; suturing of a wound; or slightly more invasive surgeries, such as the insertion of chest tubes. In this technique, a local anesthetic agent is injected into superficial tissues to produce a small area of analgesia and anesthesia. When a local anesthetic is to be administered by infiltration, epinephrine may be added to it to decrease its dosage and prolong its duration of action. However, epinephrine

(Adrenalin) should not be used to anesthetize fingers, toes, and other tissues with end arteries. Lidocaine (Xylocaine) is a popular choice for infiltration anesthesia, but bupivacaine (Marcaine, Sensorcaine) is used for longer procedures.

Field Block Anesthesia

Field block anesthesia affects a single nerve, a deep plexus, or a network of nerves. Field block anesthesia and nerve block are forms of regional anesthesia. For example, a radial nerve block may be used to anesthetize the structures innervated by the radial nerve, including portions of the forearm and hand. Intraorbital block is often used for ocular surgery. A local anesthetic is administered in a series of injections to form a wall of anesthesia encircling the operative field.

Spinal Anesthesia

During **spinal anesthesia**, an anesthetic agent is injected into the **subarachnoid** space (beneath the arachnoid membrane or between the arachnoid and pia mater and filled with cerebrospinal fluid [CSF]) through a spinal needle. Spinal anesthesia can be used for many procedures but is most often used for gynecologic, obstetric, orthopedic, and genitourinary surgery. Spinal anesthesia may cause marked vasodilation (hypotension), headaches, and respiratory depression. Lidocaine (Xylocaine), tetracaine (Xylocaine), and bupivacaine (Marcaine, Sensorcaine) are often used for spinal anesthesia.

Epidural Anesthesia

Epidural anesthesia involves the injection of the local anesthetic into the epidural (lumbar or caudal) space via a catheter that allows repeated infusions. After injection, the anesthetic agent is very slowly absorbed into the CSF. This is popular for labor and delivery. High concentrations of local anesthetic can get into the blood circulation and may increase the risk of systemic toxicity. Therefore, they can cause cardiac depression and neurotoxicity in the mother and neonate. Highly lipid-soluble locals, such as lidocaine (Xylocaine), tend to get into the blood more than the less lipid-soluble agents, such as bupivacaine (Marcaine, Sensorcaine).

Focus Point

Alleviating Headache After Spinal Block

Patients should be advised to lay flat for approximately 12 hours after a spinal block or epidural to prevent the leakage of CSF, which may increase the risk of a postanesthetic headache.

✳ Apply Your Knowledge 19.4

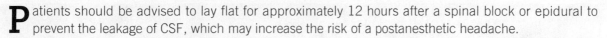

The following questions focus on what you have just learned about specific applications of anesthesia.

CRITICAL THINKING

1. What is cryoanesthesia?
2. What is field block anesthesia?
3. What is spinal anesthesia?
4. What is local infiltration anesthesia?
5. What is epidural anesthesia?

PRACTICAL SCENARIO 1

A nurse reports she was reprimanded for being late in giving a preanesthetic medication. She administered the drug 10 minutes before the patient was taken to surgery. The patient was placed under general anesthesia for the surgical procedure. Several hours after the surgery, the patient experienced complications and reported that no one told him ahead of time what to expect in the recovery room.

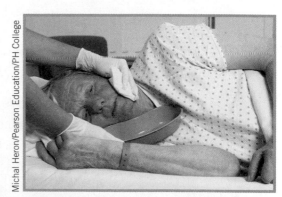

Michal Heron/Pearson Education/PH College

Critical Thinking Questions

1. Why is it important to administer the preanesthetic medication at the proper time before surgery?
2. When the nurse realized she was delayed in giving the preanesthetic, what should she have done?
3. In what way did the nurse neglect her responsibilities toward the patient?

PRACTICAL SCENARIO 2

A 31-year-old pregnant woman went into labor at the local hospital. After 12 hours, her physician ordered epidural anesthesia. A high concentration of this anesthetic caused cardiac depression in the mother and neonate.

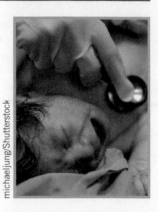

michaeljung/Shutterstock

Critical Thinking Questions

1. Besides cardiac depression, what other toxicity may manifest?
2. Explain the procedure used for epidural anesthesia.

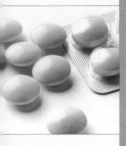

Chapter Capsule

This section repeats the objectives from the beginning of the chapter and then provides a summary of the most important concepts for that objective. Use this section as a quick review and to check your knowledge.

Objective 1: Outline the stages of anesthesia.

■ Stage 1—Analgesia: pain is abolished; consciousness is retained; sense of hearing is often enhanced

■ Stage 2—Excitement: may be unpleasant; patient may experience shaking and become violent or feel extreme fear; passage from stage 1 to stage 3 must be attained as quickly as possible because sudden death can occur during stage 2—possibly caused by vagal nerve inhibition

■ Stage 3—Surgical anesthesia: characterized by progressive muscular relaxation, which must be controlled to avoid respiratory paralysis; various body reflexes, corneal reflexes, and pupillary size are helpful indicators; patients are usually put on a respirator during this stage

■ Stage 4—Medullary paralysis: begins with respiratory failure; can lead to circulatory collapse; through careful monitoring, this stage is avoided

Objective 2: Define the importance of premedications before anesthesia.

■ Also known as *preoperative medications* or preanesthetics, premedications help to:

  ❏ Achieve sedation

  ❏ Reduce anxiety

  ❏ Induce amnesia (to minimize unpleasant surgical memories)

  ❏ Increase comfort during preoperative procedures

  ❏ Reduce gastric acidity and volume

  ❏ Increase gastric emptying

  ❏ Decrease nausea and vomiting

  ❏ Reduce incidence of aspiration by drying oral and respiratory secretions

Objective 3: Explain the action of anesthetics within the central nervous system.

- Depress the CNS to cause unconsciousness
- Create unawareness of surroundings and block pain from surgery or procedure
- Relax patients' skeletal muscles and diminish reflexes

Objective 4: List the effects of general anesthetics.

- Loss of consciousness before and during surgery
- Relief of anxiety or pain without causing unconsciousness

Objective 5: Describe the common local anesthetics and their uses.

- Ester-type agents—generally used topically
- Amide-type agents—most commonly used; used to increase patient comfort, to facilitate patient cooperation, as diagnostic aids, and for the following specific procedures:
  - Incision and drainage of abscesses
  - Laceration repair
  - Biopsy
  - Wart treatment
  - Vasectomy
  - Neonatal circumcision
  - Dental procedures
  - Labor and delivery
  - Diagnostic procedures, such as gastrointestinal endoscopy
  - Pain relief associated with pathologic conditions

Objective 6: Compare ester and amide local anesthetics.

- Ester-type agents—attributable to allergic reactions caused by para-amino benzoic acid (PABA), these agents are generally not preferred; amide-type agents are often recommended instead
- Amide-type agents—safer than ester-type agents with less allergic reaction potential; they are available in many forms, including ointments, jellies, and solutions for injection

Objective 7: List the problems associated with the use of local anesthetics.

- Allergic reactions involving the ester-type agents, caused by ingredient PABA, are common
- Toxic effects are possible and dose related
- Lightheadedness, dizziness, nystagmus, restlessness, disorientation, and psychosis may be experienced
- Slurred speech and tremors often precede seizures
- Hypotension, bradycardia, and cardiac arrest may occur

Objective 8: Explain the indications for spinal anesthesia.

- Gynecologic, obstetric, orthopedic, and genitourinary surgery

Objective 9: Discuss various techniques for local anesthetics.

■ Local anesthesia is used to provide regional or topical anesthesia to relieve pain and provide localized nerve block without a loss of consciousness. They are commonly used topically or by injection. The amide-type local anesthetics are safer than the ester-type local anesthetics.

■ Local anesthesia increases patient comfort and facilitates patient cooperation, helps to localize or identify sources of pain, and is used in all the following procedures:

❑ Incision and drainage of abscesses, laceration repair, biopsy, wart treatment, vasectomy, neonatal circumcision, dental procedures, during labor and delivery, for gastrointestinal procedures (such as endoscopy), and sometimes to relieve pain associated with pathologic conditions

Objective 10: Compare epidural anesthesia with field block anesthesia.

■ Epidural anesthesia—involves injection of the local anesthetic into the epidural space via a catheter that allows repeated infusions. It is often used in labor and delivery. Care must be taken to avoid systemic toxicity.

■ Field block anesthesia—affects a single nerve, a deep plexus, or a network of nerves. It is a form of regional anesthesia, wherein a local anesthetic is administered in a series of injections to form a wall of anesthesia encircling the operative field.

 ## Internet Sites of Interest

■ The journal of the Anesthesia & Analgesia organization can be searched at **http://www.anesthesia-analgesia.org**.

■ Excellent patient information can be found at the website of the American Society of Anesthesiologists at **http://www.asahq.org/patientEducation.htm**.

■ *Scientific American* online offers an article titled "How Does Anesthesia Work?" Search at **http://www.scientificamerican.com**.

■ Look up "anesthesia" at **http://www.myoptumhealth.com/portal/#multistory1** to find information on general and local anesthesia.

Chapter Objectives

After completing this chapter, you should be able to:

1. Describe the top two layers of the skin.
2. List five different skin disorders.
3. Identify the mainstay of treatment for acute or chronic inflammatory disorders of the skin.
4. Describe the mechanism of action of topical corticosteroids.
5. Identify the drugs used to treat psoriasis.
6. List the drugs used to treat acne.
7. Explain the action and uses of keratolytics.
8. Describe the treatments for scabies and pediculosis.

Chapter 20

Drugs Used to Treat Skin Conditions

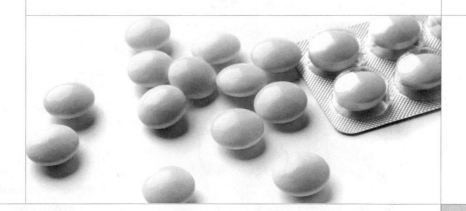

Key Terms

candidiasis (kan-dih-dy-Ay-sis) (page 350)

dermatitis (dur-mah-ty-tis) (page 344)

eczema (ECK-zih-mah) (page 344)

emollients (ee-MOLE-ee-ents) (page 347)

erythema (ear-ih-THEE-mah) (page 344)

keratinization (keh-rat-in-eh-ZAY-shun) (page 348)

keratinocytes (keh-RAT-in-oh-syts) (page 347)

keratolytic (keh-RAT-oh-lih-tik) (page 347)

pediculicides (puh-DIK-yoo-lih-sydz) (page 352)

pruritus (proo-RYE-tus) (page 347)

psoriasis (soh-RYE-uh-sis) (page 346)

scabicides (SKAY-bih-sydz) (page 352)

scabies (SKAY-beez) (page 352)

Introduction

The integumentary system is the largest of all organs in the human body. It consists of the skin, hair, nails, sweat glands, and oil glands. The skin forms a barrier between ourselves and our environment and, as such, is fundamental to the functioning of all other organs. The skin is vital in maintaining homeostasis. In addition to providing a protective covering, the skin helps regulate body temperature, retards water loss from deeper tissues, houses sensory receptors, synthesizes various biochemicals, and excretes small quantities of wastes.

The Skin

The skin consists of two distinct layers (Figure 20-1 ■). The outer layer is called the *epidermis*. The inner layer, or *dermis*, is thicker than the epidermis. Beneath the dermis are masses of loose connective and adipose tissues that bind the skin to the underlying organs. These tissues form the subcutaneous layer, which lies beneath the skin but is not a true layer of skin.

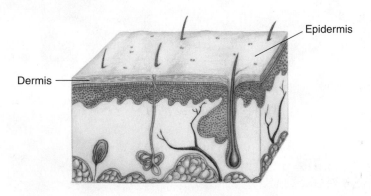

Dermis

Epidermis

Figure 20-1 ■ The two layers of the skin.

EPIDERMIS

The epidermis has either four or five sublayers. The outermost sublayer is the *stratum corneum* (horny layer). The deepest layer of epidermal cells, called the *stratum basale* or *stratum germinativum,* is close to the dermis and is nourished by dermal blood vessels. As the cells of this layer divide and grow, the older epidermal cells are pushed away from the dermis toward the skin surface. The farther the cells move, the poorer their nutrient supply becomes, and in time, they die. Specialized cells in the epidermis called *melanocytes* produce melanin, a dark pigment that provides skin color. Melanin absorbs ultraviolet (UV) radiation in sunlight, preventing mutations in the DNA of skin cells and other damaging effects. Melanocytes lie in the deepest portion of the epidermis.

DERMIS

The dermis binds the epidermis to underlying tissues. It is largely composed of dense, irregular connective tissue that gets its name from its irregular arrangement of thick protein fibers.

Dermal blood vessels supply nutrients to all skin cells. These vessels also help regulate body temperature. Nerve cell processes are scattered throughout the dermis. The dermis also contains hair follicles, oil glands, and sweat glands. Embedded in the skin are structures called *appendages,* such as the nails, hair follicles, and sweat and sebaceous glands—all of which are subject to disease.

SUBCUTANEOUS LAYER

The subcutaneous layer (hypodermis), beneath the dermal layer of the skin, consists of loose connective and adipose tissues. The adipose tissue of the subcutaneous layer insulates, helping to conserve body heat and impede the entrance of heat from the outside. The subcutaneous layer also contains the major blood vessels that supply the skin and underlying adipose tissue.

Disorders of the Skin

Disruptions in skin integrity may be precipitated by trauma, abnormal cellular function, infection and inflammation, and systemic diseases. Many of these diseases are caused by infections, and most of the drugs used to treat such infections are discussed in Chapters 12 and 13. Other common diseases of the skin are caused by inflammatory conditions resulting from allergies.

ECZEMA AND MISCELLANEOUS INFLAMMATORY DISORDERS

The most common inflammatory disorder of the skin is **eczema**, a response of the skin caused by endogenous and exogenous agents; it is often considered synonymous with **dermatitis** (inflammation of the skin). Endogenous eczemas include dermatitis and seborrheic dermatitis. Exogenous eczemas include irritant dermatitis and allergic contact dermatitis. Eczematous dermatitis is characterized by **erythema** (skin redness caused by capillary dilation), vesicles, scales, and itching.

The mainstay of treatment of acute or chronic inflammatory disorders is topical or oral corticosteroids. Systemic corticosteroids were discussed in other chapters. Only topical corticosteroids are discussed here (Table 20-1 ■).

Table 20-1 ■ Selected Topical Corticosteroids

GENERIC NAME	TRADE NAME	AVERAGE ADULT DOSAGE	ROUTE OF ADMINISTRATION
alclometasone	Aclovate	Apply 0.05% cream or ointment sparingly bid–tid.	Topical
amcinonide	Cyclocort	Apply thin film bid–tid.	Topical
betamethasone dipropionate	Diprolene, Diprosone	Apply thin film bid–tid.	Topical
betamethasone valerate	Betatrex, Psorion (cream), Valisone (scalp lotion)	Apply sparingly bid.	Topical
desoximetasone	Topicort	Apply thin layer bid.	Topical
dexamethasone	Decaderm	Apply thin layer tid–qid.	Topical
diflorasone	Florone, Maxiflor	Apply thin layer of ointment 1–3 times/d or cream 2–4 times/d.	Topical
fluocinolone	Fluonid, Flurosyn	Apply thin layer bid–qid.	Topical
fluocinonide	Lidex	Apply thin layer bid–qid.	Topical
flurandrenolide	Cordran	Apply thin layer bid–tid; apply tape 1–2 times/d q12h.	Topical
hydrocortisone	Aeroseb-HC, Alphaderm	Apply a small amount to affected area 1–4 times/d.	Topical
triamcinolone	Aristocort, Atolone	Apply sparingly bid–tid.	Topical

bid, twice a day; qid, four times a day; tid, three times a day.

Focus on Pediatrics

Eczema Common in Pediatric Patients

Atopic dermatitis (eczema) is common in pediatric patients. Eczema in some infants is believed to be traceable to sensitivity to milk, orange juice, or certain foods.

Focus On

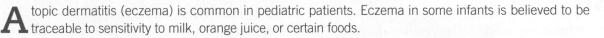

Topical Corticosteroids

The corticosteroids are potent anti-inflammatory agents. Topical administration goes directly to the site of inflammation. These drug preparations are available as lotions, creams, and aerosols in various concentrations.

How do they work?

Topical corticosteroids prevent the accumulation of inflammatory cells at sites of infection and inhibit phagocytosis. When applied to inflamed skin, they reduce itching, redness, and swelling.

(Continued)

Focus On (*Continued*)

How are they used?

Topical corticosteroids are used for the treatment of such skin disorders as eczema, dermatitis, psoriasis, insect bite reactions, and burns (first and second degree). Topical corticosteroids are the primary agents used to treat dermatitis. Potency depends on the type of drug formulation and on whether it is packaged as a cream, lotion, solution, or gel.

What are the adverse effects?

Common localized adverse effects may include dryness, redness, itching, irritation, or burning of the skin. Topical corticosteroids may also produce secondary infections.

What are the contraindications and interactions?

Topical corticosteroids are contraindicated in bacterial skin infections. They must not be used in patients with known hypersensitivity. Topical corticosteroids should be used cautiously in pregnant or lactating women. Drug interactions are not significant when administered as directed.

What are the important points patients should know?

Advise patients to follow the directions of their physician regarding covering the treated area or leaving it exposed to air. The effectiveness of certain drugs depends on keeping the area covered or leaving it open. Instruct patients to not apply medications to areas other than those specified by their physician and to use the drug as directed (for example, a thin layer or apply liberally). Topical corticosteroids must be kept away from the eyes (unless use in or around the eyes has been recommended).

✳ Apply Your Knowledge 20.1

The following questions focus on what you have just learned about the skin.

CRITICAL THINKING

1. What are the major functions of the skin?
2. What are the outermost and deepest layers of the epidermis?
3. What is the mainstay of treatment of acute or chronic inflammatory disorders of the skin?
4. What is another name for eczema?
5. What are the trade names of amcinonide, fluocinonide, and flurandrenolide?

PSORIASIS

Psoriasis is a chronic, relapsing inflammatory skin disorder that occurs at any age. The onset usually occurs by 20 years of age. The cause of psoriasis is unknown, but it has a hereditary component. The disorder is marked by a greatly increased rate of cellular proliferation, which leads to thickening of the dermis and epidermis. It is characterized by rounded plaques, covered by silvery-white scaly patches. The skin lesions of psoriasis are variably pruritic. External factors may exacerbate psoriasis, including infections, stress, and such medications as lithium, beta-blockers, and antimalarials.

The most common areas for psoriasis to occur are the elbows, knees, gluteal cleft, and scalp. Involvement tends to be symmetric. There is no cure for this disease yet, but remissions can often be produced by the available therapies, which include the use of ultraviolet (UV) light either alone or in combination with drugs and topical and systemic treatments.

Focus Point

Preventing Recurrence of Psoriasis

Keeping the skin moist and lubricated, avoiding cold and dry climates, avoiding stress and anxiety, limiting alcohol intake, and not scratching the skin help to prevent the recurrence of psoriasis.

Focus On

Topical Antipsoriatics

Treatment is related to reducing epidermal cell turnover and immunomodulations. Mild lesions are usually treated with **emollients** (skin-softening agents), **keratolytic** agents (those that separate or loosen the horny layer of the epidermis), and topical corticosteroids. Systemic medications are used for moderate to severe lesions, which may respond to methotrexate (Amethopterin), acitretin (vitamin A), and vitamin D analogues. Sometimes, for the treatment of psoriasis, various techniques are used with or without other antipsoriasis medications (Table 20-2 ■). Various forms of tar treatments (coal tar) and a material called *anthralin* are available. UV light (phototherapy) is used in cases of severe psoriasis.

How do they work?

The mechanism of action of acitretin (Soriatane), ammoniated mercury, and anthralin (Psoriatec) are unknown. Calcipotriene (Dovonex) is a synthetic vitamin D_3 that controls psoriasis by inhibiting the proliferation of **keratinocytes** (epidermal cells that produce keratin) and decreasing the number of epithelial cells. Methoxsalen (Oxsoralen) is a psoralen derivative with strong photosensitizing effects. Methoxsalen (which causes photodamage) inhibits rapid and uncontrolled epidermal psoriasis.

How are they used?

Antipsoriatic agents are used for the treatment of moderate to severe forms of psoriasis in adults.

What are the adverse effects?

The major adverse effects associated with acitretin are alopecia, skin peeling, dry skin, **pruritus** (itching), rash, skin atrophy, and abnormal skin odor. The adverse effects of calcipotriene include facial dermatitis, burning, stinging, erythema, and itching. Methoxsalen may cause severe edema, erythema, burning, peeling, and thinning of the skin.

What are the contraindications and interactions?

Topical antipsoriatics are contraindicated in hypersensitivity to these agents. Patients with hypercalcemia or vitamin D toxicity should not use calcipotriene. The antipsoriatics are also contraindicated in pregnancy or lactating women.

What are the important points patients should know?

Instruct patients to avoid additional exposure to UV light for at least 8 hours after oral drug ingestion and UVA exposure. Warn patients against mixing calcipotriene with any other topical medicines. Advise patients to discontinue the drug and immediately report visual problems.

Table 20-2 ■ Antipsoriatic Drugs

GENERIC NAME	TRADE NAME	AVERAGE ADULT DOSAGE	ROUTE OF ADMINISTRATION
acitretin	Soriatane	10–50 mg/d with main meal	PO
azelaic acid	Azelex	Apply twice daily.	Topical
calcipotriene	Dovonex	Apply twice daily.	Topical
methoxsalen	Oxsoralen, Uvadex	Give 1.5–2 h before exposure to UV light 2–3 times/wk (amounts to use range from 10–70 mg based on the weight of the patient).	PO

PO, oral; UV, ultraviolet.

ACNE

Acne vulgaris is an inflammatory disorder of the sebaceous glands that commonly occurs during puberty. The incidence of acne tends to decline with age and is unusual in adults, although it can persist for many years. Sebaceous glands secrete sebum, the natural oil of the skin. Testosterone is partially responsible for the secretion of sebum, and it may be that acne is caused by an increased responsiveness of the sebaceous glands to varying levels of this hormone during puberty. When too much sebum is produced, the duct of the gland may become blocked, and bacteria can become trapped beneath the sebum plug. The bacteria then grow in the duct, leading to a small abscess.

Focus on Natural Products

Use Caution in Treating Acne with Zinc

A variety of natural products are used to treat acne. The most common of these are zinc, niacinamide gel, and tea tree oil. It is important to note that zinc can be toxic at high dosages—primarily because it causes copper deficiency.

Focus On

Antiacne Agents

Major drugs for acne-related disorders are listed in Table 20-3 ■. Benzoyl peroxide is a powerful oxidizing agent, which at least partially relieves some cases of acne by having bacterial action, and is the main over-the-counter (OTC) drug used for this purpose. Azelaic acid (Azelex) is a naturally occurring dicarboxylic acid. Such topical antibiotics as clindamycin (Cleocin) and erythromycin (Eryc) are also prescribed.

How do they work?

The antimicrobial action of these agents may be attributable to the inhibition of microbial cellular protein synthesis. A normalization of **keratinization** (keratin formation or development of a horny layer) of some of these agents, such as azelaic acid and benzoyl peroxide, may also contribute to their clinical effectiveness.

How are they used?

These agents are used for mild to moderate inflammatory acne vulgaris. Topical applications of clindamycin are used in the treatment of acne vulgaris, and vaginal applications are used in the treatment of bacterial vaginosis in nonpregnant women.

What are the adverse effects?

Topical antiacne drugs may cause pruritus, burning, erythema, and stinging. Benzoyl peroxide can produce allergic dermatitis, excessive drying, peeling, erythema, and stinging. Topical clindamycin and erythromycin also produce dryness, burning, and excessive oil in the skin. In rare cases, clindamycin may cause bloody diarrhea and abdominal pain.

What are the contraindications and interactions?

These agents are avoided in patients with known hypersensitivity. Topical antiacne drugs are contraindicated during pregnancy and lactation.

What are the important points patients should know?

Instruct patients that proper application of these creams and gels is essential. Warn them to avoid contact with the eyes or mucous membranes and to wash out the eyes with large amounts of water if contact with the medication occurs. Advise patients to avoid breastfeeding while using these agents or to consult their physician.

Table 20-3 ■ Major Drugs Used to Treat Acne

GENERIC NAME	TRADE NAME	AVERAGE ADULT DOSAGE	ROUTE OF ADMINISTRATION
adapalene	Differin	Apply once daily to affected areas (in the evening).	Topical
azelaic acid	Azelex	Apply twice daily.	Topical
benzoyl peroxide	BenzaClin, Benzamycin	Apply 1–2 times/d.	Topical
clindamycin	Cleocin	Apply to affected areas bid.	Topical
doxycycline	Doryx, Vibramycin	100 mg q12h on Day 1 and then 100 mg/d	PO

GENERIC NAME	TRADE NAME	AVERAGE ADULT DOSAGE	ROUTE OF ADMINISTRATION
tetracycline	Achromycin	Oral: 500–1,000 mg/d in four divided doses	PO
		Topical: Apply to cleansed areas bid.	Topical
tretinoin	Retin-A	Apply once daily at bedtime.	Topical

bid, twice a day; PO, oral.

KERATOSES

Keratoses are characterized by a thickening of the keratin layer of the skin. Keratoses are benign lesions that are usually associated with aging or skin damage. *Seborrheic keratoses* result from the proliferation of epidermis, lead-ing to an oval elevation that may be smooth or rough and is often dark in color. *Actinic keratoses* occur on skin (especially fair skin) exposed to UV radiation. The lesion appears as a pigmented, scaly patch. Actinic keratoses may develop into skin cancer.

Focus On

Keratolytic Agents

Keratolytic agents promote shedding of the horny layer of the epidermis and softening of scales. The most commonly used keratolytic agents are salicylic acid (Fostex), resorcinol, and sulfur. Selected keratolytic medications are summarized in Table 20-4 ■.

How do they work?

Keratolytics act by breaking down the protein structure of the keratin layer, thereby permitting easier removal of compacted cellular material.

How are they used?

Keratolytic agents are used in the treatment of corns, calluses, and plantar warts. Some of these medications (such as sulfur and ammonium lactate) are used in the treatment of patients with acne, eczema, psoriasis, and seborrheic dermatitis.

What are the adverse effects?

The adverse effects of keratolytic agents include burning, local irritation, rash, dry skin, and scaling.

What are the contraindications and interactions?

Keratolytic drugs must be avoided in patients with known hypersensitivity. They are contraindicated on moles, warts with hair growing from them, genital or facial warts, birthmarks, or infected skin. Salicylic acid may cause salicylate toxicity (see Chapter 15) with prolonged use. These agents must be used cautiously during pregnancy and lactation.

What are the important points patients should know?

Instruct patients that keratolytic agents are for external use only. Tell them to avoid contact with the eye, face, mucous membranes, and normal skin around warts. Advise the patient to soak the area with warm water for 5 minutes before application to enhance the effect of the medication.

Table 20-4 ■ Selected Keratolytic Agents

GENERIC NAME	TRADE NAME	AVERAGE ADULT DOSAGE	ROUTE OF ADMINISTRATION
diclofenac	Solaraze	Apply to affected area bid for 60–90 d.	Topical
masoprocol cream	Actinex	Apply to lesions bid for 14–28 d.	Topical
salicylic acid	Fostex, Mediplast	Apply enough medicine to cover affected area and rub in gently or apply a patch as directed.	Topical
salicylic acid with podophyllum	Podocon-25, Podofin	Apply enough medicine to cover the affected area and rub in gently or apply a patch as directed.	Topical

bid, twice a day.

❊ Apply Your Knowledge 20.2

The following questions focus on what you have just learned about psoriasis, acne, and keratoses as well as the medications used to threat these conditions.

CRITICAL THINKING

1. What is acne? Compare it with psoriasis.
2. What is actinic keratosis and what is its complication?
3. What are the descriptions of corns and calluses?
4. What are the trade names of clindamycin, azelaic acid, tretinoin, and adapalene?
5. What are the trade names of masoprocol, diclofenac, and salicylic acid with podophyllum?

Bacterial Skin Infections

Cutaneous infections are common forms of skin disease. Most bacterial infections of the skin are caused by local invasion by pathogens. Staphylococci and beta-hemolytic streptococci are the common causative microorganisms. Examples of skin and hair bacterial infections include impetigo, cellulites, and folliculitis. These infections generally remain localized, although serious complications can occur. Impetigo is a common superficial bacterial infection of skin caused by either *Streptococcus spp.* or *Staphylococcus aureus*. The primary lesion is a superficial pustule that ruptures and forms a characteristic yellow-brown crust. Lesions caused by staphylococci may be tense, clear bullae, and this less common form of the disease is called *bulbous impetigo*. Treatment of impetigo involves gentle debridement of adherent crusts, which is facilitated by the use of soaks and topical antibiotics in conjunction with appropriate oral antibiotics. Topical antibiotic drugs are listed in Table 20-5 ■. Systemic antibiotics are discussed in Chapter 12.

FUNGAL INFECTIONS

Dermatophytes are fungi that infect skin, hair, and nails. Infection of the foot (tinea pedis) is most common and is often chronic. It is characterized by variable erythema and edema, scaling, pruritus, and occasionally vesiculation. Involvement may be widespread or localized, but almost invariably, the web space between the fourth and fifth toes is affected. Infection of the nails (tinea unguium) occurs in many patients with tinea pedis and is characterized by opacified, thickened nails and subungual debris.

The groin is the next most commonly involved area (tinea cruris), with men affected much more often than women. Dermatophyte infection of the scalp (tinea capitis) produces an inflammatory or relatively noninflammatory condition that may present with either well-defined or irregular, diffuse areas of mild scaling and hair loss.

Candidiasis is also a fungal infection caused by a related group of yeasts—mostly *Candida albicans*. This organism is a normal flora of the gastrointestinal tract, but it may overgrow (usually because of broad-spectrum antibiotic therapy) and cause disease at a number of skin sites. Other predisposing factors include diabetes mellitus, oral contraceptive use, and cellular immune deficiency. Candidiasis is a very common infection in HIV-infected individuals. The oral cavity (the tongue or buccal mucosa) is usually involved, and this type of infection is also known as *thrush*. Candida infection may involve vulvovaginal candidiasis, which is very common in women of reproductive age.

Antifungal Agents

Topical and systemic therapies may be used to treat dermatophyte infections. Treatment depends on the site involved and the type of infection (Table 20-6 ■). Systemic therapies for fungal disorders were discussed in Chapter 13.

Table 20-5 ■ Topical Antibiotic Drugs

GENERIC NAME	TRADE NAME	AVERAGE ADULT DOSAGE	ROUTE OF ADMINISTRATION
azelaic acid	Azelex	Apply a thin film to clean and dry area bid.	Topical
bacitracin	Baciguent	Apply thin layer of ointment bid–tid as solution of 250–1,000 units/mL in wet dressing.	Topical
benzoyl peroxide	Benzac, Loroxide	Apply 1–2 times/d.	Topical
clindamycin, topical	Cleocin T, Dalacin C	Apply to affected areas bid.	Topical
gentamicin	Garamycin	1–2 drops of solution in eye q4h up to 2 drops q1h or small amount of ointment bid–tid	Topical
metronidazole	MetroGel, MetroLotion	Apply thin film to affected area bid.	Topical
mupirocin	Bactroban	Apply to affected area tid; if no response in 3–5 d, re-evaluate (usually continue for 1–2 wk).	Topical
neomycin	Myciguent	Apply 1–3 times/d.	Topical
sulfacetamide	Sebizon	Apply thin film to affected area 1–3 times/d.	Topical

bid, twice a day; tid, three times a day.

Table 20-6 ■ Topical Antifungal Drugs

GENERIC NAME	TRADE NAME	AVERAGE ADULT DOSAGE	ROUTE OF ADMINISTRATION
amphotericin B	Fungizone	100 mg swish and swallow qid	PO
ciclopirox	Loprox, Penlac Nail	Massage cream into affected area and surrounding skin bid (morning and evening).	Topical
		Paint affected nails under the surface and on the nail bed once daily at bedtime (at least 8 h before washing) After 7 d, remove lacquer with alcohol and remove or trim away unattached nail. Continue for 48 wk.	Nail lacquer
		Wet hair and apply approx. 1 tsp to the scalp (up to 10 mL for long hair); leave on for 3 min and then rinse. Repeat twice/wk for 4 wk, with a minimum of 3 d between applications.	Topical on scalp
econazole	Spectazole	Apply sufficient amount of 1% cream to affected areas 1–2 times/d (morning and evening).	Topical
haloprogin	Halotex	Apply liberally to affected area bid for 2–3 wk.	Topical

(continued)

Table 20-6 ■ Topical Antifungal Drugs (*continued*)

GENERIC NAME	TRADE NAME	AVERAGE ADULT DOSAGE	ROUTE OF ADMINISTRATION
miconazole	Fungoid-HC	Apply cream sparingly to affected areas bid and once daily for tinea versicolor for 2 wk (improvement is expected in 2–3 d; tinea pedis is treated for 1 mo to prevent recurrence).	Topical
		Insert suppository or vaginal cream at bedtime for 7 d (100 mg) or 3 d (200 mg).	Intravaginal
naftifine	Naftin	Apply cream once daily or apply gel bid; may use up to 4 wk.	Topical
nystatin	Mycostatin, Nystex	Apply 100,000 units/g cream, ointment, and powder or 1–2 tablets daily for 2 wk.	Intravaginal
oxiconazole	Oxistat	Apply to affected area once daily in the evening.	Topical
terbinafine	Lamisil	Apply 1–2 times/d to affected and immediately surrounding areas until clinical signs and symptoms are significantly improved (1–7 wk).	Topical
tolnaftate	Aftate, Tinactin	Apply 0.5–1 cm (1/4–1/2 in) of cream or 3 drops of solution bid in morning and evening; powder may be used prophylactically in normally moist areas.	Topical

bid, twice a day; PO, oral; qid, four times a day.

SCABIES AND PEDICULOSIS

Scabies is a group of dermatologic conditions caused by mites that burrow into the skin, causing intense itching. Scabies may be found anywhere on the trunk or extremities. Pediculosis is a lice infestation. Lice primarily affect hairy areas of the body, including the top of the head, eyebrows, eyelids, underarms, chest, and pubic area. Lice can infest just the head or the entire body. Another species—pubic lice—is commonly referred to as *crabs*. Lice feed on human blood and lay their eggs, called *nits*, on hair shafts. When a louse has its blood meal, irritation may be produced, which can eventually lead to a severe inflammatory reaction. The condition is highly contagious and requires treatment with specially formulated insecticides.

Focus On

Antilice Drugs

Scabicides are pharmacologic drugs that kill mites; **pediculicides** kill lice. However, either treatment may be effective for both types of parasites. The choice of drug depends on where the infestation has occurred. Table 20-7 ■ summarizes the most commonly used agents.

How do they work?

The mechanism of action of antilice drugs is related to their direct absorption by parasites and ova (nits). They stimulate the nervous system of the parasites, resulting in seizures and death.

How are they used?

These agents are used topically in the treatment of *Pediculus humanus* infestations.

What are the adverse effects?

The adverse effects include irritation with repeated use, causing pruritus, burning, stinging, numbness, erythema, edema, and rash.

What are the contraindications and interactions?

Lindane (Kwell) is contraindicated in premature neonates and patients with known seizure disorders. It should not be applied to the eyes, face, mucous membranes, or open cuts. The use of pyrethrins with dyes is contraindicated. These drugs should be avoided in acute inflammation of the scalp and in pregnant or lactating women. They should be used cautiously in children younger than 2 years. There are no clinically significant interactions established with these topical agents.

What are the most important points patients should know?

Instruct patients and their families that these agents are highly toxic drugs if used in excess or if they are swallowed or inhaled. Warn patients to keep these agents out of the reach of children. Advise patients to use a fine-toothed comb (infused with medication) to remove dead lice and remaining nits or nit shells when hair is dry. Regular shampooing should be resumed after treatment; residual deposit of drug on the hair is not reduced. Warn patients not to share combs, brushes, or other grooming equipment with other people. Instruct female patients to avoid breastfeeding while using these drugs without consulting their physicians.

Table 20-7 ■ Drugs Used to Treat Lice

GENERIC NAME	TRADE NAME	AVERAGE ADULT DOSAGE	ROUTE OF ADMINISTRATION
crotamiton	Eurax	Apply directly from the neck to the toes; apply a second layer 24 h later. Bathe 48 h after the last application to remove the drug.	Topical
lindane	Kwell, Scabene	Apply to all body areas except the face; leave lotion on 8–12 h and then rinse off; leave shampoo on 5 min and then rinse thoroughly. *Do not repeat in less than 1 wk.*	Lotion, shampoo
permethrin	Acticin, Nix	Apply sufficient volume to clean, wet hair to saturate the hair and scalp; leave on 10 min and then rinse hair thoroughly.	Cream, lotion
pyrethrins	Pyrinate, Pyrinyl	Apply to affected areas and leave on 10 min and then rinse thoroughly. Reapply only as directed.	Topical

✳ Apply Your Knowledge 20.3

The following questions focus on what you have just learned about skin infections, scabies, and pediculosis.

CRITICAL THINKING

1. What are the most common bacterial infections of the skin?
2. What is impetigo?
3. What are the predisposing factors for candidiasis?
4. What is pediculosis?
5. What are scabicides?
6. What are the trade names of amphotericin B, haloprogin, oxiconazole, and nystatin?

PRACTICAL SCENARIO 1

A 45-year-old woman who has spent more than 20 summers at the beaches of Florida and goes to the tanning salon three times a week notices that a small spot has appeared on her arm. It is a different color than the surrounding skin and has a bumpy surface. She assumes that it is a skin infection or bite and applies an OTC antibiotic ointment for several weeks. Finally, she calls her physician's office and speaks to you, wondering if she should schedule an office visit for such a small matter.

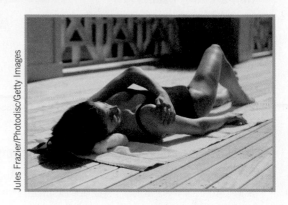
Jules Frazier/Photodisc/Getty Images

Critical Thinking Questions

1. What questions might you ask the patient about the skin spot?
2. What should you tell the patient to do about scheduling an office visit?
3. After the patient has been seen by the physician and treated, what patient education can you provide to her?

PRACTICAL SCENARIO 2

A 7-month-old infant developed sensitivity to milk and orange juice. She began to develop a skin disorder on her face.

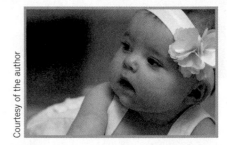
Courtesy of the author

Critical Thinking Questions

1. What is the most common skin condition caused by food allergies in infants?
2. What would be the most common type of skin medication prescribed for this condition?

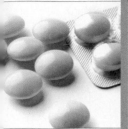

Chapter Capsule

This section repeats the objectives from the beginning of the chapter and then provides a summary of the most important concepts for that objective. Use this section as a quick review and to check your knowledge.

Objective 1: Describe the top two layers of the skin.

- Epidermis—outer layer with four or five sublayers; contains specialized cells in the called *melanocytes*, which produce melanin, a dark pigment that provides skin color

- Dermis—inner layer; thicker than the epidermis. Beneath the dermis are masses of loose connective and adipose tissues that bind the skin to the underlying organs.

Objective 2: List five different skin disorders.

- Eczema
- Dermatitis
- Psoriasis
- Acne
- Keratoses

Objective 3: Identify the mainstay of treatment for acute or chronic inflammatory disorders of the skin.

- Topical or oral corticosteroids

Objective 4: Describe the mechanism of action of topical corticosteroids.

- Prevent accumulation of inflammatory cells at sites of infection and inhibit phagocytosis; when applied to inflamed skin, they reduce itching, redness, and swelling

Objective 5: Identify the drugs used to treat psoriasis.

- Emollients
- Keratolytic agents
- Topical corticosteroids
- Systemic medications
- Tar treatments
- Anthralin
- UV light (phototherapy)

Objective 6: List the drugs used to treat acne.

- Benzoyl peroxide
- Azelaic acid
- Clindamycin
- Erythromycin

Objective 7: Explain the action and uses of keratolytics.

- Keratolytics—promote shedding of the horny layer of the epidermis and soften scales
- Used in the treatment of corns, calluses, and plantar warts; some (such as sulfur and ammonium lactate) are used in the treatment of acne, eczema, psoriasis, and seborrheic dermatitis

Objective 8: Describe the treatments for scabies and pediculosis.

- Scabicides—pharmacologic drugs that kill mites
- Pediculicides—kill lice
- Both treatments may be effective for both types of parasites; the choice of drug depends on where the infestation has occurred

Internet Sites of Interest

■ Dermatology A to Z, sun safety, and consumer information can be found at the American Academy of Dermatology's website at **http://www.aad.org**.

■ A detailed discussion of eczema, its triggers, and its treatments can be found at **http://www.webmd.com/allergies/guide/eczema**.

■ The About.com website includes an article on the use of corticosteroids in skin disorders, such as acne. The article is written by a physician. See **http://dermatology.about.com/cs/medications/a/steroidswork.htm**.

■ MedlinePlus offers a discussion of scabies, including photos, treatments, and an interactive tutorial, at **http://www.nlm.nih.gov/medlineplus/scabies.html**.

PEARSON
myhealthprofessionskit™

Go to www.myhealthprofessionskit.com to access the Companion Website created for this textbook. Simply select "Basic Health Science" from the choice of disciplines. Find this book and then log in using your username and password to access interactive learning games, assessment questions, animations, and more.

Chapter Objectives

After completing this chapter, you should be able to:

1. Identify the electrical conduction system of the heart.
2. Name the three layers of the heart and the four heart valves.
3. Define three types of angina pectoris.
4. Name the mainstays of angina therapy.
5. Describe the action of vasodilation.
6. Define calcium channel blockers.
7. Explain myocardial infarction.
8. Identify the classifications of antidysrhythmic drugs and explain their actions.
9. Describe the adverse reactions of quinidine.
10. Identify the mechanism of action of lidocaine.

Chapter 21

Drugs Used to Treat Cardiovascular Conditions

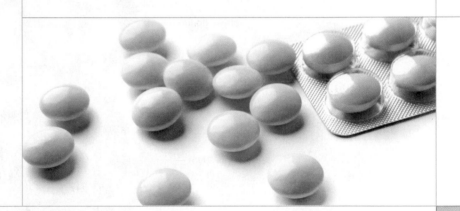

Key Terms

angina pectoris (an-JIE-nuh pek-TORE-iss) (page 359)

atrioventricular (AV) node (AY-tree-oh-ven-TRI-kyoo-ler node) (page 359)

atrium (AY-tree-um) (page 359)

automaticity (aw-toe-muh-TIH-sih-tee) (page 369)

bradycardia (bray-dee-KAR-dee-uh) (page 365)

bundle of His (page 359)

dysrhythmia (dis-RITH-mee-uh) (page 365)

electrocardiogram (ECG or EKG) (ee-lek-tro-KAR-dee-oh-gram) (page 359)

endocardium (en-do-KAR-dee-um) (page 359)

epicardium (ep-ih-KAR-dee-um) (page 359)

fibrillation (fib-rih-LAY-shun) (page 367)

flutter (page 367)

gingival hyperplasia (JIN-jih-vul hi-per-PLAY-zhuh) (page 368)

hypertension (HI-per-ten-shun) (page 358)

hypotension (HI-poe-ten-shun) (page 362)

insomnia (in-SOM-nee-uh) (page 363)

ischemia (is-KEE-mee-uh) (page 360)

myocardial infarction (my-oh-KAR-dee-ull in-FARK-shun) (page 358)

myocardium (my-oh-KAR-dee-um) (page 358)

nystagmus (nis-TAG-mus) (page 368)

platelets (PLATE-lets) (page 368)

prophylaxis (pro-fih-LAK-sis) (page 363)

Purkinje fibers (pur-KIN-jee) (page 359)

refractory (ree-FRAK-tor-ee) (page 370)

sinoatrial (SA) node (syn-oh-AY-tree-ull node) (page 359)

somnolence (SAHM-no-lents) (page 369)

sympathetic (sim-puh-THEH-tik) (page 363)

syndrome (SIN-drome) (page 365)

tachycardia (tak-ee-KAR-dee-uh) (page 362)

vasodilation (vass-oh-dy-LAY-shun) (page 364)

vasospasms (VAY-soh-spah-zims) (page 362)

ventricles (VEN-trih-kuls) (page 359)

vertigo (VER-tih-go) (page 368)

Introduction

The circulatory system is often referred to as the *cardiovascular system* and is composed of the heart and blood vessels (vasculature). Cardiovascular disease (CVD) is the most common cause of death in the United States and can result from coronary artery disease (CAD) (blockage of the arteries that supply the heart muscle itself), which can lead to a **myocardial infarction** (MI), known as a heart attack. An MI occurs when part of the heart is deprived of its blood supply to such an extent that the cells of the myocardium die. Another term for CAD is *coronary heart disease (CHD)*; the terms may be used interchangeably. Other related cardiovascular conditions that can lead to or result from CAD or MI include dysrhythmias (also called *arrhythmias*),

congestive heart failure (CHF), hyperlipidemia, and **hypertension** (blood pressure that is elevated above the normal limits). A stroke, also known as a *cerebrovascular accident (CVA)* or a *brain attack,* may be thought of as analogous to an MI except the vasculature affected is in the brain and the resulting damage occurs to brain cells.

To understand the drug therapies used to treat CVD, the health-care professional must have a solid understanding of the anatomy, physiology, and electrical properties of the heart as well as the vasculature. The medications in current use can produce their effects on the **myocardium** (the middle layer and most important structure of the heart; it contains the heart muscles that regulate cardiac output), the conduction system, and the coronary and other blood vessels (Figure 21-1 ■).

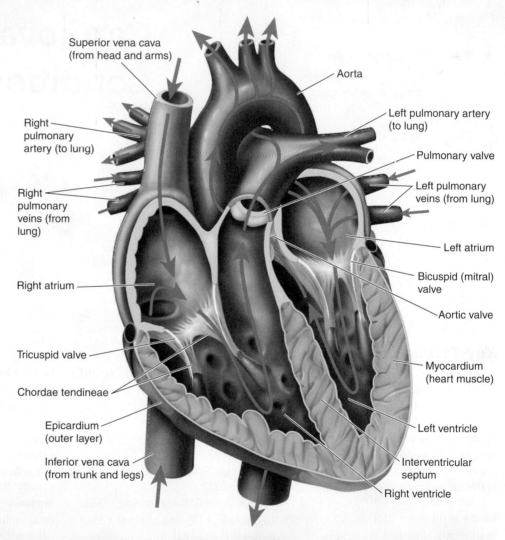

Figure 21-1 ■ Anatomy of the heart.

Focus on Geriatrics

Lifestyle and Cardiovascular Disease

CVD is most prevalent in older, sedentary individuals who are overweight or obese. With the aging of the baby boom generation, many of whom grew up on a diet of fast food rich in salt and fats, the prevalence of heart disease in the United States is increasing significantly.

Angina pectoris is a common form of ischemic heart disease and often precedes and accompanies MI. It has been described as chest pain and a squeezing pressure that can radiate to the jaw and arm. Related components of CVD and their manifestations, including CHF, hypertension, hyperlipidemia, and stroke, are discussed in Chapter 22.

Cardiac drugs to be discussed in this chapter are broadly classified according to their effects on certain parts of the cardiovascular system. These drugs can affect (1) the rate of the heart, (2) the rhythm of the heartbeat, (3) the amount of blood output, or (4) the strength of contraction.

The Cardiovascular System

The cardiovascular system begins its activity when the fetus is barely 4 weeks old and is the last system to cease activity at the end of life. This body system is so vital that it helps define the presence of life.

The heart, arteries, veins, and lymphatic system form the cardiovascular network that serves as the body's transport system. This system brings life-supporting oxygen and nutrients to cells, removes metabolic waste products, and carries hormones from one part of the body to another.

The cardiovascular, or circulatory, system is divided into two branches: pulmonary circulation and systemic circulation. In pulmonary circulation, blood picks up oxygen and liberates the waste product: carbon dioxide. In systemic circulation (which includes coronary circulation), blood carries oxygen and nutrients to all active cells and transports waste products to the kidneys, liver, and skin for excretion.

Circulation requires normal heart function to propel blood through the system by continuous rhythmic contractions of the heart. Blood circulates through three types of vessels: arteries, veins, and capillaries.

The heart is a muscular pump located within the mediastinum of the thorax. It consists of three layers:

1. The **endocardium**, which is the thin membrane lining the inside of the cardiac muscle
2. The cardiac muscle, which is called the *myocardium*
3. The **epicardium**, which is a thin membrane lining the outside of the myocardium

The heart is composed of four compartments that maintain the body's blood circulation. The two smaller upper chambers are the receiving chambers, called the left **atrium** and the right atrium; together, they are known as *atria*. The two lower chambers are called the left and right **ventricles** (the chambers that pump blood out of the heart). The upper and lower chambers are divided by a septum.

The four valves of the heart—tricuspid, pulmonary, mitral, and aortic—are located at the entrance and exit of each ventricle. Blood pumps through the four chambers of the heart with the help of the valves, which open and close via flaps, to allow blood to flow in only one direction.

The electrical conduction system contains all the wiring to initiate and maintain the rhythmic contraction of the heart (Figure 21-2 ■). The system consists of:

Sinoatrial (SA) node. Located just beneath the epicardium in the right atrium near the opening of the superior vena cava, this small, elongated mass of specialized cardiac muscle tissue initiates one impulse after another. Because it generates the heart's rhythmic contractions, it is known as the *pacemaker*.

Atrioventricular (AV) node. Located in the inferior portion of the septum, which separates the atria, and just beneath the endocardium, the AV node provides the only normal conduction pathway between the atrial and ventricular syncytia, and its fibers delay impulse transmission. This delay allows more time for the atria to completely contract so they empty all their blood into the ventricles before ventricular contraction occurs.

Bundle of His. Located between the AV node and the Purkinje fibers and also known as the *AV bundle*, the bundle of His consists of a large group of fibers that enter the upper part of the intraventricular septum and are divided into right and left bundle branches lying just beneath the endocardium.

Right and left bundle branches. Located in the heart's lower chambers (ventricles), the bundle branches divide at the bundle of His and form the right and left bundle branches. An electrical impulse travels down the right and left bundle branches at the same speed and causes the left and right ventricles to contract at the same time.

Purkinje fibers. Located about halfway down the septum, the Purkinje fibers spread from the interventricular septum into the papillary muscles toward the apex of the heart. Along this pathway, the Purkinje fibers give off many small branches, which become continuous with cardiac muscle fibers.

An **electrocardiogram** (ECG or EKG) is a tracing of the heart's electrical activity. It measures electrical activity across the myocardium. Each electrical impulse takes less than one-quarter of a second to occur. An ECG provides a visual means of examining the electrical impulses of the heart, which are labeled in a series of letters known as P, QRS, and T. An ECG graphs the atrial depolarization, ventricular depolarization, and ventricular repolarization of each electrical impulse of the heart.

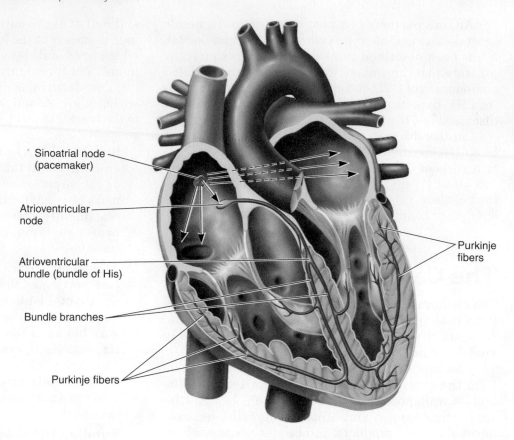

Figure 21-2 ■ Electrical conduction system of the heart.

Labels in figure:
- Sinoatrial node (pacemaker)
- Atrioventricular node
- Atrioventricular bundle (bundle of His)
- Bundle branches
- Purkinje fibers
- Purkinje fibers

✴ Apply Your Knowledge 21.1

The following questions focus on what you have just learned about the anatomy and physiology of the cardiovascular system.

CRITICAL THINKING

1. What are the major functions of the cardiovascular system?
2. What are the names of the heart wall layers?
3. What is the structure of the electrical conduction system?
4. What are the locations and names of the four valves in the heart?
5. What is the difference between pulmonary and systemic circulation?

Coronary Heart Disease

When the delivery of oxygen to the myocardium is inadequate to meet the heart's oxygen consumption needs, myocardial **ischemia** (insufficient blood flow to the myocardium) occurs. One of the major causes of ischemia is CAD, including atherosclerosis (blockage of an artery) and arteriosclerosis (hardening of an artery).

Angina pectoris is an episodic, reversible oxygen insufficiency. Oxygen demand is directly related to the strength of contraction, heart rate, and resistance to blood flow. Angina pectoris may result from the obstruction or narrowing of coronary arteries (by fatty deposits or clots), arterial spasm, pulmonary hypertension, and cardiac hypertrophy (enlargement of the heart).

Antianginal drugs are used primarily for the treatment of angina pectoris. There are several types of angina:

✳ *Classical (stable) angina* is the most common form and often occurs during exertion, emotional stress, or indigestion caused by excessive eating or a meal rich in fats and proteins. It usually causes chest discomfort, which is relieved by rest, nitroglycerin, or both. The pain typically radiates to the jaw, neck, shoulder, and left arm. Stable angina is characteristically caused by a fixed obstruction in a coronary artery.

✳ *Variant* or *vasospastic angina* is the result of a coronary artery spasm that reduces blood flow. It usually occurs at rest rather than with exertion or emotional stress.

✳ *Unstable angina* is caused by significant CAD. It occurs at rest for the first time and decreases in response to rest or nitroglycerin. It often portends an MI.

THERAPEUTIC AGENTS FOR CORONARY HEART DISEASE

Antianginal drugs are used primarily to dilate coronary blood vessels. The mainstays of treatment include the following three classes of drugs:

✳ Organic nitrates
✳ Beta-adrenergic blockers (also called beta-blockers)
✳ Calcium channel blockers

Although nitrates and calcium channel blockers dilate coronary arteries, this dilation makes a minimal contribution to their antianginal effects except in vasospastic angina.

Organic Nitrates

The oldest and most frequently prescribed drugs for the different types of angina are organic nitrates, administered to stop an acute angina attack. Inhaled amyl nitrate, translingual spray, or sublingual nitrates have a rapid onset of action and are effective for short periods. A variety of dosage forms of organic nitrates is seen in Table 21-1 ■.

Table 21-1 ■ Organonitrates and Other Anginal Medications

GENERIC NAME	TRADE NAME	USUAL DOSE FOR ADULT	ROUTES OF ADMINISTRATION
Nitrates			
nitroglycerin	Nitrolingual	0.4–0.8 mg PRN	Translingual spray
	Nitrostat	0.15–0.6 mg PRN	Sublingual
	Nitro-Bid	2.5–6.5 mg tid or qid	PO
isosorbide dinitrate	Isordil, Sorbitrate, Dilatrate-SR	2.5–40 mg tid	Sublingual
isosorbide mononitrate	Imdur, ISMO	20 mg bid	PO
erythrityl tetranitrate	Cardilate	10–30 mg tid	PO
pentaerythritol tetranitrate	Peritrate, Duotrate	10–20 mg tid or qid	30-80 mg/d
Beta-Adrenergic Blockers			
atenolol	Tenormin	25–50 mg/d; may increase to 100 mg/d	PO
propranolol	Inderal	10–90 mg bid or qid	PO
	Vascor	200–400 mg/d	PO
Calcium Channel Blockers (see Table 17-3 for other calcium channel blockers used as antidysrhythmics.)			
verapamil	Calan, Calan SR, Covera-HS, Isoptin, Isoptin SR, Verelan, Verelan PM	80 mg q6–8h; may increase up to 320–480 mg/d in divided doses (Covera-HS must be given once daily at bedtime)	PO

bid, twice a day; O, oral; PRN, as needed; qid, four times a day; tid, three times a day.

Focus On

Nitroglycerin

The classic organic nitrate nitroglycerin (Nitrostat, Nitrobid) was once the drug of choice for the treatment of patients with angina pectoris. Nitroglycerin is effective, inexpensive, and fast acting.

How does it work?

Nitroglycerin directly affects the vascular smooth muscle to dilate blood vessels. It decreases cardiac oxygen demand in stable angina, but in variant angina, it relaxes the spasms and increases oxygen supply.

How is it used?

Nitroglycerin preparations are administered by using a variety of routes, producing similar responses but differing in the time of onset and duration. Some of these preparations are rapidly effective (1–5 minutes) and last about 60 minutes, but for others, the effect is slower in onset but lasts several hours. Only a few medications have a rapid onset and long duration of action. They can be used to relieve acute anginal pain or prophylactically to prevent angina attack with extended-release forms.

Sublingual nitroglycerin is effective rapidly, lasts about 1 hour, and is an ideal preparation for acute anginal pain. By this route of administration, it avoids hepatic first-pass metabolism. If one dose is not sufficient, one or two additional doses should be taken at 5-minute intervals. The medication bottle should not be opened unless it is needed because its shelf life is longer in a dark and tightly closed container.

Transdermal nitroglycerin can release its reservoir slowly for absorption through the skin. These patches should be applied once a day to a hairless site of skin. The patch sites should be rotated daily to prevent local irritation. The patch should not be worn for more than 10 to 12 hours per day; this so-called off period is necessary to prevent the development of a tolerance to the drug and allows for continued therapeutic efficacy.

Nitroglycerin is also available as a topical ointment that must be measured on a paper provided with the prescription to ensure proper dosage. See Chapter 4 for the application of percutaneous medications.

Discontinuation of nitroglycerin should take place over time because discontinuation of long-acting nitroglycerin preparations can cause **vasospasms** (spasms of the blood vessels) and angina.

What are the adverse effects?

The most common adverse effects include headache, **hypotension** (an abnormal condition in which the blood pressure is not adequate for full oxygenation of the tissues), and **tachycardia** (an abnormally fast heartbeat). The dizziness and lightheadedness of hypotension are better tolerated with time.

What are the contraindications and interactions?

Nitroglycerin's contraindications include obstructive hypertrophic cardiomyopathy, pronounced hypovolemia (a decrease in the volume of circulating blood), inferior MI with right ventricular involvement, increased intracranial pressure, and cardiac tamponade (blockage in the heart). It should not be stopped abruptly after long therapy because there is a rebound risk of more frequent angina pectoris. Nitroglycerin (Nitrostat, Nitro-Bid) reinforces the hypotensive effect of antihypertensive agents. If combined with alcohol, a sudden decrease in blood pressure can occur. Nitroglycerin increases the bioavailability of dihydroergotamine. In smokers, nicotine antagonizes the coronary dilating effect of nitroglycerin. Nitroglycerin is also contraindicated in pregnancy and lactation.

What are the important points patients should know?

Advise patients that nitroglycerin should not be carried close to the body because heat from the body can deactivate it. Tell patients to store the medication in a cool, dark place and keep it in the original container. Advise patients to avoid alcoholic beverages when taking nitroglycerin and to take one tablet sublingually every 5 minutes, not exceeding three tablets. Tell patients that if chest pain continues, they should seek emergency medical attention. Advise patients to discard unused tablets after 6 months.

Focus Point

Nitroglycerin

Nitroglycerin may cause severe low blood pressure (marked by dizziness or lightheadedness), especially if an individual is in an upright position or has just gotten up from sitting or lying down. The heart rate can slow, and chest pain can increase. People taking diuretic medications and those who have low systolic blood pressure (less than 90 mm Hg) should use nitroglycerin with caution.

ISOSORBIDE DINITRATE AND ISOSORBIDE MONONITRATE

Isosorbide dinitrate (Cedocard Retard, Isordil, Sorbid SA) and isosorbide mononitrate (Elantan, Imdur, Ismo) are other forms of organic nitrates that provide longer durations of action than nitroglycerin. These agents are effective in the treatment of all types of angina pectoris and are available in sublingual and chewable tablet forms. The most common complaint by users is headache. Both agents should be given cautiously to patients with glaucoma (see Chapter 30). The advantage of isosorbide mononitrate over isosorbide dinitrate is that there is no first-pass metabolism.

ERYTHRITYL TETRANITRATE

The principal use of another form of organic nitrate—erythrityl tetranitrate (Cardilate)—is in the **prophylaxis** (prevention) of angina pectoris in acute situations in which an attack can be anticipated. Adverse effects include tachycardia, headache, flushing, dizziness, syncope (loss of consciousness and body tone; fainting), and nausea. It should also be given cautiously to patients with glaucoma.

PENTAERYTHRITOL TETRANITRATE

Pentaerythritol tetranitrate (Peritrate, Duotrate) is a long-acting organic nitrate. It is used in the prophylaxis of angina pectoris but not in the management of the acute attack. Transient headache and nausea may accompany its use. It should be given cautiously to patients with glaucoma.

Beta-Adrenergic Blockers

Beta-adrenergic blockers (propranolol, atenolol), known as *beta-blockers* or *β-blockers*, reduce the heart's oxygen demand by decreasing the heart rate. In the heart, **sympathetic** stimulation causes increased rate and force as well as increased oxygen use. (*Sympathetic* relates to the sympathetic part of the autonomic nervous system or the *fight-or-flight* response.) Beta-blockers prevent the development of myocardial ischemia and pain. Propranolol (Inderal) is often used for the treatment of angina, and it may be used in combination with nitrates for controlling angina. Beta-blockers should be used with caution or avoided in patients with asthma because of the potential for bronchospasm, and they may mask hypoglycemia in patients with diabetes mellitus. Beta-blockers may produce **insomnia** (inability to sleep normally), bizarre dreams, and depression. See Table 21-1 for dosages and routes of transmission. Beta-blockers are discussed in more depth later in this chapter.

Focus on Natural Products

Food and Drug Interactions

Many natural substances (including food) interact with pharmaceuticals; for example, warfarin sodium (Coumadin) interacts with such foods as beef liver, broccoli, Brussels sprouts, cabbage, spinach, and other leafy green vegetables. These foods contain large amounts of vitamin K, which decreases the effect of the drug.

Calcium Channel Blockers

Calcium channel blockers (for example, verapamil and bepridil) interfere with the movement of calcium ions through cell membranes. These drugs can affect the heart itself or the peripheral vasculature. They are used to treat the pain of angina pectoris and to lower blood pressure. Contraction of the vascular smooth muscle depends on calcium movement from extracellular to intracellular sites. The prevention of calcium action inhibits this contraction. Therefore, it decreases vascular tone and causes **vasodilation** (the dilation of blood vessels; this action relaxes the smooth muscle of the peripheral arterioles). These agents are prescribed for vasospastic angina. Calcium channel blockers are used for the treatment of angina, dysrhythmia, and hypertension (see Tables 21-1 and 21-3 for dosages and routes of delivery). Bepridil (Vascor) is a calcium channel blocker used specifically for angina pectoris. It slows the heart rate and has antidysrhythmic properties. The common adverse effects are dizziness, hypotension, fatigue, headache, and constipation. Calcium channel blockers are discussed in detail in a later section of this chapter.

✳ Apply Your Knowledge 21.2

The following questions focus on what you have just learned about CHD and related therapeutic agents.

CRITICAL THINKING

1. What are the most common types of angina?
2. What are three classes of antianginal drugs?
3. What is the mechanism of action of nitroglycerin?
4. What is the advantage of isosorbide mononitrate over isosorbide dinitrate?
5. What types of organic nitrates are used in the prophylaxis of angina pectoris?
6. What are the most common adverse effects of nitroglycerin?
7. What are three trade names of nitroglycerin?
8. Which type of angina occurs at rest for the first time?

Myocardial Infarction

Acute MI (AMI) occurs when a part of the myocardium experiences a severe and prolonged restriction of oxygenated coronary blood. Nearly 40% of all patients experiencing AMI die before reaching acute care health centers. An AMI can occur when an area of the heart muscle dies through lack of sufficient oxygen. AMI is the leading cause of death in industrialized nations, possibly because of a diet high in cholesterol and fat and a sedentary lifestyle. The insufficient oxygen supply to the myocardium is the result of (1) a decreased flow of oxygen-rich blood to the heart muscle and (2) an increased demand for oxygen by the myocardium that exceeds what the circulation can supply. CAD, clot formation in the coronary artery or spasm of these arteries, stress, heavy exertion, and an abrupt increase in blood pressure are the main causes of AMI.

Focus on Pediatrics

Acute Myocardial Infarction in Children

AMI is rare in childhood. Adults usually develop CAD from the lifelong buildup of atheroma (a yellow-tinted swelling of the arteries, characteristic of atherosclerosis) and plaque, which causes coronary artery spasm and thrombosis. Pediatric patients with AMI usually have either an acute inflammatory condition of the coronary arteries or an anomalous origin of the left coronary artery.

THERAPEUTIC AGENTS FOR MYOCARDIAL INFARCTION

The goal of treatment of patients with AMI is to limit damage to the myocardium, thereby preserving enough myocardial function to sustain life. In addition to intravenous (IV) fluids, pharmacotherapeutics are used as the first line of treatment for AMI. Treatment is designed to relieve distress, reverse ischemia, limit the size of infarct (the amount of tissue death related to lack of arterial or venous blood), reduce cardiac work, and prevent and treat complications. AMI is an acute medical emergency, and outcome is significantly influenced by rapid diagnosis and treatment. Fifty percent of deaths from AMI occur within 3 to 4 hours of onset of the clinical **syndrome** (a collection of signs and symptoms that together signify a specific disease). The outcome can be influenced by early treatment.

Nitroglycerin is administered to decrease the heart's workload and increase blood supply to the heart muscle. Aspirin and thrombolytic drugs are most effective if given within the first few minutes and hours after the onset of MI. The greatest risk of thrombolytic therapy is hemorrhage (bleeding), specifically inside the brain. Anticoagulants are discussed in Chapter 23.

Morphine sulfate—2 to 4 mg IV; repeated as needed—is a critical adjunct to nitroglycerin. Morphine is highly effective for the pain of MI. Potential side effects of morphine are the depression of respiration and reduction of myocardial contractility. Hypotension and **bradycardia** (an abnormally slow heartbeat) secondary to morphine can usually be overcome by prompt elevation of the lower extremities. Such beta-blockers as metoprolol (Toprol, Lopressor) and atenolol (Tenormin), reduce the heart's oxygen demand by decreasing the heart rate. Such calcium channel blockers as nifedipine (Procardia, Aldalat) and diltiazem (Cardizem, Dilacor) decrease myocardial oxygen demand and increase oxygen supply. Oxygen is also reasonably administered via 40% mask or nasal prongs at 4 to 6 L/min for the first few hours.

✳ Apply Your Knowledge 21.3 ▬▬▬▬

The following questions focus on what you have just learned about MI and its therapeutic agents.

CRITICAL THINKING

1. What are causes of insufficient oxygen supply to the myocardium?
2. Why is acute MI rare in childhood?
3. What is the goal of treatment in acute MI?
4. What are the mainstays of treatment in acute MI?
5. What is the definition of bradycardia?
6. What are the adverse effects of morphine to relieve pain in MI?

Dysrhythmias

The rate of heartbeat and rhythm of the heart are controlled by the SA node (sometimes termed the *pacemaker*) in the right atrium. This node generates tiny electrical impulses to the adjacent muscle of the atrium, causing the atria to contract and pump blood into the ventricles. The impulses sent out by the SA node are received by the AV node, travel down the bundle of His, and are transported to the ventricular muscles by a network of nerves. The SA node and the AV node receive autonomic innervations that control the rate of the heart to a certain extent.

Any deviation from the normal orderly sequence of impulses is a disturbance of the rhythm and is called a **dysrhythmia** or an *arrhythmia*. Sometimes, an area of muscle in one of the atria becomes more excitable than the SA node and fires more rapid impulses. The rest of the heart then responds to this new pacemaker, and the resulting dysrhythmia is known as *atrial tachycardia.* Dysrhythmias may be benign (as in atrial tachycardia) or malignant (as in ventricular tachycardia). Benign abnormalities generally have a low risk of sudden death. Malignant abnormalities have a moderate risk of sudden death. Malignant arrhythmias indicate an immediate risk for heart disease. Table 21-2 ■ summarizes different arrhythmias and beats per minute.

ANTIDYSRHYTHMIC AGENTS

Dysrhythmias can occur from heart disease or from chronic drug therapy. Dysrhythmias can also be caused by the drugs used to regulate dysrhythmia because they create an alteration of the heart's electrical

Table 21-2 ■ Various Dysrhythmias

ARRHYTHMIA	BEATS PER MINUTE
Bradycardia	Less than 60
Tachycardia	150–250
Atrial flutter	200–350
Atrial fibrillation	More than 350
Ventricular fibrillation	Variable
Premature atrial contraction	Variable
Premature ventricular contraction	Variable

impulse. When severe dysrhythmia occurs, especially in ventricular disorders, the patient can be experiencing a medical emergency requiring hospital care.

Antidysrhythmic drug therapy is the mainstay of management for most important dysrhythmias. There is no universally effective drug. All these agents have important safety limitations and can aggravate or promote arrhythmias. Drug selection is difficult and often involves trial and error (Table 21-3).

Antidysrhythmic drug actions based on cellular electrophysiologic effects have been classified into four groups. This classification is recognized internationally and provides a general logic for grouping drugs. Classifications of antidysrhythmic drugs are seen in Table 21-3 ■.

Table 21-3 ■ Antidysrhythmic Medications

GENERIC NAME	TRADE NAME	USUAL DOSE FOR ADULTS	ROUTES OF ADMINISTRATION
Class Ia			
quinidine	Cardioquin	200–600 mg tid–qid	PO
procainamide	Pronestyl, Procan-SR	1 g followed by 250–500 mg q3h	PO
		0.5–1 g q4–6h until able to take PO	IM
		100 mg q5min at a rate of 25–50 mg/min (up to 1 g)	IV
disopyramide	Norpace	400–800 mg/d in divided doses	PO
Class Ib			
lidocaine	Xylocaine	1–1.5 mg/kg; may repeat 0.5–1.5 mg/kg q5–10 min, to total of 3 mg/kg	IV
		4.3 mg/kg	IM
mexiletine	Mexitil	200–400 mg q8h	PO
phenytoin	Dilantin	100 mg q5min	PO
Class Ic			
flecainide	Tambocor	Initially, 100 mg q12h; increase in 50-mg increments twice daily q4d until effective	PO
propafenone	Rythmol	450 mg/d; increase dosage slowly if needed, up to 900 mg/d	PO
moricizine	Ethmozine	600–900 mg/d	PO
Class II			
esmolol	Brevibloc	50–500 mcg/min	IV
propranolol	Inderal	10–30 mg three to four times/d before meals and at bedtime	PO
		1–3 mg initially; repeated if necessary in 2 min	IV

GENERIC NAME	TRADE NAME	USUAL DOSE FOR ADULTS	ROUTES OF ADMINISTRATION
metoprolol	Lopressor	100 mg/d in two divided doses	PO
		5 mg q2min for three doses followed by PO	IV
acebutolol	Sectral	Initially, 200 mg bid; dose is increased gradually until the optimal response is obtained.	PO
Class III			
amiodarone	Cordarone	400–1600 mg/d	PO
		150 mg over 10 min, followed by 360 mg over the next 6h	IV loading dose
sotalol	Betapace	80–320 mg/d	PO
dofetilide	Tikosyn	125–250 mcg bid	PO
ibutilide	Corvert	Weight <60 kg, 0.01 mg/kg (0.1 mL/kg) injection	IV
		Weight >60 kg, 1 mg (10 mL)	IV
bretylium	Bretylol	5–10 mg/kg by infusion	IM
Class IV			
verapamil	Calan	240–480 mg/d divided into three to four doses	PO
		Initially, 5–10 mg as IV bolus over 2 min	IV
diltiazem	Cardizem, Tiazac	60–120 mg sustained released bid	PO
		0.25 mg/kg IV bolus over 2 min	IV

IM, intramuscular; IV, intravenous; PO, oral; qid, four times a day; tid, three times a day.

Class I—Drugs That Bind to Sodium Channels

Class I drugs are sodium channel blockers, including older antidysrhythmic drugs (for example, quinidine). These drugs reduce the maximal rate of contraction of the myocardium and slow conduction. Class I drugs are subclassified into three classes:

Class Ia—drugs with intermediate onset and offset

Class Ib—drugs with short effects

Class Ic—drugs with prolonged effects

Focus On

Quinidine (Class Ia)

Quinidine (Quinidex, Duraquin) is approved for atrial **fibrillation** (very rapid, irregular contractions or twitching of the individual muscular fibers of the atria or ventricles) and **flutter** (rapid, regular atrial contractions that often produce "sawtooth" waves in an ECG or rapid ventricular tachycardia that appears as a regular, undulating pattern in an ECG, without QRS and T waves, as would normally be found). Quinidine is related to quinine and has been used in cardiac conditions since the 1920s.

How does it work?

Quinidine depresses the myocardium and the conduction system, decreasing the contractile force of the heart and slowing the heart rate.

How is it used?

If an initial test dose of quinidine sulfate (Quinidex) is tolerated, the maintenance dosage is usually 200 to 400

(Continued)

Focus On (Continued)

mg orally every 4 to 6 hours. A salt form of quinidine gluconate is also available in intramuscular and IV forms. Sustained-release forms are also available for the sulfate and gluconate salts.

What are the adverse effects?

Adverse reactions include diarrhea, flatulence, and abdominal pain. Fever, reduced **platelets** (megakaryocyte fragments important in the clotting of blood), and liver function abnormalities can occur. Quinidine syncope (sudden ventricular fibrillation in patients taking quinidine) is potentially dangerous and can be life threatening.

What are the contraindications and interactions?

Quinidine is contraindicated in pregnancy, lactation, bacterial endocarditis, and myasthenia gravis. Quinidine

has the potential to double digoxin (Lanoxin) levels in the blood. Potentially fatal interactions can occur when quinidine is given with digoxin. Quinidine also interacts with amiodarone (Cordarone) and verapamil (Calan).

What are the important points patients should know?

Tell patients to immediately report any chest pain or change in heart rhythm to their health-care providers. Advise patients to take quinidine with food to avoid gastric upset, although this may delay absorption of the drug. A diet high in citrus fruits, vegetables, and milk may delay excretion of the drug, so advise patients not to increase their intake of these foods beyond their normal diet. Advise patients to report diarrhea to their health-care providers.

PROCAINAMIDE (CLASS Ia)

Procainamide (Pronestyl, Procan-SR) is an antidysrrhythmic drug approved for life-threatening ventricular dysrhythmias. It is related to procaine and has much less effect than quinidine on refraction (resistance to disease treatment). The usual oral dosage is 250 to 625 mg every 3 to 4 hours. Fever, arthralgia (joint pain), and pleural effusions (increased amounts of fluid accumulating in the areas surrounding the lungs) are adverse reactions of procainamide.

DISOPYRAMIDE (CLASS Ia)

Disopyramide (Norpace) decreases cardiac excitability and is a cardiac depressant. Oral dosing is usually 100 to 150 mg every 6 hours. Adverse effects are dry mouth, constipation, visual disturbances, and urine retention.

LIDOCAINE (CLASS Ib)

Lidocaine (Xylocaine) can suppress the ventricular arrhythmias that complicate MI and reduce the incidence of primary ventricular fibrillation when given prophylactically in early AMI. Its mechanism of action appears to be the blocking of activated and inactivated sodium channels, with a great effect on depolarized or ischemic tissues. Adverse effects are neurologic, such as tremor and convulsions, rather than cardiac. Drowsiness, delirium, and paresthesias (abnormal burning, pricking, tickling, or tingling) may occur with too-rapid administration. Mexiletine (Mexitil) and tocainide (Tonocard) are chemically and therapeutically related to lidocaine (Xylocaine). These two drugs have been modified for oral administration so they can be used in ambulatory care. Lidocaine (Xylocaine) has noted drug interactions with cimetidine (Tagamet).

MEXILETINE (CLASS Ib)

Mexiletine (Mexitil) has an action similar to lidocaine. It is prescribed for ventricular tachycardia but is more effective when used with another antidysrhythmic agent. Adverse effects are neurologic and gastrointestinal symptoms and increased liver enzyme levels.

PHENYTOIN (CLASS Ib)

Phenytoin (Dilantin) was used extensively for dysrhythmia management, particularly for suppressing the ventricular dysrhythmias of digitalis toxicity, until the advent of newer drugs and the decline of digoxin toxicity. Now phenytoin is most commonly used for epilepsy. The common adverse effects are **gingival hyperplasia** (an increase in the number of cells in the gums of the mouth, causing them to have a swollen appearance), blurred vision, **vertigo** (a sensation of revolving—either of the patients themselves or of their environment), and **nystagmus** (a constant, involuntary movement of the eye). Phenytoin has noted drug interactions with cimetidine (Tagamet), disulfiram (Antabuse), dopamine (Dopastat or Entropion), and fluconazole (Diflucan).

FLECAINIDE (CLASS Ic)

Flecainide (Tambocor) is an antidysrhythmic agent with electrophysiologic properties similar to those of other class Ic antidysrhythmic drugs. It is used for the treatment of patients with life-threatening ventricular dysrhythmias. Adverse effects include dizziness, headache, fatigue, chest pain, and blurred vision. Flecainide may also produce nausea, constipation, and a change in taste perception.

PROPAFENONE (CLASS Ic)

Propafenone (Rythmol) is another class Ic antidysrhythmic drug with a direct stabilizing action on myocardial membranes. It is used for the treatment and management of patients with ventricular dysrhythmias. Adverse effects include blurred vision, dizziness, fatigue, **somnolence** (sleepiness, dullness, or a deadening sensation), vertigo, and headache. It may also cause hypotension, nausea, abdominal discomfort, constipation, vomiting, dry mouth, and taste alterations.

MORICIZINE (CLASS Ic)

Moricizine (Ethmozine) is an antidysrhythmic agent with potent local anesthetic effects. It is prescribed for the treatment of ventricular tachycardia and ventricular premature depolarization (change in direction, destruction, or neutralization of polarity). Adverse effects include dizziness, lightheadedness, anxiety, euphoria, and headache. The other adverse effects may be nausea, diarrhea, dry mouth, and abdominal discomfort.

Class II—Beta-Adrenergic Blockers

Beta-blockers may be the least toxic and most powerful drugs available, but their antidysrhythmic effects are often overlooked. Relatively few dysrhythmias are caused primarily by sympathetic overactivity; most are regulated by autonomic tone (which is the firmness of muscles as controlled by the autonomic nervous system).

Overactivity of the sympathetic nerves releases norepinephrine and epinephrine. These agents increase heart rate, heart excitability, conduction velocity, and **automaticity** (the heart impulse's automatic, spontaneous initiation), particularly of the ventricles. In general, beta-blockers are well tolerated, but they may depress left ventricular function, particularly in antirrhythmic doses. They are contraindicated in people with asthma. Gastrointestinal disturbances, insomnia, and nightmares may occur. Beta-adrenergic blockers will be discussed in Chapter 22.

Focus On

Propranolol (Class II)

Propranolol (Inderal) is the most common beta-blocker used as an antidysrhythmic. Before 1978, it was the only beta-blocker approved to treat dysrhythmias. Since then, several other beta-blockers have been approved to treat dysrhythmias, but propranolol is still the mainstay of treatment.

How does it work?

Propranolol affects both types of beta receptors; because of this, it is considered a nonselective beta-blocker. It reduces or slows the heart rate and lowers blood pressure. In addition to its beta-blocking effect, it also causes a quinidine-like depression of the myocardium.

How is it used?

Propranolol is often combined with other cardiovascular drugs, such as digoxin (Lanoxin) and quinidine (Quinidex), to treat patients with CVD. It is most effective for tachycardia, but it is also approved to treat a broad range of other disorders, such as hypertension and angina, and for the prevention of MI. It is prescribed in oral form and is also administered IV. Sustained-release forms are also available.

What are the adverse effects?

Hypotension and bradycardia are the most common side effects. Patients with other cardiac disorders, such as heart failure, must be carefully monitored because propranolol can slow the heart rate. Such side effects as diminished sex drive and impotence can also occur.

What are the contraindications and interactions?

Propranolol is contraindicated in bronchial asthma or bronchospasm, severe chronic obstructive airway disease, allergic rhinitis during pollen season, and pregnancy. Propranolol interacts with clonidine (Catapres), cimetidine (Tagamet), epinephrine, and insulin.

What are the important points patients should know?

Propranolol should not be abruptly discontinued because it may cause MI or severe dysrhythmias. Tell the patient to take his or her pulse on a regular basis; if the pulse is less than 60 beats per minute, the patient's health-care provider should be notified immediately. Because of propranolol's potential to cause hypotension, advise the patient to slowly rise from a lying or sitting position.

Class III—Drugs That Interfere with Potassium Outflow

Class III antidysrhythmic agents—potassium channel blockers—interfere with potassium channels to alter the repolarization phase of the heart's contraction. This prolongs the potential contraction duration of the Purkinje fibers and the muscle fibers of the ventricles. The prolonged period decreases the frequency of heart failure.

Focus On

Amiodarone

Amiodarone (Cordarone, Pacerone) is a powerful class III antidysrhythmic agent.

How does it work?

Amiodarone blocks potassium ion channels as well as sodium ion channels. This action prolongs the resting stage of the heart's contraction as well as the refractory period, which stabilizes atrial and ventricular dysrhythmias.

How is it used?

It is used to treat atrial dysrhythmias in patients with heart failure. Oral dosage forms may take several weeks to produce an effect. However, its effects can last 4 to 8 weeks after it is discontinued because of its extended half-life. An IV form is available, but it is usually reserved for patients with serious ventricular dysrhythmias.

What are the adverse effects?

Amiodarone has few cardiovascular adverse effects, perhaps because of its modest vasodilator action, which produces little or no left ventricular depression. SA node activity is minimally affected. Amiodarone decreases automaticity, prolongs AV conduction, and can even block the exchange of sodium and potassium. Amiodarone (Cordarone, Pacerone) is too toxic for long-term use except for serious ventricular dysrhythmias. Pulmonary fibrosis can occur in some patients treated with the drug for more than 5 years and could be fatal. Other significant potential adverse effects include changes in thyroid function (hypothyroidism or hyperthyroidism) and visual disturbances as a result of optic neuritis or corneal microdeposits. Common adverse effects that may be self-limiting include dizziness, nausea, vomiting, anorexia, bitter taste, weight loss, and numbness of the fingers and toes. Weakness can also occur.

What are the contraindications and interactions?

Amiodarone is contraindicated in patients with severe liver disease, pregnancy, children, and severe sinus bradycardia. Amiodarone interacts with many other drugs, including digoxin (Lanoxin) and phenytoin (Dilantin).

What are the important points patients should know?

Tell patients to notify their health-care providers immediately if shortness of breath, cough, or a change in heart rate and rhythm occurs. Also, instruct patients to immediately report any vision changes to their health-care providers. Advise patients to change positions slowly to avoid dizziness. Advise patients, especially elderly patients, to protect their skin and eyes from the sun.

SOTALOL

Sotalol (Betapace) has class II and III antidysrhythmic properties. Although measurable class III effects can be detected in clinical use, they are largely masked by the drug's beta-blocking properties. Sotalol is used for the treatment of documented ventricular arrhythmias that, in the judgment of the physician, are life threatening.

DOFETILIDE

Dofetilide (Tikosyn) is a class III antidysrhythmic agent that prolongs the cardiac action potential by blocking the potassium channels. It is used for the treatment of symptomatic atrial fibrillation and flutter. Adverse effects on the body as a whole include flu-like syndrome and back pain. The most common adverse effects of dofetilide are headache, dizziness, insomnia, nausea, diarrhea, and abdominal pain.

IBUTILIDE

Ibutilide (Corvert) is a newly approved class III drug that differs markedly from amiodarone and sotalol. It achieves its effect by activating a slow, inward sodium current rather than by blocking outward potassium currents. Injecting ibutilide can acutely terminate atrial fibrillation and atrial flutter, particularly in patients with recent onset of dysrhythmia.

BRETYLIUM

Bretylium (Bretylo) also has antisympathetic class III action. It may cause marked hypotension and is indicated only for the management of potentially lethal **refractory** ventricular tachyarrhythmias. (*Refractory* means the period during repolarization when cells cannot respond normally to a second stimulus.) Bretylium is usually effective within 30 minutes of injection.

Class IV—Calcium Channel Blockers

Class IV drugs are termed *calcium channel blockers* because they decrease the entry of calcium into the cells of the heart and blood vessels. The SA and AV nodes require calcium for normal activity and normal sinus rhythm. Reducing calcium decreases the rate of the SA node and the conduction velocity of the AV node, and it is effective in the treatment of supraventricular tachycardia. Class IV drugs can decrease the ability of the heart to produce forceful contractions, leading to CHF. These medications also relax smooth muscle and cause vasodilation. Therefore, these agents are useful for angina and hypertension.

Focus on Geriatrics

Heart Failure and Surgery

The chance of having heart failure increases as we age. One in 15 elderly patients between the ages of 75 and 84 years (men more often than women) is diagnosed with some type of heart failure. CHD, heart failure, and clinically significant dysrhythmias require in-depth evaluation and control before any type of elective, noncardiac surgery is performed.

Focus On

Verapamil

Verapamil (Calan, Isoptin) was the first calcium channel blocker approved by the FDA.

How does it work?

Verapamil acts principally on the AV node, slowing conduction. Therefore, it causes the depression of myocardial contractibility and dilation of coronary arteries. These effects lead to decreased cardiac work and decreased cardiac energy consumption in patients with vasospastic angina. This effect increases the delivery of oxygen to myocardial cells.

How is it used?

Verapamil is used to stabilize dysrhythmias. It is also approved for use in hypertension and angina. For dysrhythmias, it is prescribed in oral forms, but sustained-release and IV forms are also available.

What are the adverse effects?

The adverse effects are dizziness, vertigo, emotional depression, sleepiness, headache, peripheral edema, hypotension, nausea, and constipation.

What are the contraindications and interactions?

Verapamil (Calan, Isoptin) is contraindicated in patients with an allergy to this agent, hypotension, pregnancy, lactation, and CHF. Verapamil interacts with carbamazepine, lithium, cyclosporine, and calcium salts. It may also increase blood levels of digoxin (Lanoxin).

What are the important points patients should know?

Instruct patients to take their blood pressure before taking verapamil. They should contact their health-care providers if their blood pressure is below 90/60 mm Hg. Advise patients to notify their health-care providers if they experience any breathing difficulty or change in heart rhythm. Also, advise patients to take verapamil with food to avoid an upset stomach and to increase their intake of fiber to avoid constipation.

Focus Point

Top 10 Prescribed Cardiovascular Drugs

1. atorvastatin (Lipitor)
2. amlodipine (Norvasc)
3. lisinopril (Zestril)
4. digoxin (Lanoxin)
5. simvastatin (Zocor)
6. enalapril (Vasotec)
7. warfarin sodium (Coumadin)
8. pravastatin (Pravachol)
9. quinapril (Accupril)
10. diltiazem (Cardizem CD)

DILTIAZEM

Diltiazem (Cardizem, Dilacor) is less potent than vera-pamil in decreasing heart rate but is more potent as a vasodilator. It is used for essential hypertension, angina pectoris caused by coronary artery spasm and such dysrhythmias as atrial fibrillation, atrial flutter, and supraventricular tachycardia. Adverse effects include headache, fatigue, dizziness, nervousness, insomnia, and confusion. It may also cause edema, flushing, hypotension, nausea, vomiting, and impaired taste. Diltiazem has noted drug interactions with cyclosporine (Nedral).

Focus Point

Look-Alike and Sound-Alike Drugs

Drug Name and Purpose	Looks Like/Sounds Like
amiodarone (antidysrhythmic)	amrinone (cardiac inotropic agent)
dopamine (heart stimulant)	dobutamine (sympathetic A and B agonist)
metoprolol (beta-blocker)	misoprostol (prostaglandin analog for ulcer therapy)
Lanoxin (digoxin-cardiac glycoside)	Lasix (diuretic)
pindolol (beta-blocker)	Parlodel (dopaminergic agonist inhibitor of prolactin)
Propulsid (stimulator of GI function)	propranolol (beta-blocker)

✳ Apply Your Knowledge 21.4

The following questions focus on what you have just learned about dysrhythmias (arrhythmias) and their therapeutic agents.

CRITICAL THINKING

1. What are the causes of dysrhythmias?
2. What is the mainstay of management for the most important dysrhythmias?
3. What are the trade names of procainamide, phenytoin, moricizine, esmolol, amiodarone, and diltiazem?
4. What class of antidysrhythmic can bind to sodium channels?
5. What are three examples of drugs in class 1A of antidysrhythmic?
6. What classes of antidysrhythmics are the least toxic and most powerful drugs available?
7. What drug is a powerful class III antidysrhythmic?
8. Which drug was the first calcium channel blocker approved by the FDA?

LABELING

Answer the following drug labeling questions by using the label depicted below. You may need to use your drug guide or the *Physicians' Desk Reference* to answer some of the questions.

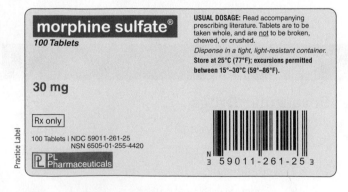

(For educational purposes only)

1. Generic name: _____

2. Drug class: _____

3. Form of drug: _____

4. Drug schedule (use "Rx" if not a scheduled drug): _____

5. Adult dosage: _____

6. Typical use: _____

7. Body system that this drug targets: _____

8. Manufacturer: _____

9. Storage requirements: _____

10. Pregnancy category: _____

PRACTICAL SCENARIO 1

A 60-year-old man called emergency medical services, complaining of severe angina and dizziness. He told the paramedic he had been prescribed nitroglycerin for angina pectoris and was taking it as needed. He stated that he always kept a little envelope of the drug in his breast pocket and the rest in his car in case he needed more. About 2 hours earlier, he reported, he had finished a large meal preceded by a cocktail and accompanied by wine. When he felt the pain begin, he slipped a nitroglycerin tablet under his tongue. When it had no effect after 10 minutes, he took another, waited, and then took another. Nothing stopped the pain, and now he was afraid he was having a heart attack. His ECG was negative for MI. The paramedic realized why the nitroglycerin did not alleviate his angina.

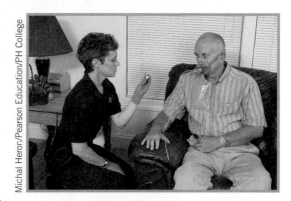

Michal Heron/Pearson Education/PH College

Critical Thinking Questions

1. What were the "clues" that helped the paramedic figure out why the nitroglycerin did not alleviate the man's angina?
2. Why did dizziness accompany the man's angina?
3. What important advice should be given to patients taking nitroglycerin?

PRACTICAL SCENARIO 2

A 52-year-old man was admitted to the intensive care unit with ventricular tachycardia. His physician ordered a class I antiarrhythmic agent.

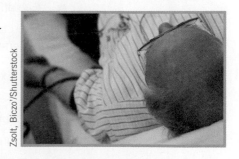

Zsolt, Biczo'/Shutterstock

Critical Thinking Questions

1. What is another name used to describe class I antiarrhythmic agents?
2. Name all drugs that are listed as class IA, IB, or IC.

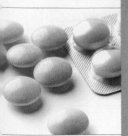

Chapter Capsule

This section repeats the objectives from the beginning of the chapter and then provides a summary of the most important concepts for that objective. Use this section as a quick review and to check your knowledge.

Objective 1: Identify the electrical conduction system of the heart.

- Sinoatrial (SA) node
- Atrioventricular (AV) node
- Bundle of His
- Right and left bundle branches
- Purkinje fibers

Objective 2: Name the three layers of the heart and the four heart valves.

- Layers of the heart—endocardium, myocardium, epicardium
- Heart valves—tricuspid, pulmonary, mitral, aortic

Objective 3: Define three types of angina pectoris.

- Classical or stable angina—caused by a fixed obstruction in a coronary artery and brought on by exertion, emotional stress, or indigestion; usually causes chest discomfort (with pain radiating to the jaw, neck, shoulder, and left arm) that is relieved by rest or nitroglycerin; the most common form
- Variant or vasospastic angina—caused by coronary artery spasm that reduces blood flow; usually occurs at rest rather than with exertion or emotional stress
- Unstable angina—caused by significant coronary artery disease; occurs at rest for the first time and decreases in response to rest or nitroglycerin; often portends myocardial infarction

Objective 4: Name the mainstays of angina therapy.

- Beta-blockers
- Calcium channel blockers

Objective 5: Describe the action of vasodilation.

- Increases the size of blood vessels to improve the circulation of the blood

Objective 6: Define calcium channel blockers.

- Drugs that decrease vascular tone and cause vasodilation by interfering with the movement of calcium ions through cell membranes, inhibiting the contraction of vascular smooth muscle
- Can affect the heart, peripheral vasculature, or both
- Used to treat dysrhythmias, the pain of angina pectoris, vasospastic angina, and hypertension

Objective 7: Explain myocardial infarction.

- Occurs when part of the myocardium experiences a prolonged restriction of oxygenated coronary blood
- Requires rapid diagnosis and treatment for a good outcome
- Is the leading cause of death in industrialized nations

Objective 8: Identify the classifications of antidysrhythmic drugs and explain their actions.

- Four classes (I to IV) of drugs are used to treat arrhythmias
- Class I includes subtypes a, b, and c
- Class I drugs bind to sodium channels, reducing the maximal rate of contraction of the myocardium and slowing conduction
- Class II drugs—beta-adrenergic blockers reduce the heart's oxygen demand by decreasing the heart rate and preventing the development of myocardial ischemias and angina
- Class III drugs—interfere with potassium channels to alter the repolarization phase; prolong the potential contraction duration of the Purkinje fibers and the muscle fibers of the ventricles, decreasing the frequency of heart failure
- Class IV drugs—calcium channel blockers decrease the vascular tone and cause vasodilation by interfering with the movement of calcium ions through cell membranes, thereby inhibiting the contraction of vascular smooth muscle

Objective 9: Describe the adverse reactions of quinidine.

- Diarrhea, flatulence, abdominal pain, and fever
- Reduced platelets
- Liver function abnormalities
- Quinidine syncope

Objective 10: Identify the mechanism of action of lidocaine.

- Blocks activated and inactivated sodium channels, affecting depolarized or ischemic tissues

Objective 11: List the adverse effects of phenytoin.

- Gingival hyperplasia
- Blurred vision
- Vertigo
- Nystagmus

 ## Internet Sites of Interest

- At the InteliHealth website at **http://www.intelihealth.com**, experience an interactive look at the heart and its functions. Click "Interactive Tools" on the left and then choose "Heart Basics."
- Search for "heart and circulatory disorders" at **http://www.intelihealth.com**.

PEARSON
myhealthprofessionskit™

Go to www.myhealthprofessionskit.com to access the Companion Website created for this textbook. Simply select "Basic Health Science" from the choice of disciplines. Find this book and then log in using your username and password to access interactive learning games, assessment questions, animations, and more.

Chapter 22

Drugs Used to Treat Vascular Conditions

Chapter Objectives

After completing this chapter, you should be able to:

1. Describe primary and secondary hypertension.

2. Identify the different types of antihypertensive agents and their actions.

3. Explain the effects of angiotensin-converting enzyme (ACE) inhibitors.

4. Describe the newest and oldest drugs that are used for congestive heart failure.

5. Explain the most common side effects of digitalis.

6. Describe disorders that are related to hyperlipidemia.

7. Define statin drugs (HMG-CoA reductase inhibitors).

8. Identify the adverse effects of niacin.

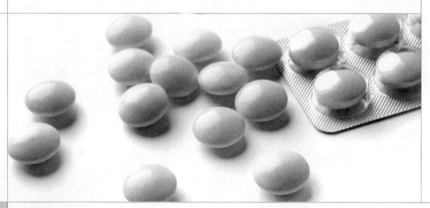

Key Terms

blood pressure (page 377)
blood volume (page 377)
cardiac output (page 377)
congestive heart failure (CHF) (page 377)
connective tissue (page 377)

cutaneous flush (kew-TAY-nee-us) (page 395)
diastole (dye-AH stoh-lee) (page 377)
hypercholesterolemia (hy-per-koh-lester-rawl-LEE-mee-uh) (page 392)
hypertensive crisis (page 378)

peripheral resistance (page 377)
primary hypertension (page 378)
steatorrhea (stee-at-oh-REE-ah) (page 394)
stroke volume (page 377)
systole (SIS-toh-lee) (page 377)

Introduction

It is estimated that nearly 60 million people in the United States have hypertension (signified by a systolic blood pressure more than 140 mm Hg and diastolic above 90 mm Hg or those taking antihypertensive medication). Whereas *Prehypertension* is classified as blood pressure 120/80 to 140/90 mm Hg, *normal* blood pressure is 119/79 mm Hg or less. Hypertension—the most common of the CVDs—occurs more often in black adults than in white adults, and morbidity and mortality are greater in blacks. Men experience more hypertension than women. The actual level of pressure that can be considered hypertensive is difficult to define; it depends on a number of factors, including the patient's age, gender, race, and lifestyle.

Uncontrolled hypertension can damage small blood vessels, causing narrowing of the arteries, which can result in kidney failure, strokes, and cardiac arrest. Chronic hypertension causes the heart to work harder pumping blood to organs and tissues and can result in **congestive heart failure (CHF)**, which develops when plasma volume increases and fluid accumulates in the lungs, abdominal organs (especially the liver), and peripheral tissues.

Hyperlipidemia—an elevation of lipoprotein levels in the plasma—is also a strong risk factor for cardiovascular disease (CVD). The major plasma lipids are cholesterol, and the triglycerides that are bound to proteins and transported as macromolecular complexes are called *lipoproteins*. These help to form the fatty material (plaque) that builds up in the lining of blood vessels and can cause angina, stroke, and myocardial infarction (MI). Hyperlipidemias are linked to specific genetic mutations, and most have a multifactorial basis that can respond to lifestyle changes or drug therapy.

Such lifestyle changes as the reduction of body weight; decreased intake of dietary total fat, cholesterol, saturated fatty acids, and salt; smoking cessation; increased exercise; and stress management can be effective for minor hypertension and hyperlipidemias. Pharmacologic methods combined with healthy lifestyle habits are usually necessary to treat patients with chronic hypertension and serious hyperlipidemias.

The Vascular System

Circulatory pressure within the vascular system is divided into three components: (1) arterial pressure, (2) capillary pressure, and (3) venous pressure. **Blood pressure**, which commonly means arterial pressure, is created by the pumping action of the heart and varies from one vessel to another within the systemic circuit. Systemic pressures are highest in the aorta, peaking at around 120 mm Hg, and lowest at the venae cavae, averaging about 2 mm Hg. Blood pressure in large and small arteries rises and falls—rising during ventricular **systole** (when the ventricles of the heart contract and eject blood) and falling during ventricular **diastole** (when the ventricles relax and the heart stops ejecting blood).

Three main factors affect blood pressure:

1. **Cardiac output:** the volume of blood pumped per minute, which is determined by heart rate, and **stroke volume**, the amount of blood pumped by a ventricle in one contraction. The higher the cardiac output, the higher the blood pressure.

2. **Peripheral resistance:** the friction in the arteries as blood flows through the vessels. The smooth muscle in artery walls can constrict, causing the inside diameter of the artery to narrow, creating more resistance and higher pressure.

3. **Blood volume:** the total amount of blood in the vascular system; more blood creates added pressure on the artery walls, increasing blood pressure.

Many of the drugs used to treat hypertension target one of these three factors.

The body regulates blood pressure through the vasomotor center, a cluster of neurons in the medulla oblongata, that signals the smooth muscle of the arteries to constrict (raising blood pressure) or relax (lowering blood pressure). Baroreceptors—one type of clusters of neurons in the aorta and internal carotid artery—sense pressure within the large vessels of the vascular system and send this information to the vasomotor center. Another type—chemoreceptors—sends information to the vasomotor center about levels of oxygen, carbon dioxide, and the acidity or pH of the blood. The vasomotor center raises or lowers blood pressure based on the information it receives.

The walls of arteries and veins contain three distinct layers (Figure 22-1 ■):

1. Tunica interna: the innermost layer of blood vessels, including the endothelial lining of the vessel and an underlying layer of **connective tissue** (elastic fibers)

2. Tunica media: the middle layer, which contains smooth muscle tissue in a framework of collagen and elastic fibers

3. Tunica externa: the outer layer, which is a sheath of connective tissue around the vessel

These multiple layers give arteries and veins considerable strength, and the muscular and elastic components permit controlled alterations in diameter as blood pressure or blood volume changes. Under normal circumstances, blood flow is equal to cardiac output. When cardiac output increases, so does capillary blood flow; when cardiac output declines, blood flow is reduced. Two factors—pressure and resistance—affect the flow rates of blood through the capillaries.

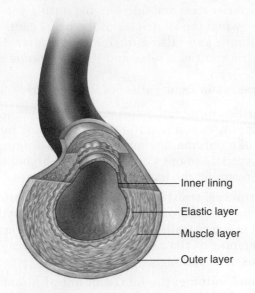

Figure 22-1 ■ The structure of an artery, showing the outer protective layer, muscle layer, elastic layer, and inner lining. © Dorling Kindersley.

Inner lining
Elastic layer
Muscle layer
Outer layer

Hypertension

Hypertension is the most prevalent cardiovascular disorder in the United States and is the result of chronically elevated pressure throughout the vascular system. Atherosclerosis, arteriosclerosis, renal disease, and any condition that creates increased vascular pressure cause the heart to work harder as it pumps against the increased resistance. The cause of **primary hypertension** (also called *essential hypertension*), which accounts for 90% of cases, is unknown. Heredity is a predisposing factor, but the exact mechanism is unclear. Such environmental factors as dietary sodium, obesity, and stress seem to act only in genetically susceptible people. *Secondary hypertension* is associated with such renal diseases as chronic glomerulonephritis, pyelonephritis, polycystic renal disease, or endocrine disorders, which include Cushing's syndrome, pheochromocytoma, and myxedema. It may also be associated with the use of excessive alcohol, oral contraceptives, corticosteroids, and cocaine. Table 22-1 ■ summarizes the classifications of blood pressure in adults.

Hypertension is a major cause of cerebrovascular accident, cardiac disease, and renal failure. The prognosis is good if this disorder is detected early and treatment begins before complications develop. Severely elevated blood pressure (**hypertensive crisis**) may be fatal.

The values shown in Table 22-1 should not be considered as absolutes, but they are representative as models for treatment of hypertension. In general terms, hypertension can be defined as the level of blood pressure at which there is risk. The ultimate judgment concerning the severity of hypertension in any given patient must also include a consideration of factors other than diastolic or systolic pressure, such as age and comorbid conditions.

Table 22-1 ■ **Classification of Blood Pressure in Adults**

CLASSIFICATION	SYSTOLIC (mm Hg)		DIASTOLIC (mm Hg)
Normal	<120	and	<80
Prehypertension	120–139	or	80–89
Stage I hypertension	140–159	or	90–99
Stage II hypertension	≥160	or	≥100

✳ Apply Your Knowledge 22.1

The following questions focus on what you have just learned about the vascular system and hypertension.

CRITICAL THINKING

1. What is prehypertension?
2. What are complications of uncontrolled hypertension?
3. What are lipoproteins?
4. What factors may reduce the risk of hypertension?
5. What are the three main factors affecting blood pressure?
6. What are the three walls of an artery?
7. What is the description of *hypertensive crisis*?
8. Which type of hypertension is the most prevalent cardiovascular disorder in the United States?

ANTIHYPERTENSIVE AGENTS

Antihypertensive agents are used to reduce blood pressure to within the normal levels. If the cause of hypertension is known, such as secondary hypertension, therapy is directed toward correction of the etiology. Unfortunately, the cause of about 90% of cases of hypertension is unknown.

Primary hypertension has no cure, but treatment can modify its course. The basic approach for antihypertensive therapy starts with changes in lifestyle. These changes include controlling weight by diet and exercise, stopping smoking, decreasing alcohol intake, decreasing sodium intake, exercising on a regular basis, resting and avoiding stress, and taking prescribed medications. Long-term therapy is essential to prevent the morbidity and mortality

associated with uncontrolled hypertension. Drug therapy used in the treatment of hypertension includes diuretics (to reduce circulating blood volume), beta-adrenergic blockers (to slow the heartbeat and dilate vessels), vasodilators (to dilate vessels), calcium channel blockers (to slow the heartbeat, reduce conduction irritability, and dilate vessels), and angiotensin-converting enzyme (ACE) inhibitors (to produce vasodilation and increase renal blood flow.) These medications may be prescribed singly or in combination. The administration of drug therapy is designed to fit each patient's needs and response. Noncompliance is associated with poor prognosis; compliance with an individualized regimen is associated with good prognosis. Table 22-2 ■ lists the most commonly used agents for hypertension.

Table 22-2 ■ Most Commonly Prescribed Antihypertensive Agents

GENERIC NAME	TRADE NAME	AVERAGE ADULT DOSAGE	ROUTE OF ADMINISTRATION
Diuretics (see Table 22-3)			
Beta-Blockers			
acebutolol	Sectral	200–800 mg bid	PO
atenolol	Tenormin	25–100 mg/d	PO
betaxolol	Kerlone	10–20 mg/d	PO
bisoprolol	Zebeta	2.5–20 mg/d	PO
carteolol	Cartrol	2.5–10 mg/d	PO
metoprolol	Lopressor	50–450 mg/d	PO
nadolol	Corgard	40–320 mg/d	PO
penbutolol	Levatol	20–80 mg/d	PO
pindolol	Visken	up to 60 mg/d	PO
propranolol	Inderal	10–240 mg/d	PO
timolol	Blocadren	20–60 mg/d	PO
Alpha- and Beta-blockers			
labetalol	Normodyne	100–400 mg PO bid (maximum: 1,200–2,400 mg/d)	PO
		20 mg slowly over 2 min, with 40–80 mg q10min if needed (maximum: 300 g total dose)	IV
Centrally Acting Blockers			
clonidine	Catapres	0.1–0.8 mg bid	PO
		Apply patch q7d.	Transdermal
guanabenz	Wytensin	4–32 mg bid	PO

(continued)

Table 22-2 ■ Most Commonly Prescribed Antihypertensive Agents (*continued*)

GENERIC NAME	TRADE NAME	AVERAGE ADULT DOSAGE	ROUTE OF ADMINISTRATION
guanfacine	Tenex	1–3 mg bid	PO
methyldopa	Aldomet	250 mg bid–tid (maximum: 3 g/d in divided doses)	PO
		250–500 mg q6h, increased up to 1 g q6h	IV
Peripherally Acting Blockers			
doxazosin	Cardura	1–16 mg/d	PO
guanadrel	Hylorel	10–75 mg/d	PO
guanethidine	Ismelin	10–50 mg/d	PO
prazosin	Minipress	1–20 mg/d	PO
reserpine	Serpalan, Serpasil	0.1–0.25 mg/d	PO
terazosin	Hytrin	1–20 mg/d	PO
Calcium Channel Blockers			
amlodipine with benazepril	Norvasc	5–10 mg/d	PO
diltiazem	Cardizem	80–120 mg tid	PO
felodipine	Plendil	5–10 mg/d	PO
isradipine	DynaCirc	1.25–10 mg bid	PO
nicardipine	Cardene	20–40 mg tid	PO
nifedipine	Procardia, Adalat	10–20 mg tid	PO
nisoldipine	Nisocor, Sular	10–20 mg tid	PO
verapamil	Calan, Verelan	40–80 mg tid	PO
Angiotensin II Receptor Blockers			
bisoprolol	Zebeta	2.5–5 mg/d (maximum: 20 mg/d)	PO
candesartan	Atacand	8–32 mg/d	PO
eprosartan	Teveten	400–800 mg/d	PO
irbesartan	Avapro	150–300 mg/d	PO
losartan	Cozaar	25–50 mg 1–2 times/d	PO
olmesartan	Benicar	20–40 mg/d	PO
valsartan	Diovan	80–160 mg/d	PO
telmisartan	Micardis	40–80 mg/d	PO
Angiotensin-Converting Enzyme Inhibitors			
benazepril	Lotensin	4–50 mg/d	PO
captopril	Capoten	25/100 mg/d	PO

GENERIC NAME	TRADE NAME	AVERAGE ADULT DOSAGE	ROUTE OF ADMINISTRATION
enalapril	Vasotec	5–40 mg/d	PO
fosinopril	Monopril	10–40 mg/d	PO
lisinopril	Prinivil, Zestril	10–40 mg/d	PO
moexipril	Univasc	7.5–30 mg/d	PO
perindopril	Aceon	2.5–20 mg/d	PO
quinapril	Accupril	2–8 mg/d	PO
ramipril	Altace	2.5–5 mg/d	PO
trandolapril	Mavik	1–4 mg/d	PO
Vasodilators			
fenoldopam	Corlopam	0.025–0.3 mcg/kg/min by continuous infusion for up to 48h	IV
hydralazine	Apresoline	10–50 mg qid	PO
		10–50 mg q4–6h	IM
		10–20 mg q4–6h	IV
minoxidil	Loniten, Rogaine	5 mg/d, increased q3–5d up to 40 mg/d in single or divided doses as needed (maximum: 100 mg/d)	PO

bid, twice a day; IM, intramuscular; IV, intravenous; PO, oral; qid, four times a day; tid, three times a day.

Diuretics

Diuretics reduce circulating blood volume by blocking the reabsorption of sodium and chloride, which results in more water being retained in the kidneys and the excretion of excess fluid. Diuretics are mainstays of hypertensive therapy and can be used alone or in combination with other antihypertensive agents. The four major groups of diuretics are thiazide diuretics, thiazide-like diuretics, loop diuretics, and potassium-sparing diuretics. These agents are discussed in more detail in Chapter 24.

Diuretic drugs—either alone or in combination with other agents—are frequently used in the management of mild to moderate hypertension. Diuresis and restriction of salt intake are often sufficient for many hypertensive patients except those with severe, malignant, or complicated hypertension. Table 22-3 ■ lists commonly used diuretics.

Table 22-3 ■ Diuretics

GENERIC NAME	TRADE NAME	AVERAGE ADULT DOSAGE	ROUTE OF ADMINISTRATION
Thiazide Diuretics			
chlorothiazide	Diuril, Duragen	500 mg 1–2 times/d	PO
hydrochlorothiazide	Esidrix, HydroDIURIL	25–100 mg/d	PO
indapamide	Lozol	2.5–5 mg/d	PO

(continued)

Table 22-3 ■ Diuretics (*continued*)

GENERIC NAME	TRADE NAME	AVERAGE ADULT DOSAGE	ROUTE OF ADMINISTRATION
polythiazide	Renese	1–4 mg/d	PO
hydroflumethiazide	Diucardin	25–200 mg 1–2 times/d	PO
Thiazide-Like Diuretics			
chlorthalidone	Hygroton	12.5–25 mg/d (maximum: 100 mg/d)	PO
indapamide	Lozol	1.25–5 mg/d	PO
metolazone	Zaroxolyn	5–20 mg/d	PO
quinethazone	Hydromox	50 mg 1–2 times/d	PO
Loop Diuretics			
furosemide	Lasix	20–80 mg/d, up to 600 mg/d	PO
		20–40 mg in 1 or more divided doses (maximum: 600 mg/d)	IM, IV
ethacrynic acid	Edecrin	50–100 mg 1–2 times/d	PO
		0.5–1 mg/kg or 50 mg, up to 100 mg	IV
torsemide	Demadex	5–20 mg/d up to 200 mg/d	PO, IV
bumetanide	Bumex	0.5–2 mg/d; may repeat at 4–5-h intervals (maximum: 10 mg/d)	PO
		0.5–1 mg over 1–2 min; repeated q2–3h PRN (maximum: 10 mg/d)	IM, IV
Potassium-Sparing Diuretics			
amiloride	Midamor	5 mg/d	PO
spironolactone	Aldactone	50–100 mg bid	PO
triamterene	Dyrenium	50–100 mg bid	PO

bid, twice a day; IM, intramuscular; IV, intravenous; PO, oral; PRN, as needed.

Focus On

Beta-Adrenergic Blockers

Beta-blockers are very popular antihypertensive drugs. They competitively antagonize the responses to catecholamines that are mediated by beta receptors.

(See Chapter 18 for a detailed discussion of beta-adrenergic blockers.)

Alpha- and Beta-Blockers

Alpha- and beta-blockers are indicated for severe hypertension. Alpha- and beta-blocking actions contribute to the blood pressure–lowering effect.

How do they work?

Alpha- and beta-blockers act as adrenergic-receptor blocking agents that combine selective alpha activity and nonselective beta-adrenergic blocking actions. Both actions contribute to blood pressure reduction.

How are they used?

Alpha- and beta-blockers, such as labetalol (Normodyne), are used in the treatment of mild, moderate, and severe hypertension. They may be used alone or in combination with other antihypertensive agents, especially thiazide diuretics.

What are the adverse effects?

The adverse effects include postural hypotension, dizziness, vertigo, headache, bronchospasm, and dyspnea. Alpha-receptor blockade causes vasodilation and decreased peripheral vascular resistance that is added to the beta-blocking mechanisms (see Table 22-2).

What are the contraindications and interactions?

Alpha- and beta-blockers are contraindicated in bronchial asthma, uncontrolled cardiac failure, cardiogenic shock, and severe bradycardia. Safe use during pregnancy, lactation, or in children is not established.

Labetalol should be used cautiously in patients with impaired liver function, jaundice, and diabetes mellitus. Cimetidine (Tagamet) may increase the effects of labetalol, and glutethimide (Doriglute) decreases its effects.

What are the important points patients should know?

Inform patients who are taking alpha- and beta-blockers that hypotension may occur. Instruct them to make all position changes slowly and in stages, particularly from a lying to an upright position. Advise patients to avoid driving and engaging in other potentially hazardous activities until their responses to the drug are known.

Focus on Geriatrics

Alpha- and Beta-Blocker Use in Older Adults

Older adults are especially sensitive to the hypotensive effects of alpha- and beta-blockers. They must be careful not to engage in any activity that could be especially dangerous because of low blood pressure.

Focus On

Centrally Acting Adrenergic Blockers

Centrally acting adrenergic blockers, such as clonidine hydrochloride (Catapres) and methyldopa (Aldomet), are not regarded as first-line therapies in hypertension. These drugs tend to be used in cases in which the affected person has not responded to other therapies.

How do they work?

These agents are able to reduce the hyperactivity in the medulla oblongata of the brain. Sympathetic outflow from the medulla is diminished, and as a result, either systemic vascular resistance or cardiac output is decreased.

How are they used?

Centrally acting adrenergic blockers are used for the management of hypertension, especially in combination with a diuretic.

(Continued)

Focus On (*Continued*)

What are the adverse effects?

The adverse effects include drowsiness, sedation, headache, nightmares, anxiety, orthostatic hypotension, and CHF (see Table 22-2). Centrally acting agents may also cause peripheral edema, tachycardia, bradycardia, flushing, and hepatitis.

What are the contraindications and interactions?

Centrally acting blockers are contraindicated in pregnancy, lactation, hepatitis, cirrhosis of the liver, and blood dyscrasias. These agents should be used cautiously in kidney disease, angina pectoris, and a history of mental depression.

What are the important points patients should know?

Advise patients to avoid potentially hazardous tasks, such as driving, until response to these drugs is known. Instruct them to check with their physicians before taking over-the-counter (OTC) medications. Tell women they should not breastfeed while taking these drugs without consulting their physicians.

Peripherally Acting Adrenergic Blockers

Peripherally acting adrenergic blockers, such as doxazosin (Cardura), phenoxybenzamine (Dibenzyline), and reserpine (Serpalan), lower blood pressure in supine or standing individuals, with the most pronounced effect on diastolic blood pressure.

How do they work?

Peripherally acting blockers are antihypertensive in that their effects depend on the inhibition of norepinephrine release and the depletion of norepinephrine from nerve terminals. These drugs reduce blood pressure by reducing vascular tone, primarily in the veins and the arteries.

How are they used?

Peripherally acting adrenergic blockers are used for severe hypertension or as adjunctive therapy with other antihypertensive agents in the more severe form of hypertension.

What are the adverse effects?

The adverse effects of these drugs are drowsiness, fatigue, headache, confusion, palpitation, dry mouth, dyspnea, nausea, and vomiting (see Table 22-2).

What are the contraindications and interactions?

Contraindications include hypersensitivity to reserpine (Serpalan), a history of mental depression, acute peptic ulcer, and ulcerative colitis. Safe use during pregnancy and lactation and in children is not established. Peripherally acting adrenergic blockers should be used cautiously in patients with diabetes mellitus, impaired renal or hepatic function, coronary disease with insufficiency, and recent heart attack. Alcohol intensifies orthostatic hypotension and sedation. Reserpine may enhance the action of epinephrine (Bronkaid Mist), norepinephrine (Levarterenol), and antidepressants.

What are the important points patients should know?

Inform patients about the possibility of orthostatic hypotension and advise them to have assistance getting out of bed during initial dosage adjustment. Tell them to take the drug at the same time(s) each day in relation to a daily routine activity. OTC drugs for treatment of colds, allergy, asthma, or appetite suppressants should not be used without consulting a physician or pharmacist.

Angiotensin-Converting Enzyme Inhibitors

ACE inhibitors, such as enalapril maleate (Vasotec) and ramipril (Altace), are drugs that prevent ACE from producing angiotensin II. ACE inhibitors are used to treat patients with hypertension and CHF.

How do they work?

ACE inhibitors decrease the formation of angiotensin II, which lowers blood volume and blood pressure. Renin is an enzyme that is secreted by the kidneys in response to reduced renal blood circulation or lower sodium in the blood. The renin–angiotensin system controls blood pressure and fluid balance and is one of the body's primary homeostatic mechanisms. Figure 22-2 ■ shows the renin–angiotensin system.

How are they used?

ACE inhibitors are a very popular class of drugs for the treatment of patients with severe hypertension. They are becoming the drugs of choice in the treatment of those with primary hypertension. These agents are also used to treat those with CHF.

What are the adverse effects?

Although ACE inhibitors as a group are relatively free of side effects in the majority of patients, they do occur, and some can be life threatening. The adverse effects include loss of taste, photosensitivity, severe hypotension, hyperkalemia, renal impairment, blood dyscrasias, dizziness, and angioedema. ACE inhibitors are contraindicated in angioedema, pregnant women, renal impairment, scleroderma, and lupus erythematosus.

What are the contraindications and interactions?

ACE inhibitors are contraindicated in patients with hypersensitivity to these agents. Safety during pregnancy and lactation and in children is not established. ACE inhibitors should be used cautiously in renal impairment and renal-artery stenosis and in patients with hypovolemia, receiving diuretics, undergoing dialysis, with hepatic impairment, or with diabetes mellitus.

Potassium-sparing diuretics may increase the risk of hyperkalemia. Aspirin and other nonsteroidal anti-inflammatory drugs may antagonize hypotensive effects. ACE inhibitors may increase lithium (Eskalith) levels and toxicity.

What are the important points patients should know?

Instruct patients who are using ACE inhibitors to consult their physicians promptly if vomiting or diarrhea occurs. OTC medications should be used only with the approval of a physician. When applicable, advise patients to inform their surgeons or dentists that they are taking ACE inhibitors.

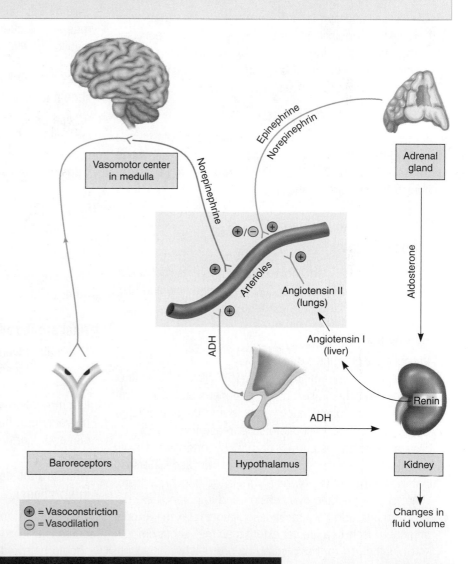

Figure 22-2 ■ The renin–angiotensin system.

⊕ = Vasoconstriction
⊖ = Vasodilation

Focus Point

Angiotensin-Converting Enzyme Inhibitors and Diabetes

ACE inhibitors can produce hypoglycemia in diabetic patients. Monitoring blood glucose is important during the first few weeks of therapy.

Focus On

Angiotensin II Receptor Blockers

Angiotensin receptor blockers antagonize the effects of angiotensin II.

How do they work?

Angiotensin II receptor blockers inhibit the binding of angiotensin II to the angiotensin I receptor in vascular smooth muscle. By blocking these receptors, angiotensin II cannot raise blood pressure. This action blocks the vasoconstriction and aldosterone secretion stimulated by angiotensin II.

How are they used?

These agents have beneficial effects on patients with CHF. Angiotensin II receptor blockers have been one of the fastest-growing groups of agents for the management of hypertension. The most common angiotensin II receptor blockers are listed in Table 22-2.

What are the adverse effects?

The adverse effects of these drugs are similar to those of ACE inhibitors. One effect that is absent with these drugs but present with ACE inhibitors is a persistent cough, which can be annoying to patients.

What are the contraindications and interactions?

These drugs are contraindicated in known sensitivity to angiotensin II receptor blockers, bilateral artery stenosis, overt cardiac failure, cardiogenic shock, pregnancy, and lactation. Angiotensin II receptor blockers must be used cautiously in patients with asthma, chronic obstructive pulmonary disease, peripheral vascular disease, diabetes mellitus, hyperthyroidism, and renal or hepatic insufficiency.

Angiotensin II receptor blockers may interact with amiodarone (Cordarone) and cause significant bradycardia. Beta-blockers may interact with angiotensin II receptor blockers and reduce glucose tolerance, inhibit insulin secretion, and produce hypertension.

What are the important points patients should know?

Advise patients to report episodes of dizziness, especially when making position changes. Inform female patients to immediately report pregnancy to their physicians. Women should not breastfeed while taking these drugs.

Vasodilators

Vasodilators (listed in Table 22-2) are agents that cause blood vessels to expand, increasing blood flow and lowering blood pressure in the affected area.

How do they work?

Vasodilators produce a direct relaxation of vascular smooth muscle, and these actions result in vasodilation. This effect is called *direct* because it does not depend on the innervation of the vascular smooth muscle and is not mediated by receptors. The vasodilators decrease total peripheral resistance and thus correct primary hypertension. Unlike many other antihypertensive agents, the vasodilators do not inhibit the activity of the sympathetic nervous system; therefore, orthostatic hypotension and impotence are not problems. In addition, most vasodilators relax the arterial smooth muscle to a greater extent than the venous smooth muscle, thereby further minimizing postural hypotension.

How are they used?

The vasodilators are generally inadequate as the sole therapy for hypertension and produce many side effects.

However, the administration of beta-blockers and diuretics is more useful than vasodilators alone.

What are the adverse effects?

The main adverse effects of vasodilators include headache, dizziness, tachycardia, nausea, and vomiting. The specific adverse effects of fenoldopam (Corlopam), a commonly prescribed vasodilator, include insomnia, nervousness, flushing, postural hypotension, bradycardia, and heart failure.

What are the contraindications and interactions?

Vasodilators are contraindicated in patients with hypersensitivity to these agents. Fenoldopam (Corlopam) should be avoided if beta-blockers are being used. Hydralazine (Apresoline) is contraindicated in coronary artery disease, mitral valvular rheumatic heart disease, and MI. Safety during pregnancy and lactation for vasodilators has not been established.

Vasodilators should be used cautiously in cerebrovascular accident, advanced renal impairment, and coronary artery disease. Drug interactions occur with epinephrine (Bronkaid Mist) and norepinephrine (Levarterenol), which can cause excessive cardiac stimulation. If used with guanethidine (Ismelin), these agents cause profound orthostatic hypotension.

What are the important points patients should know?

Instruct patients to monitor their weight, check for edema, make position changes slowly, and avoid standing still. Advise them to avoid excessive alcohol intake and driving and engaging in other potentially hazardous activities until their responses to these drugs are known. Female patients should not breastfeed while taking these drugs without consulting their physicians.

✳ Apply Your Knowledge 22.2

The following questions focus on what you have just learned about antihypertensive agents.

CRITICAL THINKING

1. What is the effect of diuretics in the treatment of hypertension?
2. What is the role of beta-adrenergic blockers in the management of hypertension?
3. What are the trade names of nadolol, bisoprolol, clonidine, methyldopa, and doxazosin?
5. What are the 10 most commonly prescribed ACE inhibitors for hypertension?
6. What are the classifications of diuretics?
7. What is the mechanism of action of centrally acting adrenergic blockers?
8. What are the indications of peripherally acting adrenergic blockers?
9. What are the adverse effects of ACE inhibitors?
10. What are the indications of angiotensin II receptor blockers?

Congestive Heart Failure and Treatment

Heart failure is defined as an inability of the heart, under normal filling conditions, to pump blood at a rate sufficient to meet the metabolic demands of the tissues. The inability to pump blood can be caused by various abnormalities in the myocardium. When the heart pumps blood at an insufficient rate, the kidneys retain salt and water, and fluid accumulates in interstitial spaces. Thus, the term *congestive heart failure* is used to describe this condition. Figure 22-3 ■ shows normal blood flow through the heart.

CHF occurs when the heart pumps less blood than it receives, which results in blood accumulating in the heart chambers and the stretching of the heart walls. CHF is accompanied by abnormal increases in blood volume and interstitial fluid; the heart, veins, and capillaries are generally dilated with blood. As a result of CHF, organs receive less blood circulation.

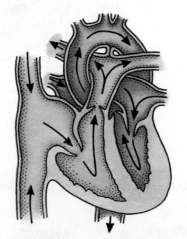

Figure 22-3 ■ Human heart with atria and ventricles highlighted to illustrate the flow of blood through the chambers and pulmonary blood vessels. Arrows depict the path of blood through the open valves. © Dorling Kindersley.

Therefore, less oxygen reaches the kidneys and water is retained, increasing blood volume. Edema of the lower limbs is a common symptom. Other symptoms include pulmonary congestion with left heart failure and peripheral edema with right heart failure. The underlying causes of CHF include arteriosclerotic heart disease, hypertensive heart disease, valvular heart disease, dilated cardiomyopathy, and congenital heart disease. Left systolic dysfunction secondary to coronary artery disease is the most common cause of heart failure. Figure 22-4 ■ shows signs and symptoms of patients with heart failure.

The therapeutic goal for CHF is to increase cardiac output. Three classes of drugs have been shown to be clinically effective in reducing symptoms and prolonging life: inotropic, diuretics, and vasodilators. The treatment of CHF may include combinations of inotropic drugs, diuretics, and vasodilators, including ACE inhibitors. Table 22-4 ■ lists the main classes of drugs used for CHF.

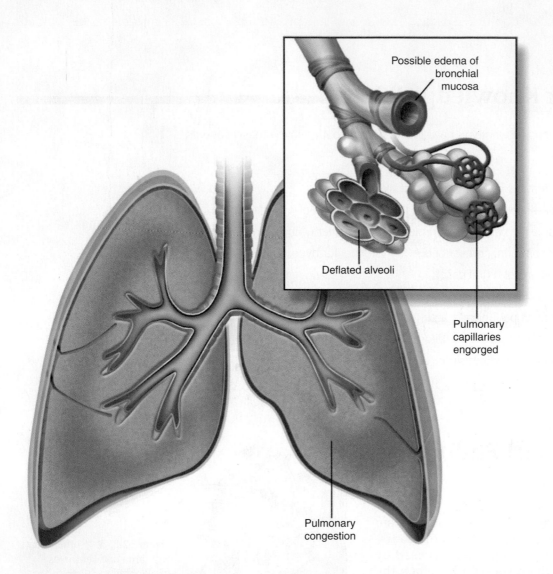

Possible edema of
bronchial
mucosa

Deflated alveoli

Pulmonary
capillaries
engorged

Pulmonary
congestion

Figure 22-4 ■ Signs of congestive heart failure with pulmonary congestion.

Table 22-4 ■ Main Classes of Drugs Used for Congestive Heart Failure

GENERIC NAME	TRADE NAME	AVERAGE ADULT DOSAGE	ROUTE OF ADMINISTRATION
Inotropic Drugs			
Cardiac Glycosides			
digitoxin	Crystodigin	150 mcg daily (maximum: 0.3 mg/d)	PO

GENERIC NAME	TRADE NAME	AVERAGE ADULT DOSAGE	ROUTE OF ADMINISTRATION
digoxin	Lanoxin	10–15 mcg/kg in divided doses over 24–48 h and then 0.1–0.375 mg/d	PO
		10–15 mcg/kg in divided doses over 24 h and then 0.1–0.375 mg/d	IV
Beta-Adrenergic Antagonists			
propranolol	Inderal	40 mg bid (usually need 160–480 mg/d in divided doses)	PO
Phosphodiesterase Inhibitors			
inamrinone lactate	Amrinone	0.75 mg/kg bolus given slowly over 2–3 min and then start infusion at 5–10 mcg/kg/min; may repeat bolus in 30 min (maximum: 10 mg/kg/d)	IV
milrinone lactate	Primacor	Loading dose: 50 mcg/kg over 10 min; maintenance dose: 0.375–0.75 mcg/kg/min	IV
Diuretics (see Table 22-3)			
Vasodilators (see Table 22-2)			

bid, twice a day; IV, intravenous; PO, oral; qid, four times a day.

Focus On

Inotropic Drugs

Inotropic agents increase the cardiac muscle's strength of contraction. These drugs relieve the symptoms of cardiac insufficiency but do not reverse the underlying pathologic condition. Knowledge of the physiology of heart muscle contraction is essential to an understanding of the compensatory responses evoked by the failing heart as well as the actions of drugs used to treat CHF.

Inotropic drugs act by different mechanisms; in each case, the inotropic action is the result of an increased cell calcium concentration that enhances the contractility of cardiac muscle. Inotropic drugs include cardiac glycosides and beta-adrenergic agonists (see Table 22-4). Cardiac glycosides, such as digitoxin (Crystodigin) and digoxin (Lanoxin), are obtained from the plant leaves of *Digitalis pupurea* and *Digitalis lanata*, respectively. They all are derived from natural sources whose medicinal qualities have been recognized for centuries. The cardiac glycosides are popular and effective drugs for the treatment of patients with CHF. They act by exerting a positive inotropic action on the heart, which increases the force of myocardial contraction, thereby

improving the mechanical efficiency of the heart as a blood-pumping organ. This ultimately results in a reduced heart size and increased blood flow to the kidneys.

How do they work?

Cardiac glycosides act by increasing the force and velocity of myocardial systolic contraction and decreasing conduction velocity through the atrioventricular node. Cardiac glycosides inhibit the enzyme *ATPase*, which is associated with the sodium pump, and the exchange between sodium and calcium is impaired. Stores of calcium within the myocardium are released, and the membrane becomes more permeable to this ion. As a result, intracellular calcium levels are elevated. Because calcium is necessary for normal muscle contraction, the elevated calcium levels result in a stronger force of contraction (Figure 22-5 ■).

How are they used?

Digoxin (Lanoxin) is the most commonly prescribed digitalis preparation for treating patients with CHF. It is used

(Continued)

Focus On (Continued)

for rapid digitalization and maintenance therapy in CHF as well as for atrial fibrillation and flutter. Digoxin and digitoxin (Crystodigin)—the two primary cardiac glycosides—are similar in efficacy. The main difference between the two drugs is digitoxin's more prolonged half-life.

What are the adverse effects?

Common adverse effects of cardiac glycosides include fatigue, muscle weakness, headache, mental depression, visual disturbances, anorexia, nausea, vomiting, and diarrhea.

What are the contraindications and interactions?

Cardiac glycosides are contraindicated in patients with digitalis hypersensitivity, ventricular fibrillation, and ventricular tachycardia (unless it is caused by CHF). These drugs should be used cautiously in patients with renal insufficiency, hypokalemia, advanced heart disease, acute MI, hypothyroidism, pregnancy, and lactation and in older adults.

Antacids, cholestyramine (LoCholest), and colestipol (Colestid) decrease digoxin absorption. Diuretics, corticosteroids, amphotericin B (Amphocin), and laxatives may cause hypokalemia.

What are the important points patients should know?

Advise patients who are taking digoxin (Lanoxin) for atrial fibrillation to report to their physicians a pulse rate that falls below 60 or rises above 110 beats per minute. Inform patients of the occurrence of anorexia, nausea, vomiting, diarrhea, or visual disturbances because these adverse effects may be caused by toxicity. They must report these adverse effects to their physicians.

Digoxin must be taken exactly as prescribed and at the same time each day; be sure to tell patients to not skip or double a dose or change dose intervals. Patients should not take OTC medications, especially those for coughs, colds, allergies, GI upset, or obesity without the approval of their physicians.

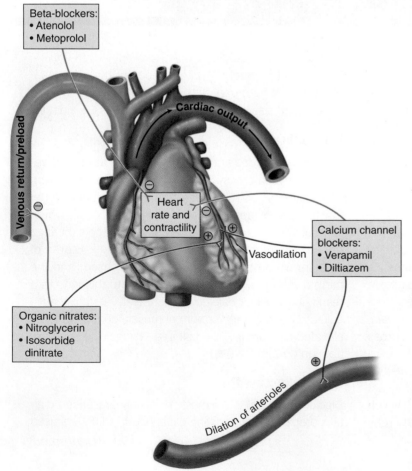

Figure 22-5 ■ Mechanisms of action of drugs used for congestive heart failure, including cardiac glycosides.

Focus on Natural Products

Foxglove and Digoxin

The cardiac drug digoxin is derived from foxglove, a purple flowering plant that has been described in the medical literature for more than 200 years as a treatment for heart disease. English physician William Withering is credited with discovering in 1775 that the foxglove plant could help those with a condition of abnormal fluid buildup, which, at that time, was called *dropsy*. In 1930, the glycosides of the woolly foxglove (*Digitalis lanata*) were isolated, and the drug digoxin was born. Similar to foxglove, other plants, such as oleander and lily of the valley, also have cardiac glycoside properties. Patients must be aware of taking digoxin and these herbs together because they may receive a toxic dose. Reports of digoxin toxicity are often linked with extracts and teas containing the foxglove, oleander, and lily of the valley herbs.

Focus Point

Cardiac Glycosides and Low Pulse

If the apical pulse falls below a set parameter in a patient taking cardiac glycosides, administration of the drug should be withheld and a physician notified.

Beta-Adrenergic Agonists

Beta-adrenergic stimulation improves cardiac performance by positive inotropic effects and vasodilation (see Chapter 28 for a detailed discussion of beta-adrenergic agonists). See Table 22-4 for beta-adrenergic agonists.

Phosphodiesterase Inhibitors

Phosphodiesterase inhibitors, such as inamrinone lactate (Amrinone) and milrinone lactate (Primacor), increase the force of the heart's contraction and cause vasodilation. They work by blocking the enzyme phosphodiesterase in cardiac and smooth muscle, resulting in a positive inotropic response and vasodilation. They are commonly used for the short-term control of acute heart failure, and they have high toxicity.

Diuretics

Diuretics relieve the pulmonary congestion and peripheral edema common in CHF. These agents are useful in reducing the symptoms of volume overload, including orthopnea and paroxysmal nocturnal dyspnea. Diuretics decrease plasma volume and subsequently decrease venous return to the heart (preload). This decreases the cardiac workload and oxygen demand. Diuretics also decrease afterload by reducing plasma volume, thus decreasing blood pressure. Diuretics are discussed in detail in Chapter 24.

* Apply Your Knowledge 22.3

The following questions focus on what you have just learned about CHF and its treatment.

CRITICAL THINKING

1. What is the pathophysiology of congestive heart failure?
2. What are the causes of congestive heart failure?
3. What is the mechanism of action of inotropic drugs?
4. What is the most commonly prescribed digitalis preparation for treating congestive heart failure?
5. What are the trade names of inamrinone, milrinone, digoxin, and digitoxin?

Hyperlipidemia and Related Disorders

Hyperlipidemia is characterized by an increase in plasma cholesterol or triglycerides containing lipoprotein particles. These particles, which are key to the development of atherogenesis, are initially synthesized by the intestinal mucosa and the liver and undergo extensive metabolism in the plasma. They also play an essential role in the transport of lipids between tissues. The lipoproteins differ in density and are referred to as very-low-density lipoprotein (VLDL), low-density lipoprotein (LDL), high-density lipoprotein (HDL), and chylomicrons. Each lipoprotein includes different amounts of triglycerides and cholesterol in the core. The size of the core varies with the size of the lipoprotein. When carried as circulating lipoprotein, cholesterol is the predominant core of LDL and HDL. Chylomicrons produced by the intestines transport dietary cholesterol and triglycerides. Triglycerides are the predominant makers of chylomicrons and the VLDL secreted by the liver.

A patient with high serum cholesterol and increased LDL is at risk for atherosclerotic coronary disease, MI, and hypertension. Disorders of hyperlipidemia are characterized by an elevation in triglycerides and an elevation of cholesterol. Elevated triglycerides can produce life-threatening pancreatitis.

Although **hypercholesterolemia** (higher-than-normal levels of cholesterol in the blood) are linked to specific genetic mutations, most have a multifactorial basis that can respond to lifestyle changes. These changes include the reduction of body weight; decreased dietary total fat, cholesterol, and saturated fatty acids; increased exercise; and stress management.

There are several different types of hypercholesterolemia. Type IIa is associated with high levels of both cholesterol and LDL in the blood. Ischemic heart disease is common in this type. The condition may be hereditary and is then termed *familial hypercholesterolemia.*

Type IIb is associated with high VLDL and LDL and, therefore, high triglycerides and cholesterol blood levels. Ischemic heart disease may result. This type may be related to high alcohol intake, obesity, diabetes mellitus, and overeating. Dietary modification is usually all that is required, but drugs may be necessary in resistant cases.

Type IV is characterized by high VLDL and hypertriglyceridemia. Causes are similar to that of type IIb, but peripheral vascular disease and ischemic heart disease can be found in people with this type. The treatment is the same as for type IIb.

ANTIHYPERLIPIDEMICS

Antihyperlipidemic medications should be used if diet modification and exercise programs fail to lower LDL to normal levels. When medications are started, diet therapy must continue. Whereas some of the antihyperlipidemic drugs decrease production of the lipoprotein carriers of cholesterol and tricylcerol, others increase lipoprotein degradation. Still others directly increase cholesterol removal from the body. These drugs may be used singly or in combination but are always accompanied by the requirement that dietary lipid intake be significantly low, especially cholesterol and saturated fats, and the caloric content of diet must be closely monitored. The major drugs for reduction of LDL cholesterol levels are bile acid sequestrants and nicotinic acid. The fibric acid derivatives, such as clofibrate, are less effective in reducing LDL cholesterol. The most effective drugs for lowering plasma LDL levels are the HMG-CoA reductase inhibitors, or statins. Antihyperlipidemic drugs are listed in Table 22-5 ∎.

Table 22-5 ∎ Antihyperlipidemic Drugs

GENERIC NAME	TRADE NAME	AVERAGE ADULT DOSAGE	ROUTE OF ADMINISTRATION
Bile Acid Sequestrants			
cholestyramine resin	LoCholest, Questran	4–6 g/d	PO
colestipol	Colestid	15–30 g/d	PO
HMG-CoA Reductase Inhibitors (Statins)			
atorvastatin	Lipitor	10–80 mg qid	PO
fluvastatin	Lescol	20–40 mg/d	PO
lovastatin	Altoprev, Mevacor	20–80 mg/d	PO
pravastatin	Pravachol	10–40 mg/d	PO
rosuvastatin	Crestor	5–40 mg/d	PO

GENERIC NAME	TRADE NAME	AVERAGE ADULT DOSAGE	ROUTE OF ADMINISTRATION
simvastatin	Zocor	10–80 mg/d	PO
simvastatin/ezitimibe	Vytorin	10/10 mg/d to 10/80 mg/d (ezitimibe is 10 mg)	PO
Miscellaneous Drugs			
nicotinic acid (niacin)	Niac, Nicobid	1–2 g bid–tid	PO
Fibric Acid Derivatives			
clofibrate	Atromid-S	2 g/d	PO
gemfibrozil	Lopid	1,200 mg/d	PO
dextrothyroxine	Choloxin	4–8 mg/d	PO

bid, twice a day; IMPO, oral; qid, four times a day; tid, three times a day.

Focus Point

Alcohol and Cholesterol

Moderate alcohol intake increases HDL cholesterol (the "good" cholesterol) but does not reduce LDL cholesterol (the "bad" cholesterol).

Focus On

Bile Acid Sequestrants

Bile acid sequestrants, such as cholestyramine resin (LoCholest, Questran) and colestipol (Colestid), are drugs that chemically combine with bile acids in the intestine, causing these bile acids to be excreted from the body.

How do they work?

Bile acid sequestrants are used for their cholesterol-lowering effect. They *bind* with bile salts in the intestinal tract to form an insoluble complex that is excreted in the feces, thus reducing circulating cholesterol and increasing serum LDL removal rates.

How are they used?

Bile acid sequestrants are nonabsorbable drugs prescribed for decreasing serum cholesterol. Lowering the bile acid concentration causes the liver to increase the conversion of cholesterol to bile acids, resulting in a replenished supply of these compounds, which are essential components of the bile. Because the bile acids are lost in feces, LDLs and serum cholesterol are reduced. The bile acid binding resins are prescribed for primary hyperlipidemias.

What are the adverse effects?

The adverse effects of bile acid sequestrants include constipation, nausea, flatulence, and the impaired absorption of fat-soluble vitamins.

What are the contraindications and interactions?

Bile acid sequestrants should be avoided in patients with bowel obstruction, and their safety is not established for patients with dysphagia, swallowing disorders, and major gastrointestinal tract surgery. Safety during pregnancy and lactation and in children younger than 6 years of age is not established. These agents should be used

(Continued)

Focus On (*Continued*)

cautiously in patients with bleeding disorders, hemorrhoids, peptic ulcer, and malabsorption states, such as **steatorrhea** (elimination of large amounts of fat in the stool).

Cholestyramine resin and colestipol interfere with the intestinal absorption of many drugs—for example, tetracycline (Achromycin), phenobarbital (Barbital), digoxin (Lanoxin), warfarin (Coumadin), aspirin, and thiazide diuretics.

What are the important points patients should know?

Advise patients to report promptly to their physicians if they develop severe gastric distress with nausea and vomiting, unusual weight loss, black stools, severe hemorrhoids, and sudden back pain. A high-bulk diet with adequate fluid intake is an essential adjunct to resolve constipation.

HMG-CoA Reductase Inhibitors (Statin Drugs)

This powerful group of antihyperlipidemic agents includes the most effective drugs for reducing LDL and cholesterol levels. They share the generic name of *statin* and are described as *the statins*.

How do they work?

Statin drugs reduce LDL and total triglyceride production. These agents are inhibitors of reductase (HMG-CoA), which is essential to hepatic production of cholesterol.

How are they used?

The statins are the most widely used drugs for lowering hyperlipidemia. Lovastatin (Altoprev), simvastatin (Zocor), pravastatin (Pravachol), and fluvastatin (Lescol) are completely effective in inhibiting HMG-CoA reductase, which is the enzyme needed in cholesterol production. These drugs are often given in combination with other antihyperlipidemic drugs. It should be noted that despite the protection afforded by cholesterol lowering, about 25% of patients treated with these drugs still present with coronary events. Thus, such additional strategies as diet, exercise, or additional agents may be warranted.

What are the adverse effects?

Some patients may have muscle pain. A severe but rare adverse effect is life-threatening rhabdomyolysis (degeneration of skeletal muscle tissue, with possible renal failure). Other adverse effects may include abdominal pain, flatulence, constipation, dyspepsia, headache, and cramping. Liver function and serum transaminase levels must be measured periodically. If there is muscle pain, creatine kinase levels should be monitored to rule out rhabdomyolysis. The HMG-CoA reductase inhibitors may increase coumarin levels. Thus, it is important to evaluate prothrombin times frequently.

What are the contraindications and interactions?

Statins are contraindicated for patients who are hypersensitive to these agents and in myopathy, active liver disease, unexplained persistent transaminase elevations, and during pregnancy and lactation. Statin drugs may increase levels of digoxin (Lanoxin), norethindrone (Micronor), and the oral contraceptive ethinyl estradiol (Estinyl).

What are the important points patients should know?

Instruct patients they cannot interrupt, increase, decrease, or omit dosage without the advice of their physicians. They should notify their physicians promptly about muscle tenderness or pain, especially if accompanied by fever or malaise. Alcohol consumption should be avoided or reduced. Advise women that they should not breastfeed while taking these drugs without consulting their physicians.

Focus on Pediatrics

Statin Drugs and Children

Statin drugs should not be prescribed for children or teenagers. The safety and effectiveness of these drugs in children and adolescents has not been established.

Focus on Natural Products

Food Interactions and Statins

Grapefruit and grapefruit juice should be avoided by patients who are taking the statin drug simvastatin (Zocor). Regular consumption of the fruit or juice can lead to high levels of the drug in the blood. This is not true of other statin drugs.

MISCELLANEOUS ANTIHYPERLIPIDEMIC DRUGS

Some other antihyperlipidemic drugs lower serum lipids in primary and secondary hyperlipidemias. Nicotinic acid (Niac) and the fibrates, such as clofibrate (Atromid-S) and gemfibrozil (Lopid), are included in this category.

Focus On

Nicotinic Acid (Niacin)

Nicotinic acid, or niacin (Niac), has a broad lipid-lowering ability, but its clinical use is limited because of its unpleasant side effects. Derivatives of this drug, which are not available in the United States, appear to have fewer adverse effects.

How does it work?

Niacin (Niac) appears to reduce the level of the VLDL, LDL, and total cholesterol. Combination drug therapy, such as nicotinic acid, bile acid binding sequestrants, and a statin, may decrease LDL cholesterol levels by 70% or more. Niacin causes a decrease in liver triacylglycerol synthesis, which is required for VLDL production. LDL is derived from VLDL in the plasma. Therefore, a reduction in the VLDL concentration also results in a decreased plasma LDL concentration.

How is it used?

Niacin (Niac) is used in the adjuvant treatment of hypercholesterolemias in patients who do not respond adequately to diet or weight loss. It is the most potent antihyperlipidemic agent for raising plasma HDL levels.

What are the adverse effects?

The most common adverse effects of niacin therapy are an intense **cutaneous flush** (skin reddening) and pruritus. The administration of aspirin before taking niacin decreases the flush. Some patients also experience nausea and abdominal pain, syncope, nervousness, and blurred vision. Hyperuricemia, gout, impaired glucose tolerance, and hepatotoxicity have also been reported.

What are the contraindications and interactions?

Niacin is contraindicated in patients with hypersensitivity to this agent. It must be avoided in hepatic impairment, severe hypotension, active peptic ulcer, pregnancy, lactation, and in children younger than 16 years of age.

Niacin should be used cautiously in patients with a history of gallbladder disease, liver disease, and peptic ulcer, glaucoma, coronary artery disease, and diabetes mellitus. Niacin is able to potentiate the hypotensive effects of antihypertensive agents.

What are the important points patients should know?

Alert patients to the possibility of feeling warm and flushed in the face, neck, and ears within the first 2 hours after oral ingestion and immediately after parenteral administration. This may last for several hours. Effects are usually transient and subside as therapy continues. Instruct patients to sit or lie down, avoiding sudden posture changes if they feel weak or dizzy. These symptoms as well as persistent flushing should be reported to their physicians. Relief may be obtained by reducing the dosage, increasing subsequent doses in small increments, or changing to a sustained-release formulation. Alcohol and large doses of niacin cause increased flushing and sensations of warmth. Tell patients to avoid exposure to direct sunlight until lesions have entirely cleared if they have skin manifestations. Women should not breastfeed while taking niacin.

(Continued)

Focus On *(Continued)*

· ·

Fibric Acid Derivatives

Gemfibrozil (Lopid) and clofibrate (Atromid-S) are derivatives of fibric acid that lower triglycerides and VLDL and increase HDL.

How do they work?

Both drugs cause a decrease in plasma triglyceride levels by blocking lipolysis of stored triglycerides in adipose tissue and inhibiting hepatic uptake of fatty acids. In addition to inhibiting the breakdown of fats into triglycerides, liver production of triglycerides is inhibited.

How are they used?

Fibric acid derivatives are approved for use in patients with hypertriglyceridemia who do not respond to diet—those in whom triglyceride levels can exceed 1,000 mg/dL (reference range, 10–190 mg/dL). They can also be prescribed in combination with other drugs to facilitate a reduction in triglycerides that complements the cholesterol-lowering action of the antihyperlipidemic agent. These agents are also used for severe familial hypercholesterolemia (type IIa or IIb) that develops early in childhood and has failed to respond to dietary control or to other cholesterol-lowering drugs.

What are the adverse effects?

The most common adverse effects are mild gastrointestinal disturbances, dizziness, and blurred vision.

Gemfibrozil (Lopid) may increase cholesterol excretion into the bile, leading to gallstone formation. Treatment with clofibrate (Atromid-S) has resulted in significant occurrences of cancer. Inflammation of the skeletal muscle can occur with both drugs; thus, muscle weakness or tenderness should be evaluated.

What are the contraindications and interactions?

Fibric acid derivatives are contraindicated in patients with gallbladder disease, biliary cirrhosis, or hepatic or severe renal dysfunction and during pregnancy and lactation. Safety and efficacy in children younger than age 18 years are not established. These drugs should be used cautiously in patients with diabetes mellitus, hypothyroidism, renal impairment, and cholelithiasis (gallstones).

Fibric acid derivatives may potentiate the hypoprothrombinemic effects of oral anticoagulants. Lovastatin (Altoprev) increases the risk of myopathy and rhabdomyolysis and may increase repaglinide (Prandin) levels and duration of action.

What are the important points patients should know?

Instruct patients to notify their physicians promptly if unexplained bleeding occurs. This includes easy bruising, epistaxis (nosebleed), and hematuria (blood present in the urine).

✳ Apply Your Knowledge 22.4

The following questions focus on what you have just learned about bile acid sequestrants, HMG-CoA reductase inhibitors, and fibric acid derivatives.

CRITICAL THINKING

1. What are the mechanisms of action of bile acid sequestrants?
2. What are the indications of HMG-CoA reductase inhibitors?
3. What are the trade names of colestipol, clofibrate, dextrothyroxine, and gemfibrozil?
4. What are the seven generic and trade names of the HMG-CoA reductase inhibitors?
5. What is the mechanism of action of nicotinic acid?
6. What drugs are derivatives of fibric acid that lower triglycerides and increase HDL?

PRACTICAL SCENARIO 1

The husband of an elderly woman, who had become incoherent over the past day, called emergency medical services (EMS). When they arrived at the house and asked the woman's husband for her history, he told them his wife had has diabetes and hypertension for many years. Before calling EMS, he had checked her medicines, and based on the number of pills still left in the bottle, he estimated she had not been taking her antihypertensive medication for about 2 weeks. On examination, the EMS team found that she was afebrile, her pulse rate was 112 beats/min, her respirations were 24 breaths/min, and her blood pressure was 230/160 mm Hg.

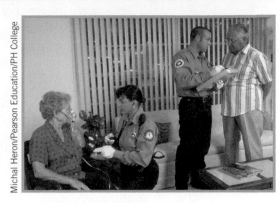

Michal Heron/Pearson Education/PH College

Critical Thinking Questions

1. What might be the results of this patient stopping her antihypertensive medications so abruptly?
2. What consequences could a long-term blood pressure of 230/160 mm Hg have for this patient?
3. What questions would you ask the patient and her family to help guide ongoing treatment and adherence to the medication regimen?

PRACTICAL SCENARIO 2

A 33-year-old African American woman went to her family practitioner for a physical examination. She is overweight, with a history of hypertension.

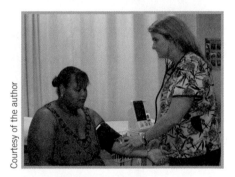

Courtesy of the author

Critical Thinking Questions

1. If her cholesterol and triglycerides are elevated, what medications could the physician order to lower her cholesterol and triglycerides?
2. List the complications of hypercholesterolemia.

Chapter Capsule

This section repeats the objectives from the beginning of the chapter and then provides a summary of the most important concepts for that objective. Use this section as a quick review and to check your knowledge.

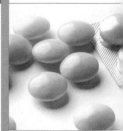

Objective 1: Describe primary and secondary hypertension.

- Primary (essential) hypertension—unknown etiology; heredity is a predisposing factor, but the exact mechanism is unclear; environmental and lifestyle factors (dietary sodium, obesity, stress) seem to act only in genetically susceptible people

■ Secondary hypertension—associated with such renal diseases as chronic glomeru-lonephritis; pyelonephritis; polycystic renal disease; or endocrine disorders, which include Cushing's syndrome, pheochromocytoma, and myxedema; may also be associated with the use of excessive alcohol, oral contraceptives, corticosteroids, and cocaine

Objective 2: Identify the different types of antihypertensive agents and their actions.

■ Diuretics (reduce circulating blood volume)

■ Beta-adrenergic blockers (slow the heartbeat and dilate vessels)

■ Vasodilators (dilate vessels)

■ Calcium channel blockers (slow the heartbeat, reduce conduction irritability, and dilate vessels)

■ Angiotensin-converting enzyme (ACE) inhibitors (produce vasodilation and increase renal blood flow)

Objective 3: Explain the effects of angiotensin-converting enzyme (ACE) inhibitors.

■ ACE inhibitors decrease the formation of angiotensin II, which lowers blood volume and blood pressure.

■ The renin–angiotensin system controls blood pressure and fluid balance and is one of the body's primary homeostatic mechanisms; renin is an enzyme that is secreted by the kidneys in response to reduced renal blood circulation or lower sodium in the blood.

Objective 4: Describe the newest and oldest drugs used for congestive heart failure.

■ Combinations of inotropic drugs, diuretics, and vasodilators that include ACE inhibitors are the newest treatments

■ Cardiac glycosides, derived from natural plant sources, have been recognized for centuries for their medicinal qualities

Objective 5: Explain the most common side effects of digitalis.

■ Fatigue, muscle weakness, headache, mental depression, visual disturbances, anorexia, nausea, vomiting, and diarrhea

Objective 6: Describe disorders that are related to hyperlipidemia.

■ Atherosclerotic coronary disease

■ Myocardial infarction

■ Hypertension

■ Pancreatitis caused by elevated triglycerides

Objective 7: Define statin drugs (HMG-CoA reductase inhibitors).

■ Inhibitors of reductase (HMG-CoA), which is essential to hepatic production of cholesterol

■ Most effective drugs for reducing low-density lipoprotein (LDL) and cholesterol levels

■ Reduce LDL and total triglyceride production

Objective 8: Identify the adverse effects of niacin.

- Intense cutaneous flush (skin reddening) and pruritus (very common)
- Nausea and abdominal pain, syncope, nervousness, and blurred vision (less common)
- Hyperuricemia, gout, impaired glucose tolerance, and hepatotoxicity (uncommon)

Internet Sites of Interest

- The American Heart Association at **http://www.americanheart.org** is one of the best websites for information for patients and professionals on all topics related to heart diseases as well as medications and lifestyle changes to treat or prevent them. Take a look around the site.

- A site dedicated to heart disease in women is Heart Healthy Women at **http://www.hearthealthywomen.org**, where information for patients and professionals can be found.

- Cardiovascular Physiology Concepts offers information about secondary hypertension at **http://www.cvphysiology.com**. Click "Hypertension" in the left column.

- Everything you have always wanted to know about hypertension is available at **http://www.hypertension-facts.org**.

- MedicineNet.com, a pharmacists' website, discusses ACE inhibitors at **http://www.medicinenet.com/ace_inhibitors/article.htm**.

- MedlinePlus, a service of the National Institutes of Health and National Library of Medicine, presents an in-depth look at digitalis drugs at **http://www.nlm.nih.gov/medlineplus**. Click the "Drugs and Supplements" tab and then search for "digitalis."

- The Health Illustrated Encyclopedia of About.com offers information about high blood cholesterol and triglycerides at **http://adam.about.com/encyclopedia**. Search for "cholesterol."

Chapter 23

Anticoagulants

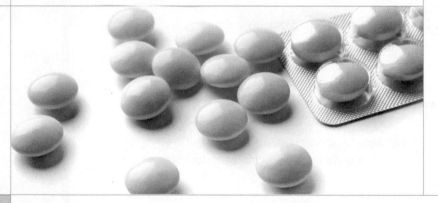

Key Terms

coagulation (ko-ag-yew-LAY-shun) (page 401)

embolus (EM-bo-lus) (page 403)

hemostasis (hee-mo-STAY-sis) (page 401)

platelet plug (PLAY-tel-let) (page 401)

serotonin (sayr-uh-TO-nin) (page 401)

thrombi (THROM-beye) (page 404)

thromboembolism (throm-bo-EM-bo-liz-im) (page 406)

Introduction

The blood transports blood cells, gases, hormones, immune cells, metabolic wastes, and nutrients. Normal blood clotting protects against excessive hemorrhaging, but the development of certain clots may obstruct the flow of blood and ultimately cause a myocardial infarction (MI), or stroke, and necrosis (death) of tissue. Hemorrhagic and thrombotic disorders may be treated with a variety of medications.

This chapter focuses on anticoagulant drug therapy, which is aimed at reducing the occurrences of thrombosis. Anticoagulants decrease the blood's ability to clot. There are two main types of anticoagulants: parenteral and oral. Often, both types are used together. Caution must be taken by health-care professionals because many conditions cause an increased risk of hemorrhaging. Anticoagulants should not be used or should be used only in severely limited quantities in treating patients who have these types of conditions, such as hemophilia or thrombocytopenia (low platelet count).

Hemostasis

Limited intravascular coagulation of blood occurs in normal physiologic conditions. The circulatory system has to be self-sealing; otherwise, continued blood loss from even the smallest injury would be life threatening. Bleeding usually stops spontaneously when an injury is minor. However, a more serious bleeding episode can be life threatening and often requires medical intervention. Normally, all but the most catastrophic bleeding is rapidly stopped through a physiologic progression of several steps, known as **hemostasis** (Figure 23-1 ■).

Hemostasis involves three events:

1. *Vascular spasms.* The platelets release the neurotransmitter **serotonin**, which causes the blood vessel to go into spasms. The spasms decrease blood loss until clotting can occur.

2. *Formation of a platelet plug.* When a blood vessel is torn, the inner lining of the vessel stimulates, or activates, the platelets. The platelets become sticky and adhere to the inner lining of the injured vessel and to each other. By sticking together, they form a **platelet plug**. Over several minutes, the plug is invaded by activated blood-clotting factors and eventually evolves into a stable and strong blood clot.

3. *Blood clotting.* Vascular spasm and a platelet plug alone are not sufficient to prevent the bleeding caused by a larger tear in a blood vessel. With a more serious injury to the vessel wall, bleeding stops only if a blood clot forms. Blood clotting, or **coagulation**, is the third event in the process of hemostasis. A blood clot is formed by a series of chemical reactions that result in the formation of a netlike structure. The net is composed of protein fibers called *fibrin*, which seals off the opening in the injured blood vessel and stops the bleeding. The three basic steps of hemostasis are shown in Figure 23-2 ■.

HEMOSTASIS MECHANISM OF ACTION

The mechanism of action of hemostasis is complex and involves 11 different plasma proteins called *clotting factors*. The process of blood clotting occurs in a series of sequential steps that are referred to as a *cascade*.

Normal coagulation cannot occur unless the plasma contains the necessary clotting factors. Most of the circulating clotting proteins are synthesized by the liver. The injured vessel releases a chemical called *prothrombin activator* (prothrombinase). Prothrombin activator converts the clotting factor prothrombin to an enzyme called *thrombin*. Thrombin then converts *fibrinogen* to *fibrin*. Normal blood clotting occurs in about 6 minutes. The primary steps in the coagulation cascade are shown in Figure 23-3 ■.

✳ Apply Your Knowledge 23.1

The following exercises focus on what you have just learned about the physiology of hemostasis.

CRITICAL THINKING

1. What are the three events of hemostasis?

2. What is serotonin and its effect on blood vessels?

3. What is fibrin and its effect on blood clotting?

4. Where is the site of formation of the circulating clotting proteins in the human body?

5. What are clotting factors?

6. How many clotting factors are involved in the mechanism of action of hemostasis?

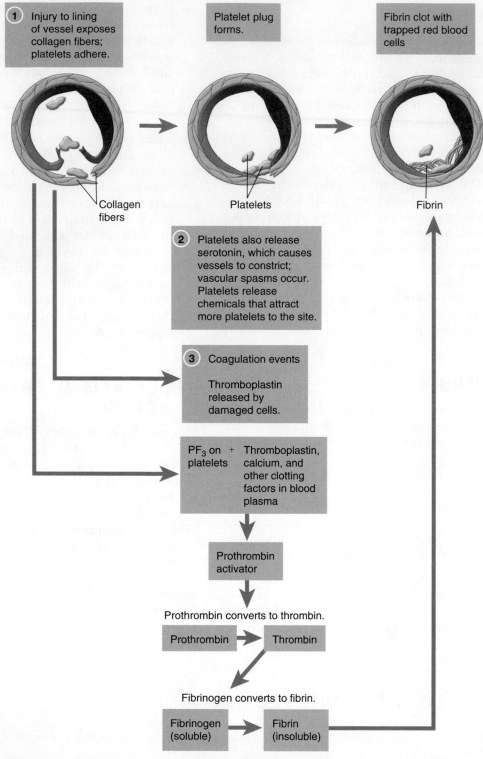

Figure 23-1 ■ Hemostasis begins when a blood vessel is damaged and ends when the fibrin threads trap blood cells, forming a clot that seals the injured vessel.

Anticoagulant Agents

Anticoagulants are medications used to prolong bleeding time; therefore, they help to prevent harmful clots from forming in the blood vessels. These medications are sometimes called *blood thinners,* although they do not actually thin the blood. Anticoagulants do not dissolve clots that have already formed, but they may prevent the clots from becoming larger and causing more serious problems. They are often used as treatment for certain cardiovascular (CV)

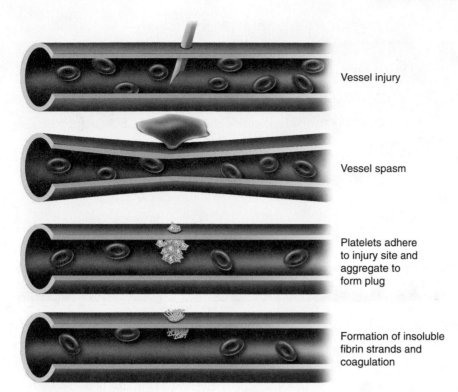

Vessel injury

Vessel spasm

Platelets adhere
to injury site and
aggregate to
form plug

Formation of insoluble
fibrin strands and
coagulation

Figure 23-2 ■ Basic steps of hemostasis.

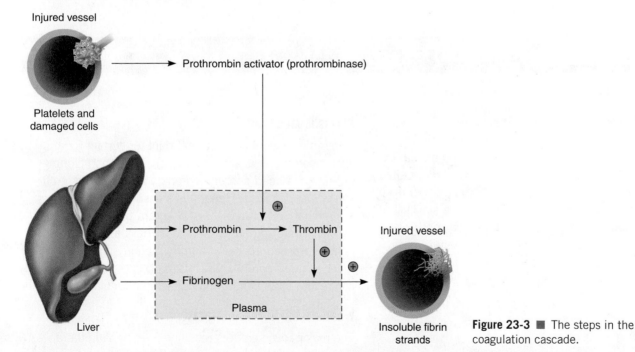

Injured vessel

Prothrombin activator (prothrombinase)

Platelets and
damaged cells

Prothrombin → Thrombin

Injured vessel

Fibrinogen

Plasma

Liver

Insoluble fibrin
strands

Figure 23-3 ■ The steps in the
coagulation cascade.

and lung conditions, such as MI, venous thrombosis, peripheral arterial **embolus** (an abnormal particle circulating in blood, such as an air bubble or blood clot), and pulmonary emboli. Anticoagulants have been used to prevent transient ischemic attacks and to reduce the risk of recurrent MI. There are two main groups of anticoagulants: (1) drugs that are administered orally and (2) drugs that are administered parenterally. Warfarin (Coumadin) is an example of an oral anticoagulant, and heparin is an anticoagulant only given parenterally. Table 23-1 ■ lists the primary anticoagulants.

Drugs that dissolve preformed clots (thrombolytic agents or tissue plasminogen activators), including streptokinase (Streptase, Kabikinase) and urokinase (Abbokinase), are not referred to as anticoagulants.

Table 23-1 ■ Anticoagulants

GENERIC NAME	TRADE NAME	ADULT DOSE	ROUTE OF ADMINISTRATION
heparin sodium*	Hep-Lock	15,000–20,000 units bid	IV infusion
		5,000–40,000 units/d subcutaneously	Subcutaneous
pentoxifylline	Trental	400 mg tid	PO
warfarin sodium	Coumadin	2–15 mg/d	PO

*For low-molecular-weight heparins, see Table 23-2.
bid, twice a day; IV, intravenous; PO, oral; tid, three times a day.

Focus on Geriatrics

Anticoagulants in Elderly Patients

Older adults are more susceptible to the effects of anticoagulants. Signs of overdose include nosebleeds, blood in the stool or urine, excessive bruising, and prolonged bleeding from the gums after brushing or from cutting the face while shaving. Elderly patients especially should limit use of alcohol to only 1 drink per day while using anticoagulants.

Focus On

Heparin

Heparin is an anticoagulant and a protein. Two types of heparin are used clinically. The first and older of the two, standard (unfractionated) heparin is an animal extract (from pork). The second and newer type, called *low-molecular-weight heparin (LMWH),* is derived from unfractionated heparin. The two classes are similar but not identical in their actions and pharmacokinetic characteristics. Standard heparin (heparin sodium) is produced by and can be released from mast cells located throughout the body. It is especially abundant in the liver, lung, and intestines.

How does it work?

Similar to other anticoagulants, heparin is a drug that increases the length of clotting time and prevents thrombi from forming or growing larger. The anticoagulation action of heparin depends on the inhibition of **thrombi** (blood clots that form within a blood vessel and attach to the site of formation) and clot formation by blocking the conversion of prothrombin to thrombin and fibrinogen to fibrin, which is the final step in the clotting process. Figure 23-4 ■ shows the mechanisms of action of anticoagulants.

How is it used?

Heparin is prescribed as a treatment for certain CV and lung disorders. It is also used to prevent blood clotting during open-heart surgery, coronary artery bypass graft surgery, and dialysis. Heparin is measured on a unit (international unit) rather than milligram basis. The dose must be determined on an individual basis. Heparin is not absorbed after oral administration and therefore must be given parenterally. Intravenous (IV) administration results in an almost immediate anticoagulant effect.

What are the adverse effects?

The major adverse effect resulting from heparin therapy is hemorrhage. Bleeding can occur in the urinary or gastrointestinal (GI) tract. Other types of hemorrhages and related conditions that may occur include subdural hematoma (bleeding into the areas below the dura mater, which encases the brain and central nervous system), acute hemorrhagic pancreatitis, hemarthrosis (blood in a joint), and ecchymosis (blood that has pooled in the skin). Additional adverse effects of heparin treatment include hypersensitivity reactions, fever, alopecia, osteoporosis, and ostealgia.

What are the contraindications and interactions?

Absolute contraindications include serious bleeding and intracranial bleeding. Heparin is also contraindicated in severe liver or kidney disease as well as malignant hypertension. It has not been shown to cause birth defects or bleeding problems in infants. It does not pass into breast milk.

Drugs that inhibit platelet function (for example, aspirin) or produce thrombocytopenia increase the risk of bleeding when heparin is administered. Other drugs that interact with heparin include nonsteroidal anti-inflammatory drugs (NSAIDs), anesthetics, valproic acid, sulfinpyrazone, cefamandole, cefoperazone, cefotetan, plicamycin, methimazole, propylthiouracil, probenecid, and various thrombolytics.

What are the most important points patients should know?

Teach patients how to correctly administer heparin subcutaneously if they are discharged from the hospital while on heparin. Advise patients to protect themselves from injury (for example, by using an electric shaver instead of a razor). Warn patients against taking aspirin and other over-the-counter (OTC) medications. Instruct them to notify their health-care providers if urine is pink, red, dark brown, or cloudy; if vomitus is red or dark brown; and/or if stools are red or black. Also, instruct patients to report bleeding gums or oral mucosa; bruising; hematoma; epistaxis; bloody sputum; chest, abdominal, lumbar, or pelvic pain; an unusual increase in menstrual flow; and severe or continuous headache, faintness, or dizziness.

Focus Point

Heparin

Overdosage of heparin can be treated by the administration of a slow infusion of 1% protamine sulfate solution. A dose of 0.5 to 1 mg of protamine is required to antagonize the action of each 100 units of heparin.

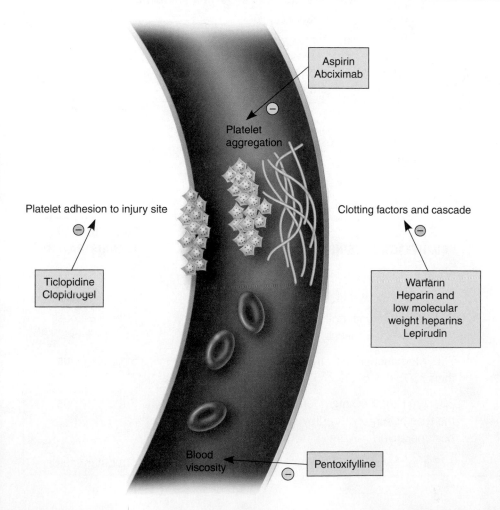

Figure 23-4 ■ Mechanism of action of anticoagulants.

Focus On

Low-molecular-weight Heparin

LMWH is a relatively new class of anticoagulant that has been used in Europe and is now being used more often in the United States.

How do they work?

LMWHs are derived from standard heparin (hence, from pork). Low-molecular-weight fragments have greater bioavailability (the proportion of a drug's dose that is absorbed into the bloodstream) than standard heparin, a longer-lasting effect, and dose-independent clearance pharmacokinetics.

How are they used?

LMWHs are more effective than standard heparin in preventing and treating venous **thromboembolism** (blockage of blood vessel by a part of a thrombus that has broken away from its formation site and is circulating in the blood), such as deep venous thrombosis (DVT). The incidence of thrombocytopenia after administration of LMWHs is lower than with standard heparin. LMWHs can be given according to body weight once or twice daily without laboratory monitoring. LMWHs are superior for preventing venous thrombosis in patients undergoing hip replacement. They are administered by subcutaneous injection, and they offer the option of treatment on an outpatient basis for patients with DVT. The

clinical advantages of LMWHs include predictability, dose-dependent plasma levels, a long half-life, and less bleeding for a given antithrombotic effect. The standard treatment of DVT with IV heparin administered in the hospital offers no advantages over LMWH administered in the outpatient setting.

What are the adverse effects?

Adverse effects like those caused by standard heparin have been seen during therapy with LMWH, and overdose is treated with protamine. The most common LMWHs are shown in Table 23-2 ■.

What are the contraindications and interactions?

Although safer than regular heparin, LWMHs are contraindicated for use in children and in patients with unstable angina, allergy to heparin or pork, active bleeding, and thrombocytopenia. Drug interactions occur with oral anticoagulants, antiplatelets, and thrombolytics.

What are the most important points patients should know?

The points to teach patients who are taking LMWHs are the same as those for regular heparins. See the previous section on patient teaching.

Table 23-2 ■ Common Low-Molecular-Weight Heparins

GENERIC NAME	TRADE NAME	PROPHYLACTIC DOSING	ROUTE OF ADMINISTRATION
ardeparin	Normiflo	50 international units/kg following surgery and then q12h for 14 d or until ambulatory	Subcutaneous
dalteparin	Fragmin	2,500 international units 1–2 h before surgery and then 2,500 international units/d for 5–10 d	Subcutaneous
danaparoid	Orgaran	750 international units 1–4 h before surgery and then 750 units q12h for 7–10 d	Subcutaneous
enoxaparin	Lovenox	30 mg q12h or 40 mg/d for 7–10 d depending on the type of surgery; therapy should begin postoperatively	Subcutaneous
tinzaparin	Innohep	175 international units/kg/d	Subcutaneous

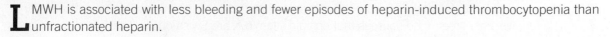

Focus Point

Low-Molecular-Weight Heparin

LMWH is associated with less bleeding and fewer episodes of heparin-induced thrombocytopenia than unfractionated heparin.

Focus On

Warfarin

Orally effective anticoagulant drugs are fat-soluble derivatives of coumarin or indandione, and they resemble vitamin K. Warfarin (Coumadin) is the oral anticoagulant of choice. It is the most widely used anticoagulant drug because of its potency and reliable bioavailability. It is the fourth-most prescribed CV agent and, overall, the 11th-most prescribed drug in the United States, with annual sales of approximately $500 million. The indandione anticoagulants have greater toxicity than the coumarin drugs. Table 23-1 lists the primary anticoagulants.

How does it work?

Warfarin interferes with the hepatic synthesis of vitamin K–dependent clotting factors (factors II [prothrombin], VII, IX, and X), resulting in their eventual depletion and prolongation of clotting times. Warfarin is rapidly and almost completely absorbed after oral administration (its onset of action is from 12 hours to 3 days), and it is bound extensively to plasma proteins. Although these drugs do not cross the blood–brain barrier, they can cross the placenta and may cause teratogenicity (the capability of producing malformations) and hemorrhage in fetuses. Therefore, warfarin carries a strong warning against its use during pregnancy.

How is it used?

Warfarin is used on an inpatient and outpatient basis when long-term anticoagulant therapy is indicated. Warfarin is administered in conventional doses or mini-doses to reduce bleeding. The dose range is adjusted to provide the desired endpoint. The duration of action of warfarin is 2 to 5 days.

What are the adverse effects?

The major adverse effect of warfarin is hemorrhage that occurs at a predisposing abnormality, such as an ulcer or tumor. Prolonged therapy with the coumarin-type anticoagulants is relatively free of untoward effects. Bleeding may occur in the skin, mucous membranes, GI tract, kidneys, brain, liver, uterus, or lungs. However, close monitoring of the degree of anticoagulation is important. Practitioners are advised to keep treatment periods at a minimum to reduce risks. Rare adverse effects include diarrhea, urticaria (eruption of itching hives), alopecia, skin necrosis, and dermatitis.

What are the contraindications and interactions?

Oral anticoagulants are ordinarily contraindicated in the presence of active or past GI ulceration, hepatic or renal disease, malignant hypertension, bacterial endocarditis, chronic alcoholism, and pregnancy. Warfarin is an antagonist of vitamin K, a necessary element in the synthesis of clotting factors II, VII, IX, and X. Drug interactions occur with hepatic enzyme inhibitors, aspirin, NSAIDs, and thrombolytics.

What are the most important points patients should know?

Instruct patients to report signs of bleeding, including blood in the urine, red or black tarry stools, vomiting of blood, bleeding with toothbrushing, blue or purple spots on the skin or mucous membranes, pinpoint purplish red spots, nosebleeds, and bloody sputum. Chest, abdominal, lumbar, and pelvic pain should also be reported. Advise patients to stop the drug immediately if they have signs of hepatitis (dark urine, itchy skin, jaundice, light stools, and abdominal pain) or a hypersensitivity reaction. Instruct patients to avoid changing brands of warfarin and to take the same dose of drug at the same time each day. Advise female patients to use a barrier contraceptive to avoid pregnancy. Breastfeeding is not advised.

Focus on Natural Products

Anticoagulants and Natural Products

Dietary or supplemental intake of vitamin K can potentiate or inhibit the actions of oral anticoagulants. The top five leafy green food sources that contain vitamin K are Swiss chard, kale, parsley, Brussels sprouts, and spinach. Mineral oil and other laxatives may reduce the absorption of warfarin.

Focus Point

Warfarin

Approximately 5 days are required for the antithrombotic effects of warfarin to occur. It should not be used in patients who must undergo dental procedures.

✳ Apply Your Knowledge 23.2

The following exercises focus on what you have just learned about anticoagulant agents.

CRITICAL THINKING

1.   What are three primary anticoagulants?
2.   What is the major adverse effect of heparin therapy?
3.   What is the treatment for an overdose of heparin?
4.   What is the mechanism of action of anticoagulants?
5.   What are the trade names of dalteparin, enoxaparin, ardeparin, and danaparoid?
6.   What is the difference between standard and low-molecular-weight heparin?
7.   When long-term anticoagulant therapy is indicated, what type of anticoagulant should be used?
8.   What is an antagonist of warfarin?

Focus On

Antiplatelet Agents

Antiplatelets are medications that help to prevent the formation of blood clots by keeping platelets from binding together—a process called *platelet aggregation*. Unlike the anticoagulants, which are used primarily to prevent thrombosis in veins, antiplatelet drugs are used to prevent clot formation in arteries. Antiplatelet drugs include aspirin, ticlopidine (Ticlid), clopidogrel (Plavix), abciximab (ReoPro), eptifibatide (Integrilin), and tirofiban (Aggrastat) (Table 23-3 ■).

How do they work?

The role platelets play in blood clotting is essential when the body has been cut. Without platelets to stop the bleeding, a person would bleed to death. However, there are times when blood clotting is harmful. The size and location of blood clots may increase the person's risk of an MI or stroke. Therefore, antiplatelets may be prescribed for patients with heart disease to reduce the likelihood that the platelets will aggregate and form potentially harmful blood clots.

Aspirin in low doses inhibits platelet aggregation and prolongs bleeding time. It remains the first choice in antiplatelet therapy. Aspirin is useful in preventing coronary thrombosis in patients with unstable angina, serving as an adjunct to thrombolytic therapy, and reducing recurrence of thrombotic stroke.

Ticlopidine (Ticlid) and clopidogrel (Plavix) are structurally related drugs that irreversibly inhibit platelet activation, leading to inhibition of platelet aggregation. Clopidogrel is preferred to ticlopidine because of its better safety profile and its lack of the serious life-threatening side effects (leukopenia and thrombocytopenia) that can occur with ticlopidine. Clopidogrel is also more potent, is better tolerated, and can be administered as a loading dose.

Abciximab (ReoPro), eptifibatide (Integrilin), and tirofiban (Aggrastat), which interrupt the interaction of fibrinogen with clotting factors, are capable of inhibiting the aggregation of platelets activated by a wide variety of stimuli. Abciximab is used in conjunction with angioplasty and stent procedures, and it is an adjunct to fibrinolytic therapy. Eptifibatide is approved for the treatment of acute coronary disease and for use in patients undergoing percutaneous transluminal coronary angioplasty (PTCA), commonly known as *stenting*.

How are they used?

Drugs that inhibit platelet function are administered for the relatively specific prophylaxis of arterial thrombosis and for the prophylaxis or therapeutic management of MI and stroke. The antiplatelet drugs are administered as adjuncts to thrombolytic therapy, along with heparin, to maintain perfusion (blood flow per unit volume of tissue) and to limit the size of MI. Recently, antiplatelet drugs have found new importance in preventing thrombosis in PCTA. The administration of an antiplatelet drug increases the risk of bleeding.

What are the adverse effects?

Antiplatelet agents may be associated with epigastric pain, heartburn, nausea, diarrhea, and major or minor bleeding events. Abciximab may also be associated with cardiac arrhythmias, abnormal thoughts, and dizziness.

What are the contraindications and interactions?

Antiplatelet drugs are generally contraindicated in patients with a history of GI ulceration, hypertension, asthma, allergies, and nasal polyps. Patients should consult their physicians before taking any other medication (either prescription or OTC), nutritional supplements, and/or herbal remedies. Some of these substances can interact with antiplatelets. Interactions occur with anticoagulants, platelet aggregation inhibitors, thrombolytic agents, dextran, abciximab, anagrelide, and dipyridamole.

What are the most important points patients should know?

Instruct patients to report nausea, diarrhea, rash, sore throat, or infection; signs of bleeding; yellow skin; dark urine; and clay-colored stools. Advise patients to not take aspirin or antacids and to keep appointments for blood tests.

Table 23-3 ■ Antiplatelet Agents

GENERIC NAME	TRADE NAME	ADULT DOSE	ROUTE OF ADMINISTRATION
abciximab	ReoPro	0.25 mg/kg initially over 5 min and then 10 mcg/min for 12 h	IV
aspirin	Ecotrin	80 mg/d–650 mg bid	PO
clopidogrel	Plavix	75 mg/d	PO
dipyridamole	Persantine	75–100 mg qid	PO
eptifibatide	Integrilin	180 mcg/kg initial bolus over 1–2 min and then 2 mcg/kg/min for 24–72 h	IV
ticlopidine	Ticlid	250 mg bid	PO
tirofiban	Aggrastat	0.4 mcg/kg/min for 30 min and then 0.1 mcg/kg/min for 12–24 h	IV

bid, twice a day; IV, intravenous; PO, oral; qid, four times a day.

Focus on Natural Products

Garlic as an Anticoagulant

Garlic has long been studied as a natural alternative to antiplatelet drugs because it has been shown to decrease platelet aggregation. Proponents of garlic claim it can reduce heart disease and the incidence of stroke. Garlic is also used by many people to treat colds, coughing, infections, bronchitis, arteriosclerosis, high blood cholesterol levels, and hypertension. It is wise to alert patients that using garlic concomitantly with anticoagulants may cause bleeding complications.

Focus Point

Antiplatelets During Pregnancy

Taking antiplatelets in the last 2 weeks of pregnancy may cause bleeding problems in the baby—before and after delivery. When taken in the last 3 months of pregnancy, antiplatelets may prolong the length of the pregnancy and the delivery.

✳ Apply Your Knowledge 23.3

The following exercises focus on what you have just learned about antiplatelet agents.

CRITICAL THINKING

1. What is the description of platelet aggregation?
2. What is the effect of low doses of aspirin on platelets?
3. What is the difference between ticlopidine (Ticlid) and clopidogrel (Plavix)?
4. What is another name for percutaneous transluminal coronary angioplasty?
5. What are the trade names of abciximab, dipyridamole, eptifibatide, and tirofiban?

Focus On

Thrombolytic Agents

Thrombolytic agents (also called *thrombolytics*) are the small group of drugs used to dissolve blood clots. Five thrombolytic drugs are available: streptokinase (Streptase, Kabikinase), alteplase (Activase), urokinase (Abbokinase), reteplase (Retavase), and anistreplase (Eminase). These drugs are prescribed in a hospital setting. Table 23-4 ■ lists thrombolytic drugs.

How do they work?

Thrombolytics facilitate the conversion of plasminogen to plasmin, which subsequently hydrolyzes fibrin to dissolve blood clots, or thrombi, that have already formed. Thrombolytic agents are plasminogen activators. The ideal thrombolytic drug is one that can be administered IV to produce clot-selective fibrinolysis without activating plasminogen to plasmin in plasma.

Newer thrombolytic agents bind to fibrin and activate fibrinolysis (breakdown of fibrin) more than fibrinogenolysis (breakdown of fibrinogen).

How are they used?

Thrombolytic drugs are indicated for the management of severe pulmonary embolism, DVT, and arterial thromboembolism; they are especially important for therapy after MI and acute ischemic stroke. Thrombolysis must be accomplished quickly after MI or cerebral infarction because clots become more difficult to dissolve (or lyse) as they age. Adjunctive anticoagulant and antiplatelet drugs may contribute to bleeding during thrombolytic therapy.

What are the adverse effects?

The principal adverse effect associated with thrombolytic therapy is bleeding caused by fibrinogenolysis or fibrinolysis at the site of vascular injury. The incidence of bleeding occurs at a similar rate for all agents.

Life-threatening intracranial bleeding may necessitate stopping therapy.

What are the contraindications and interactions?

The contraindications to the use of thrombolytic drugs are similar to those for anticoagulant drugs. Absolute contraindications include active bleeding, pregnancy, lactation, intracranial trauma, vascular disease, and cancer.

Anticoagulants and aspirin can cause interactions with thrombolytics and increase the risk of bleeding. Such herbs as feverfew, galling, ginger, and ginkgo may increase the risk of bleeding.

What are the most important points patients should know?

Instruct patients to immediately report signs of bleeding (blood in urine, tarry stools, or oozing from cuts) or changes in consciousness to their health-care providers. Advise women to not breastfeed while taking urokinase.

Table 23-4 ■ Thrombolytics

GENERIC NAME	TRADE NAME	ADULT DOSE	ROUTE OF ADMINISTRATION
alteplase recombinant	Activase	Begin with 60 mg and then infuse 20 mg/h over next 2 h	IV
anistreplase	Eminase	30 units over 2–5 min	IV
reteplase recombinant	Retavase	10 units over 2 min; repeat dose in 30 min	IV
streptokinase	Streptase, Kabikinase	250,000–1.5 million units over a short period	IV
tenecteplase recombinant	TNKase	Up to 50 mg bolus over 5 seconds based on patient weight	IV
urokinase	Abbokinase	4,400–6,000 units administered over several min to 12 h	IV

IV, intravenous.

Focus Point

Thrombocytopenia

Platelet deficiency (thrombocytopenia) is the most common cause of abnormal bleeding. The term *hemophilia* applies to several different hereditary bleeding disorders that result from a lack of any of the factors needed for clotting.

Focus Point

Top Five Prescribed Anticoagulants

1. warfarin (Coumadin, Panwarfin)
2. clopidogrel (Plavix)
3. ticlopidine (Ticlid)
4. alteplase (Activase)
5. dipyridamole (Persantine)

✳ Apply Your Knowledge 23.4

The following exercises focus on what you have just learned about thrombolytic agents.

CRITICAL THINKING

1. What is the term for platelet deficiency?
2. What is the mechanism of action of thrombolytics?
3. What are the indications for thrombolytic drugs?
4. What are the top five prescribed anticoagulants?
5. What are the trade names of anistreplase, urokinase, streptokinase, and tenecteplase recombinant?

PRACTICAL SCENARIO 1

A 65-year-old patient with a history of deep vein thrombosis has been admitted to the hospital with chest pain. He is having trouble breathing. His physician orders an electrocardiogram, a Doppler ultrasonography, a ventilation-perfusion scan, and a computed tomography scan. The diagnosis is a pulmonary embolus.

Michal Heron/PH College

Critical Thinking Questions

1. What medicine will the physician likely immediately prescribe for this patient while he is hospitalized?
2. What teaching will you provide the patient and family about the reasons he is taking this medication and the precautions he needs to take during therapy?
3. Do you think the patient will be released from the hospital while taking this medication or will his medication be switched? If the medication is changed when the patient is discharged, what is a likely alternative medicine that will be prescribed?
4. What teaching will you provide the patient when he leaves the hospital, especially regarding his medication?

PRACTICAL SCENARIO 2

A 23-year-old pregnant woman underwent a caesarean section for delivery. Her physician ordered anticoagulants to prevent complications that could potentially occur.

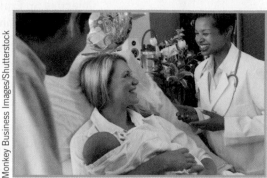

Critical Thinking Questions

1. What is the most common complication after this type of surgery that requires the use of anticoagulants?
2. Name the common medication used after surgery for preventing clots.

Chapter Capsule

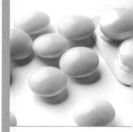

This section repeats the objectives from the beginning of the chapter and then provides a summary of the most important concepts for that objective. Use this section as a quick review and to check your knowledge.

Objective 1: Explain hemostasis.

- Hemostasis encompasses three events that occur in a cascade:
  - Blood vessel spasm
  - Formation of platelet plug
  - Blood clotting

Objective 2: Explain the mechanisms of action of heparin and warfarin.

- Heparin (parenteral anticoagulant)—increases the length of clotting time and prevents thrombi from forming or growing larger; action depends on inhibition of thrombus and clot formation by blocking conversion of prothrombin to thrombin and fibrinogen to fibrin
- Warfarin (oral anticoagulant)—interferes with hepatic synthesis of vitamin K–dependent clotting factors (factors II [prothrombin], VII, IX, and X), resulting in eventual depletion and prolongation of clotting times

Objective 3: Describe the advantages of low-molecular-weight heparin.

- Greater bioavailability and longer lasting effect than standard heparins, and dose-independent clearance pharmacokinetics

Objective 4: Name the class of drugs that can be used to induce bleeding or delay coagulation and explain individual drug mechanisms of action.

- Antiplatelets:
  - aspirin (Ecotrin)—inhibits platelet aggregation and prolongs bleeding time
  - ticlopidine (Ticlid) and clopidogrel (Plavix)—structurally related to aspirin; irreversibly block platelet activation, leading to inhibition of platelet aggregation
  - abciximab (ReoPro), eptifibatide (Integrilin), and tirofiban (Aggrastat)—interrupt interaction of fibrinogen with clotting factors and inhibit aggregation of platelets activated by a wide variety of stimuli

Objective 5: Explain the mechanism of action of thrombolytic drugs and list five drugs in this class.

■ Facilitate conversion of plasminogen to plasmin, which subsequently hydrolyzes fibrin to dissolve blood clots that have already formed; they are plasminogen activators that include:

- ❒ alteplase recombinant (Alteplase)
- ❒ anistreplase (Eminase)
- ❒ reteplase recombinant (Retavase)
- ❒ streptokinase (Streptase, Kabikinase)
- ❒ urokinase (Abbokinase)

 Internet Sites of Interest

■ The American Heart Association offers information about anticoagulants and antiplatelet agents in acute ischemic stroke at **http://stroke.ahajournals.org/content/33/7/1934.full?ck=nck**.

■ HealthCenter Online offers a discussion and illustrations of thrombus formation. with patient information on anticoagulants and antiplatelets at **http://heart.healthcentersonline.com/bloodclot/anticoagulants.cfm**. Considerations for use of these drugs in children, pregnant women, and elderly patients are included. Also available is a list of questions that patients can ask their health-care providers.

■ A discussion of coronary heart disease is available on WebMD at **http://www.webmd.com/heart-disease/antiplatelet-drugs**. The site offers information on many drug therapies for heart disease, including anticoagulants and antiplatelets. You will also find information on this site about the drug classes discussed in Chapter 21.

■ MedicineNet explains deep venous thrombosis and pulmonary embolism at **http://www.medicinenet.com**. Search for "DVT" for symptoms, diagnosis, treatment, and lifestyle considerations.

PEARSON myhealthprofessionskit™

Go to www.myhealthprofessionskit.com to access the Companion Website created for this textbook. Simply select "Basic Health Science" from the choice of disciplines. Find this book and then log in using your username and password to access interactive learning games, assessment questions, animations, and more.

Chapter Objectives

After completing this chapter, you should be able to:

1. Describe the structure of the nephron and the processes involved in the formation of urine.
2. Explain the processes of urine formation.
3. List the ways that electrolytes are lost from the body.
4. Describe how antidiuretic hormone and aldosterone levels influence the volume and concentration of urine.
5. Explain the indications for the use of diuretics in various conditions and disorders of the human body.
6. Classify the five major types of diuretics.
7. Describe the mechanism of action for osmotic diuretics.
8. List the major adverse effects of potassium-sparing diuretics.

Chapter 24

Drugs Used to Treat Fluid and Electrolyte Imbalances

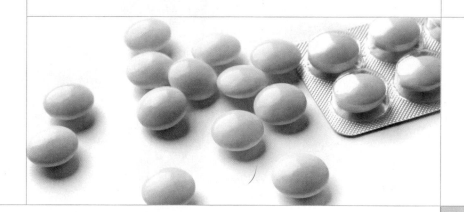

Key Terms

anions (AN-eye-ons) (page 422)
antidiuretic hormone (ADH) (page 418)
cations (KAT-eye-ons) (page 422)
creatinine (kree-AT-tih-neen) (page 417)
dehydration (dee-hy-DRAY-shun) (page 424)
diuretics (dy-yoo-REH-tiks) (page 423)
edema (eh-DEE-muh) (page 423)
glomerular capsule (glah-MAYR-yoo-lar KAP-sool) (page 416)
glomerular filtration (page 418)
glomerulus (glo-MAYR-yoo-lus) (page 416)

hyperkalemia (hi-per-kah-LEE-mee-uh) (page 428)
hypokalemia (hi-po-kah-LEE-mee-uh) (page 425)
hyponatremia (hi-po-nuh-TREE-mee-uh) (page 425)
loop of Henle (loop of HEN-lee) (page 416)
nephrons (NEH-fronz) (page 416)
osmolality (oz-moh-LAL-ih-tee) (page 421)
renal corpuscle (REE-nul KOR-pus-sul) (page 416)

renal tubule (REE-nul TOO-byool) (page 416)
renin (REE-nin) (page 416)
total body water (page 418)
tubular reabsorption (TOO-byoo-lar ree-ab-SORP-shun) (page 418)
tubular secretion (TOO-byoo-lar seh-KREE-shun) (page 418)
urea (yoo-REE-uh) (page 417)
uric acid (YOO-rik) (page 417)
water deficit (page 421)
water of metabolism (page 421)

Introduction

The primary function of the kidneys is to maintain a stable internal environment for optimal cell and tissue metabolism. The kidneys accomplish these life-sustaining tasks by balancing solute and water transport, excreting metabolic waste products, conserving nutrients, and regulating acids and bases. The kidneys also have an endocrine function and secrete the hormones **renin** (a hormone that converts angiotensinogen to angiotensin I), erythropoietin, and vitamin D$_3$ for the regulation of blood pressure, red blood cell (RBC) production, and calcium metabolism, respectively. The formation of urine is achieved through the process of filtration, reabsorption, and secretion by the glomeruli and tubules within the kidneys. The bladder stores the urine that is received from the kidneys by way of the ureters. Urine is then removed from the body through the urethra. Figure 24-1 ■ illustrates the urinary system.

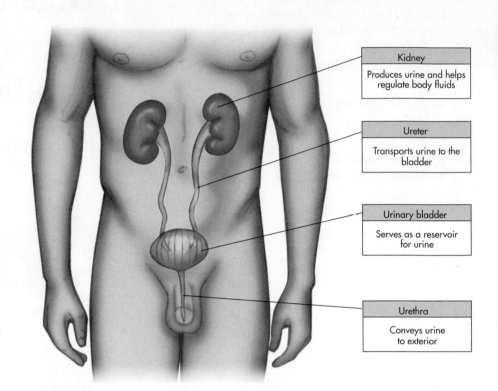

| Kidney |
| Produces urine and helps regulate body fluids |

| Ureter |
| Transports urine to the bladder |

| Urinary bladder |
| Serves as a reservoir for urine |

| Urethra |
| Conveys urine to exterior |

Figure 24-1 ■ The urinary system.

Kidney Structure and Functions

The kidneys include two distinct regions: an inner medulla and an outer cortex. The renal *cortex* is the superficial portion of the kidney. The renal *medulla* consists of 6 to 18 distinct triangular structures called *renal pyramids*. The base of each pyramid faces the cortex, and the tip of each pyramid—a region known as the *renal papilla*—projects into the renal sinus. The basic unit of the kidney is the nephron. The main function of the kidneys is to regulate the volume, composition, and pH of body fluids. The kidneys remove metabolic wastes from the blood and excrete them to the outside.

NEPHRONS

Each kidney contains about 1 million functional units called **nephrons**. Nephrons are located in the renal cortex. Each nephron consists of a **renal corpuscle** and a renal tubule. A renal corpuscle consists of a filtering unit composed of a cluster of blood capillaries called a **glomerulus** and a surrounding thin-walled, sac-like structure called a **glomerular capsule**. The renal tubule leads away from the glomerular capsule and becomes highly coiled. This coiled portion of the tubule is the *proximal convoluted tubule*. Following the proximal convoluted tubule is the *nephron loop* (**loop of Henle**). The ascending limb of this loop becomes highly coiled again and is called the *distal convoluted tubule* (DCT). This portion of the nephron then forms a *collecting duct* (collecting tubule), which is technically not part of the nephron (Figure 24-2 ■).

PRINCIPLES OF RENAL PHYSIOLOGY

The aim of urine production is to maintain homeostasis by regulating the volume and composition of blood. This process involves the excretion of solutes—specifically, metabolic waste products. Three organic

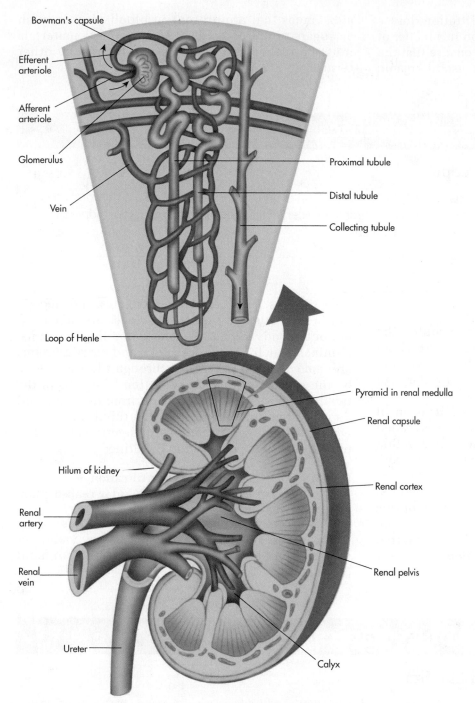

Figure 24-2 ■ The kidney with an expanded view of the nephron.

waste products are very important: urea, creatinine, and uric acid.

✳ **Urea** is the most abundant organic waste. Each person generates about 21 g of urea each day, which results in the breakdown of amino acids.

✳ **Creatinine**—a chemical waste molecule—is produced in skeletal muscle tissue by the breakdown of *creatine phosphate*, a high-energy compound that plays an important role in muscle contraction. The body generates roughly 1.8 g of creatinine each day, and virtually all of it is excreted in urine.

✳ **Uric acid**—another type of waste molecule—is formed by recycling a nitrogenous base from RNA molecules. Humans produce approximately 480 mg of uric acid each day.

These waste products are dissolved in the bloodstream and can be eliminated only while dissolved in the bloodstream or urine. As a result, their removal is accompanied by an unavoidable water loss. The kidneys are usually capable of producing more than four times the amount of concentrated urine than plasma. If the kidneys were not able to concentrate the filtrate produced by glomerular filtration, losses of fluid would lead to fatal dehydration in a matter of hours. At the same time, the kidneys ensure that the fluid lost does not contain potentially useful organic substances that are present in blood plasma, such as sugars or amino acids. These valuable materials must be reabsorbed and retained for use by other tissues.

Focus on Geriatrics

Diuresis in Elderly People

Older adults have a decreased ability to concentrate urine and are less able to tolerate dehydration or water loads because they have fewer nephrons. In older adults, drugs eliminated by the kidneys can accumulate in the plasma, causing toxic reactions.

URINE FORMATION

The main function of the nephrons is to control the composition of the body fluids and remove wastes from the blood. The product is urine, which is excreted from the body. It contains wastes, excess water, and electrolytes.

Urine formation begins with the filtration of plasma by the glomerular capillaries—a process called **glomerular filtration**. However, glomerular filtration produces 180 L of fluid, which is more than four times the amount of **total body water** (TBW; total water content of the body), every 24 hours. Glomerular filtration could not continue for very long unless most of this filtered fluid was returned to the internal environment.

The kidneys return filtered fluid to the internal environment through **tubular reabsorption**, selectively reclaiming just the right amounts of substances that the body requires, such as water, electrolytes, and glucose. Waste products and excess substances are processed out of the body. Some substances that the body must eliminate, such as hydrogen ions and certain toxins, are removed even faster than through filtration alone by the process of **tubular secretion** (the cells of the tubules remove certain substances from the blood and deposit them into the fluid in the tubules). In other words, the following relationship determines the volume of substances excreted in the urine:

Urinary excretion = Glomerular filtration + Tubular secretion − Tubular reabsorption

The final product of these processes is urine. The kidneys contribute to homeostasis by maintaining the composition of the internal environment (see Figure 24-3 ■).

Focus on Pediatrics

Fluid Imbalances in Children

The urine of infants and children is more dilute than that of adults because of pediatric higher blood flow and shorter loops of Henle. Pediatric patients are more affected by fluid imbalances resulting from diarrhea, infection, or improper feeding because their systems have a limited ability to quickly regulate changes in pH or osmotic pressure.

CONTROL OF URINE VOLUME

Urine volume is regulated by controlling the reabsorption of water. Water is reabsorbed by osmosis in the proximal convoluted tubule and the descending limb of the loop of Henle—a long, U-shaped part of the *renal tubule* extending through the *medulla* from the end of the *proximal convoluted tubule* to the beginning of the DCT. The ascending limb of the loop of Henle is impermeable to water. The DCT and collecting duct are also impermeable to water except in the presence of **antidiuretic hormone** (ADH). ADH is a hormone (also called *vasopressin*) that is released

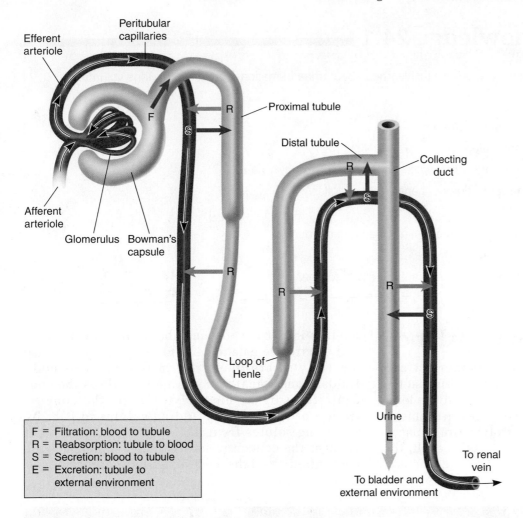

F = Filtration: blood to tubule
R = Reabsorption: tubule to blood
S = Secretion: blood to tubule
E = Excretion: tubule to external environment

Figure 24-3 ■ Sites of resorption and secretion in a nephron.

from the posterior lobe of the pituitary gland. The higher the circulating levels of ADH, the greater water permeability of these segments of the urinary system. In the absence of ADH, water is not reabsorbed in the DCT or the collecting system. Therefore, large amounts of very dilute urine are produced, which can cause diabetes insipidus. Failure of the posterior pituitary to produce ADH, or hypophysectomy (removal of the pituitary gland), may cause diabetes insipidus.

Focus Point

Medications and Urine Retention

Several medications cause urine retention and require careful consideration of use in certain patients. These include:

■ Anticholinergic and antispasmodic medications, such as atropine and papaverine

■ Antidepressant and antipsychotic agents, such as phenothiazines and monoamine oxidase inhibitors

■ Antihistamine preparations, such as pseudoephedrine (Sudafed and Actifed)

■ Antihypertensives, such as hydralazine (Apresoline) and methyldopa (Aldomet)

■ Beta-adrenergic blockers, such as propranolol (Inderal)

■ Opioids, such as hydrocodone (Vicodin)

Apply Your Knowledge 24.1

The following questions focus on what you have just learned about urine formation and control of urine volume.

CRITICAL THINKING

1. What are the functions of renin and erythropoietin?
2. What is the process of urine formation?
3. What is meant by the terms *urea* and *creatinine*?
4. Why do elderly people have fewer nephrons than younger adults?
5. What is tubular reabsorption?
6. Why is the urine of infants and children more dilute than that of adults?
7. What is another name for antidiuretic hormone?
8. What disorder may result from the absence of antidiuretic hormone?

Fluid and Electrolyte Balance

The term *balance* suggests a state of equilibrium, and in the case of water and electrolytes, it means that the quantities entering the body equal the quantities leaving it. Maintaining such a balance requires mechanisms to ensure that lost water and electrolytes are replaced and that any excesses are excreted. As a result, the levels of water and electrolytes in the body remain relatively stable at all times.

It is important to remember that water balance and electrolyte balance are interdependent because electrolytes are dissolved in the water of body fluids. Consequently, anything that alters the concentrations of the electrolytes alters the concentration of the water by adding solutes to it or by removing solutes from it. Likewise, anything that changes the concentration of the water changes the concentrations of the electrolytes by concentrating or diluting them.

Focus on Pediatrics

Threat of Dehydration in Infants

At birth, TBW represents about 75% to 80% of body weight and decreases to about 67% during the first year of life. Infants are particularly susceptible to significant changes in TBW because of a high metabolic rate and greater body surface area. Renal mechanisms of fluid and electrolyte conservation may not be mature enough to counter losses, thereby allowing dehydration to occur.

Focus Point

Water Deficit

Dehydration describes water deficit but is also commonly used to indicate sodium and water loss. Pure water deficits are rare because most people have access to water. Patients who are comatose or paralyzed have insensible water loss through the skin and lungs, with minimal obligatory formation of urine, and must be monitored closely for water deficit.

WATER BALANCE

Water balance exists when water intake equals water output. Homeostasis requires control of water intake and water output. Ultimately, maintenance of the internal environment depends on thirst centers in the brain to vary water intake and on the kidneys' ability to vary water output. Water balance is regulated by the secretion of ADH and the perception of thirst. Thirst stimulates water drinking and is experienced when water loss equals 2% of an individual's body weight or when there is an increase in **osmolality** (concentration of particles in plasma). ADH is secreted when plasma osmolality increases or when circulating blood volume decreases and blood pressure decreases. Increased plasma osmolality occurs with **water deficit** (low levels of water in the body) or sodium excess in relation to water.

Focus on Geriatrics

Fluctuating Total Body Water Content in Elderly Patients

The decline in the percentage of TBW content in elderly patients results, in part, because of increased body fat and decreased muscle as well as the kidneys' reduced ability to regulate sodium and water balance. Kidneys are less efficient in producing concentrated urine, and sodium-conserving responses are sluggish. With stress or when disease is present, this normal decrease in TBW can become life threatening.

Water intake: The volume of water gained each day varies among individuals (Table 24-1 ■). An average adult living in a moderate environment takes in about 2,500 mL per day. Approximately 60% is obtained from drinking water or other beverages, and another 30% comes from moist foods. The remaining 10% is a byproduct of the oxidative metabolism of nutrients, which is called **water of metabolism**.

Water output: Water normally enters the body only through the mouth, but it can be lost by a variety of routes. These include obvious losses in urine (the largest amount), feces, and sweat as well as evaporation from the skin and from the lungs during breathing (insensible water loss).

If an average adult takes in 2,500 mL of water each day, then 2,500 mL must be eliminated to maintain water balance. Of this volume, perhaps 60% is lost in urine, 6% in feces, and 6% in sweat. About 28% is lost by evaporation from the skin and lungs. These percentages vary with such environmental factors as temperature and relative humidity and with physical exercise. Therefore, the primary means of regulating water output is the control of urine production.

Table 24-1 ■ Normal Water Gains and Losses*

DAILY INTAKE	(mL)	DAILY OUTPUT	(mL)
Drinking	1,400–1,800	Urine	1,400–1,800
Water in food	700–1,000	Stool	100
Water of oxidation	300–400	Skin	300–500
		Lungs	600–800
Total	**2,000–3,200**	**Total**	**2,400–3,200**

*Based on a 70-kg adult man.

Focus Point

Maintaining Fluid and Electrolyte Balance

Remind patients of the following points to promote fluid and electrolyte balance:

- Consume six to eight glasses of water daily.
- Avoid excess amounts of foods or fluids high in salt, sugar, and caffeine.
- Eat a well-balanced diet.
- Limit alcohol intake because it has a diuretic effect.
- Increase fluid intake before, during, and after strenuous exercise.
- Maintain normal body weight.

ELECTROLYTE BALANCE

An *electrolyte* is any compound that, in solution, conducts electricity or is decomposed by it. An electrolyte balance exists when the quantities of electrolytes (molecules that release ions in water) gained and lost are equal (Figure 24-4 ■).

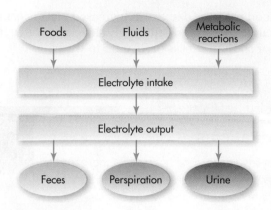

Figure 24-4 ■ Electrolyte balance. Electrolyte intake occurs through the ingestion of foods and fluids through metabolic reactions. Electrolyte output occurs through the excretion of feces, sweat, and urine.

Electrolyte intake: The electrolytes of greatest importance to cellular functions release sodium, potassium, calcium, magnesium, chloride, sulfate, phosphate, bicarbonate, and hydrogen ions. These electrolytes are primarily obtained from foods, but they may also be found in drinking water and other beverages. In addition, some electrolytes are by-products of metabolic reactions.

Electrolyte output: The body loses some electrolytes by perspiring (sweat has about half the solute concentration of plasma). The quantities of lost electrolytes vary with the amount of perspiration. More electrolytes are lost in sweat on warmer days and during strenuous exercise. Varying amounts of electrolytes are lost in the feces. The greatest electrolyte output occurs because of kidney function and urine production. The kidneys alter renal electrolyte losses to maintain the proper composition of body fluids.

The concentrations of positively charged ions, such as sodium (Na^+), potassium (K^+), and calcium (Ca^{+2}), are particularly important. For example, certain concentrations of these ions are vital for nerve impulse conduction, muscle fiber contraction, and the maintenance of cell membrane permeability. Potassium is especially important in maintaining the resting potential of nerve and cardiac muscle cells, and abnormal potassium levels may cause these cells to function abnormally.

Sodium ions account for nearly 90% of the **cations** (positively charged ions) in extracellular fluid (ECF). Primarily, the kidneys and the hormone aldosterone regulate these ions. Aldosterone, which the adrenal cortex secretes, increases sodium ion reabsorption in the DCTs and collecting ducts of the nephrons. A decrease in sodium ion concentration in the ECF stimulates aldosterone secretion.

Aldosterone also regulates potassium ions. An important stimulus for aldosterone secretion is an increasing potassium ion concentration, which directly stimulates cells of the adrenal cortex. This hormone enhances the renal tubular reabsorption of sodium ions and, at the same time, stimulates the renal tubular secretion of potassium ions.

Generally, the regulatory mechanisms that control positively charged ions secondarily control the concentrations of **anions** (negatively charged ions). For example, chloride ions (Cl^-)—the most abundant negatively charged ions in the ECF—are passively reabsorbed from the renal tubules in response to the active reabsorption of sodium ions. That is, the negatively charged chloride ions are electrically attracted to the positively charged sodium ions and accompany them as they are reabsorbed. The main electrolytes in the body are listed in Table 24-2 ■.

Table 24-2 ■ The Main Electrolytes in the Body

CATIONS	IONS	ANIONS	IONS
calcium	Ca^{++}	phosphate	PO^{4-} or HPO^{4-}
magnesium	Mg^{++}	sulfate	SO^{4-}
potassium	K^+	bicarbonate	HCO_3^-
sodium	Na^+	chloride	Cl^-

Focus on Geriatrics

Threats to Fluid and Electrolyte Imbalance in Elderly Patients

Certain changes related to aging cause elderly people to be at higher risk for serious problems with fluid and electrolyte imbalance if homeostatic mechanisms are compromised. Some of these changes include:

- Decreased thirst sensation
- Decreased ability of the kidneys to concentrate urine
- Decreased intracellular fluid and total body water
- Decreased response to body hormones that help regulate fluid and electrolytes
- Increased use of diuretics for hypertension and heart disease
- Decreased fluid and food intake

✳ Apply Your Knowledge 24.2

The following questions focus on what you have just learned about fluid and electrolyte balance.

CRITICAL THINKING

1. What is osmolality?
2. What is water of metabolism?
3. What are the most important electrolytes for cellular functions?
4. What are the definitions of *cations* and *anions*?
5. What is the percentage of total body water at birth?

DIURETICS

Diuretics are a group of drugs that promote water loss from the body into the urine. Because urine formation takes place in the kidneys, it is not surprising that diuretics have their principal action at the level of the nephrons. Diuretics remove the excess ECF from the body that can result in **edema** (abnormal fluid accumulation) of the tissues, ascites, and hypertension. These conditions occur in diseases of the heart, kidneys, and liver.

Each human kidney has about 1 million nephrons. More than 120 mL of ultrafiltrate is formed per minute, but only 1 mL of urine is produced. Thus, more than 99% of ultrafiltrate is reabsorbed. Diuretics increase the rate of urine flow. Clinically useful diuretics increase the rate of excretion of sodium (Na^+) and chloride (Cl^-).

NaCl is the major determinant of the ECF volume; therefore, most clinical applications of diuretics are directed toward reducing ECF volume by decreasing total body NaCl content. Sustained positive Na^+ balance causes volume overload with pulmonary edema. Sustained negative Na^+ balance causes volume depletion and cardiovascular collapse. The five major classes of diuretics are:

1. Osmotic diuretics
2. Carbonic anhydrase inhibitors
3. Thiazide diuretics
4. Loop diuretics
5. Potassium-sparing diuretics

Focus Point

Contraindications of Diuretics in Pregnancy

Diuretics are not recommended during pregnancy because they may interfere with the normal expansion of fluid that occurs during pregnancy and disrupt neurodevelopment of the fetus. Diuretic use increases the fetus's risk of such conditions as schizophrenia, jaundice, blood problems, and potassium depletion. Most diuretics pass into breast milk and can cause dehydration in nursing babies.

Focus On

Osmotic Diuretics

The capacity of the renal tubule to reabsorb various electrolytes and nonelectrolytes is limited and varies for each ionic species. If large amounts of these substances are administered to an individual, their concentration in the body fluids and subsequently in the glomerular filtrate exceeds the reabsorption capacity of the tubules. The excess then appears in the urine, accompanied by an increased volume of water.

Generally, substances that increase urine formation in this manner are called *osmotic diuretics*. This group of diuretics includes osmotic electrolytes (potassium and sodium salts), osmotic nonelectrolytes (urea,

(Continued)

Focus On (Continued)

. . . .

glycerin, and mannitol), and acid-forming salts (ammonium chloride) (Table 24-3 ■).

How do they work?

Osmotic agents may have multiple sites of action. Nevertheless, their major component is a decrease in solute content, resulting in less water reabsorption from the descending loop of Henle and collecting duct and less sodium chloride reabsorption in the proximal tubule and ascending limb of Henle.

How are they used?

Osmotic diuretics are highly effective treatments for cerebral edema and are used primarily for this purpose.

What are the adverse effects?

The major adverse effects of osmotic diuretics are related to the amount of solute administered and the effect on the volume and distribution of body fluids. They may cause headache, tremor, convulsions, dizziness, hypotension or hypertension, and thrombophlebitis. They may also produce blurred vision, dry mouth, nausea, vomiting, chills, fever, and allergic reactions.

What are the contraindications and interactions?

Osmotic diuretics are contraindicated in patients with anuria, marked pulmonary congestion or edema, severe congestive heart failure (CHF), metabolic edema, organic central nervous system disease, intracranial bleeding, shock, severe **dehydration** (excessive loss of body water), history of allergy, pregnancy, and lactation.

What are the important points patients should know?

Advise patients to report thirst, muscle cramps or weakness, paresthesia, dyspnea, and headache and to keep follow-up appointments for laboratory tests. Instruct female patients to avoid breastfeeding while taking these drugs.

Table 24-3 ■ Osmotic Diuretics

GENERIC NAME	TRADE NAME	AVERAGE ADULT DOSAGE	ROUTE OF ADMINISTRATION
glycerin	Osmoglyn	1–2 g/kg	PO
isosorbide	Ismotic	1–3 mg/kg bid–qid	PO
mannitol	Osmitro	150–100 g as 10–20% solution over 2–6h	IV for edema or ascites
urea	Ureaphil	1–1.5 g/kg/d	IV

bid, twice a day; IV, intravenous; PO, oral; qid, four times a day.

Focus On

Carbonic Anhydrase Inhibitors

Carbonic anhydrase inhibitors stop the conversion of carbon dioxide to carbonic acid and bicarbonate ions. They are generally used to treat glaucoma and epilepsy and to lessen the effects of high altitudes on the body (Table 24-4 ■).

How do they work?

The enzyme carbonic anhydrase catalyses the conversion of carbon dioxide into bicarbonate ions and vice versa according to the following equation:

$$CO_2 + H_2O \; H_2CO_3^- \leftrightarrow H_2CO_3 \; H^+ + HCO_3^-$$

This reaction occurs in the kidneys as well as other parts of the body. In the kidneys, the reaction occurs mainly in the proximal tubule, and because it involves bicarbonate loss, it affects acid–base balance. The tubular cells are not very permeable to bicarbonate ions or carbonic acid, but they are very permeable to carbon dioxide. Under normal conditions, carbonic anhydrase in the tubular cell converts the carbonic acid into carbon dioxide and water, which are promptly reabsorbed. If the enzyme is inhibited, there will be a net loss of bicarbonate from the body, with a consequent loss of water.

The drug acetazolamide (Diamox) is a noncompetitive inhibitor of this enzyme and has been used as a diuretic.

How are they used?

Carbonic anhydrase inhibitors are used in the treatment of absence, generalized tonic–clonic, and focal seizures. They can also be used for the reduction of intraocular pressure in glaucoma (see Chapter 30) and to treat acute high-altitude sickness.

What are the adverse effects?

The adverse effects of carbonic anhydrase inhibitors include anorexia, nausea, vomiting, weight loss, dry mouth, thirst, diarrhea, and bone marrow depression. Other adverse effects are fatigue, dizziness, drowsiness, hyperglycemia, exacerbation of gout, and hepatic dysfunction.

What are the contraindications and interactions?

Carbonic anhydrase inhibitors are contraindicated in patients with hypersensitivity to sulfonamides and derivatives such as thiazides. They should be avoided in marked renal and hepatic dysfunction, Addison's disease or other types of adrenocortical insufficiency, **hyponatremia** (an abnormally low concentration of sodium ions in blood), **hypokalemia** (an abnormally low concentration of potassium ions in blood), or hypochloremic acidosis. Safety during pregnancy and lactation is not established.

Carbonic anhydrase inhibitors should be used cautiously in patients with a history of hypercalciuria, diabetes mellitus, gout, obstructive pulmonary disease, and respiratory acidosis and in patients receiving digitalis. Carbonic anhydrase inhibitors, such as acetazolamide (Diamox), may cause renal excretion of amphetamines, ephedrine, quinidine, and procainamide. They may decrease the effects of tricyclic antidepressants. Renal excretion of lithium is increased. Excretion of phenobarbital may be increased. Amphotericin B and corticosteroids may accelerate potassium loss.

What are the important points patients should know?

Instruct patients taking carbonic anhydrase inhibitors to avoid driving and operating heavy machinery if drowsiness or dizziness occurs.

Table 24-4 ■ Carbonic Anhydrase Inhibitors

GENERIC NAME	TRADE NAME	AVERAGE ADULT DOSAGE	ROUTE OF ADMINISTRATION
acetazolamide	Diamox Sequels	250 mg/d 1–4 times/d; 500 mg sustained release bid	PO
	Diamox Parenteral	500 mg, may repeat in 2–4 h	IV, IM
dichlorphenamide	Daramide, Oratrol	100–200 mg followed by 100 mg q12h until desired response is obtained	PO
methazolamide	Neptazane	50–100 mg bid–tid	PO

bid, twice a day; IM, intramuscular; IV, intravenous; PO, oral; tid, three times a day.

Focus Point

The Threat of Hypokalemia

Hypokalemia is a potentially life-threatening condition that occurs most often as a side effect of diuretic therapy or prolonged diarrhea. Hypokalemia may be caused by inappropriate or excessive use of such drugs as corticosteroids, penicillin, aminoglycosides, cardiac glycosides, laxatives, and vitamin B_{12} therapy.

Focus On

Thiazide and Thiazide-Like Diuretics

Thiazides are a group of drugs that are chemically similar. The thiazide-like drugs are chemically dissimilar from the thiazides but have an identical mode of action. Thiazides are the most commonly used diuretic drugs influencing the function of the urinary tract (Table 24-5 ■).

How do they work?

The thiazide diuretics increase the urinary excretion of sodium and water by inhibiting sodium reabsorption on the DCTs and collecting ducts. They also increase the excretion of chloride, potassium, and bicarbonate ions.

How are they used?

The thiazide drugs are commonly used in the treatment of patients with hypertension and can add to the effectiveness of other antihypertensive drugs, reversing fluid retention caused by some of these agents.

Thiazide diuretics are also used as adjunctive therapy in edema associated with CHF, hepatic cirrhosis, and corticosteroids or estrogen therapy; edema caused by acute glomerulonephritis; and chronic renal failure.

What are the adverse effects?

The common adverse effects of thiazide diuretics include anorexia, gastric irritation, nausea, vomiting, cramping, diarrhea, constipation, jaundice, hypokalemia, and pancreatitis. Other adverse effects are headache, dizziness, vertigo, leukopenia, aplastic anemia, orthostatic hypotension, fever, respiratory distress, anaphylactic reactions, and hyperglycemia.

What are the contraindications and interactions?

Thiazide diuretics are contraindicated in patients with diabetes, a history of gout, severe renal disease, and impaired liver function and in elderly patients. Thiazide diuretics are not recommended for use by nursing mothers. Drug interactions may occur with corticosteroids, lithium, probenecid, and antidiabetic agents.

What are the important points patients should know?

Instruct patients with diabetes to monitor their blood glucose levels with extra care because thiazide, loop, and potassium-sparing diuretics can cause hyperglycemia.

Table 24-5 ■ Thiazides and Thiazide-like Diuretics

GENERIC NAME	TRADE NAME	AVERAGE ADULT DOSAGE	ROUTE OF ADMINISTRATION
Thiazide Diuretics			
chlorothiazide	Diuril, Duragen	250–500 mg 1–2 times/d	PO
cyclothiazide	Anhydron	2 mg/d	PO
hydrochlorothiazide	HydroDIURIL, Esidrix	12.5–100 mg/d	PO
hydroflumethiazide	Diucardin, Saluron	25–100 mg 1–2 times/d	PO
methyclothiazide	Aquatensen, Enduron	2.5–10 mg/d	PO
polythiazide	Renese	1–4 mg/d	PO
Thiazide-Like Diuretics			
chlorthalidone	Hygroton	50–100 mg/d	PO
indapamide	Lozol	2.5–5 mg/d	PO

PO, oral.

Focus on Natural Products

Gossypol and Diuretics

When used concomitantly with diuretics, gossypol (an herbal supplement used as a vaginal spermicide, to induce labor and delivery, and to treat dysmenorrhea) may result in hypokalemia.

Focus On

Loop Diuretics

The loop diuretics are sometimes referred to as high-ceiling diuretics. In high doses, loop diuretics can increase urine output astronomically, leading to severe hypovolemia (decreased blood volume) and death (Table 24-6 ■).

How do they work?

Loop diuretics act directly on the loop of Henle in the kidneys to inhibit sodium and chloride reabsorption. Potent diuretics, such as furosemide (Lasix), bumetanide (Bumex), and ethacrynic acid (Edecrin), are not thiazides but act in a similar way to increase the excretion of water, sodium, chloride, and potassium. Their action is more rapid and effective than that of thiazides with greater diuresis.

How are they used?

The loop diuretics are the drugs of choice in patients with acute pulmonary edema, resulting in CHF. Because of their rapid onset of action, the drugs are useful in emergencies, such as acute pulmonary edema. They are also useful in treating patients with hypercalcemia because they stimulate tubular calcium ion secretion. Loop diuretics are used in hypertension when other diuretics and other antihypertensives do not result in satisfactory response. In edema of nephrotic syndrome, only loop diuretics are capable of reducing edema.

What are the adverse effects?

The adverse effects of the loop diuretics include abnormalities of fluid and electrolyte balance, hyponatremia, hypotension, circulatory collapse, thromboemboli, and hepatic encephalopathy. They may cause hypokalemia (which may induce cardiac dysrhythmias in patients taking glycosides) and hypocalcemia (which can lead to tetany).

Loop diuretics are toxic to the ear, particularly when used in conjunction with the aminoglycosides (antibiotics). Ethacrynic acid (Edecrin) is the most ototoxic. Irreversible damage may result with continued treatment. Furosemide (Lasix) and ethacrynic acid compete with uric acid for the renal and biliary secretory systems. This results in the blocking of secretions, resulting in hyperuricemia and causing gout attacks. Other adverse effects of loop diuretics may be skin rashes, photosensitivity, hypotension, shock, cardiac arrhythmias, and bone marrow depression.

What are the contraindications and interactions?

Loop diuretics are contraindicated in patients with hypersensitivity to these drugs. They are not recommended for use in infants or lactating women. They should be avoided in patients with severe diarrhea, dehydration, electrolyte imbalance, and hypotension.

Loop diuretics should be used cautiously in patients with hepatic cirrhosis, diabetes mellitus, pulmonary edema, pregnancy, and a history of gout. They may cause drug interactions with aminoglycosides, anticoagulants, lithium, propranolol, sulfonylureas, nonsteroidal anti-inflammatory drugs (NSAIDs), probenecid, and thiazide diuretics.

What are the important points patients should know?

Instruct patients to follow their physician's orders to take diuretic medications early in the morning and not at bedtime. Advise women to avoid this drug when breastfeeding.

Table 24-6 ■ Loop Diuretics

GENERIC NAME	TRADE NAME	AVERAGE ADULT DOSAGE	ROUTE OF ADMINISTRATION
bumetanide	Bumex	0.5–2 mg/d	PO
		0.5 1 mg over 1–2 min, repeated q2–3h PRN (maximum: 10 mg/d)	IV, IM
ethacrynic acid	Edecrin	50–100 mg 1–2 times/day (maximum: 400 mg/d)	PO
		0.5–1 mg/kg	IV
furosemide	Lasix	20–80 mg/d in 1 or several divided doses (maximum: 600 mg/d)	PO
		20–40 mg in one or several divided doses, up to 600 mg/d	IM, IV
torsemide	Demadex	4–20 mg/d	PO, IV

IM, intramuscular; IV, intravenous; PO, oral; PRN, as needed.

Focus On

Potassium-Sparing Diuretics

The potassium-sparing diuretics include spironolactone (Aldactone), triamterene (Dyrenium), and amiloride (Midamor). The potassium-sparing diuretics are able to produce a mild diuresis without affecting blood potassium levels. The effects of these agents on urine electrolyte composition are similar in that they decrease potassium and hydrogen ion excretion. Despite this similarity, these agents actually comprise two groups with respect to mechanism of action. Spironolactone—the prototype agent of the aldosterone antagonists—is a specific competitive inhibitor of aldosterone at the receptor site level; hence, it is effective only when aldosterone is present. The other two potassium-sparing diuretics—triamterene and amiloride—exert their effects independently of the presence or absence of aldosterone (Table 24-7 ■).

How do they work?

Spironolactone (Aldactone) is a synthetic aldosterone antagonist that competes with aldosterone for intracellular cytoplasmic receptor sites. The spironolactone receptor complex cannot translocate into the nucleus of the target cell. Therefore, this prevents sodium reabsorption in the distal tubule.

How are they used?

The potassium-sparing agents are used in the treatment of edema associated with CHF, hepatic cirrhosis with ascites, and the nephrotic syndrome. Because these diuretics have little antihypertensive action of their own, they are used mainly in combination with other drugs in the management of hypertension and to correct hypokalemia often caused by other diuretic agents. Spironolactone is also used in primary hyperaldosteronism.

What are the adverse effects?

Potassium-sparing diuretics may cause life-threatening **hyperkalemia** (an abnormally high amount of potassium ions in blood). The main adverse effects of these agents include hyperkalemia, acute renal failure, and kidney stones. Because spironolactone chemically resembles some of the sex steroids, it has minimal hormonal activity and may cause gynecomastia (development of mammary glands) in men and menstrual irregularities in women. At low doses, spironolactone can be used chronically with few adverse effects. Potassium-sparing diuretics may cause nausea, lethargy, headache, and mental confusion.

What are the contraindications and interactions?

Potassium-sparing diuretics are contraindicated in patients with anuria, acute renal insufficiency, impaired renal function, or hyperkalemia. They should be used cautiously in patients with cirrhosis of the liver or who are pregnant or lactating. Potassium supplements, NSAIDs, and lithium may interact with potassium-sparing diuretics.

What are the important points patients should know?

Teach patients taking potassium-sparing diuretics about the symptoms of hypokalemia, such as muscle cramps and weakness, lethargy, anorexia, irregular pulse, and confusion. Instruct them about the symptoms of hyperkalemia, such as thirst, dry mouth, and drowsiness. Caution patients to maintain normal potassium levels while taking combination digoxin and diuretic therapy.

Table 24-7 ■ **Potassium-Sparing Diuretics**

GENERIC NAME	TRADE NAME	AVERAGE ADULT DOSAGE	ROUTE OF ADMINISTRATION
amiloride	Midamor	5–20 mg/d	PO
spironolactone	Aldactone	Up to 400 mg/d	PO
triamterene	Dyrenium	Up to 300 mg/d	PO

PO, oral.

✳ Apply Your Knowledge 24.3

The following questions focus on what you have just learned about diuretics and their effects on fluid and electrolyte balance.

CRITICAL THINKING

1. What are the major classes of diuretics?
2. What are the risks to the fetus when diuretics are used during pregnancy?
3. What are the indications for osmotic diuretics?
4. What are three examples of carbonic anhydrase inhibitors?
5. What is the mechanism of action of thiazide diuretics?
6. What are two examples of thiazide-like diuretics?
7. What are the trade names of furosemide, acetazolamide, mannitol, chlorothiazide, and bumetanide?
8. What are the indications of potassium-sparing agents?
9. What are the major adverse effects of potassium-sparing diuretics?
10. Which diuretics are the drugs of choice in acute pulmonary edema, resulting in chronic heart failure?

PRACTICAL SCENARIO 1

A middle-aged man who is being treated with hydrochlorothiazide for control of mild edema presents to the physician complaining of malaise, fatigue, muscular weakness, and muscle cramps. In response to the physician's questions about how he is taking his medication, he reports that he takes the medication daily but that causes constipation. Therefore, he has been taking laxatives. The physician orders electrocardiography (ECG) and blood tests to check the patient's levels of creatinine, blood urea nitrogen, uric acid, and electrolytes.

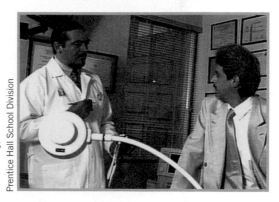

Prentice Hall School Division

Critical Thinking Questions

1. What do you think might be the result of the man's use of diuretics and laxatives together?
2. Why do you think the physician ordered the ECG and blood tests and what is he looking for?
3. What blood test results do you expect to find?
4. When providing patient education for this man, what would you tell him?

PRACTICAL SCENARIO 2

A 58-year-old woman who had congestive heart failure was admitted to the hospital. She had a history of hypertension and liver disease.

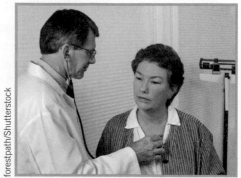

forestpath/Shutterstock

Critical Thinking Questions

1. What type of diuretics is more appropriate for this patient?
2. If the physician prescribes potassium-sparing diuretics, what adverse effects may be caused?

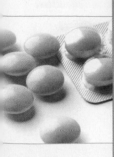

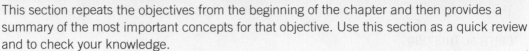

Chapter Capsule

This section repeats the objectives from the beginning of the chapter and then provides a summary of the most important concepts for that objective. Use this section as a quick review and to check your knowledge.

Objective 1: Describe the structure of the nephron and the processes involved in the formation of urine.

- Nephrons—consist of a renal corpuscle and renal tubule.
- The renal corpuscle has a filtering unit composed of a cluster of blood capillaries called a *glomerulus* and a surrounding thin-walled, sac-like structure called a *glomerular capsule.*
- The renal tubule leads away from the glomerular capsule and becomes highly coiled (the proximal convoluted tubule).
- Next is the loop of Henle, the ascending limb of which becomes highly coiled again (the distal convoluted tubule), forming a collecting duct (tubule).
- Urinary excretion = Glomerular filtration + Tubular secretion − Tubular reabsorption.

Objective 2: Explain the processes of urine formation.

- Urine formation—maintains homeostasis by regulating the volume and composition of blood.
- Involves the excretion of such solutes (specifically, metabolic waste products) as urea, creatinine, and uric acid.
- Valuable materials, such as sugars or amino acids, are reabsorbed and retained for use by other tissues.

Objective 3: List the ways that electrolytes are lost from the body.

- Sweat, feces, urine.

Objective 4: Describe how antidiuretic hormone and aldosterone levels influence the volume and concentration of urine.

- ADH—controls water permeability; when absent, water is not reabsorbed in the distal convoluted tubules and the collecting system, producing large amounts of very dilute urine, which can cause diabetes insipidus.
- Aldosterone—increases sodium ion reabsorption in the distal convoluted tubules and collecting ducts of the nephrons.

Objective 5: Explain the indications for the use of diuretics in various conditions and disorders of the human body.

- Diuretics are indicated for edema (cerebral, acute pulmonary edema or congestive heart failure), hepatic cirrhosis with or without ascites, use with corticosteroids or estrogen therapies, acute glomerulonephritis, hypercalcemia, nephrotic syndrome, and chronic renal failure), various seizures, for the reduction of intraocular pressure in glaucoma, acute high-altitude sickness, and hypertension (including the reversal of fluid retention caused by some antihypertensive drugs).

Objective 6: Classify the five major types of diuretics.

- Osmotic diuretics—affect the capacity of the renal tubule to reabsorb electrolytes and nonelectrolytes.
- Carbonic anhydrase inhibitors—stop the conversion of carbon dioxide to carbonic acid and bicarbonate ions.
- Thiazide and thiazide-like diuretics—inhibit sodium reabsorption on distal convoluted tubules and collecting ducts.
- Loop diuretics—work on the loop of Henle to inhibit sodium and chloride reabsorption
- Potassium-sparing diuretics—decrease potassium and hydrogen ion excretion.

Objective 7: Describe the mechanism of action for osmotic diuretics.

- Decrease solute content, resulting in less water reabsorption from the descending loop of Henle and collecting duct and less sodium chloride reabsorption in the proximal tubule and ascending loop of Henle.

Objective 8: List the major adverse effects of potassium-sparing diuretics.

- Hyperkalemia, acute renal failure, and kidney stones.

Internet Sites of Interest

- Answers to your questions about diuretics can be found at **http://www.rxlist.com/script/main/art.asp?articlekey=94169**.
- A description of kidneys and how they work can be found on the National Kidney and Urologic Diseases (a service of National Institute of Diabetes and Digestive and Kidney Diseases [NIDDK]) website at **http://kidney.niddk.nih.gov**. Search for "your kidneys."
- Medical tests to determine kidney function are explained on the NIDDK's website at **http://kidney.niddk.nih.gov**. Search for "medical tests kidneys."

PEARSON
myhealthprofessionskit™

Go to www.myhealthprofessionskit.com to access the Companion Website created for this textbook. Simply select "Basic Health Science" from the choice of disciplines. Find this book and then log in using your username and password to access interactive learning games, assessment questions, animations, and more.

Chapter 25

Drugs Used to Treat Endocrine Conditions

Chapter Objectives

After completing this chapter, you should be able to:

1. Describe the main functions of a hormone.
2. Explain the endocrine functions of the hypothalamus.
3. List six types of hormones that are secreted from the anterior pituitary gland.
4. Describe the role of the thyroid gland and its replacement and antithyroid drugs.
5. Explain the pharmacotherapy of diabetes insipidus.
6. Identify the role of hypoglycemic medications in treating diabetes mellitus.
7. Describe the adverse effects of insulin and corticosteroids.
8. Identify the two major classes of steroids.

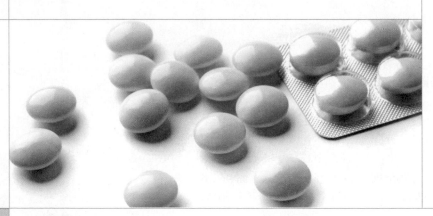

Key Terms

acromegaly (ak-roh-MEHG-uh-lee) (page 433)

Addison's disease (ADD-iss-uns) (page 439)

adenohypophysis (ADD-eh-no-hy-PO-fih-sis) (page 433)

congenital hypothyroidism (kun-JEN-i-tul hi-po-THY-royd-i-zum) (page 438)

Cushing's disease (KUSH-ings) (page 435)

Cushing's syndrome (page 435)

diabetes insipidus (dy-uh-BEE-tees in-SIP-uh-dus) (page 437)

diabetes mellitus (dy-uh-BEE-tees MEL-uh-tiss) (page 442)

dwarfism (DWARF-izm) (page 433)

gestational diabetes mellitus (jeh-STAY-shuh-nul) (page 443)

gigantism (jy-GANT-izm) (page 433)

glucagon (GLOO-kuh-gon) (page 442)

Graves's disease (page 434)

hyperglycemia (hi-per-GLI-seem-ee-uh) (page 443)

hyperthyroidism (hy-per-THY-royd-izm) (page 438)

hypoglycemia (hy-po-gli-SEE-mee-uh) (page 444)

hypoparathyroidism (hy-po-par-uh-THY-royd-izm) (page 441)

hypopituitarism (hy-po-pih-TOO-ih-tair-izm) (page 433)

hypothyroidism (hi-po-THIE-royd-izm) (page 440)

iatrogenic (eye-a-troh-JEH-nik) (page 452)

islets of Langerhans (EYE-lits of LANG-ur-hans) (page 433)

lithium (LITH-ee-um) (page 439)

myxedema (mix-uh-DEEM-uh) (page 438)

neurohypophysis (noor-oh-hy-PO-fih-sis) (page 433)

oxytocin (awk-see-TOH-sin) (page 437)

parafollicular cells (par-uh-fo-LIK-u-lur) (page 437)

thyrotoxicosis (thy-ro-toks-ih-KOH-sis) (page 438)

vasopressin (vaz-oh-PRESS-in) (page 437)

Introduction

Hormones are chemical substances secreted directly into the blood by endocrine glands—generally in response to a change in the internal condition of the body and with the goal of maintaining homeostasis. This chapter focuses on hormones that regulate growth, blood glucose, and intermediary metabolism. The synthesis and secretion of many hormones are controlled by other hormones or changes in the concentration of essential chemicals or electrolytes in the blood. The interrelationships among the peptide hormones of the hypothalamus, the trophic hormones of the anterior pituitary, and other endocrine glands are examples of elegant feedback regulation—positive feedback, in which one hormone stimulates the secretion of another, or negative feedback, in which one hormone turns off the action of the previous hormone. Drugs and diseases can modify hormone secretion as well as specific hormone effects at target organs.

Pharmacologic preparations are used to detect and treat disorders involving any of the following glands: pituitary, thyroid, adrenal cortex, pancreas, or gonads. The effects of these drugs are derived from the physiological actions of the endogenous hormones that they stimulate if they are activators (agonists) or block if they are antagonists.

Endocrine System

The endocrine system secretes hormones that control the body by maintaining its internal environment within certain narrow ranges, which is known as *homeostasis*. The maintenance of homeostasis involves growth, maturation, reproduction, metabolism, and human behavior. Responsibility for homeostasis is shared by the endocrine system and the nervous system, working in tandem in a unique partnership. The hypothalamus of the brain (a part of the nervous system) sends directions via chemical signals (the releasing of hormones) to the pituitary gland (a part of the endocrine system). It also controls the release of corticotropin-releasing hormone (CRH), growth hormone–releasing hormone (GHRH), gonadotropin-releasing hormone (GnRH), thyrotropin-releasing hormone (TRH), and anterior–pituitary hormones. The pituitary stimulates the other endocrine glands to secrete their hormones. The endocrine glands include the pituitary gland, pineal gland, thyroid gland, parathyroid glands, thymus gland, adrenal glands, **islets of Langerhans** (small clusters of cells within the pancreas), ovaries in women, and testes

in men (see Figure 25-1 ■). The ovarian and testicular hormones are discussed in Chapter 26. Hormone secretion is precisely regulated by the hypothalamus, the anterior pituitary gland, and other groups of glands that respond to the hypothalamus and pituitary glands (see Figure 25-2 ■).

Pituitary Gland

The pituitary gland—sometimes called the *master gland* because of its regulatory effects on the other endocrine glands—consists of an anterior lobe (**adenohypophysis**) and a posterior lobe (**neurohypophysis**) that are under the influence of hypothalamic hormones. The hypothalamic hormones control the secretion of specific trophic hormones; they in turn regulate other endocrine gland secretions and target tissues. Table 25-1 ■ lists the pituitary gland and other endocrine glands and their functions.

Anterior Pituitary Hormones

The anterior lobe of the pituitary secretes at least six separate hormones: growth hormone (somatotropin, GH), adrenocorticotropin hormone (ACTH), thyroid-stimulating hormone (TSH), follicle-stimulating hormone (FSH), luteinizing hormone (LH), and prolactin (PRL). Clinically, an abnormal level of activity of the pituitary gland causes two conditions: *hyperpituitarism*—overactivity of the pituitary gland (causing gigantism or acromegaly)—and **hypopituitarism**—underactivity of the pituitary gland (causing dwarfism). The relationships between hypothalamic hormones, pituitary hormones, and target organs are shown in Table 25-2 ■.

GROWTH HORMONE

GH causes an increase in the weight and length of the body. The increase in length is especially prominent GH bone growth, but its effect is manifested in nearly all the tissues of the body. Excessive secretion of GH before puberty—usually the result of a tumor of the anterior pituitary—causes **gigantism** (a condition in which the entire body or any of its parts is abnormally large). If excessive production of GH occurs after puberty, it can result in **acromegaly** (a disorder in which the extremities, such as the hands, feet, and head, are greatly enlarged). GH insufficiency during childhood causes **dwarfism** (a condition in which the body is abnormally undersized).

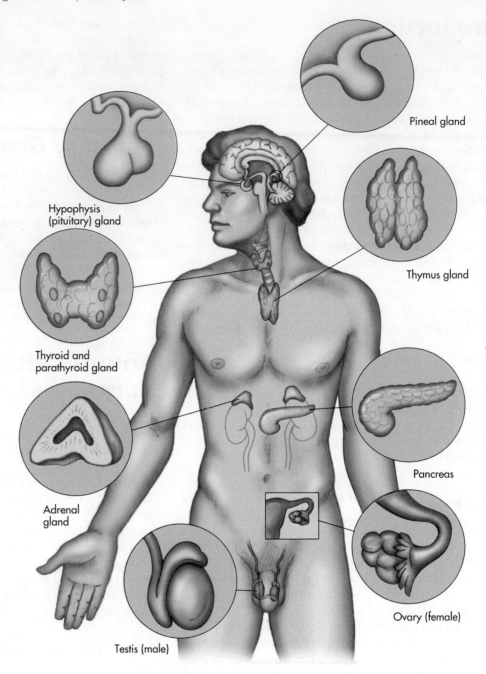

Figure 25-1 ■ Primary glands of the endocrine system.

Labels in figure:
- Pineal gland
- Hypophysis (pituitary) gland
- Thymus gland
- Thyroid and parathyroid gland
- Pancreas
- Adrenal gland
- Ovary (female)
- Testis (male)

THYROID-STIMULATING HORMONE

TSH—another hormone of the anterior lobe of the pituitary gland—controls the secretion of the thyroid hormone and is important for the growth and function of the thyroid gland. TSH stimulates the thyroid gland to increase the uptake of iodine and increase the synthesis and release of thyroid hormones.

In the absence of TSH, the thyroid gland atrophies, producing only small amounts of thyroid hormone, which can have numerous multisystem negative effects on the body. An excess of TSH causes hypertrophy and hyperplasia of the thyroid and a severe form of hyperthyroidism called **Graves's disease** (an overactive thyroid condition characterized by numerous eye problems).

ADRENOCORTICOTROPIC HORMONE

Adrenocorticotropic hormone (ACTH) is released by the anterior lobe of the pituitary gland and by the placenta during pregnancy. It stimulates the growth

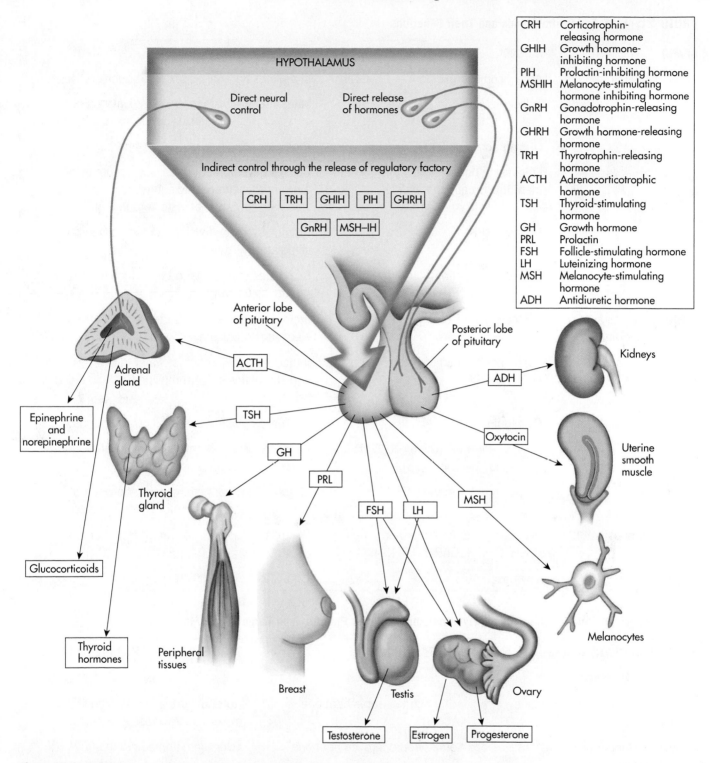

CRH	Corticotrophin-releasing hormone
GHIH	Growth hormone-inhibiting hormone
PIH	Prolactin-inhibiting hormone
MSHIH	Melanocyte-stimulating hormone inhibiting hormone
GnRH	Gonadotrophin-releasing hormone
GHRH	Growth hormone-releasing hormone
TRH	Thyrotrophin-releasing hormone
ACTH	Adrenocorticotrophic hormone
TSH	Thyroid-stimulating hormone
GH	Growth hormone
PRL	Prolactin
FSH	Follicle-stimulating hormone
LH	Luteinizing hormone
MSH	Melanocyte-stimulating hormone
ADH	Antidiuretic hormone

Figure 25-2 ■ Pituitary hormones and their target cells, tissues, and organs.

of the adrenal gland cortex and the secretion of corticosteroids. Hypersecretion of ACTH can cause **Cushing's syndrome** (a condition that affects the trunk of the body, in which a pad of fat develops between the shoulders, producing a "buffalo hump," and the face becomes round and moon shaped). Cushing's syndrome is called **Cushing's disease** when it is caused by a tumor in the pituitary gland.

GONADOTROPIC HORMONES

The gonadotropic hormones include FSH and LH, which are produced by gonadotroph cells in the anterior pituitary. These two hormones affect the target gonadal tissue in men and women. The principal function of FSH is to stimulate gametogenesis and follicular development in women and

Table 25-1 ■ Endocrine Glands and Their Functions

GLAND	HORMONE	MAJOR FUNCTIONS
Anterior pituitary	Adrenocorticotropic hormone (ACTH)	Stimulates adrenal cortex to produce cortisol
	Follicle-stimulating hormone (FSH)	Stimulates follicular growth, secretion of estrogen, growth of testes; promotes development of sperm cells
	Growth hormone (GH)	Promotes growth of soft tissue and bone
	Luteinizing hormone (LH); in men, this is called *interstitial cell-stimulating hormone* (ICSH)	Causes development of corpus luteum at site of a ruptured ovarian follicle in women; can also stimulate secretion of testosterone in men
	Prolactin (PRL)	Promotes breast development in women and stimulates milk secretion
	Thyroid-stimulating hormone (TSH)	Stimulates thyroid gland to produce thyroid hormones (T3 and T4)
Posterior pituitary (hormone storage site)	Oxytocin	Increases contractility of uterus and causes milk ejection postpartum
	Vasopressin (antidiuretic hormone [ADH])	Increases reabsorption of water in kidney tubules and stimulates smooth muscle tissue in blood vessels to constrict
Thyroid	Calcitonin	Decreases plasma calcium concentrations
	Thyroid hormone (thyroxine [T4] and triiodothyronine [T3])	Increase metabolic rate; are essential for normal growth and nerve development
Parathyroid	Parathyroid hormone (PTH)	Regulates exchange of calcium between blood and bones; increases calcium level in blood
Hypothalamus	Releasing and inhibiting hormones (CRH, GHRH, GnRH, TRH)	Controls release of anterior pituitary hormones
Thymus	Thymosin	Enhances proliferation and function of T lymphocytes

Table 25-2 ■ Relationships Among Hypothalamic, Anterior Pituitary, and Target Organ Hormones

HYPOTHALAMIC HORMONE	PITUITARY HORMONE	TARGET ORGAN (HORMONE PRODUCT)
Stimulatory Hormones		
Corticotropin-releasing hormone (CRH)	Adrenocorticotropic hormone (ACTH)	Adrenal cortex (glucocorticoids, mineralocorticoids, androgens)
Growth hormone–releasing hormone (GHRH)	Somatotropin, growth hormone (GH)	Liver (somatomedins)
Gonadotropin-releasing hormone (GnRH)	Follicle-stimulating hormone (FSH), luteinizing hormone (LH)	Gonads (estrogen, progesterone, testosterone)
Thyrotropin-releasing hormone (TRH)	Thyroid-stimulating hormone (TSH)	Thyroid (thyroxine)
Inhibitory Hormones		
Dopamine	Prolactin (PRL)	Breast (none)
Somatostatin	GH	Liver (Insulin-like growth factor)
		Pancreas (insulin)

spermatogenesis in men. LH is primarily responsible for the regulation of gonadal steroid hormone production.

PROLACTIN

PRL is a hormone with many different actions. By itself, PRL does not cause breast development, but in concert with estrogens, progesterone, hydrocortisone, and insulin, it is mammotropic. In humans, it also stimulates milk secretion by the mammary glands. Other effects in humans include the increase in testicular steroidogenesis and the development of the male accessory sex organs. It is also involved in the regulation of gonadotropin release. PRL deficiency is associated with disorders of the hypothalamus or pituitary gland.

Posterior Pituitary Hormones

The posterior pituitary gland is also called the *neurohypophysis* and contains two peptide hormones: **vasopressin** and **oxytocin**. Neither is made in the posterior pituitary; rather, they are synthesized in neurons in the hypothalamus.

VASOPRESSIN

Vasopressin is also called *antidiuretic hormone* (ADH), which stimulates water reabsorption from the nephrons (collecting ducts) of the kidneys back into the bloodstream. It plays a significant role in concentrating urine to conserve water. When there is a defect in the hypothalamic–pituitary secretion of ADH, **diabetes insipidus** (chronic increased thirst and urination caused by damage of the hypothalamus) results in a water diuresis. Vasopressin is used mainly for its antidiuretic effects in this disease rather than for its vasoconstrictor actions, from which the name vasopressin is derived.

OXYTOCIN

Oxytocin stimulates the contraction of smooth muscle in the uterus and alveoli of the lactating breast. The hormone enhances uterine contractions during labor and stimulates the release of milk during breastfeeding.

✳ Apply Your Knowledge 25.1

The following questions focus on what you have just learned about the endocrine system.

CRITICAL THINKING

1. What are the islets of Langerhans?
2. What are the names of the hormones of the anterior pituitary glands?
3. What is the effect of growth hormone insufficiency during childhood?
4. What is Cushing's syndrome?
5. What is the influence of hypothalamic hormones on neurohypophysis?
6. When do gigantism and acromegaly occur?

Thyroid Gland

The thyroid gland lies in the neck just below the larynx and in front of the trachea. It plays a vital role in regulating the body's metabolic processes.

THYROID HORMONES

Thyroid hormone is secreted from follicular cells in the thyroid gland and includes two different hormones: thyroxine (tetraiodothyronine, or T4) and triiodothyronine (T3). Iodine is vital for the synthesis of these hormones and is provided through the dietary intake of common iodized salt. Another hormone releases from **parafollicular cells** in the thyroid gland—calcitonin—which is involved with calcium homeostasis. Calcitonin inhibits bone reabsorption and the release of calcium ions into the blood while promoting the uptake of these ions back into bone. Its effects on blood calcium levels are rapid but short acting.

In the absence of the thyroid gland and thus thyroid hormones, the basal metabolic rate is less than half its normal rate, and growth and development are impaired. In the presence of a hyperactive gland, the metabolic rate is much higher than normal, resulting in tachycardia, nervousness, and other symptoms. An enlargement of the thyroid gland is called a *goiter*. Simple (nontoxic) goiter results from a shortage of iodine in the diet. A goiter also can be caused by constant stimulation of an underactive or nonfunctioning thyroid to release more hormones.

The two most common thyroid disorders are Graves's disease and Hashimoto's thyroiditis of the immune system, an autoimmune disease that attacks the thyroid

Focus on Geriatrics

Myxedema Coma

Myxedema coma is a medical emergency that is indicated by a diminished level of consciousness associated with severe hypothyroidism. Symptoms include hypothermia without shivering, hypoventilation, hypotension, and hypoglycemia. Older patients with severe vascular disease and moderate or untreated hypothyroidism are particularly at risk. Myxedema coma can be caused by overuse of narcotics or sedatives or, in hypothyroid patients, by an acute illness.

gland, causing hypothyroidism. Graves's disease—an autoimmune disease in which antibodies overstimulate the thyroid gland—is characterized by **hyperthyroidism** (overactive thyroid), usually associated with an enlarged thyroid gland and exophthalmos (protrusion of the eyeballs). Graves's disease is also known as **thyrotoxicosis**.

Deficiency of thyroid hormones (hypothyroidism) during infancy causes **congenital hypothyroidism**, resulting in dwarfism and severe mental retardation. **Myxedema** is the most severe hypothyroidism, developing in older children or adults. It is characterized by swelling of the hands, feet, and face (especially around the eyes) and can lead to coma and death. In older adults, severe hypothyroidism can cause myxedema coma.

Focus on Pediatrics

Thyroid Hormone Essential to Fetal Development

Congenital hypothyroidism is the absence of thyroid tissue during fetal development or caused by defects in hormone synthesis. Absence of the thyroid occurs more often in female infants, with permanent abnormalities in one of every 4,000 live births. Because thyroid hormone is essential for embryonic growth, particularly of brain tissue, the infant will be mentally retarded if there is no T4 during fetal life.

Antithyroid Drugs

Disorders of the thyroid gland are quite common, and treatment of individuals with these conditions indicates drug therapy. In the case of hyperthyroidism, a number of organic compounds inhibit the production of thyroid hormone by the thyroid gland. Iodine drugs, such as potassium iodide, radioactive iodine, and thioamide derivatives, are the drugs of choice for antithyroid therapy (see Table 25-3 ■) and are discussed here.

Table 25-3 ■ Common Thyroid and Antithyroid Agents

GENERIC NAME	TRADE NAME	AVERAGE ADULT DOSAGE	ROUTE OF ADMINISTRATION
Thyroid Agents			
levothyroxine	Synthroid, Levothroid, Levoxyl	100–400 mcg/d	PO (Synthroid IV available)
liothyronine	Cytomel	25–75 mcg/d	PO
thyroid	Thyroid, Thyrar	60–180 mg/d	PO
Antithyroid Agents			
methimazole	Tapazole	5–15 mg/d	PO
potassium iodide	Lugol's solution	0.1–1.0 mL tid	PO
propylthiouracil	PTU	100–150 mg tid	PO
radioactive iodide	^{131}I, Iodotope	0.8–150 millicurie (mCi)*	PO

*Based on radiation quantity; millicurie stands for 1/1,000? of a curie—a measurement of radiation intensity.

PO, oral; PTU, propylthiouracil

Focus On

Potassium Iodide

Iodine drugs, such as potassium iodide (Pima, SSKI), may be administered to inhibit thyroid hormones by saturating the thyroid gland.

How does it work?

The exact mechanism of action is not clear, but excess iodide ions cause minimal change in thyroid gland mass. Conversely, when the thyroid gland is hyperplastic, excess iodide ions temporarily inhibit the secretion of thyroid hormone.

How is it used?

Iodide is used alone for hyperthyroidism or in conjunction with antithyroid drugs and propranolol in the treatment of thyrotoxic crisis. It is also prescribed for the treatment of persistent or recurring hyperthyroidism that occurs in patients with Graves's disease. Iodide can be administered as a radiation protectant.

What are the adverse effects?

Iodide may cause diarrhea, nausea, vomiting, and stomach pain. Fever, joint pain, lymph node enlargement, and weakness are also seen. Iodide can produce irregular heartbeat, mental confusion, productive cough, and pulmonary edema.

What are the contraindications and interactions?

Iodide is contraindicated in patients with hypersensitivity to this agent. It must be avoided in patients with hypothyroidism, hyperkalemia (excessive potassium in the blood), and acute bronchitis. Safety during pregnancy, lactation, and in children younger than 1 year of age is not established. Iodide must be used cautiously in patients with renal impairment, cardiac disease, pulmonary tuberculosis, and **Addison's disease** (adrenocortical insufficiency caused by an autoimmune response to the adrenal gland).

Drug interactions include antithyroid drugs; **lithium** (a drug that reduces the activity of certain neurotransmitters and is used in the treatment of bipolar disorder), which may potentiate hypothyroid and goitrogenic actions; potassium-sparing diuretics; and potassium supplements, which increase the risk of hyperkalemia.

What are the important points patients should know?

Instruct patients about the effects of iodine and its presence in shellfish, iodized salt, and certain over-the-counter cough preparations. Advise patients about the manifestations of hyperthyroidism and hypothyroidism and about the fact that each of them can occur as a result of treatment for the other. Teach patients how to monitor their pulse rate and to report any marked increase or decrease.

Focus Point

Graves's Disease

Every year, approximately 5 in 10,000 people in the United States develop Graves's disease, which is related to hyperthyroidism. There are four to eight times more female patients than male patients with Graves's disease. Most patients who develop this disease are between 20 and 45 years of age. Besides the prevalent eye problems, signs of Graves's disease also include rapid heartbeat, palpitations, nervousness, excitability, weight loss, profuse perspiration, and insomnia.

Focus On

Methimazole

Methimazole (Tapazole) is an antithyroid drug that is approximately 10 times as potent as propylthiouracil (PTU) and is faster in eliciting an antithyroid response.

How does it work?

Methimazole inhibits the synthesis of thyroid hormones as the drug accumulates in the thyroid gland. It does not affect existing T3 or T4 levels.

(Continued)

Focus On (Continued)

How is it used?

Methimazole is used for hyperthyroidism and before surgery or radiotherapy of the thyroid. It may be used cautiously to treat hyperthyroidism in pregnancy.

What are the adverse effects?

The adverse effects of methimazole include hypothyroidism, pancytopenia (a blood disorder), aplastic anemia, arthralgia (joint pain), peripheral neuropathy, drowsiness, vertigo, rash, alopecia, and pruritus.

What are the contraindications and interactions?

Methimazole is contraindicated in pregnancy and lactation. It should be used cautiously with other drugs known to cause agranulocytosis. Methimazole can reduce the anticoagulant effects of warfarin (Coumadin). It may increase serum levels of digoxin and alter theophylline levels. Methimazole may require decreased doses of beta-blockers.

What are the important points patients should know?

Instruct patients to take methimazole at the same time each day—preferably before breakfast. Food tends to inhibit the absorption rate.

Focus On

Propylthiouracil

PTU is an antithyroid agent that has no effect on hormone release, and the antithyroid action cannot be observed until the thyroid stores of T3 and T4 become depleted.

How does it work?

PTU belongs in the thioamide family. It interferes with the use of iodine and blocks the synthesis of T3 and T4. It does not interfere with the release and utilization of stored thyroid hormone. Therefore, antithyroid action of PTU is delayed days and weeks until preformed T3 and T4 are degraded.

How is it used?

PTU is prescribed for hyperthyroidism, iodine-induced thyrotoxicosis, and hyperthyroidism associated with thyroiditis. It is also used to shrink the size of the thyroid before surgery.

What are the adverse effects?

PTU may cause headache, vertigo, drowsiness, nausea, vomiting, diarrhea, loss of taste, and hepatitis. Other adverse effects include agranulocytosis, hypothyroidism, periorbital edema, puffy hands and feet, bradycardia, cool and pale skin, sleepiness, fatigue, mental depression, changes in menstrual periods, and unusual weight gain.

What are the contraindications and interactions?

PTU is contraindicated in the last trimester of pregnancy and during lactation. It should not be concurrently administered with sulfonamides or coal tar derivatives, such as aminopyrine or antipyrine. Thyroid hormones can reverse the efficacy of amiodarone, potassium iodide, and sodium iodide.

What are the important points patients should know?

Remind patients with Graves's disease who are taking PTU about the drug's side effects. Patients taking PTU often complain about a sore throat and fever, but agranulocytosis is the most serious adverse effect of this drug. Stress the importance of reporting agranulocytosis symptoms to these patients. Instruct patients to avoid foods that can inhibit thyroid secretion, such as strawberries, peaches, pears, cabbage, turnips, radishes, peas, and spinach, and to take medication early in the day to prevent nighttime insomnia. Advise female patients to keep a record of menstruation because menstrual irregularities may occur.

Thyroid Drugs

Hypothyroidism (low or absent thyroid function) is a common disorder caused by the deficient secretion of TSH or other thyroid hormones. Replacement therapy with natural or synthetic thyroid hormone is required. Periodic testing and adjustment of the drug level may be necessary.

Focus On

Levothyroxine

Levothyroxine (Synthroid) is a commonly prescribed synthetic form of T4.

How does it work?

The actions of levothyroxine replicate those of natural thyroid hormone, which regulates the body's basal metabolic rate.

How is it used?

Levothyroxine is used in cases of low thyroid function. It is generally taken orally, and an intravenous form is also available.

What are the adverse effects?

Too high a dose level of levothyroxine can cause symptoms resembling hyperthyroidism, including tachycardia, weight loss, insomnia, anxiety, and intolerance of heat. Women can experience menstrual irregularities, and long-term use can cause osteoporosis. Serious adverse effects include chest pain (angina) and a rapid or irregular heartbeat or pulse.

What are the contraindications and interactions?

People with allergies to povidone-iodine or tartrazine (a yellow dye in some processed foods and drugs) should inform their doctors because levothyroxine contains these ingredients.

Patients taking amphetamines; anticoagulants such as warfarin (Coumadin); antidepressants or antianxiety agents; arthritis medicine; aspirin; such beta-blockers as metoprolol (Lopressor, Toprol), propranolol (Inderal), or timolol (Blocadren, Timoptic); cancer chemotherapy agents; diabetes medications (insulin); digoxin (Lanoxin); estrogens; iron; methadone; oral contraceptives; phenytoin (Dilantin); steroids; or theophylline (TheoDur) should inform their doctors. Caution should be used in prescribing the drug for women who are pregnant or may become pregnant or are breastfeeding.

What are the important points patients should know?

Instruct patients to see their physicians regularly so their blood can be tested to be sure the prescribed dose is therapeutic. There is a fine line between the proper dose and one that produces adverse effects, and a periodic adjustment of the dose level may be needed. Tell patients to take levothyroxine on an empty stomach with a full glass of water (first thing in the morning is generally best) and to not eat for an hour after. Antacids, calcium carbonate (Tums), cholestyramine (Questran), colestipol (Colestid), iron, sodium polystyrene sulfonate (Kayexalate), simethicone (Phazyme, Gas X), or sucralfate (Carafate) should be taken at least 4 hours before or 4 hours after taking levothyroxine. Advise patients to call their physicians immediately if chest pain (angina) and rapid or irregular heartbeat or pulse are experienced.

PARATHYROID HORMONE

The four tiny parathyroid glands are located in the neck, behind the thyroid gland. Spontaneous atrophy or injury (as in thyroidectomy) of the parathyroid glands is followed by a decrease in the concentration of serum calcium and an increase in serum phosphorus. These changes can be reversed by the parenteral administration of suitably prepared extracts of the parathyroids of domestic animals. **Hypoparathyroidism** is a rare disorder in which the body produces little or no parathyroid hormone (PTH), resulting in an abnormally low level of blood calcium (hypocalcemia).

Secretion of PTH is stimulated by a decrease in the free calcium ion concentration of the plasma. The hormone then acts to restore calcium concentration by:

✳ Increasing the reabsorption of calcium and the excretion of phosphate

✳ Decreasing the absorption of bicarbonate by the kidney

✳ Increasing the reabsorption of bone, with release of calcium ions

✳ Increasing the absorption of calcium and phosphate from the gastrointestinal (GI) tract

The GI tract mediates calcitriol (a metabolite of vitamin D_3), which may be considered a hormone. PTH is a tropin for the renal synthesis of calcitriol. Vitamin D_2 (calciferol) can stimulate the hypercalcemic effect of PTH. Overdosage with any of these compounds can lead to dangerously high calcium concentrations in the blood, which may cause the calcification of kidneys and blood vessels.

✱ Apply Your Knowledge 25.2

The following questions focus on what you have just learned about the thyroid hormones, PTH, and antithyroid drugs.

CRITICAL THINKING

1. What are the two most common thyroid disorders?
2. What are the results of hypothyroidism during infancy and adulthood?
3. What are the indications of iodide as antithyroid drugs?
4. What is the effect of PTH on the metabolism of calcium and vitamin D_3?
5. What are the trade names of methimazole, propylthiouracil, levothyroxine, and potassium iodide?

Pancreas

The *pancreas* is found beneath the great curvature of the stomach and is connected by a duct to the duodenum of the small intestine. The pancreas is composed of clusters of glandular epithelial cells. One group of these clusters—the *islets of Langerhans*—forms the endocrine portions of the gland (and are therefore part of the endocrine system), regulating blood glucose levels and playing a vital role in metabolism.

PANCREATIC HORMONES

Some of the islets of Langerhans cells consist of alpha cells that secrete the hormone **glucagon**, which is secreted when blood glucose levels are low. The function of glucagon is to maintain adequate levels of glucose in the blood between meals. Other clusters consist of beta cells that secrete the hormone *insulin*, which is essential for the maintenance of normal blood sugar. Insulin promotes the use of glucose in cells (so it can used as fuel), thereby lowering the blood glucose level, and in the metabolism of carbohydrates, proteins, and fats. The dysregulation of beta cell function can lead to a disorder known as *diabetes mellitus* (see Figure 25-3 ■).

Diabetes mellitus is a serious endocrine disorder characterized by hyperglycemia (high glucose levels in the blood) and resulting from deficient insulin secretion or decreased sensitivity of insulin receptors on target cells. This condition affects approximately 17 million people in the United States. Diabetes mellitus exists in three forms: type 1, type 2, and gestational diabetes mellitus. Diabetes is more prevalent in the African American and Hispanic populations, and a genetic predisposition may increase susceptibility (especially with type 2 diabetes).

Type 1 diabetes—also called *insulin-dependent diabetes mellitus*—comprises about 10% of the diabetic population and is still sometimes referred to as *juvenile-onset diabetes* even though a significant percentage

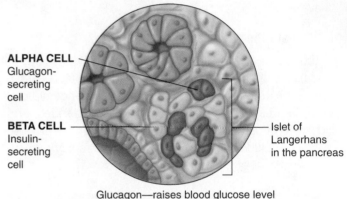

ALPHA CELL
Glucagon-secreting cell

BETA CELL
Insulin-secreting cell

Islet of Langerhans in the pancreas

Glucagon—raises blood glucose level
Insulin—lowers blood glucose level

A

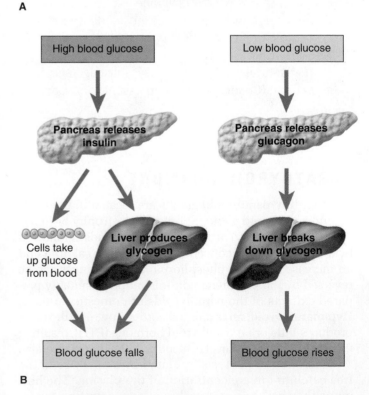

High blood glucose

Low blood glucose

Pancreas releases insulin

Pancreas releases glucagon

Cells take up glucose from blood

Liver produces glycogen

Liver breaks down glycogen

Blood glucose falls

Blood glucose rises

B

Figure 25-3 ■ A: Diabetes mellitus can be caused by dysregulation of beta-cell function. **B:** Interaction of blood glucose levels, insulin, and glucagon.

of people are diagnosed with the disease after age 20. It results from a lack of insulin secretion by the pancreas, often occurs between the ages of 11 to 13 years, and has an abrupt onset. Within 5 to 10 years after diagnosis, the beta cells of the pancreas have been destroyed, and even minute amounts of insulin are no longer produced. The treatment of patients with type 1 diabetes involves drug therapy with insulin or other hypoglycemics—the goal being maintenance of proper blood glucose levels.

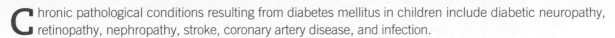

Focus on Pediatrics

Diabetes in Children

Chronic pathological conditions resulting from diabetes mellitus in children include diabetic neuropathy, retinopathy, nephropathy, stroke, coronary artery disease, and infection.

Type 2 diabetes is also called *noninsulin-dependent diabetes mellitus* and makes up approximately 90% of all cases of diabetes mellitus. It occurs mainly in adults older than 40 years of age, although the incidence has been increasing in younger patients because of physical inactivity and obesity. The onset is gradual and is often diagnosed by a routine physical examination, with the patient unaware of any signs and symptoms. Type 2 diabetics may secrete small amounts of insulin, but the greater problem is that insulin receptors in the target cells have become resistant to the hormone. Type 2 diabetes mellitus can be treated through diet and exercise (which can sometimes increase the sensitivity of the receptors) and, if needed, through the use of oral antidiabetic medications or even insulin.

Gestational diabetes mellitus develops during pregnancy, and symptoms may be similar to type 2 diabetes. Generally temporary, it ends when the pregnancy is over. The treatment is through diet and exercise. In some cases, low doses of insulin are appropriate, but oral hypoglycemics are not given.

Complications from diabetes are a leading cause of suffering, disability, and premature death. The following disorders are associated with long-term diabetes, especially with poorly controlled hyperglycemia: retinopathy, nephropathy, depressed immune function, elevated blood lipid levels, and vascular disease. The consequences of these complications are blindness, renal impairment and kidney failure, neuropathic pain, opportunistic infections, wounds and sores that do not heal, loss of limbs, atherosclerosis, hypertension, and myocardial infarction.

Focus Point

Diabetes and Obesity

Seventeen million Americans have diabetes. Forty million are obese—a major cause of type 2 diabetes. These conditions are among the top public health problems in the United States today. Usually, type 2 diabetes affects people older than age 40 years, but because of increased obesity in children and other young patients, more of them than ever before are being diagnosed with this condition. African Americans have the highest rates of obesity and diabetes compared with other ethnic groups. For good health, 30 minutes of moderate physical activity most days of the week is recommended, and 60 minutes is recommended to achieve significant weight loss.

HYPOGLYCEMIC DRUGS

The purpose of hypoglycemic drugs is to treat **hyperglycemia** (abnormally high blood glucose level) by lowering glucose levels in the blood. There are two types of hypoglycemic drugs; they are classified according to the manner in which they are administered: parenteral and oral. Insulin is the sole representative of the parenteral type.

Insulin Injection

Insulin is an antidiabetic hormone that lowers blood glucose levels by facilitating glucose uptake into body cells. Insulin cannot be taken orally because it is destroyed by digestive enzymes. Several types of insulin are available for subcutaneous or intramuscular injection (Table 25-4 ■). Patient participation is an essential component of comprehensive insulin care.

Table 25-4 ■ Classifications of Insulin

GENERIC NAME	TRADE NAME	AVERAGE ADULT DOSAGE	ROUTE OF ADMINISTRATION
Rapid-Acting Insulin Analogs			
lispro	Humalog	5–10 U 0–15 min ac	Subcutaneous
aspart	NovoLog	0.25–0.7 U/kg/d 5–15 min ac	Subcutaneous
glulisine	Apidra	Individualized doses	Inhalation
Short-Acting Insulin			
regular insulin	Humulin R, Novolin R	5–10 U 15–30 min ac and at bedtime	Subcutaneous
insulin (regular) (from pork pancreas)	Iletin	5–10 U 15–30 min ac and at bedtime	Subcutaneous
Intermediate-Acting Insulin			
isophane insulin suspension	NPH, Humulin N, Novolin N	2–4 hours	Subcutaneous
insulin zinc suspension (Lente)	Lente L, Humulin L, Novolin L	3–4 hours	IM, subcutaneous
Extended Zinc Suspension			
insulin zinc suspension, extended	Humulin U Ultralente	Individualized doses	IM, Subcutaneous

Focus Point

Insulin Therapy

Insulin controls the level of blood glucose but does not cure diabetes. Therefore, insulin therapy is required long term.

Focus On

Rapid-Acting Insulin: Lispro

Lispro insulin (Humalog) is one of this class that has a rapid onset (5–10 minutes) and short duration of effect (2–4 hours). It is used to achieve glycemic control if taken immediately before or after meals, which reduces the danger of **hypoglycemia** (abnormally low blood glucose level). Rapid-acting insulins must be used in combination with longer-acting preparations.

How does it work?

Lispro—a human insulin of recombinant DNA origin—is a rapid-acting and glucose-lowering agent that increases peripheral glucose uptake, especially by skeletal muscle and fat tissue, by inhibiting the liver from changing glycogen to glucose.

How is it used?

Lispro is used in the treatment of diabetes mellitus.

What are the adverse effects?

Most adverse effects are related to hypoglycemia, which results from either an overdose of insulin or a mismatch in blood glucose levels with the appropriate dose of insulin. Lipodystrophy, allergic reactions, and insulin resistance are other complications of insulin therapy.

What are the contraindications and interactions?

Insulin is contraindicated during episodes of hypoglycemia and in patients sensitive to any ingredient in the formulation. It must be used cautiously with insulin-resistant patients, with those with hyperthyroidism or hypothyroidism, with patients with renal or hepatic impairment, with women who are lactating or pregnant, and with older adults. Safety and efficacy in children younger than 3 years old are not established.

Alcohol, anabolic steroids, and salicylates may potentiate hypoglycemic effects. Corticosteroids, epinephrine, and dextrothyroxine may antagonize hypoglycemic effects.

What are the important points patients should know?

Instruct patients to recognize the manifestations of a hypoglycemic reaction (nervousness, sweating, tremors, rapid pulse, hunger, and weakness) as well as manifestations of a hyperglycemic reaction (thirst, sweating, a "fruity" breath odor, abdominal pain, increased urine output, nausea, and vomiting). Eating a sugary snack or taking glucose tablets followed by a food containing complex carbohydrates (milk, crackers, fruit) will reverse a hypoglycemic reaction. However, if not treated, the result can be coma and even death.

Focus on Natural Products

Garlic and Ginseng

Garlic and ginseng may potentiate the hypoglycemic effects of insulin lispro (Humalog).

Focus On

Short-Acting Insulins: Regular Insulin

Regular (natural) insulin (Humulin R, Novolin R) is an example of a short-acting insulin that is injected before a meal. The onset is 30 to 60 minutes, and the duration of action is 5 to 7 hours. Short-acting insulins are highly soluble, and their solutions have a clear appearance. Regular insulin may be administered either subcutaneously or intravenously.

How does it work?

Regular insulin lowers blood glucose levels by increasing peripheral glucose uptake, especially by skeletal muscle and fat tissue, and by inhibiting the liver from changing glycogen to glucose.

How is it used?

Regular insulin is used in the emergency treatment of patients with diabetic ketoacidosis or coma, to initiate therapy in patients with type 1 diabetes, and in combination with intermediate-acting or long-acting insulins to provide better control of blood glucose concentrations in diabetic patients.

What are the adverse effects?

The most common adverse effects are hypoglycemic reactions, especially when diabetes is newly diagnosed, and the correct insulin dosage, which is highly individualized for each patient, has not yet been established. Symptoms of hypoglycemia include headache, hunger, weakness, sweating, tachycardia, confusion, and emotional disturbances as well as coma and death.

What are the contraindications and interactions?

Regular insulin is contraindicated in patients with hypersensitivity to any ingredient of the product and when a patient is hypoglycemic. Insulin is used cautiously during pregnancy and in patients with kidney or liver impairments. It should be avoided during lactation. Certain drugs, such as contraceptives, corticosteroids, diuretics, epinephrine, lithium, niacin, thyroid hormones, albuterol, and dobutamine, may interact with the administration of insulin and increase or decrease blood sugar.

What are the important points patients should know?

Advise patients to drink orange juice and sugar-containing drinks and foods when a hypoglycemic reaction occurs.

Focus On

Intermediate-Acting Insulins

Insulin isophane—an NPH (neutral protamine Hagedorn) insulin (Humulin N, Novolin N)—and insulin Lente—an insulin zinc suspension (Humulin L, Novolin L)—are classified as intermediate-acting insulins. NPH insulin is a sterile suspension of zinc–insulin crystals and protamine sulfate in buffered water for injection. It is typically injected twice daily. NPH insulin has an onset of action of 1 to 2 hours, a peak of 6 to 14 hours, and a duration of action of approximately 10 to 16 hours.

Lente insulin is a sterile suspension in buffered water for injection and is modified by the addition of zinc chloride. Lente insulin is also an intermediate-acting insulin that is typically injected twice daily. It has an onset of action of 1 to 2 hours, a peak of 6 to 14 hours, and a duration of action of approximately 10 to 16 hours.

How do they work?

The mechanism of action of intermediate-acting insulins is similar to that of rapid-acting insulins.

How are they used?

NPH insulin and other intermediate-acting insulins are used to control hyperglycemia in patients with diabetes. Mixtard and Novolin 70/30 are fixed combinations of purified regular insulin 30% and NPH 70%.

What are the adverse effects?

The adverse effects of intermediate-acting insulins occur in fewer than 1% of patients and are similar to those of rapid-acting insulins.

What are the contraindications and interactions?

Intermediate-acting insulins are contraindicated during episodes of hypoglycemia and in patients sensitive to any ingredient in the formulation. They must be used cautiously in insulin-resistant patients, those with hyperthyroidism or hypothyroidism, patients with renal or hepatic impairment, women who are lactating or pregnant, and in older adults. Safety and efficacy in children younger than 3 years of age are not established. Drug interactions are similar to those of rapid-acting insulins.

What are the important points patients should know?

Teach patients how to check their blood glucose levels by using a blood glucose monitoring machine. These levels should be checked about four times daily. More frequent monitoring is required if levels are not within the normal range. Stress the importance of maintaining a well-balanced diet with the dietary restrictions specified by the health-care team. Delaying or missing a meal may lead to hypoglycemia. Advise patients to avoid alcohol.

Focus On

Extended Insulin in Zinc Suspension

This type of suspension consists of sterile insulin (Humulin U) suspended in buffered water for injection modified by the addition of zinc chloride. Large particle size and a high zinc content delay absorption and prolong action. The brand name is Ultralente, and it has an onset of action of 4 to 8 hours, a peak of 10 to 30 hours, and a duration usually in excess of 36 hours. A theoretical advantage is that it is free of protamine and other foreign proteins, so the incidence of allergic reactions may be minimized. This type of insulin is obtained from pig pancreas.

How does it work?

The mechanism of action of extended-insulin zinc suspension is similar to other types of insulin (see "Rapid-Acting Insulin: Lispro").

How is it used?

Ultralente is used for diabetes mellitus type 1. It is composed of 70% Ultralente and 30% Semilente (prompt-release) insulin.

What are the adverse effects?

The adverse effects of extended-insulin zinc suspension are similar to rapid-acting insulins.

What are the contraindications and interactions?

Extended-insulin zinc suspension is contraindicated during episodes of hypoglycemia or in patients sensitive to any ingredient in the formulation. Drug interactions and cautioned uses are similar to those of other types of insulin.

What are the important points patients should know?

Advise patients to recognize the manifestations of a hypoglycemic reaction, and instruct them to use orange juice and sugar-containing foods when a hypoglycemic reaction occurs. Educate patients with diabetes mellitus about nutrition, exercise, care of diabetes during illness, and medications to lower plasma glucose.

Focus Point

Patient Education about Diabetes

Patient education is a continuing process; regular visits are needed for reinforcement.

COMBINATION INSULIN PRODUCTS

Combinations of different types of insulins can increase the onset of effects while maintaining a long duration of glycemic control. The following combination insulin products are examples:

✳ Insulin 70/30: 70% NPH and 30% regular (Humulin 70/30, Novolin 70/30)

✳ Insulin 50/50: 50% NPH and 50% regular (Humulin 50/50)

✳ Insulin 75/25: 75% insulin lispro protamine (intermediate acting) and 25% lispro (Humalog mix 75/25)

Focus Point

Hypoglycemic Reactions

Patient participation is an essential component of comprehensive diabetes care. Patients with type 1 or type 2 diabetes who are receiving insulin should be taught to be cautious about hypoglycemic reactions. Signs and symptoms include hunger, nausea, pale and cool skin, and sweating.

ORAL ANTIDIABETIC DRUGS

Patients with type II diabetes mellitus have a defect in insulin secretion from the pancreas, inappropriate hepatic glucose production, tissue insulin resistance, or a combination of any of these as a major cause of glucose dysregulation. Drugs that improve insulin secretion, decrease hepatic glucose production, and improve insulin sensitivity at the tissue receptors are therefore effective in treating patients with type 2 diabetes.

There are now four chemical categories of orally administered agents that act on lower blood sugar levels: sulfonylureas, biguanides, thiazolidinediones, and alpha-glucosidase inhibitors. The sulfonylureas and biguanides have been available the longest and are the traditional initial treatment choices for type 2 diabetes. Table 25-5 ■ lists common oral antidiabetic drugs.

Table 25-5 ■ Common Oral Antidiabetic Drugs

GENERIC NAME	TRADE NAME	AVERAGE ADULT DOSAGE	ROUTE OF ADMINISTRATION
Sulfonylureas: First Generation			
acetohexamide	Dymelor	250–750 mg/d	PO
chlorpropamide	Diabinese, Glucamide	100–250 mg/d	PO
tolazamide	Tolamide, Tolinase	100–500 mg bid	PO
tolbutamide	Orinase	250–1500 mg bid	PO
Sulfonylureas: Second Generation			
glimepiride	Amaryl	1–4 mg/d	PO
glipizide	Glucotrol	2.5–20 mg bid	PO
glyburide	DiaBeta, Micronase, Glynase	1.25–5 mg/d with breakfast	PO
Biguanides			
metformin	Glucophage, Fortamet	500–850 mg tid	PO
Thiazolidinediones			
pioglitazone	Actos	15–30 mg/d	PO
rosiglitazone	Avandia	4 mg/d	PO
Alpha-Glucosidase Inhibitors			
acarbose	Precose	25–100 mg tid	PO
miglitol	Glyset	25–100 mg tid	PO
Other			
pramlintide acetate	Symlin	Initially: 60 mcg before meals; insulin dose must be reduced; increase to 120 mcg as directed by physician	Subcutaneous
exenatide (incretin mimetic)	Byetta	Individual dosing according to size of meal and amount of exercise	Subcutaneous
sitagliptin (dipeptidyl peptidase inhibitor)	Januvia	100 mg/d in a single dose	PO

bid, twice a day; PO, oral; tid, three times a day.

Focus On

Sulfonylureas

The sulfonylurea drugs have been available in the United States since 1954 and have been the mainstay of oral anti-diabetic therapy for many years. They are classified as either first generation—acetohexamide (Dymelor), tolbutamide (Orinase), tolazamide (Tolamide, Tolinase), and chlorpropamide (Diabinese, Glucamide)—or second generation—glipizide (Glucotrol), glyburide (DiaBeta, Micronase), and glimepiride (Amaryl)—based on their pharmacokinetic profiles. Second-generation sulfonylureas tend to be prescribed more frequently because of their tolerability and dosing schedules.

How do they work?

The sulfonylureas act in three ways: (1) by stimulating the release of insulin from the pancreas, (2) by inhibiting the process of forming glucose from amino acids and fatty acids in the liver, and (3) by increasing the number of insulin receptors to target cells.

How are they used?

The sulfonylureas are used for the treatment of mild to moderately severe type 2 diabetes that cannot be controlled by diet alone and in patients who do not have complications of diabetes.

What are the adverse effects?

The adverse effects of the sulfonylureas include hypoglycemia caused by an overdosage, allergic skin reactions, fainting, confusion, blurred vision, depression of bone marrow, and GI disturbances.

What are the contraindications and interactions?

The sulfonylureas are contraindicated in hypersensitivity to these agents. They should be avoided in patients with diabetes complicated by severe infection; acidosis; and severe renal, hepatic, or thyroid insufficiency. Safe use of the sulfonylurea drugs during pregnancy, in nursing mothers, and in children has not been established. These agents should be used cautiously in older adult patients and in those with Addison's disease or hepatic porphyria.

What are the important points patients should know?

Teach patients that oral hypoglycemic drugs are not the same as insulin. They enhance the effectiveness of insulin. Instruct patients taking sulfonylureas to avoid alcohol because a disulfiram-like reaction may occur. Symptoms of this reaction include fever, chills, diarrhea, abdominal pain, and severe nausea and vomiting.

Focus On

Biguanides

Metformin (Fortamet, Glucophage) is a biguanide compound that keeps the blood sugar levels from increasing too high or too fast after meals. This agent does not necessarily decrease blood glucose levels.

How do they work?

Biguanides act by promoting glucose uptake into cells through enhanced insulin-receptor binding and by decreasing the production of glucose in the liver. They slow glucose absorption and increase glucose removal from the blood without causing hypoglycemia. They may also reduce glucagon levels.

How are they used?

Biguanides are used for type 2 diabetes when no response occurs to sulfonylureas. They may be combined with sulfonylureas, in which case dose reduction of the biguanide agent would be needed.

What are the adverse effects?

Common adverse effects of biguanides include anorexia, GI upset (such as diarrhea, nausea, and vomiting), and lactic acidosis (rare).

What are the contraindications and interactions?

The biguanides are contraindicated in patients with renal disease, alcoholism, hepatic disease, and chronic cardiopulmonary dysfunction. Biguanides interact with amiloride, calcium channel blockers, cimetidine, digoxin, furosemide, morphine, procainamide, quinidine, quinine, ranitidine, trimethoprim, triamterene, and vancomycin.

What are the important points patients should know?

Instruct patients that biguanides should be taken with meals to minimize the effect of gastric irritation. Because these agents have a slow onset, glucose control may take up to 2 weeks to establish. Instruct patients to limit alcohol intake because the combination can increase the risk of lactic acidosis.

Focus On

Thiazolidinediones

Two thiazolidinediones are currently available: pioglitazone (Actos) and rosiglitazone (Avandia). A third compound—troglitazone—was withdrawn from the market because of hepatic toxicity.

How do they work?

The thiazolidinediones improve cell sensitivity to insulin via the stimulation of a receptor in skeletal muscle, liver, and fat cells.

How are they used?

These agents are used as adjuncts to diet in the treatment of type 2 diabetes.

What are the adverse effects?

Common adverse effects include edema, anemia, headache, back pain, fatigue, weight gain, and hypoglycemia. Hepatic function needs to be closely monitored during therapy for signs of hepatic impairment.

What are the contraindications and interactions?

The thiazolidinediones are contraindicated in patients who have hypersensitivity to these agents. These drugs should be avoided in patients who have active liver impairment or during pregnancy and lactation. Safety and efficacy in children younger than 18 have not been established. Drug interactions between insulin and the thiazolidinediones may increase risk of heart failure or edema or enhance hypoglycemia with oral antidiabetic agents. Ketoconazole and such herbs as garlic and ginseng may potentiate hypoglycemic effects.

What are the important points patients should know?

Advise patients to contact their physicians if any of the following symptoms develop during thiazolidinedione therapy because these symptoms may indicate hepatic dysfunction: dark urine, jaundice, abdominal pain, nausea, vomiting, anorexia, or fatigue.

Focus On

Alpha-Glucosidase Inhibitors

Dietary carbohydrates require enzymatic degradation by alpha-glucosidase to monosaccharides within the GI tract to enable absorption. Alpha-glucosidase inhibitors, such as acarbose (Precose) and miglitol (Glyset), make up a unique class of drugs that act on this enzyme in the small intestine.

How do they work?

Alpha-glucosidase inhibitors inhibit or delay the absorption of sugar from the GI tract.

How are they used?

Alpha-glucosidase inhibitors are used as monotherapy or in combination with a sulfonylurea in patients with type 2 diabetes mellitus.

What are the adverse effects?

Prominent adverse effects include flatulence, diarrhea, and abdominal pain; they result from the appearance of undigested carbohydrate in the colon that is then fermented into short-chain fatty acids, releasing gas. Hypoglycemia may occur with concurrent sulfonylurea treatment.

What are the contraindications and interactions?

Alpha-glucosidase inhibitors are contraindicated in patients with inflammatory bowel disease and any intestinal condition that could be worsened by gas and distention. Because miglitol (Glyset) and acarbose (Precose) are absorbed from the gut, these medications should not be prescribed in patients with renal impairment. Acarbose has been associated with reversible hepatic enzyme elevation and should be used with caution in the presence of hepatic disease.

What are the important points patients should know?

Instruct patients that insulin might be needed instead of or to supplement oral hypoglycemic drugs in times of infection, stress, or surgery.

❋ Apply Your Knowledge 25.3

The following questions focus on what you have just learned about the pancreatic hormones and hypoglycemic drugs.

CRITICAL THINKING

1. How many types of diabetes are known?
2. What hormones are released by the islets of Langerhans cells?
3. What are the contraindications of insulin?
4. What are the three examples of combination insulin products?
5. What are the trade names of glipizide, rosiglitazone, tolbutamide, and metformin?

Adrenal Glands

The adrenal glands sit on top of each kidney. The cortex— or outer portion of the adrenal gland—is one of the endocrine structures most vital for normal metabolic function. It is impossible for life to continue in the complete absence of adrenal cortical function.

ADRENOCORTICAL STEROIDS

The adrenal cortex secretes three types of steroid hormones: the glucocorticoids (also called adrenocortical hormones), mineralocorticoids, and gonadal corticoids. As a group, these hormones are called *corticosteroids*. In humans, *hydrocortisone* (cortisol) is the main glucocorticoid and *aldosterone* is the main mineralocorticoid. Gonadal corticoids are a group of androgens that mostly contain testosterone, estrogen, and progesterone. They are discussed in detail in Chapter 26.

ACTH is the primary stimulus to hydrocortisone secretion. ACTH is released in response to CRH. Adrenocortical hormones (glucocorticoids) and their effects on the human body are listed in Table 25-6 ■.

Table 25-6 ■ Adrenocortical Hormones and Their Effects

HORMONE	EFFECTS
Glucocorticoids	
Cortisone, hydrocortisone	Increase blood sugar levels, stimulate protein catabolism, mobilize fats, and decrease immunity and inflammatory responses
Mineralocorticoids	
Aldosterone	Cause sodium and water retention, increase blood pressure and blood volume
Gonadal Corticoids	
Androgens	Stimulate activity of the accessory male sex organs, promote development of male sex characteristics, or prevent changes in the latter after castration

Focus On

Glucocorticoids

Glucocorticoids, such as cortisone (Cortistan, Cortone) and prednisone (Deltasone), have diverse effects, including alterations in carbohydrate, protein, and lipid metabolism; maintenance of fluid and electrolyte balance; and preservation of normal function of the cardiovascular system, immune system, kidneys, skeletal muscle, endocrine system, and nervous system. One of the major pharmacological uses of this class of drugs is based on their anti-inflammatory and immunosuppressive actions. A protective role for cortisol is apparent in the physiological response to severe stress that can increase daily production more than tenfold.

The relative or complete absence of adrenocortical function, known as Addison's disease, is accompanied by a loss of sodium chloride and water, retention of potassium, lowering of blood glucose and liver glycogen levels, increased sensitivity to insulin, nitrogen retention, and lymphocytosis. The disturbances in electrolyte metabolism are the causes of morbidity and mortality in most cases of severe adrenal insufficiency. Disorders caused by adrenal insufficiency can be corrected by the administration of adrenal cortical extract or the pure adrenal cortical steroids now available. Overproduction of or overtreatment with glucocorticoids may cause Cushing's syndrome.

(Continued)

Focus On (*Continued*)

Major adrenal corticosteroids (glucocorticoids) are listed in Table 25-7 ■.

How do they work?

The major actions of glucocorticoids are to suppress an acute inflammatory process and for immunosuppression.

How are they used?

Glucocorticoids are used for replacement therapy in adrenal insufficiency, such as Addison's disease and congenital adrenal hyperplasia. Glucocorticoids are also used to treat rheumatic, inflammatory, allergic, neoplastic, and other disorders. Glucocorticoids are of value in decreasing some cerebral edemas. Their value in the treatment of bacterial meningitis is probably caused by the decreasing of edema. Topical or systemic glucocorticoids are used to treat such certain skin diseases as pruritus, psoriasis, and eczema.

What are the adverse effects?

When the glucocorticoids are used for short periods (less than 2 weeks), serious adverse effects are unusual even with moderately large doses. However, insomnia, behavioral changes, and acute peptic ulcers are occasionally observed even after only a few days of treatment.

Most patients who are given daily doses of 100 mg of hydrocortisone (Aeroseb-HC, Alphaderm) or more for longer than 2 weeks undergo a series of changes that have been termed **iatrogenic** (that is, produced inadvertently by medication or another treatment). Cushing's syndrome, acne, insomnia, and increased appetite are noted. In the treatment of dangerous or disabling disorders, these changes may not require the cessation of therapy. However, the underlying metabolic changes accompanying them can be very serious by the time they become obvious, and eventually, osteoporosis, diabetes, and aseptic necrosis of the hip bone may develop. Wound healing is also impaired under these circumstances.

What are the contraindications and interactions?

The corticosteroids are contraindicated in patients with peptic ulcer, heart disease, hypertension with heart failure, certain infectious illnesses (such as varicella and tuberculosis), psychoses, diabetes, osteoporosis, and glaucoma.

Patients receiving these drugs must be monitored carefully for the development of hypoglycemia, glycosuria, sodium retention with edema or hypertension, hypokalemia, peptic ulcer, osteoporosis, and hidden infections. Glucocorticoids decrease the hypoglycemic activity of insulin and oral hypoglycemics, so a change in dose of the antidiabetic drugs may be necessitated.

What are the important points patients should know?

Advise patients to take glucocorticoids as ordered. These drugs should not be stopped abruptly. Instead, the physician will organize the dose to be reduced over 1 to 2 weeks. Warn patients that they should not have any immunizations while taking these drugs unless they have been approved by their physicians. Advise patients to take oral drugs with food to prevent gastric irritation. Antacids or other anti-ulcer drugs may be prescribed to lessen the risk of ulceration.

Large doses of steroids may increase the patient's susceptibility, to infection. Warn patients about this possibility, and instruct them to notify their physicians of fever, cough, sore throat, or injuries that do not heal. They should inform other health-care professionals about their use of these drugs, especially before surgery.

Table 25-7 ■ Major Adrenal Corticosteroids (Glucocorticoids)

GENERIC NAME	TRADE NAME	AVERAGE ADULT DOSAGE	ROUTE OF ADMINISTRATION
betamethasone	Celestone, Betacort	0.6–7.2 mg/d	PO
cortisone	Cortistan, Cortone	20–300 mg/d in divided doses	PO
dexamethasone	Decadron	0.25–4 mg bid–qid	PO
hydrocortisone	Cetacort, Cortaid	0.5% cream applied daily qid	Topical
		10–320 mg tid–qid	PO
prednisolone	Delta-Cortef, Key-Pred, Prelone	5–60 mg/d qid	PO
prednisone	Deltasone	5–60 mg/d qid	PO
triamcinolone	Kenalog, Azmacort	4–48 mg/d qid	PO

PO, oral; qid, four times a day; tid, three times a day.

Focus Point

Glucocorticoids

A patient who is taking glucocorticoids should understand the benefits and possible side effects of long-term use and be advised to report any new side effects. The patient should also be instructed to take oral doses with meals, avoid alcohol, limit sodium intake, and increase potassium intake.

Focus On

Mineralocorticoids

Mineralocorticoids are a group of hormones secreted from the adrenal cortex. The most important mineralocorticoid in humans is aldosterone. Small amounts of desoxycorticosterone are also formed and released, although the amount is normally insignificant.

The rate of aldosterone secretion is subject to several influences. ACTH produces a moderate stimulation of its release, but this effect is not sustained for more than a few days in normal individuals.

How do they work?

Aldosterone and other steroids with mineralocorticoid properties regulate sodium and potassium balance in the blood by promoting the reabsorption of sodium from the distal convoluted and collecting ducts of the kidneys, which results in the excretion of potassium. Mineralocorticoids act by binding to the mineralocorticoid receptor in the cytoplasm of target cells, especially principal cells of the distal convoluted and collecting tubules.

How are they used?

Mineralocorticoids are used for replacement therapy for primary and secondary adrenocortical deficiency.

What are the adverse effects?

The adverse effects of mineralocorticoids can occur if the dosage is too high or prolonged or if withdrawal is too rapid. They can cause edema, hypertension, congestive heart failure, increased sweating, or skin rashes. They can also cause hypokalemia, muscular weakness, and headache.

What are the contraindications and interactions?

The mineralocorticoids are contraindicated in patients with hypersensitivity to these agents and those with systemic fungal infections. They must be used cautiously in patients with Addison's disease or infection and during pregnancy and lactation. Mineralocorticoids can decrease the effects of barbiturates, rifampin, and hydantoins.

What are the important points patients should know?

Advise patients to maintain a low-sodium and high-potassium diet if weight gain is an issue. Teach patients to recognize the adverse effects of these drugs, which may include edema, hypertension, congestive heart failure, increased sweating, and skin rashes.

Focus Point

Addison's Disease

Addison's disease is caused by adrenocortical insufficiency, which is characterized by an insidious onset of fatigue, weakness, lack of appetite, nausea and vomiting, weight loss, skin pigmentation, and hypotension.

Apply Your Knowledge 25.4

The following questions focus on what you have just learned about adrenocortical steroids.

CRITICAL THINKING

1. What are the adrenocortical hormones and their effects?
2. What are the major actions of glucocorticoids?
3. What class of adrenocortical hormones includes aldosterone?
4. What are the trade names of prednisolone, prednisone, and dexamethasone?
5. What is the result of adrenocortical insufficiency?

PRACTICAL SCENARIO 1

Perhaps the greatest example of an endocrine system run amok was the case of Robert Wadlow (b. 2/22/1918; d. 7/15/1940), who attained the height of 8 feet, 11.1 inches and a weight of 490 pounds. Although a normal size at birth, by 6 months of age, he weighed 30 pounds and continued to grow at an astounding rate. At age 13 years, he was the tallest Boy Scout in the world, standing 7 feet, 4 inches high. At his death at age 22 years, he was still growing. His 1,000-pound casket required 12 pallbearers and eight assistants. During his lifetime, his condition was untreatable.

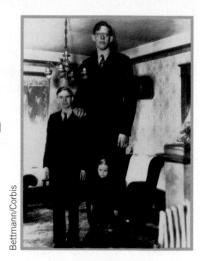

Bettmann/Corbis

Critical Thinking Questions

1. What are the name and criteria of Wadlow's condition and what part of the endocrine system was responsible for them?
2. What was the probable cause of Wadlow's condition?
3. How would physicians treat such a problem today?

PRACTICAL SCENARIO 2

A 45-year-old woman developed hypertension, a moon-shaped face, and a "buffalo hump" on her upper back. She was diagnosed with Cushing's syndrome.

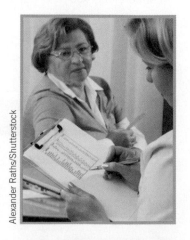

Alexander Raths/Shutterstock

Critical Thinking Questions

1. Explain the causes of Cushing's syndrome.
2. What is the treatment for Cushing's syndrome?

Chapter Capsule

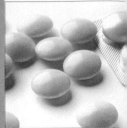

This section repeats the objectives from the beginning of the chapter and then provides a summary of the most important concepts for that objective. Use this section as a quick review and to check your knowledge.

Objective 1: Describe the main functions of a hormone.

- Regulate growth
- Regulate blood glucose
- Regulate intermediary metabolism
- Maintain homeostasis

Objective 2: Explain the endocrine functions of the hypothalamus.

- Sends directions via hormones to the pituitary gland
- Controls the release of corticotropin-releasing hormone (CRH), growth hormone–releasing hormone (GHRH), gonadotropin-releasing hormone (GnRH), and thyrotropin-releasing hormone (TRH)
- Controls the release of anterior pituitary hormones

Objective 3: List six types of hormones that are secreted from the anterior pituitary gland.

- Growth hormone (GH)
- Adrenocorticotropin hormone (ACTH)
- Thyroid-stimulating hormone (TSH)
- Follicle-stimulating hormone (FSH)
- Luteinizing hormone (LH)
- Prolactin (PRL)

Objective 4: Describe the role of the thyroid gland and its replacement and antithyroid drugs.

- It secretes thyroxine (T4) and triiodothyronine (T3), which require iodized salt in the diet for synthesis, and calcitonin, which is involved with calcium homeostasis.
- Its absence or dysfunction can result in low to nonexistent levels of thyroid hormone (hypothyroidism), which lowers the basal metabolic rate, impairing growth and development.
- Its overactivity (hyperthyroidism) results in increased body metabolism, which can cause tachycardia, anxiety, weight loss, and other problems.
- Disorders of the thyroid gland are quite common; treatment indicates drug therapy.
- Levothyroxine is a commonly prescribed synthetic thyroid replacement hormone.
- Iodine or potassium iodide, radioactive iodine, and thioamide derivatives are the drugs of choice for antithyroid therapy.

Objective 5: Explain the pharmacotherapy of diabetes insipidus.

- Vasopressin is most often used to treat patients with this disease—mainly for its antidiuretic effects.

Objective 6: Identify the role of hypoglycemic medications in treating diabetes mellitus.

- Insulin—lowers blood glucose levels by facilitating glucose uptake into body cells; controls the level of blood sugar but does not cure diabetes; insulin therapy required long term; insulin used parenterally

- Oral antidiabetic drugs—sulfonylureas, biguanides, thiazolidinediones, and alpha-glucosidase inhibitors; these drugs are indicated for type 2 diabetes

- Sulfonylureas—stimulate the release of insulin; inhibit glucose formation; increase the number of insulin receptors to target cells

- Biguanides—promote glucose uptake into cells and decrease glucose production in the liver; slow glucose absorption and increase glucose removal from the blood without causing hypoglycemia; can also reduce glucagon levels

- Thiazolidinediones—improve body cell sensitivity to insulin via the stimulation of a receptor in skeletal muscle, liver, and fat cells

- Alpha-glucosidase inhibitors—delay or inhibit the absorption of sugar from the intestinal tract

Objective 7: Describe the adverse effects of insulin and corticosteroids.

- Insulin—lipodystrophy, allergic reactions, insulin resistance, hypokalemia, injection site reaction, pruritus, rash, hypoglycemic reactions (headache, hunger, weakness, sweating, tachycardia, confusion, emotional disturbances, coma, and death)

- Corticosteroids—insomnia, behavioral changes, acute peptic ulcers, Cushing's syndrome, acne, increased appetite, osteoporosis, diabetes, aseptic necrosis of the hip bone, impaired wound healing, edema, hypertension, congestive heart failure, increased sweating, skin rashes, hypokalemia, muscular weakness, and headache

Objective 8: Identify the two major classes of steroids.

- Glucocorticoids
- Mineralocorticoids

 ## Internet Sites of Interest

- For an overview of diabetes, first click "Diabetes" in the right-hand column and then click on images that provide illustrations of the endocrine glands, islets of Langerhans, pancreas, insulin production, glucose testing, insulin pump, and diabetes circulation in the foot, visit **http://health.allrefer.com**.

- WebMD.com offers an in-depth look at diabetes prevention, treatment, and research at **http://www.webmd.com**. Search for "diabetes."

- To read an article about hypothyroidism diagnosis and treatment by a UCLA School of Medicine (Endocrinology Division) professor, visit: **http://thyroid.about.com**. Search for "Hashimoto."

- The Nemours Foundation sponsors a website that provides information about thyroid disease in children and adolescents at **http://www.kidshealth.org**. Enter the Parents Site and then search for "thyroid disease."

PEARSON
myhealthprofessionskit™

Go to www.myhealthprofessionskit.com to access the Companion Website created for this textbook. Simply select "Basic Health Science" from the choice of disciplines. Find this book and then log in using your username and password to access interactive learning games, assessment questions, animations, and more.

Chapter Objectives

After completing this chapter, you should be able to:

1. Describe the male and female reproductive structures.
2. Discuss the male and female sex hormones and their effects on the reproductive system.
3. Explain the contraindications of estrogens.
4. Describe how oral contraceptives work to prevent pregnancy.
5. Discuss menopause and hormone therapy.
6. Provide information about androgens and anabolic steroids.
7. Explain the indications of androgens.
8. Discuss the major adverse effects of progestins.
9. Describe the contraindications of oral contraceptives.
10. Explain the mechanism of action for oxytocic drugs.

Chapter 26

Drugs Used to Treat Reproductive Conditions

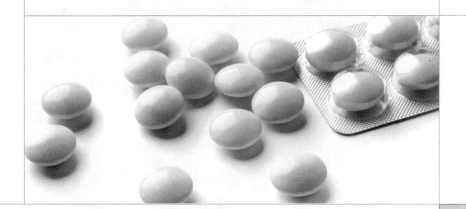

Key Terms

androgens (page 459)
estrogens (page 461)
menorrhagia (men-no-RAH-jee-uh) (page 467)
metrorrhagia (mee-tro-RAH-jee-uh) (page 467)

oocytes (OO-oh-sites) (page 458)
oxytocin (OK-see-TO-sin) (page 470)
priapism (PRY-uh-pizm) (page 460)
progesterones (page 461)
ptosis (TOE-sis) (page 465)

puberty (page 459)
salpingitis (sal-pin-JY-tis) (page 465)
sperm (page 458)
testosterone (page 459)

Introduction

The male and female reproductive systems are a connected series of organs and glands that produce and nurture sex cells and transport them to sites of fertilization. Male sex cells are called **sperm**. Female sex cells are called eggs, or **oocytes**. Some of the reproductive organs secrete hormones vital to the development and maintenance of secondary sex characteristics and the regulation of reproductive physiology. These hormones are also the main drugs that affect the reproductive system. Some agents stimulate the secretions of hormones, and others block these same secretions. Drug therapy for disorders or conditions of the reproductive system can be very complicated, although the names of the drugs are familiar to many people.

Male Reproductive System

Organs of the male reproductive system produce and maintain male sex cells, or *sperm cells*; transport these cells and supporting fluids to the outside; and secrete male sex hormones. A male's *primary sex organs* (gonads) are the two testes in which sperm cells and male sex hormones form. The accessory sex organs of the male reproductive system are the internal and external reproductive organs, including the epididymis, vas deferens, seminal vesicle, prostate gland, bulbourethral glands (Cowper's glands), scrotum, and penis (see Figure 26-1 ■). Table 26-1 ■ summarizes the functions of the male reproductive organs.

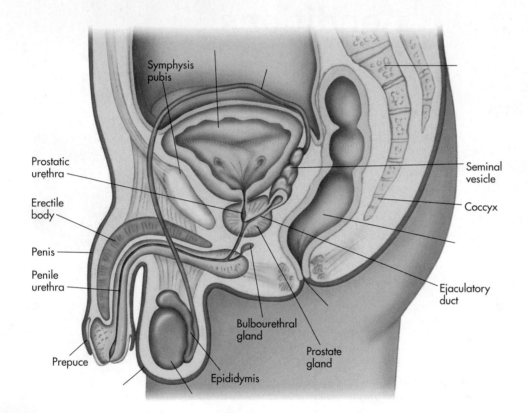

Figure 26-1 ■ The male reproductive system.

Table 26-1 ■ Functions of the Male Reproductive System

ORGAN	FUNCTION
Testes	
Interstitial cells	Produce and secrete testosterone
Seminiferous tubules	Produce sperm cells
Epididymis	Stores sperm cells
Vas deferens	Conveys sperm cells to ejaculatory duct

ORGAN	FUNCTION
Seminal vesicles	Secrete an alkaline fluid containing nutrients and prostaglandins
Prostate gland	Secretes an alkaline fluid and enhances sperm cell motility
Bulbourethral glands	Secrete fluid that lubricates the end of the penis
Scrotum	Encloses, protects, and regulates the temperature of the testes
Penis	Conveys semen into the vagina during sexual intercourse

MALE SEX HORMONES

Male sex hormones are called **androgens**. Testicular interstitial cells produce most of them, but the adrenal cortex also synthesizes small amounts. **Testosterone** is the most abundant androgen. Its secretion begins during fetal development and continues for several weeks after birth and then it nearly ceases during childhood. Between the ages of 13 and 15 years, a young man's androgen production usually increases rapidly. The phase in development when an individual becomes reproductively functional is known as **puberty**. After puberty, testosterone secretion continues throughout the life of a male. The chief drugs that affect the male reproductive system are androgens and anabolic steroids (see Table 26-2 ■).

Table 26-2 ■ Male Hormones

GENERIC NAME	TRADE NAME	AVERAGE ADULT DOSAGE	ROUTE OF ADMINISTRATION
Androgens			
fluoxymesterone	Halotestin	5–20 mg/d	PO
methyltestosterone	Android, Virilon	10–50 mg/d in divided doses	PO (Buccal)
testosterone cypionate	Depo-Testosterone, Duratest	200–400 mg q2wk	IM
testosterone enanthate	Delatest, Delatestryl	50–400 mg q2–4wk	IM
testosterone (transdermal)	Androderm, Testoderm	Start with 6 mg/d; apply patch daily	Transdermal
Anabolic Steroids			
nandrolone	Durabolin	50–200 mg/wk	IM
oxandrolone	Oxandrin	1–5 mg/kg/d	PO
oxymetholone	Anadrol-50	2.5 mg bid–qid	PO
stanozolol	Winstrol	2 mg tid and then reduce to 2 mg/d or to 2 mg every other day	PO

bid, twice a day; IM, intramuscular; PO, oral; qid, four times a day; tid, three times a day.

Focus On

Synthetic Androgens

Androgen therapy is often given to correct hypogonadism or to increase sperm production.

How do they work?

Synthetic steroids compound with androgenic and anabolic activity to control the development and maintenance of secondary sexual characteristics. Androgenic activity is responsible for the growth spurt of adolescents and for growth termination by epiphyseal closure. Anabolic activity increases protein metabolism and decreases its catabolism. Large doses suppress spermatogenesis, thereby causing testicular atrophy. Androgens antagonize the effects of estrogen excess in the female breasts and endometrium.

How are they used?

Testosterones are given to men and women for therapeutic purposes in various conditions. Their main indications in men are to supplement low levels of testosterone to correct hypogonadism (abnormally decreased gonadal function that results in retarded sexual development) or cryptorchidism (undescended testes). Androgens are also used to increase sperm production in cases of infertility. In women, they can be used in the palliative treatment of metastatic breast cancer. Androgens are also prescribed in women for the treatment of postpartum breast engorgement, endometriosis, and fibrocystic breast disorder. These agents are able to stimulate the increased production of red blood cells, protein synthesis, and muscle mass. Therefore, athletes may use androgens to improve athletic performance.

What are the adverse effects?

The common adverse effects of androgens include insomnia, excitation, skin flushing, nausea, vomiting, anorexia, diarrhea, and jaundice. Hypercalcemia, hypercholesterolemia, sodium retention, and water retention (especially in older adults) with edema are seen. The adverse effects of testosterone may also cause renal calculi, bladder irritability, and increased libido.

What are the contraindications and interactions?

Androgens are contraindicated in patients with hypersensitivity or toxic reactions. These agents should be avoided in patients with serious cardiac, liver, or kidney diseases. Androgens must not be prescribed in male patients with known or suspected prostatic or breast cancer. Testosterone (Androderm, Testopel) and other androgens cannot be used during pregnancy or lactation because of the possibility of virilization (the changes that occur as the male body develops, which are different from the development of the female body); that is, these substances would have undesired effects on women. Androgens must be used cautiously in people with cardiac, liver, and kidney diseases; prepubertal boys; geriatric patients; and people with acute intermittent porphyria. Testosterone alters glucose tolerance tests and may increase creatinine and creatinine secretion. Androgens may suppress some clotting factors and may increase or decrease serum cholesterol.

What are the important points patients should know?

Advise patients about skin hygiene measures to reduce the severity of acne. Oral androgens should be taken with meals to reduce gastric upset. Instruct patients taking androgens to report a **priapism** (painful and prolonged erection) because the dose would need to be reduced and to also report decreased flow of urine because androgens can cause prostatic hypertrophy.

Focus on Geriatrics

Anabolic Steroids and Elderly Men

When anabolic steroids are given to elderly men, their risk of prostate cancer is increased.

✱ Apply Your Knowledge 26.1

The following questions focus on what you have just learned about the male reproductive system.

CRITICAL THINKING

1. What hormones are essential to the development and maintenance of secondary sex characteristics?
2. What are the functions of the prostate gland and seminal vesicles?
3. What are the main indications of testosterone in men and women?
4. What are four examples of anabolic steroids?
5. What are the trade names of oxandrolone, fluoxymesterone, nandrolone, and stanozolol?
6. What is the definition of priapism?

Female Reproductive System

The organs of the female reproductive system produce and maintain the female sex cells: the egg cells (or oocytes); transport these cells to the site of fertilization; provide a favorable environment for developing fetuses; propel the fetus outside the body during birth; and produce female sex hormones. A female's *primary* sex organs (gonads) are the two ovaries, which produce the female sex cells and sex hormones. The *accessory sex organs* of the female reproductive system are the internal and external reproductive organs. They include the ovaries, uterine tubes, uterus, vagina, labia majora, labia minora, clitoris, and vestibule (Figure 26-2 ■). Table 26-3 ■ summarizes the functions of the female reproductive organs.

FEMALE SEX HORMONES

The female body is reproductively immature until about age 10. Then, the hypothalamus begins to secrete increasing amounts of gonadotropin-releasing hormone (GnRH). GnRH, in turn, stimulates the anterior pituitary to release the gonadotropins follicle-stimulating hormone (FSH) and luteinizing hormone (LH). These hormones play primary roles in controlling female sex cell maturation and in producing female sex hormones. Several tissues, including the tissues of the ovaries, adrenal cortices, and placenta (during pregnancy), secrete female sex hormones that belong to two major groups: **estrogens** and **progesterones**. Estradiol is the most abundant of the estrogens, which also include *estrone* and *estriol*.

The ovaries are the primary source of estrogens (in nonpregnant females). At puberty, under the influence of the anterior pituitary, the ovaries secrete increasing amounts of estrogens. Estrogens stimulate enlargement of accessory organs, including the vagina, uterus, uterine tubes, ovaries, and external reproductive structures. Estrogens also develop and maintain the *female secondary sex characteristics*.

The ovaries are also the primary source of progesterone (in nonpregnant females). This hormone promotes changes in the uterus during the female reproductive cycle, affects the mammary glands, and helps regulate the secretion of gonadotropins from the anterior pituitary. Androgen (male sex hormone) concentrations produce certain other changes in young women at puberty. For example, increased hair growth in the pubic and axillary regions is caused by androgens secreted by the adrenal cortices. Conversely, development of the female skeletal configuration, which includes narrow shoulders and broad hips, is a response to a low androgen concentration. Estrogens support the development and maintenance of reproductive organs and the secondary sex characteristics. Table 26-4 ■ summarizes the major synthetic estrogens.

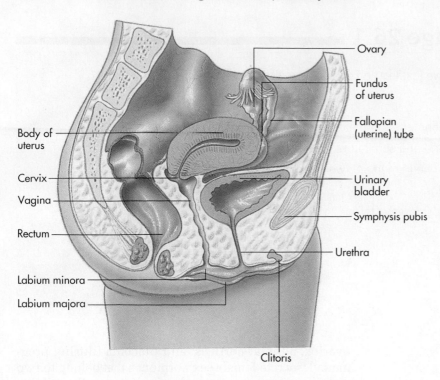

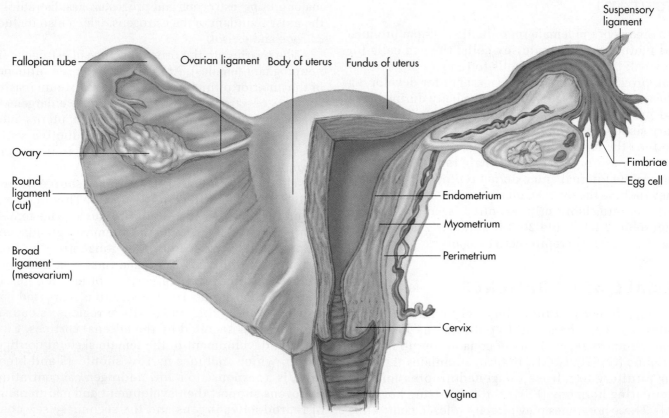

Figure 26-2 ■ The female reproductive system.

Table 26-3 ■ Functions of the Female Reproductive System

ORGAN	FUNCTION
Ovaries	Produce oocytes and female sex hormones
Uterine tubes	Convey oocytes toward the uterus and site of fertilization
Uterus	Protects and sustains the embryo during pregnancy
Vagina	Conveys uterine secretions to outside the body; receives the erect penis during sexual intercourse
Labia majora	Enclose and protect other external reproductive organs
Labia minora	Form margins of the vestibule; protect the openings of the vagina and urethra
Clitoris	Produces feelings of pleasure and sexual stimulation
Vestibule	Space between the labia minora that contains vaginal and urethral openings

Table 26-4 ■ Major Synthetic Estrogens

GENERIC NAME	TRADE NAME	AVERAGE ADULT DOSAGE	ROUTE OF ADMINISTRATION
conjugated estrogens	Premarin	0.3–2.5 mg/d in cycles; 25 mg by injection	PO, IM, IV
estradiol	Estrace	05–2 mg/d in cycles	PO
estradiol hemihydrate	Vagifem	25 mcg/d for 2 wk and then 25 mcg 2 times/wk	Vaginal
estradiol transdermal system	Alora, Estraderm	0.05–0.1 mg patch 2 times/wk	Transdermal
estradiol valerate	Delestrogen	5–20 mg q2–3wk	IM
esterified estrogens	Estratab, Menest	0.3–1.25 mg/d	PO
estrone	Kestrone 5	0.1–0.5 mg 2–3 times/wk	IM
estropipate	Ogen, Ortho-Est	1–2 mg tid	PO

IM, intramuscular; IV, intravenous; PO, oral.

Focus On

Synthetic Estrogens

The best known synthetic estrogen is diethylstilbestrol (Stilbestrol), which possesses most of the therapeutic and untoward actions of the natural estrogenic hormones. Because nonsteroidal estrogens lose little activity after oral administration, they have advantages over the natural estrogens, but the comparative toxicities are not clear.

How do they work?

Estrogens bind to intracellular receptors that stimulate DNA and RNA to synthesize proteins responsible for the effects of these hormones.

How are they used?

The estrogens are used in both genders, including replacement estrogen therapy in women who have had their

(*Continued*)

Focus On (*Continued*)

ovaries removed during the reproductive years, in older women for the prevention and treatment of osteoporosis, and as palliative therapy for breast and prostatic carcinomas in men. Estrogens are also prescribed for abnormal bleeding (hormonal imbalance) and atrophic vaginitis.

What are the adverse effects?

The adverse effects of estrogen therapy include anorexia, nausea, vomiting, stomach cramping, flatulence, headaches, changes in libido (in females), edema of the lower extremities, and breast discomfort or enlargement. In males, feminization may occur, including changes in the fat deposit sites, atrophy of the sex organs, and loss of facial or body hair. Estrogens can cause the retention of sodium and water, resulting in weight gain, edema, and hypertension.

What are the contraindications and interactions?

The estrogens are contraindicated in women with breast cancer and those who are pregnant or lactating. Estrogens should be used with caution in patients with liver disease, gallbladder disease, endometriosis, pancreatitis, diabetes mellitus, heart failure, and kidney dysfunction.

Estrogens may interact with barbiturates, phenytoin, and rifampin, possibly causing decreased estrogen effects by increasing its metabolism. Estrogens may interfere with the effects of bromocriptine (Parlodel). They may also increase the levels and toxicity of cyclosporine (Restasis) and theophylline (Bronkodyl), and they may decrease the effectiveness of clofibrate (Atromid-S).

What are the important points patients should know?

Advise patients to take the drug exactly as prescribed and to not omit, increase, or decrease doses without the advice of their physicians. Instruct patients about what to do when a dose is missed. Advise patients to review the package inserts to ensure the understanding of estrogen therapy. Patients should not breastfeed while taking this drug.

Focus Point

Testosterone Use During Pregnancy

The use of testosterone during pregnancy can cause the masculinization of the fetus, particularly if testosterone (androgen) therapy is provided during the first trimester of pregnancy.

Focus on Pregnancy

Estrogens During Pregnancy

Use of conjugated estrogens during the first trimester of pregnancy may increase the risk of fetal malformations, including cleft palate, heart defect, dislocated hips, absent tibiae, and polydactylia (the presence of more than five digits on the hands or feet).

Focus on Geriatrics

Hormonal Therapy After Menopause

In women taking an estrogen preparation on a long-term basis after menopause, a progestin should be added to estrogen preparations to prevent endometrial hyperplasia and endometrial carcinoma. This practice is not necessary for women who have had a hysterectomy.

Focus On

Progestins

Progesterone is the primary progestational substance that is naturally produced by ovarian cells of the corpus luteum. It has a physiological action that is unique and distinct from estrogen. Progestin derivatives are synthetic drugs. Table 26-5 ■ provides a summary of several progestins and combination products.

How do they work?

Progesterone transforms the endometrium from a proliferative to a secretory state; it suppresses pituitary gonadotropin secretion, thereby blocking follicular maturation and ovulation. Acting with estrogen, it promotes mammary gland development without causing lactation, and it increases body temperature 1°F at the time of ovulation. The synthetic progestins are usually preferred for clinical use because of the decreased effectiveness of progesterone when administered orally.

How are they used?

The progestins are prescribed for women with secondary amenorrhea, functional uterine bleeding, endometriosis, and premenstrual syndrome. As an intrauterine agent (Progestasert) and in combination with estrogens, a progestin provides fertility control, largely supplanted by new progestins, which have longer action and may be taken orally.

What are the adverse effects?

Use of progestins may result in many adverse effects, and the incidence and intensity of these reactions may be varied. They may cause vaginal candidiasis, chloasma, cervical erosion, breakthrough bleeding, dysmenorrhea, amenorrhea, breast tenderness, edema, acne, pruritus, and mental depression. Thromboembolic disorder, pulmonary embolism, changes in vision, nausea, vomiting, and abdominal cramps are also seen.

What are the contraindications and interactions?

Progestins are contraindicated in patients who are hypersensitive to these agents. Progestins must be avoided in patients with known or suspected breast or genital malignancies. These agents are contraindicated in patients with impaired liver disease, undiagnosed vaginal bleeding, miscarriage, thrombophlebitis, and thromboembolic disorders. Progestins should be used cautiously in patients with anemia, diabetes mellitus, a history of psychic depression, previous ectopic pregnancy, presence or history of **salpingitis** (an inflammation or infection of a fallopian tube), and unresolved abnormal Pap smear result. Barbiturates, carbamazepine (Tegretol), phenytoin (Dilantin), and rifampin (Rifadin) may alter contraceptive effectiveness. Ketoconazole (Nizoral) may inhibit progesterone metabolism.

What are the important points patients should know?

Advise patients to avoid exposure to ultraviolet light and prolonged periods of time in the sun. Tell patients to inform their physicians promptly if any of the following occurs: sudden severe headache or vomiting, dizziness or fainting, numbness in an arm or leg, and acute chest pain. Advise patients to also report an unexplained, sudden, gradual, partial, or complete loss of vision, **ptosis** (drooping eyelid), or diplopia (double vision). The physician should be notified if the patient becomes pregnant or suspects pregnancy. Patients should not breastfeed while taking these drugs.

Table 26-5 ■ Progestins

GENERIC NAME	TRADE NAME	AVERAGE ADULT DOSAGE	ROUTE OF ADMINISTRATION
hydroxyprogesterone caproate in oil	Hylutin	375 mg q4 weeks	IM
medroxyprogesterone	Amen, Provera	2–10 mg/d × 5–10 days	PO
	Depo-Provera	150 mg q3 mo or 400–1000 mg/wk	IM
megestrol	Megace	40–30 mg 1–4 times/d in divided doses	PO
norethindrone	Micronor, Norlutin	2.5–10 mg in cycles	PO

(continued)

Table 26-5 ■ Progestins *(continued)*

GENERIC NAME	TRADE NAME	AVERAGE ADULT DOSAGE	ROUTE OF ADMINISTRATION
Combination Products			
estrogen and androgen	Estratest	Tablets of 1.25 mg estrogen/2.5 mg androgen	PO
estrogen and androgen	Depo-Testadiol	2 mg estrogen/50 mg/mL androgen	IM
estrogens and progestins combined	Activelle	Tablets of 1 mg estradiol/0.5 mg norethindrone acetate	PO

IM, intramuscular; PO, oral.

Focus Point

Estrogen–Progestin Combinations for Postmenopausal Women

The use of estrogen–progestin combinations for postmenopausal women is very controversial. There are benefits in protection against osteoporosis and colon cancer, but there is an increased relative risk of cardiovascular disease, breast cancer, and thromboembolism.

CONTRACEPTION

The contraceptive methods most commonly used in the United States are (in order of popularity) oral contraceptives (hormones), condoms, withdrawal (coitus interruptus), progestin injections, spermicides, diaphragms, progestin subdermal implants, and intrauterine devices. Each method has advantages and disadvantages. In this chapter, only contraceptive hormones are discussed.

Focus On

Contraceptive Hormones

Oral contraceptives usually consist of combinations of estrogen and progesterone derivatives to prevent pregnancy. Oral contraceptives are also available that contain only progesterone (progestin). Progestin-only contraceptives have a slightly higher failure rate (pregnancy) than do the combination agents. Table 26-6 ■ lists the various types of oral contraceptives.

How do they work?

Oral contraceptives provide negative feedback to the hypothalamus and inhibit GnRH. Therefore, the pituitary does not secrete FSH to stimulate ovulation. The endometrium of the uterus becomes thin, and the cervical mucus becomes thick and impervious to sperm. The mechanism of action is not fully understood.

How are they used?

Oral contraceptives are based on hormonal contraception. Combination tablets are taken every day for 3 weeks and then not taken during the fourth week to allow for withdrawal bleeding. Progestin alone is given in a small dose every day and is recommended only when estrogen is contraindicated (for example, during breastfeeding).

What are the adverse effects?

The adverse effects of oral contraceptives include nausea, abdominal pain, gallbladder disease, hepatic adenomas, breast tenderness or pain, weight gain, thromboembolism, stroke, headache, nervousness, dizziness, hypertension, myocardial infarction, and thrombophlebitis. Oral contraceptives may also cause amenorrhea, dysmenorrhea, menorrhagia (abnormally heavy or prolonged menstruation), and metrorrhagia (uterine bleeding that occurs independent of the normal menstrual period). Other adverse effects include a decreased libido and vaginal candidiasis (fungal infection).

What are the contraindications and interactions?

Oral contraceptives are contraindicated in patients with hypersensitivity to any component of the products. These agents should be avoided in pregnant women; in women who suspect pregnancy; and in women with genital bleeding of unknown etiology, thrombophlebitis, or history of thrombophlebitis. Oral contraceptives must be avoided in patients with coronary artery disease; liver dysfunction; carcinoma of the endometrium, breast, or other known estrogen-dependent neoplasia; severe hypertension; and diabetes with vascular involvement. Antibiotics, barbiturates, carbamazepine (Tegretol), fosphenytoin (Cerebyx), griseofulvin (Fulvicin), modafinil (Provigil), phenytoin (Dilantin), and rifampin (Rifadin) may decrease contraceptive effectiveness.

What are the important points patients should know?

Instruct women who are using oral contraceptives to follow the schedule for receiving these agents and to use alternative forms of barrier contraception while taking antibiotics. Over-the-counter drugs, including vitamin C and acetaminophen, should not be used without consulting a physician. Instruct patients to report episodes of calf pain or tenderness, shortness of breath, chest pain, visual disturbances, drooping eyelids, and double vision.

Table 26-6 ■ Types of Oral Contraceptives

GENERIC NAME	TRADE NAME	AVERAGE PRESCRIBED DOSAGE
Monophasic Combinations		
estinyl estradiol/desogestrel	Desogen, Mircette	1 active tablet/d; for 21 d and then none for 7 d
estinyl estradiol/ethynodiol	Demulen	1 active tablet/d; for 21 d and then none for 7 d
estinyl estradiol/levonorgestrel	Alesse, Levlen	30 mcg ethinyl estradiol/0.15 mg levonorgestrel in cycles
estinyl estradiol/norgestimate	Levora, Ortho-cyclin	1 active tablet/d; for 21 d and then none for 7 d
estinyl estradiol/norgestrel	Lo-Ovral, Ovral	30 mcg estinyl estradiol/0.3 mg norgestrel in cycles
estrogen/progestin	Alesse-28, Necon 1/35	1 active tablet/d; for 21 d and then none for 7 d
ethinyl estradiol/drospirenone	Yasmin	1 active tablet/d; for 21 d and then none for 7 d
ethinyl estradiol/norethindrone	Brevicon, Genora	35 mcg ethinyl estradiol/0.5 mg norethindrone in cycles
mestranol/norethindrone	Genora 1/50, Nelova 1/50	50 mcg mestranol/1 mg norethindrone in cycles
Biphasic Combinations		
ethinyl estradiol/norethindrone	Nelova 10/11, Ortho-Novum 10/11	35 mcg ethinyl estradiol/0.5 mg norethindrone (×10 tablets) or 1 mg norethindrone (×11 tablets) in cycles
Triphasic Combinations		
ethinyl estradiol/levonorgestrel	Tri-Levlen, Triphasil	30 mcg ethinyl estradiol (×6 or 10 d) or 40 mcg ethinyl estradiol (×5 days)/0.05 mg levonorgestrel (×6 d) or 0.075 mg levonorgestrel (×5 d) or 0.125 mg levonorgestrel (×10 d) in cycles

(continued)

Table 26-6 ■ Types of Oral Contraceptives (*continued*)

GENERIC NAME	TRADE NAME	AVERAGE PRESCRIBED DOSAGE
ethinyl estradiol/ norethindrone	Ortho-Novum 7/7/7, Tri/Norinyl	35 mcg ethinyl estradiol/0.5 mg norethindrone (×5 or 7 d) or 1 mg norethindrone (×9 d) in cycles
ethinyl estradiol/norgestimate	Ortho TriCyclen	1 active tablet/d for 21 d and then none for 7 d
Estrophasic Combination		
ethinyl estradiol/ norethindrone	Estrostep	1 active tablet/d for 21 d and then none for 7 d
Progestin-Only Medications		
norethindrone	Micronor, Nor-Q.D.	0.35 mg/d starting on day 1 of menstrual flow, continuing indefinitely
norgestrel	Ovrette	0.075 mg/d starting on day 1 of menstrual flow, continuing indefinitely

Focus Point

Oral Contraceptives and Surgery

Oral contraceptives should be discontinued at least 4 weeks before a surgical procedure because of the risk for postoperative thromboembolic complications.

Injectable Contraceptives

Injectable contraceptives contain hormonal drugs that provide reversible contraceptive protection. They are safe and highly effective. There are two types of injectable contraceptives:

✳ Progestogen-only formulations, which contain a progestogen hormone. They are effective for 2 to 3 months. These formulations consist of depot medroxyprogesterone acetate (DMPA) or norethisterone enanthate (NET-EN). DMPA is the most widely used injectable contraceptive throughout the world. The most common trade names for DMPA formulations include Depo-Provera and Depo-Clinovir. DMPA formulations are injected every 3 months. NET-EN is injected every 2 months. The most common trade names for NET-EN formulations include Noristerat, Norigest, and Doryxas. The most common adverse effects of these formulations include amenorrhea, prolonged menses, spotting between periods, heavy bleeding, and weight gain. These formulations are contraindicated in women with a confirmed or suspected pregnancy, malignant disease of the breast, diabetes with vascular disease or of more than 20 years' duration, cerebrovascular or coronary artery disease, acute liver disease, liver tumors, and severe hypertension or with vascular disease. Drugs that may interact with any form of injectable contraceptives include rifampicin, griseofulvin, phenytoin, carbamazepine, and barbiturates.

✳ Combined formulations, which contain both a progestogen and an estrogen. They are effective for 1 month. The most common combined formulations are sold under the trade names Mesigyna and Norigynon. They are injected once per month and contain norethisterone enanthate as well as an added estrogen. Combined formulations are administered as deep intramuscular injections into the arm or buttock. They are slowly absorbed into the bloodstream. Adverse effects of combined formulations are much less common than those caused by progestogen-only formulations. When they do occur, they include irregular or heavy bleeding, amenorrhea, prolonged bleeding, headaches, dizziness, and weight changes. Contraindications for injectable combined formulations are based on data from oral combined formulations.

Focus Point

Combined Formulations of Injectable Contraceptives

Combined formulations are effective immediately if administered at specific times after menses.

Focus Point

Implantable Contraceptives

Contraceptive devices may be implanted either surgically or by a physician. They contain contraceptive hormones that are released regularly for 3 to 5 years.

✳ Apply Your Knowledge 26.2

The following questions focus on what you have just learned about the female reproductive system and female sex hormones.

CRITICAL THINKING

1. What are the functions of the ovaries?
2. What is the function of GnRH?
3. What are the actions of the gonadotropins FSH and LH on the female reproductive system?
4. How do estrogens work?
5. What are the indications of progestins?
6. What is salpingitis?
7. What are the most commonly used contraceptive methods in the United States?
8. What are the meanings of the terms *menorrhagia* and *metrorrhagia*?

Focus on Natural Products

Kelp for Menorrhagia

Kelp is seaweed found in the Atlantic and Pacific oceans that in traditional herbal medicine has been used to treat menorrhagia. It is available as a fluid or soft extract, as tablets or gel tabs, and in dried whole plant form. Until more research is done, kelp should not be used during pregnancy and lactation and should not be given to children, elderly adults, or persons with cardiac disorders. It may decrease the effects of thyroid hormones.

Focus Point

Smoking and Oral Contraceptives

Women must avoid smoking while using oral contraceptives. Smoking greatly increases the risk of serious cardiovascular adverse effects.

LABOR AND DELIVERY

Pregnancy usually continues for 38 weeks after conception. Pregnancy ends with the *birth process*. A period of rapid changes and intense physical demands on the pregnant woman begins hours or days before the birth.

The declining progesterone concentration plays a major role in initiating birth. During pregnancy, progesterone suppresses uterine contractions. As the placenta ages, the progesterone concentration within the uterus declines. This stimulates the synthesis of a prostaglandin that promotes uterine contractions. At the same time, the cervix begins to thin and then open. Changes in the cervix may begin a week or 2 weeks before other signs of labor occur.

Another stimulant of the birth process is the stretching of uterine and vaginal tissues late in the pregnancy. This initiates nerve impulses to the hypothalamus, which in turn signals the posterior pituitary gland to release the hormone **oxytocin**. Oxytocin stimulates powerful uterine contractions and aids labor in its later stages.

Uterine relaxants are useful in the process of preterm labor. These agents decrease uterine contraction and prolong the pregnancy to permit the fetus to develop more fully, therefore promoting neonatal survival. Oxytocic agents and uterine relaxants are listed in Table 26-7 ■.

Table 26-7 ■ Effects of Drugs on Labor and Delivery

GENERIC NAME	TRADE NAME	AVERAGE ADULT DOSAGE	ROUTE OF ADMINISTRATION
Oxytocics			
ergonovine	Ergotrate	0.2 mg q2–4h	IM, IV
methylergonovine	Methergine	0.2–0.4 mg q6–12 h until the danger of atony passes (2–7 d)	PO
		0.2 mg q2–4 h (maximum: 5 doses)	IM, IV
oxytocin	Pitocin	Antepartum: 1 mU/min; increase by 1 mU/min q15min (maximum: 20 mU/min)	IV
		Postpartum: infuse a total of 10 U at a rate of 20–40 mU/min after delivery	
Uterine Relaxants			
ritodrine	Yutopar	0.05–0.35 mg/min	IV
terbutaline	Brethaire	10 mcg/min q10min to 80 mcg/min	IV
		250 mg/h until contractions stop	SC
		2.5 mg q4–6h until delivery	PO

IM, intramuscular; IV, intravenous; PO, oral.

Focus On

Oxytocic Agents

Oxytocic drugs are able to induce uterine contractions before birth in normal labor. These agents are desirable in early vaginal delivery to stimulate the uterus.

How do they work?

Oxytocic drugs are identical pharmacologically to the oxytocic principle of the posterior pituitary gland. By direct action on uterine muscle, this produces phasic contractions characteristic of normal delivery. These agents also promote the milk ejection (letdown) reflex in nursing mothers, thereby increasing the flow of milk. Uterine sensitivity to oxytocin (Pitocin) increases during the gestation period and peaks sharply before birth.

How are they used?

Oxytocic drugs are used to initiate or improve uterine contractions at term only in carefully selected patients, only after the cervix is dilated, and after presentation of the fetus has occurred. These drugs are also used to stimulate the letdown reflex in nursing mothers and to relieve pain from breast engorgement. Oxytocic drugs are prescribed for the management of inevitable, incomplete, or missed abortion; the control of postpartum hemorrhage; and the promotion of postpartum uterine involution. Oxytocic drugs are also used to induce labor in cases of maternal diabetes and preeclampsia or eclampsia.

What are the adverse effects?

The adverse effects of oxytocic drugs are varied. Generally, they cause nausea, vomiting, maternal cardiac arrhythmias, hypertensive episodes, chest pain, dizziness, headache, and intracranial (within the cranium) hemorrhage. Allergic reactions may also occur.

What are the contraindications and interactions?

The oxytocic preparations are contraindicated in hypersensitive patients. Ergonovine (Ergotrate) and methylergonovine (Methergine) must be avoided in patients with hypertension and preeclampsia. They are not to be used to induce labor or before delivery of the placenta. Oxytocin injection is contraindicated in patients with significant cephalopelvic disproportion (the fetal head is too large to pass through the mother's pelvis), an unfavorable fetal position or presentation (undeliverable without conversion before delivery), obstetric emergencies in which the benefit-to-risk ratio for mother or fetus favors surgical intervention, and fetal distress in which delivery is not imminent. Oxytocin should be avoided in placenta previa and in women with previous cesarean section.

Oxytocic drugs may interact with vasoconstrictor drugs, causing severe hypertension. They may also interact with cyclopropane anesthesia, causing hypotension, maternal bradycardia, and arrhythmias. Some herbal supplements, such as ephedra and ma huang, may cause hypertension.

What are the important points patients should know?

Instruct patients to report severe cramping, increased bleeding, cold or numb fingers or toes, nausea, vomiting, chest pain, and sudden, severe headache immediately to their health-care providers. Advise patients to avoid breastfeeding while taking ergonovine or methylergonovine.

Uterine Relaxants

Uterine relaxants are beta$_2$-adrenergic agonists that are prescribed as uterine relaxants in the management of preterm (premature) labor. Ritodrine (Yutopar) and terbutaline (Bricanyl) are two drugs currently used as uterine relaxants.

How do they work?

Beta$_2$-adrenergic agonists are clinically effective in preventing or delaying preterm labor because of their tocolytic effect. Uterine contractions decrease in frequency and intensity during treatment.

How are they used?

Beta$_2$-adrenergic agonists are used to manage premature labor in selected patients.

What are the adverse effects?

Ritodrine and terbutaline alter maternal and fetal heart rates and maternal blood pressure (dose related). They can also cause chest pain, palpitations, arrhythmias, and pulmonary edema. Additional common adverse effects of beta$_2$-adrenergic agonists include headache, nausea, vomiting, nervousness, restlessness, sweating, and emotional upset.

What are the contraindications and interactions?

Ritodrine should be avoided in patients with antepartum hemorrhage, eclampsia, uncontrolled diabetes mellitus, bronchial asthma, and pulmonary hypertension. Terbutaline is contraindicated in patients with severe cardiac disorders, digital toxicity, and hypertension. Both ritodrine and terbutaline are given cautiously in patients with cardiac disease, hyperthyroidism, seizure disorders, and migraine headaches.

Corticosteroids may interact with ritodrine and may precipitate pulmonary edema. Epinephrine (Bronkaid Mist) and other sympathomimetic bronchodilators may increase the effects of terbutaline.

What are the important points patients should know?

Advise patients about the potential adverse effects and drug interactions of these agents. Instruct women to avoid breastfeeding while taking beta$_2$-adrenergic agonist drugs. Patients must be instructed to review instructions for the use of inhalators and how to take their own pulses.

✸ Apply Your Knowledge 26.3

The following questions focus on what you have just learned about labor and delivery and the drugs that affect labor and delivery.

CRITICAL THINKING

1. What are three examples of oxytocic drugs?
2. What are the indications of oxytocic agents?
3. What are the names of two uterine relaxants?
4. What medications are used to manage premature labor in selected patients?
5. What are the trade names of ritodrine, ergonovine, and terbutaline?

PRACTICAL SCENARIO 1

A 34-year-old mother of three children has just been prescribed a combination oral contraceptive because she wants to avoid having any more children. She has never taken oral contraceptives before. Her physician told her about the possible side effects of the hormones and what symptoms she should report immediately. She is now talking with you and says that she works in a bar on the weekends, and her coworkers smoke. She says that her husband hates the smell of smoke on her clothes when she gets home from work. She also starts rummaging through her purse, looking for her car keys. She says that she can be very forgetful and loses everything, but she just attributes that to her crazy schedule and the kids.

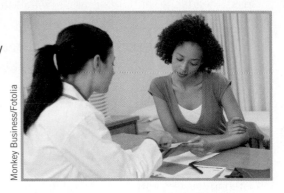

Monkey Business/Fotolia

Critical Thinking Questions

1. What are some key areas of concern to raise in your discussion with this patient?
2. What teaching should you provide to her?

PRACTICAL SCENARIO 2

A 25-year-old pregnant woman in her first pregnancy went into labor. She had only 1 cm dilation of the cervix after 8 hours.

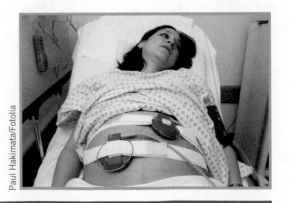

Paul Hakimata/Fotolia

Critical Thinking Questions

1. What are the most common drugs given intravenously to induce delivery?
2. What are the most common adverse effects of these drugs?

Chapter Capsule

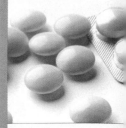

This section repeats the objectives from the beginning of the chapter and then provides a summary of the most important concepts for that objective. Use this section as a quick review and to check your knowledge.

Objective 1: Describe the male and female reproductive structures.

- Male—testes, epididymis, vas deferens, seminal vesicle, prostate gland, bulbourethral (Cowper's) glands, scrotum, penis
- Female—ovaries, uterine tubes, uterus, vagina, labia majora, labia minora, clitoris, and vestibule

Objective 2: Discuss the male and female sex hormones and their effects on the reproductive system.

- Male sex hormones—androgens
- Testosterone—most abundant
- Between 13 and 15 years of age, a young man's androgen production usually increases rapidly as he reaches puberty.
- After puberty, testosterone secretion continues throughout the life of a man.
- Female sex hormones: estrogen and progesterone
- Several tissues, including the tissues of the ovaries, adrenal cortices, and placenta (during pregnancy), secrete female sex hormones
- Estradiol—most abundant estrogen
- At puberty, under the influence of the anterior pituitary, the ovaries secrete increasing amounts of estrogens, which stimulate the enlargement of accessory organs, including the vagina, uterus, uterine tubes, ovaries, and external reproductive structures.
- Estrogens—develop and maintain *female secondary sex characteristics*
- Progesterone promotes changes in the uterus during the female reproductive cycle, affects the mammary glands, and helps regulate the secretion of gonadotropins from the anterior pituitary.

Objective 3: Explain the contraindications of estrogens.

- Contraindicated in women with breast cancer or who are pregnant or lactating
- Used with caution in women with liver disease, gallbladder disease, endometriosis, pancreatitis, diabetes mellitus, heart failure, and kidney dysfunction

Objective 4: Describe how oral contraceptives work to prevent pregnancy.

- Provide negative feedback to the hypothalamus and inhibit gonadotropin-releasing hormone
- Pituitary does not secrete follicle-stimulating hormone to stimulate ovulation; the endometrium of the uterus becomes thin; cervical mucus becomes thick and impervious to sperm

Objective 5: Discuss menopause and hormone therapy.

- Postmenopausal patients who are on long-term estrogen therapy should also be given progestin, to prevent endometrial hyperplasia and endometrial carcinoma.
- Progestin is not given to women who have had a hysterectomy.

Objective 6: Provide information about androgens and anabolic steroids.

- Chief drugs that affect the male reproductive system
- Synthetic steroids that compound with androgenic and anabolic activity to control the development and maintenance of secondary sexual characteristics
- Androgenic activity: responsible for the growth spurt of adolescents and the growth termination by epiphyseal closure
- Anabolic activity: increases protein metabolism and decreases its catabolism; large doses suppress spermatogenesis, thereby causing testicular atrophy
- Androgens: antagonize effects of estrogen excess in the female breasts and endometrium

Objective 7: Explain the indications of androgens.

- Main indications in men: to supplement low levels of testosterone to correct hypogonadism or cryptorchidism
- Also used to increase sperm production in cases of infertility
- Indications in women: palliative treatment of metastatic breast cancer; for treatment of postpartum breast engorgement, endometriosis, and fibrocystic breast disorder
- Able to stimulate increased production of red blood cells, protein synthesis, and muscle mass; athletes may use androgens to improve athletic performance

Objective 8: Discuss the major adverse effects of progestins.

- Vaginal candidiasis, chloasma, cervical erosion, breakthrough bleeding, dysmenorrhea, amenorrhea, breast tenderness, edema, acne, pruritus, and mental depression
- Thromboembolic disorder, pulmonary embolism, changes in vision, nausea, vomiting, and abdominal cramps also seen

Objective 9: Describe the contraindications of oral contraceptives.

- Hypersensitivity of any component of the products; should be avoided in pregnant women, women who suspect pregnancy, women with genital bleeding of unknown etiology, thrombophlebitis, or a history of thrombophlebitis
- Must be avoided in patients with coronary artery disease; liver dysfunction; carcinoma of the endometrium, breast, or another known estrogen-dependent neoplasia; severe hypertension; and diabetes with vascular involvement

Objective 10: Explain the mechanism of action for oxytocic drugs.

- Identical pharmacologically to the oxytocic principle of posterior pituitary
- By direct action on uterine muscle, they produce phasic contractions characteristic of normal delivery.
- They also promote a milk ejection (letdown) reflex in nursing mothers, thereby increasing the flow of milk.
- Uterine sensitivity to oxytocin (Pitocin) increases during the gestation period and peaks sharply before birth.

Internet Sites of Interest

- Further information about contraceptive options can be found at **http://womenshealth.about.com**. Search for "prevent pregnancy."

- Personal stories of menopause and hormone therapy are available at **http://www.womenshealth.gov/Menopause**.

- Visit the National Institute on Drug Abuse at **http://www.nida.nih.gov/Infofacts/Steroids.html** for information on anabolic steroids.

- Information about the safety, availability, and efficacy of emergency contraception is available at **http://www.contraceptiononline.org**. Click "The Contraception Report."

PEARSON myhealthprofessionskit™

Go to www.myhealthprofessionskit.com to access the Companion Website created for this textbook. Simply select "Basic Health Science" from the choice of disciplines. Find this book and then log in using your username and password to access interactive learning games, assessment questions, animations, and more.

Chapter 27

Drugs Used to Treat Gastrointestinal Conditions

Chapter Objectives

After completing this chapter, you should be able to:

1. Describe the major parts of the digestive system.

2. Explain how medications are absorbed from the gastrointestinal tract and metabolized.

3. Describe the use of histamine-2 (H_2)-receptor antagonists in the treatment of peptic ulcers.

4. Describe the use of antacids for the treatment of peptic ulcers.

5. Explain the effects of prostaglandins on the digestive tract.

6. List four generic names and trade names for proton pump inhibitors.

7. Explain the problems associated with laxative use.

8. Describe the drug treatment for diarrhea.

9. Describe the mechanism of action for bulk-forming laxatives, osmotic laxatives, and laxative stimulants.

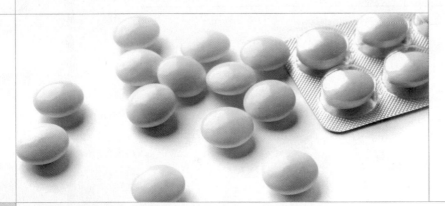

Key Terms

alimentary canal (page XX)
aluminum hydroxide (page XX)
amylase (AM-mil-lace) (page XX)

magnesium carbonate (page XX)
melanosis (page XX)
osmosis (oz-MOH-sis) (page XX)

paralytic ileus (par-uh-LIT-tik ILL-ee-us) (page XX)
ulcers (page XX)

Introduction

Growth of the body depends on the consumption, absorption, and metabolism of food. The gastrointestinal (GI) tract is involved in the first essential components of these processes and is subject to many disease conditions—some of which are very common. It is not surprising that a number of drugs are used to treat these varying conditions. Because of the number of drugs available, it is helpful for discussion to divide the GI tract into two parts: the upper part (from the mouth to the stomach) and the lower part (from the duodenum to the anus). Some problems of the GI tract, specifically nausea and vomiting, are sometimes associated with the central nervous system (CNS).

The Digestive System

The digestive system consists of the alimentary canal, which extends about 8 m from the mouth to the anus, and several accessory organs that secrete substances used in the process of digestion into the canal. The **alimentary canal** includes the mouth, pharynx, esophagus, stomach, small intestine, large intestine, rectum, and anus; the accessory organs include the salivary glands, liver, gallbladder, and pancreas (Figure 27-1 ■).

Organ	Primary Functions
Salivary Glands	Provide lubrication; produce buffers and the enzymes that begin digestion
Pharynx	Passageway connected to the esophagus
Esophagus	Delivers food to the stomach
Stomach	Secretes acids and enzymes
Small Intestine	Secretes digestive enzymes; absorbs nutrients
Liver	Secretes bile; regulates blood chemistry
Gallbladder	Stores bile for release into the small intestine
Pancreas	Secretes digestive enzymes and buffers; contains endocrine cells
Large Intestine	Removes water from fecal material; stores waste

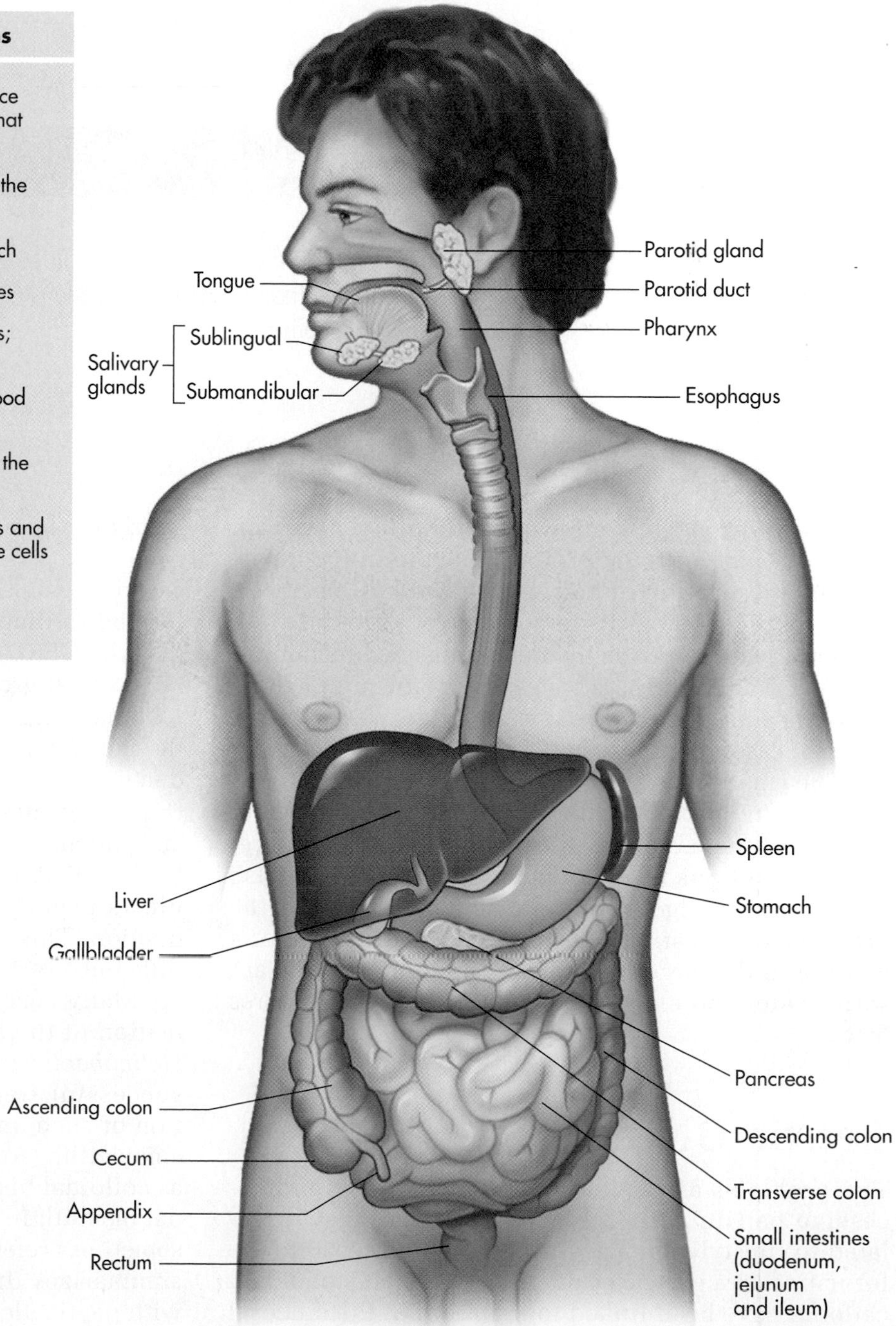

Figure 27-1 ■ The digestive system.

Overall, the digestive system is a tube, open at both ends, that has a surface area of 186 m². It supplies nutrients for body cells. Therefore, digestion changes food into its simpler constituents before absorption.

Primary digestion occurs in the mouth. When food is ingested in the mouth, it is chewed and mixed with saliva that is excreted from the three major pairs of salivary glands: the parotid, submandibular, and sublingual glands. Saliva contains the digestive enzyme **amylase**. The three processes—digestion, absorption, and metabolism—begin here in the mouth.

The 25-cm-long esophagus is a straight tube through which food passes from the pharynx to the stomach. When food enters the stomach from the mouth and esophagus, it is mixed with stomach juices that include hydrochloric acid and some enzymes, such as pepsin, which breaks it into much smaller, digestible pieces. The final stages of chemical digestion occur in the small intestine, where almost all nutrients from the ingested food are absorbed. Excessive secretions of hydrochloric acid, under certain conditions, may break down the gastric surface and cause sores or **ulcers** (breaks in mucous membranes with loss of surface tissue, disintegration, and necrosis). The term *gastric ulcer* is used interchangeably with *peptic ulcer* for this condition. Peptic ulcer disease (PUD) is the most common disorder of the stomach.

Focus Point

Gastric Juice

The 40 million cells that line the stomach's interior can secrete 2 to 3 qt (about 2 to 3 L) of gastric juice per day—no wonder PUD is so common!

The liver is the center of metabolic activity in the body, playing a very important role in the digestion and absorption of nutrients as well as metabolic activities. The detoxification (removal of toxins from the blood) and secretion of bile are the key functions of the liver. The pancreas secretes pancreatic juice, which contains such digestive enzymes as amylase, lipase, and nucleases, to aid in digestion.

The small intestine is a tubular organ that extends from the pyloric sphincter of the stomach to the beginning of the large intestine. The small intestine receives secretions from the pancreas and liver. It also completes the digestion of nutrients and absorbs the products of digestion. The small intestine transports residue to the large intestine. The large intestine absorbs water and electrolytes. It also forms and stores feces.

Peptic Ulcers

The problems associated with hyperacidity and excessive pepsin activity—some of which may be related to lifestyle choices—may eventually lead to the formation of a gastric or duodenal ulcer. Alcohol and caffeine have been linked to irritation of the mucosal lining of the esophagus and stomach. Smoking has been linked to greater volume and concentration of gastric acid. Upper GI radiography is usually performed to diagnose PUD or gastroesophageal reflux disease (GERD).

Several groups of drugs have revolutionized the pharmacologic treatment of ulcers. Three receptors in the stomach wall need to be stimulated to cause the production of hydrochloric acid. These are the histamine-2 (H_2)-receptors, muscarinic cholinergic receptors, and gastrin receptors. Gastric ulcers are caused mainly by a defect in mucus production, and duodenal ulcers usually result from an increase in acid production. This makes the treatment of each somewhat different.

Many cases of gastric ulcer or gastritis (inflammation of the stomach) are caused by the bacterium *Helicobacter pylori*. In bacteria-related peptic ulcers, successful treatment usually includes a combination of such antibacterials as metronidazole (Flagyl), amoxicillin (Amoxil), or tetracyclines with such agents as colloidal bismuth or omeprazole (Prilosec). Colloidal bismuth in combination with two antibacterials is sometimes referred to as "triple therapy." Table 27-1 ■ summarizes drugs commonly used to treat patients with peptic ulcers.

Table 27-1 ■ Drugs Commonly Used in Peptic Ulcer Disease

GENERIC NAME	TRADE NAME	AVERAGE ADULT DOSAGE	ROUTE OF ADMINISTRATION
Antacids			
aluminum hydroxide	Amphojel	600 mg tid–qid	PO
calcium carbonate	Titralac, Tums	1–2 g bid–tid	PO
calcium carbonate with magnesium hydroxide	Mylanta Gel-caps, Rolaids	2–4 capsules or tablets PRN (maximum: 12 tablets/d)	PO
magaldrate	Riopan	480–1,080 mg (5–10 mL suspension or 1–2 tablets) 4 times/d (maximum: 20 tablets or 100 mL/d)	PO
magnesium hydroxide	Milk of Magnesia	2.4–4.8 g (30–60 mL)/d in one or more divided doses	PO
magnesium hydroxide/ aluminum hydroxide with simethicone	Mylanta, Maalox Plus	10–20 mL PRN (maximum: 120 mL/d) or 2–4 tablets PRN (maximum: 24 tablets/d)	PO
sodium bicarbonate	Alka-Seltzer, baking soda	0.3–2 g 1–4 times/d or 1/2 tsp of powder in a glass of water	PO
H₂-Receptor Antagonists			
cimetidine	Tagamet	800 mg/d in divided doses	PO
		300 mg q6–8h	IM, IV
famotidine	Pepcid	20–40 mg/d in divided doses	PO
		20 mg q12h	
nizatidine	Axid	300 mg at bedtime or in two divided doses	PO
ranitidine	Zantac	300 mg/d in two divided doses	PO
		50 mg q6–8h; 150–300 mg/24 h by continuous infusion	IV
Proton Pump Inhibitors			
esomeprazole	Nexium	20–40 mg/d	PO
lansoprazole	Prevacid	15–30 mg/d	PO
omeprazole	Prilosec	20–40 mg/d	PO
pantoprazole	Protonix	40 mg/d for 8–16 wk	PO
		40 mg/d for 7 10 d	IV
rabeprazole	AcipHex	20 mg/d	PO
Combination Medications			
bismuth-tetracycline-metronidazole	Helidac	1 blister pack/d for 14 d	PO
bismuth-ranitidine	Tritec	1 blister pack/d for 14 d	PO
Prostaglandins			
misoprostol	Cytotec	100–200 mcg qid with food	PO

bid, twice a day; PO, oral; PRN, as needed; qid, four times a day; tid, three times a day.

Focus On

Antacids

Antacids are alkaline compounds that may be used to neutralize hydrochloric acid in the stomach, thereby relieving the pain of hyperacidity or even peptic ulcer.

How do they work?

The antacids are weak bases that readily combine with and neutralize hydrochloric acid. The combination of an antacid with digestive acid produces water and carbon dioxide gas.

How are they used?

The bases used in antacid preparations are usually basic compounds of aluminum, magnesium, sodium, calcium, and potassium. Of these, the most common are **aluminum hydroxide** (Amphojel) and **magnesium carbonate**—usually used in combination. Antacids counteract hyperacidity of the stomach, protect from peptic ulcers, and promote ulcer healing.

What are the adverse effects?

Depending on the type of antacid, the most common adverse effects may be diarrhea or constipation. For example, the magnesium- and sodium-containing antacids may cause diarrhea. Calcium- and aluminum-containing products can produce constipation. The other adverse effects that are less common but more serious include anorexia, weakness, bone pain, and tremors (aluminum-containing antacids). Hypermagnesemia may produce nausea, vomiting, confusion, renal calculi, metabolic alkalosis, and headache. Neurologic disorders sometimes occur with the use of calcium-containing antacids.

What are the contraindications and interactions?

The contraindications of antacids depend on their compounds: For example, calcium carbonate (Tums) should not be used in hypercalcemia and hyperparathyroidism, vitamin D overdosage, and decalcifying tumors. Calcium carbonate is also contraindicated in patients with severe renal disease, renal calculi, ventricular fibrillation, and pregnancy. Magnesium-containing antacids are contraindicated in patients with hypermagnesemia and pregnant women.

Antacids should be used cautiously in patients with impaired kidney function, lactation, and dialysis of the kidneys. Calcium carbonate should be used with caution in older adults and in lactating patients. Some antacids may interact with digoxin (Lanoxin). Calcium-containing antacids may decrease the absorption of tetracyclines and ciprofloxacin (Cipro).

What are the important points patients should know?

Instruct patients to take antacids 1 to 3 hours after meals and at bedtime. Patients must avoid taking antacids within 1 to 2 hours of other oral medications. Advise them to increase fluid intake to about 3,000 mL per day to prevent kidney stones. Instruct those with heart disease and those on sodium-restricted diets to avoid antacids high in sodium content. Teach patients to alternate an aluminum or calcium salt antacid with a magnesium salt antacid to prevent diarrhea or constipation. Remind patients that antacids should be used only for symptomatic relief and that they should notify their physicians if relief does not occur in 1 or 2 days.

Focus on Geriatrics

Cautious Use of Tums in Older Adults

Calcium carbonate (Tums) should be used with caution in older adults because it is contraindicated in a wide variety of diseases and conditions that affect elderly adults, including calcium loss caused by immobilization, renal disease, renal calculi, ventricular fibrillation, and cardiac disease.

Focus On

H₂-Receptor Antagonists

The H₂-receptor antagonists, of which cimetidine (Tagamet) is the prototype, were a huge discovery in the treatment of patients with PUD and GERD.

How do they work?

Acid secretion is stimulated by H₂-receptor activation. H₂-receptor antagonists reduce the secretion of gastric acid from stomach cells by blocking these receptors.

How are they used?

H₂-receptor antagonists are used in short-term treatment of active duodenal ulcer and prevention of ulcer recurrence (at reduced dosage). They are also used for the short-term treatment of active benign gastric ulcer, pathologic hypersecretory conditions, such as Zollinger-Ellison syndrome, and heartburn.

What are the adverse effects?

The most common adverse effects are GI disturbances, headache, drowsiness, confusion, agitation, hallucinations, and reversible impotence. H₂-receptor antagonists may also cause cardiac arrhythmias and cardiac arrest after a rapid intravenous bolus dose.

What are the contraindications and interactions?

These medications are contraindicated in patients with known hypersensitivity to cimetidine (Tagamet) or other H₂-receptor antagonists. They must not be used in lactating or pregnant patients or in children younger than 16 years.

What are the important points patients should know?

Warn patients to avoid smoking and drinking alcohol while taking H₂-receptor antagonists because these substances can impede the effectiveness of the drug.

Proton Pump Inhibitors

Several compounds have been investigated because of their ability to block hydrochloric acid production.

How do they work?

The formation of hydrochloric acid depends on the production of hydrogen ions (protons) in the parietal cells, and proton pump inhibitors (PPIs) block this production.

How are they used?

PPIs are used to heal stomach and duodenal ulcers and to relieve symptoms of GERD and esophagitis.

What are the adverse effects?

The common adverse effects of PPIs include headache, dizziness, fatigue, diarrhea, abdominal pain, nausea, skin rash, and, rarely, hematuria.

What are the contraindications and interactions?

Long-term use of PPIs for GERD or duodenal ulcers is contraindicated. These drugs should not be used in hypersensitive patients or in children younger than 18 years. PPIs should be avoided in pregnancy and in patients with GI bleeding.

What are the important points patients should know?

Advise patients that treatment with PPIs is for a short course of therapy only. Treatment is usually limited to about 4 to 8 weeks.

Focus on Pediatrics

Use Care in Choosing Over-the-Counter Medications for Children

Over-the-counter (OTC) formulations of omeprazole, such as Prilosec and Zegerid, must not be used in children younger than 18 years of age. Omeprazole has not been significantly tested in children.

Focus On

Prostaglandins

The prostaglandins are perhaps the most versatile and powerful substances used to treat patients with GI disorders. They affect GI motility and gastric acid secretions.

How do they work?

Prostaglandins produce a variety of actions on the body. The effects of these substances (related to the stomach) include the inhibition of gastric acid and gastrin production, the stimulation of mucus, and the secretion of bicarbonate. The prostaglandin analogue misoprostol (Cytotec) is most commonly used, and although not as effective as the H_2-receptor antagonists, it has been effective in some cases when treatment with the latter has not been effective.

How are they used?

Prostaglandins tend to be antagonistic to ulcer formation in the stomach and the duodenum. This avenue seems to offer a promising new approach to ulcer therapeutics in certain cases. Prostaglandins are used to prevent complications of gastric ulcers that result from nonsteroidal anti-inflammatory drugs (NSAIDs), especially in patients at high risk for complications from a gastric ulcer (for example, older adults and patients with a concomitant debilitating disease or a history of ulcers). These drugs are taken for the duration of NSAID therapy and do not interfere with the efficacy of the NSAID.

What are the adverse effects?

Prostaglandins, such as misoprostol (Cytotec), can cause diarrhea in some patients, which is usually mild and of short duration. The only other significant adverse effect is menorrhagia in women.

What are the contraindications and interactions?

Prostaglandins should not be used in pregnant women because they may induce premature labor by increasing uterine tone and contractility. Prostaglandins are contraindicated in lactation and in a history of allergies to prostaglandins.

What are the important points patients should know?

Ask female patients if they are or might be pregnant because prostaglandins are contraindicated in pregnant women. Tell female patients that these agents may cause women of childbearing age to experience spontaneous abortion, so they should use reliable contraception. Advise patients that diarrhea may occur with these drugs but will disappear after the first month of therapy.

✳ Apply Your Knowledge 27.1

The following questions focus on what you have just learned about the digestive system, peptic ulcers, and related medications.

CRITICAL THINKING

1. Where do the processes of digestion, absorption, and metabolism begin?
2. Which organ of the GI tract receives secretions from the liver and pancreas?
3. What are the four generic names of PPIs?
4. What are the four trade names of H_2-receptor antagonists?
5. What is the mechanism of action of the prostaglandins in treating GI disorders?
6. What are the trade names of ranitidine, famotidine, pantoprazole, omeprazole, and esomeprazole?
7. What is the treatment of gastric ulcers when caused by *H. pylori*?
8. What is the mechanism of action of PPIs?

Diarrhea

Diarrhea is defined as an increase in the volume, fluidity, or frequency of bowel movements relative to a particular individual's usual pattern. The causes of this condition are numerous, and consequently, the treatments are varied. In many instances, drug intervention is not required. For example, antidiarrheals are not used in the case of infective gastroenteritis, in which the diarrhea is a protective mechanism used by the body to flush out the offending pathogen. Clearly, the use of drugs to slow down GI motility in such circumstances would be inadvisable. Similarly, the use of antibiotics in diarrhea-causing bacterial infections of the GI tract may kill the offending pathogen but also kill off some normal bacterial flora. Indeed, the World Health Organization recommends that the first-line emergency treatment for diarrhea should be rehydration and electrolyte replacement therapy. Diarrhea is usually self-limiting and resolves without further effects. The antidiarrheal drugs may be classified as opioids, synthetic opioid medications, and adsorbents (Table 27-2 ■).

Table 27-2 ■ Classifications of Antidiarrheal Drugs

GENERIC NAME	TRADE NAME	TYPE	COMMENTS
bismuth subsalicylate	Pepto-Bismol	Adsorbent	OTC
camphorated opium tincture (paregoric)	(generic)	Opioid	Schedule III
difenoxin hydrochloride with atropine sulfate	Motofen	Opioid	Schedule IV
diphenoxylate hydrochloride with atropine sulfate	Logen, Lomanate, Lomotil, Lonox	Opioid	Schedule V
kaolin and pectin	Kao-Span, Kaolin with Pectin, K-C	Adsorbent	OTC
loperamide	Imodium, Kaopectate III, Maalox Antidiarrheal	Opioid	OTC (abuse is very low, and it is not classified as a controlled substance)

OTC, over the counter.

Focus Point

Acute Diarrhea in Adults

Acute diarrhea in adults is usually self-limiting. Treatment with an antidiarrheal agent is usually unnecessary. However, symptomatic control may help some adults.

Focus On

Opioid and Synthetic Opioid Drugs

These drugs require a prescription and are controlled substances. Opioid antidiarrheals are the most effective drugs for controlling diarrhea. Table 27-3 ■ lists the most common antidiarrheals.

How do they work?

Most of the narcotic analgesics can act on opioid receptors in the GI tract and are actually stimulants at these receptors. The stimulus increases the segmentation or mixing movements of the gut and simultaneously decreases the peristaltic movements. These effects in turn slow down forward movement and at the same time reabsorption.

How are they used?

The most commonly used opioid antidiarrheal drug is camphorated opium tincture (paregoric; generic only). This is a Schedule III drug and requires a prescription. When paregoric is combined with another drug, the medication

(Continued)

Focus On *(Continued)*

becomes a Schedule V product (that is, if the combination contains less than 25 mL of paregoric per 100 mL of preparation).

What are the adverse effects?

The main adverse effect of these drugs is a reversal in the movement of the bowels that results in constipation. Other possible adverse effects include nausea, vomiting, agitation, drowsiness, tachycardia, and numbness of the hands and feet.

What are the contraindications and interactions?

Opioid preparations are contraindicated in patients with intestinal obstruction and should be avoided in children younger than 6 years. In patients who have chronic diarrhea, treatment with opioids is not recommended.

What are the important points patients should know?

Encourage patients to keep a record of bowel movements while they are taking these medications to determine its effectiveness and possible constipating effect. Advise patients to ingest a clear fluid diet for a few days, avoid fruit juices, and maintain fluid intake of about 3,000 mL per day. Patients should avoid the use of alcohol because it promotes diuresis.

Table 27-3 ■ The Most Common Antidiarrheals

GENERIC NAME	TRADE NAME	AVERAGE ADULT DOSAGE	ROUTE OF ADMINISTRATION
bismuth subsalicylate	Pepto-Bismol	30 mL or 2 tablets q30–60 min PRN (maximum, 8 doses/d)	PO
camphorated opium tincture (paregoric)	(Schedule III generic)	5–10 mL after loose stool and then q2h up to 4 times PRN	PO
difenoxin hydrochloride with atropine sulfate	Motofen	Initial dose: 2 tablets (1 mg each) and then 1 tablet after each loose stool or 1 tablet q3–4 h, PRN (maximum: 8 mg/d)	PO
diphenoxylate hydrochloride with atropine sulfate	Logen, Lomanate, Lomotil, Lonox	Initial dose: 2.5–5 mg tid–qid Maintenance: 2.5 mg bid–tid	PO (solution or tablets)
kaolin and pectin	Kao-Span, Kaolin w/Pectin, K-C	60–120 mL of regular suspension or 45–90 mL of concentrated suspension after each loose stool	PO
loperamide	Imodium, Kaopectate III, Maalox Antidiarrheal	Initial dose: 4 mg and then 2 mg after each loose stool (maximum: 16 mg/d)	PO

bid, twice a day; PO, oral; PRN, as needed; qid, four times a day; tid, three times a day.

Focus on Geriatrics

Elderly Patients and Opioid Antidiarrheals

Vital signs should be monitored regularly in older patients taking opioid antidiarrheals. These drugs may cause respiratory depression and decreased blood pressure in elderly individuals.

Focus On

Adsorbents

The other class of antidiarrheals is adsorbents (see Table 27-3). These preparations are still used in some parts of the world because they are inexpensive and relatively effective.

How do they work?

Adsorbents act by coating the walls of the GI tract and adsorbing the toxins that might be implicated in causing diarrhea.

How are they used?

These medications are usually taken after each loose bowel movement until the diarrhea is controlled.

What are the adverse effects?

Adsorbents may cause constipation, which is usually mild and transient.

What are the contraindications and interactions?

The contraindications of adsorbents include a suspected obstructive bowel lesion, pseudomembranous colitis, diarrhea (associated with bacterial toxins), and the presence of fever. They should not be used for more than 48 hours without medical direction. Safety during pregnancy or lactation is not established. Adsorbents may interact with chloroquine (Aralen), digoxin (Lanoxin), penicillamine (Cuprimine), tetracycline (Achromycin), ciprofloxacin (Cipro), and many other drugs.

What are the important points patients should know?

Instruct patients not to exceed prescribed dosages and to notify their physicians if diarrhea is not controlled within 48 hours or if fever develops. Women taking these drugs should not breastfeed without consulting their physicians.

✳ Apply Your Knowledge 27.2

The following questions focus on what you have just learned about antidiarrheals.

CRITICAL THINKING

1. Which antidiarrheals are the most effective drugs for controlling diarrhea?
2. What are the trade names of difenoxin hydrochloride with atropine sulfate?
3. What is the generic name for Imodium?
4. What are the contraindications of opioid antidiarrheals?
5. What is the significant adverse effect of absorbents?

Constipation

Many people misunderstand the meaning of the word *constipation* and therefore resort to the use of laxatives in cases of what could be termed as "perceived" constipation—that is, slow gut transit time. A common cause of constipation is dehydration caused by inadequate liquid ingestion, especially in hot weather and among elderly individuals. Nondietary constipation can be caused by **paralytic ileus** (no peristaltic movements in the intestines), which can occur after abdominal surgery. Many drugs, particularly those with antimuscarinic activity, can slow down peristalsis and lead to constipation.

Laxatives, which are used to combat constipation, are among the most misused drugs because of misperceptions about constipation. Individuals tend to self-treat with easily available OTC drugs. Overuse of laxatives can in turn cause constipation. Laxatives are classified into several different categories depending on their mechanism of action: osmotic (saline) laxatives, stool softeners, stimulants, and bulk-forming laxatives. Table 27-4 ■ presents the characteristics of different laxative categories.

Table 27-4 ■ Categories of Laxatives

GENERIC NAME	TRADE NAME	AVERAGE ADULT DOSAGE	ROUTE OF ADMINISTRATION
Osmotic Laxatives			
lactulose	Cephulac, Chronulac	30–60 mL/d PRN	PO
magnesium citrate	Citrate of Magnesia, Citroma	240 mL/d in 8 oz of water	PO
magnesium hydroxide	Magnesia Magma, Milk of Magnesia	2.4–4.8 g (30–60 mL)/d in 1 or more divided doses	PO
magnesium sulfate	Epsom Salt	10–15 g/d in 8 oz of water	PO
Stool Softeners			
docusate calcium	DCS, Surfak	50–500 mg/d	PO
docusate potassium	Dialose, Diocto-K	50–500 mg/d	PO
docusate sodium	Colace, Dio-Sul	50–500 mg/d	PO
		50–100 mg added to enema fluid	Rectal
glycerin	Glycerol, Osmoglyn	Insert 1 suppository of 5–15 mL of enema high into rectum and retain for 15 min	Rectal
Stimulant Laxatives			
bisacodyl	Apo-Bisacodyl, Dulcolax	5–15 mg PRN (maximum: 30 mg for special procedures)	PO
		10 mg PRN	Rectal
cascara sagrada	Cascara Sagrada Aromatic Fluidextract, Cascara Sagrada Fluidextract	Tablets: 325–1,000 mg/d Aromatic Fluidextract: 2–6 mL/d; Fluidextract: 0.5–1.5 mL/d	PO
senna (sennosides)	Black-Draught, Senokot	Standard concentrate: 1–2 tablets or ½–1 tsp at bedtime (maximum: 4 tablets or 2 tsp bid); syrup: 10–15 mL at bedtime	PO
Bulk-Forming Laxatives			
polycarbophil	FiberCon, Mitrolan	1 g qid PRN (maximum: 6 g/d)	PO
psyllium hydrophilic mucilloid	Metamucil, Serutan	1–2 rounded tsp or 1 packet 1–3 times/d PRN	PO

bid, twice a day; PO, oral; PRN, as needed; qid, four times a day.

Focus On

Osmotic Laxatives

Osmotic (or saline) laxatives are a mixture of sodium and magnesium salts.

How do they work?

These drugs work via **osmosis**, in which sodium and magnesium ions attract water into the bowel, causing a more liquid stool to be formed. The contents are hypertonic, causing water to be retained, and if the osmotic pressure is great enough, it can pull water from the bowel's capillaries back into the bowel lumen. This results in an increase in pressure and volume in the colon and rectum, leading to stimulation of the defecation reflex.

How are they used?

Osmotic laxatives are used for the short-term treatment of occasional constipation. They have also been used in the treatment of poisoning by mineral acids and arsenic or as mouthwash to neutralize acidity.

What are the adverse effects?

Common adverse effects include nausea, vomiting, abdominal cramps, diarrhea, weakness, lethargy, and electrolyte imbalance. In severe cases, they may cause hypotension, bradycardia, mental depression, and coma.

What are the contraindications and interactions?

The use of osmotic laxatives is contraindicated in patients with renal impairment and hypertension because sodium ions can be absorbed and accumulate in the blood.

What are the important points patients should know?

Instruct patients that the action of osmotic laxatives does not occur until the drugs reach the colon; therefore, about 24 to 48 hours are needed before an effect results. Advise patients not to self-medicate with another laxative while waiting for the onset of action. Patients should notify their physicians if diarrhea (more than two to three soft stools per day) persists more than 24 to 48 hours after taking a laxative. Diarrhea is a sign of overdosage. Dose adjustment may be indicated. Women should not breastfeed while taking these drugs without consulting their physicians.

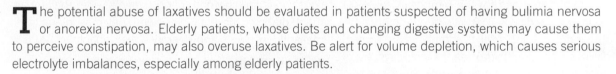

Focus Point

Laxative Abuse

The potential abuse of laxatives should be evaluated in patients suspected of having bulimia nervosa or anorexia nervosa. Elderly patients, whose diets and changing digestive systems may cause them to perceive constipation, may also overuse laxatives. Be alert for volume depletion, which causes serious electrolyte imbalances, especially among elderly patients.

Focus On

Stool Softeners

Stool softeners are sometimes known as emollients or surfactants. Few of these compounds are in common use. One of them is docusate sodium (Colace).

How do they work?

Docusate sodium has detergent-like properties and seems to act mainly by holding water molecules in the fecal material, thus rendering them softer and easier to pass. Because the main mechanism of action is the softening process, these laxatives do not work quickly. Their effect usually takes several days to become apparent.

How are they used?

Stool softeners are used to ease bowel movements in constipated patients. They are used prophylactically in patients who should avoid straining during defecation and for the treatment of constipation associated with hard and dry stools.

What are the adverse effects?

Stool softeners may cause mild abdominal cramps, diarrhea, nausea, and a bitter taste.

What are the contraindications and interactions?

Stool softeners are contraindicated in patients with atonic constipation, nausea, vomiting, abdominal pain, and intestinal obstruction or perforation. These drugs should be used cautiously in patients with a history of congestive heart failure, edema, and diabetes mellitus. Docusate may interact with and increase the systemic absorption of mineral oil (Milkinol), which is also commonly used as a lubricant to treat constipation.

What are the important points patients should know?

Instruct patients to take sufficient liquids with each dose and increase fluid intake during the day. Advise them that docusate should not be taken for prolonged dietary management.

Focus Point

Diabetes and Laxatives

The blood glucose levels of patients with diabetes must be carefully monitored while taking laxatives that contain high amounts of lactose and galactose.

Focus On

Laxative Stimulants

Laxative stimulants include cascara sagrada (Cascara Sagrada Fluidextract) and senna (Senokot).

How do they work?

Laxative stimulants are true purgatives in that they directly affect the walls of either the small or large intestine. They cause an increase in peristaltic movements, leading to defecation.

How are they used?

Laxative stimulants are used for the temporary relief of constipation in various disease conditions and to prevent straining during defecation. Laxative stimulants are sometimes used with magnesium hydroxide (Milk of Magnesia).

What are the adverse effects?

Common adverse effects of laxative stimulants include anorexia, nausea, gripping, abnormally loose stools, constipation rebound, and **melanosis** (abnormal dark pigmentation) of the colon. They may cause the discoloration of urine and hypokalemia.

What are the contraindications and interactions?

Laxative stimulants are contraindicated in patients with abdominal pain, fecal impaction, GI bleeding, ulcerations, appendicitis, and intestinal obstruction. They should not be used during pregnancy or in patients with congestive heart failure. Laxative stimulants should be used cautiously in lactating women and patients with renal impairment, diabetes, or rectal bleeding. They may interact with oral anticoagulants and decrease their effect.

What are the important points patients should know?

Instruct patients that the frequent or prolonged use of irritant cathartics disrupts normal reflex activity of the colon and rectum, leading to drug dependence for evacuation.

Bulk-Forming Laxatives

The proper functioning of the bowel depends on the presence of adequate amounts of liquids as well as dietary fiber. Dietary fiber consists of such plant products as cellulose, hemicellulose, and lignin, which are all found in high quantities in the outer coating of seeds and grains. Many vegetables and fruits also contain high amounts of fiber. These substances are not digestible (to any great extent) in humans and therefore add bulk to the colonic contents, which stimulates forward-propulsive movements and the defecation reflex. Examples of bulk-forming laxatives are psyllium hydrophilic mucilloid (Metamucil) and polycarbophil (FiberCon).

How do they work?

Bulk-forming laxatives absorb free water in the intestinal tract and oppose the dehydrating forces of the bowel by forming a gelatinous mass.

How are they used?

Bulk-forming laxatives are used in chronic atonic or spastic constipation and constipation associated with rectal disorders or anorectal surgery.

What are the adverse effects?

Common adverse effects include nausea and vomiting, diarrhea (with excessive use), and abdominal cramps.

What are the contraindications and interactions?

Bulk-forming laxatives are contraindicated in patients with esophageal and intestinal obstruction, nausea, vomiting, fecal impaction, undiagnosed abdominal pain, and appendicitis and in children younger than age 2 years. They should be used cautiously in patients with diabetes, pregnant women, and during lactation. Bulk-forming laxatives may decrease absorption and clinical effects of antibiotics, warfarin (Coumadin), digoxin (Lanoxin), nitrofurantoin (Nitrofan), and salicylates.

What are the important points patients should know?

Instruct patients who are on a low-sodium or low-calorie diet to note the sugar and sodium content of these preparations. Some of them contain natural sugars, but others contain artificial sweeteners. Be sure that patients understand that these drugs work to relieve both diarrhea and constipation by restoring a more normal moisture level to the stool. These drugs may reduce appetite if taken before meals. Women should not breastfeed while taking these drugs without consulting their physician.

✳ Apply Your Knowledge 27.3

The following questions focus on what you have just learned about laxatives.

CRITICAL THINKING

1. What are the classifications of laxatives?
2. What are the adverse effects of stool softeners?
3. What are two examples of laxative stimulants?
4. What is the mechanism of action for bulk-forming laxatives?
5. What is the mechanism of action for osmotic laxatives?

Vomiting

Vomiting is an act of disgorging the contents of the stomach through the mouth. It is also called *emesis*. Infectious diseases can directly irritate vomiting centers to inhibit impulses going to the stomach. Certain drugs, radiation, and chemotherapy may irritate the GI tract or stimulate the chemoreceptor trigger zone and vomiting center in the brain (medulla). After surgery, particularly abdominal surgery, nausea and vomiting are common. The main neurotransmitters that produce nausea and vomiting include dopamine, serotonin, and acetylcholine.

Focus On

Emetics

Emetic drugs can induce vomiting. Vomiting is a reflex primarily controlled by the medulla oblongata of the brain (often affected by such drugs as morphine and digitalis).

How do they work?

Ipecac syrup has central and peripheral emetic actions, but after oral administration, the peripheral action is predominant. Vomiting is triggered by intense irritation of the mucosal layer of the intestinal wall. Not surprisingly, the central action comprises the stimulation of the vomiting center via the chemoreceptor trigger zone in the medulla.

How are they used?

Ipecac syrup is used as an emergency emetic to remove unabsorbed ingested poisons. The use of ipecac syrup as an emetic is controversial and in decline. In some regions, its use has been completely abandoned in the clinical setting, and it is not recommended for the treatment of poisoning in the home.

What are the adverse effects?

The adverse effects of ipecac syrup may include stiff muscles, severe myopathy, convulsions, and coma. Cardiac arrhythmias, chest pain, dyspnea, hypotension, and fatal myocarditis may also occur. Diarrhea and mild GI upset are seen in some cases.

(Continued)

Focus On (Continued)

What are the contraindications and interactions?

Ipecac syrup is contraindicated in comatose, semicomatose, or deeply sedated patients. It should not be used in patients who are in shock or having seizures or in patients with impaired cardiac function. Ipecac syrup must be used cautiously during pregnancy and lactation and in infants younger than 6 months old.

What are the important points patients should know?

Instruct patients or their families to call an emergency department, poison control center, or physician before using ipecac syrup. Patients should not breastfeed after using this drug without consulting their physicians.

Focus Point

Ipecac Toxicity

The misuse of ipecac has occurred in persons with eating disorders, such as bulimia, and may result in ipecac toxicity. Patients must immediately report to their physicians if vomiting persists longer than 2 to 3 hours after ipecac syrup is given.

Focus On

Antiemetics

Antiemetics are agents used to prevent or relieve nausea and vomiting that may be caused by many different disorders. Table 27-5 ■ shows the most commonly used antiemetics.

How do they work?

The mechanism of action of antiemetics is largely unknown except that they help to relax the portion of the brain controlling the muscles that cause vomiting.

How are they used?

The antiemetics are used for the prevention or treatment of patients with nausea and vomiting, especially to treat those with motion sickness and radiation or postchemotherapy vomiting.

What are the adverse effects?

Drowsiness is a common adverse effect of antiemetics. Additional adverse effects include confusion, dry mouth, headache, hypotension, hypersensitivity reactions, and blurred vision.

What are the contraindications and interactions?

Antiemetic drugs should be avoided in patients with known hypersensitivity to these medications, coma, and severe CNS depression. Antiemetics are contraindicated during pregnancy or lactation, especially during the first trimester. Antiemetics are also contraindicated if there is nausea and vomiting with an undiagnosed condition. This is especially true in patients with suspected appendicitis, intestinal obstruction, brain tumors, or drug toxicity. Different types of antiemetics may have different drug interactions. For example, whereas serotonin antagonists usually have no drug interactions, the effects of dopamine are altered by antiemetics.

What are the important points patients should know?

Advise patients who are taking antiemetics to avoid driving a car and operating heavy machinery. Instruct them to avoid alcohol because it intensifies the sedative effects of antiemetics. Pregnant women should avoid antiemetics during the first trimester. Nonpharmacological measures for nausea are safer and more appropriate. These measures include small, frequent meals; dry biscuits; and a quiet environment. Advise patients with motion sickness to take antiemetics 30 minutes before travel.

Focus on Natural Products

Ginger for Nausea

For thousands of years, the Chinese have used ginger medicinally to treat people with nausea, vomiting, morning sickness, and motion sickness. Studies have shown ginger to be about as effective as OTC medications sold for these purposes. It is also said to have anti-inflammatory properties and is given to patients who have arthritis. Ginger is also used to soothe coughing or for fever. Because ginger may affect blood clotting, it should be avoided by patients who are taking anticoagulants.

Table 27-5 ■ The Most Commonly Used Antiemetics

GENERIC NAME	TRADE NAME	AVERAGE ADULT DOSAGE	ROUTE OF ADMINISTRATION
Dopamine Antagonists			
haloperidol	Haldol	1–2 mg q12 h	PO
chlorpromazine	Thorazine	10–25 mg q4–6 h	PO, IM, IV
perphenazine	Trilafon	8–16 mg/d	PO, IM, IV
prochlorperazine	Compazine	5–10 mg tid–qid	PO, IM, IV, rectal
promethazine	Phenergan	25 mg q4–6 h	PO, IM, IV, rectal
thiethylperazine	Torecan	10 mg 1–3 times/d	PO, IM, rectal
Other			
metoclopramide	Reglan	1–2 mg/kg 30 min before chemotherapy and q2–4 h PRN	IV
Serotonin Antagonists			
granisetron	Kytril	1 mg 1 h before chemotherapy	PO, IV
ondansetron	Zofran	4–8 mg tid	PO, IV
Antihistamines			
dimenhydrinate	Dramamine	50–100 mg q4–6 h PRN	PO, IM, IV
diphenhydramine	Benadryl	10–50 mg q4–6 h PRN	PO, IM, IV
hydroxyzine	Atarax, Vistaril	25–100 mg q6h PRN	PO, IM
meclizine	Antivert, Bonine	25–50 mg/d	PO
Anticholinergics			
scopolamine	Transderm-Scop	0.5 mg q72h	Transdermal
trimethobenzamide	Tigan	250 mg tid–qid	PO, rectal

IM, intramuscular; IV, intravenous; PO, oral; PRN, as needed; qid, four times a day; tid, three times a day.

Apply Your Knowledge 27.4

The following questions focus on what you have just learned about vomiting, emetics, and antiemetics.

CRITICAL THINKING

1. Where is the vomiting center in the human body?
2. What are the causes of vomiting?
3. What is the mechanism of action of ipecac syrup?
4. What are the indications of antiemetics?
5. What are the contraindications of ipecac syrup?
6. What are the trade names of chlorpromazine, promethazine, and dimenhydrinate?

PRACTICAL SCENARIO 1

A 26-year-old woman in graduate school visits the family physician because for the past 3 to 4 months, she has been experiencing gnawing pains in her upper-middle abdomen. When you ask her what seems to precipitate the pain, she is unable to say for sure. She says she feels the best in the early morning before eating. As the day progresses, she usually feels worse and worse and takes Mylanta or Milk of Magnesia to relieve the pain. Sometimes, her pain is accompanied by severe diarrhea, and she has been tired, weak, and nauseous. In response to your question about stress, she tells you she is under extreme stress because she is preparing to defend her thesis for her Ph.D. She has been smoking more cigarettes than usual and drinking 6 to 8 cups of coffee each morning. In the evening, she often has a few glasses of wine to help her relax.

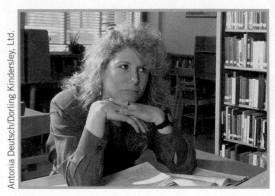

Antonia Deutsch/Dorling Kindersley, Ltd.

Critical Thinking Questions

1. Based on this patient's complaints, lifestyle, and use of OTC medications, what do you expect may be the cause of her initial complaint of upper-middle abdomen pain and her symptoms of fatigue, weakness, and nausea?
2. What diagnostic tests do you anticipate the physician ordering and for what possible diagnoses?
3. Instead of OTC antacids, what are the other choices for this patient to relieve her symptoms? Is there a class of medications you think might be the better choice for her. If so, why?

PRACTICAL SCENARIO 2

A 75-year-old man complained about constipation, telling the physician assistant that he only had a bowel movement every 4 or 5 days. The physician assistant gave him laxatives.

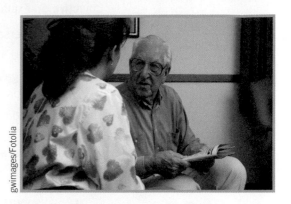

gwimages/Fotolia

Critical Thinking Questions

1. Explain the classifications of laxatives.
2. Explain the mechanism of action of stimulant laxatives.

Chapter Capsule

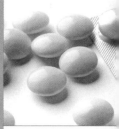

This section repeats the objectives from the beginning of the chapter and then provides a summary of the most important concepts for that objective. Use this section as a quick review and to check your knowledge.

Objective 1: Describe the major parts of the digestive system.

- Alimentary canal, including the mouth, pharynx, esophagus, stomach, small intestine, large intestine, rectum, and anus
- Accessory organs, including the salivary glands, liver, gallbladder, and pancreas

Objective 2: Explain how medications are absorbed in the gastrointestinal tract and metabolized.

- Stomach juices mix with a substance and break it down for absorption.
- Chemical digestion occurs in the small intestine.
- The liver is the center of metabolic activity and is very important in digestion, absorption, and metabolic activities.

Objective 3: Describe the use of histamine-2 (H_2)-receptor antagonists in the treatment of peptic ulcers.

- Short-term treatment of active duodenal ulcer and the prevention of ulcer recurrence (at reduced dosage) after it is healed
- Short-term treatment of active benign gastric ulcer, pathologic hypersecretory conditions, such as Zollinger-Ellison syndrome, and heartburn

Objective 4: Describe the use of antacids for the treatment of peptic ulcers.

- For hyperacidity of the stomach, to protect from peptic ulcers, and to promote peptic ulcer healing

Objective 5: Explain the effects of prostaglandins on the digestive tract.

- Most versatile and powerful substances used to treat gastrointestinal (GI) disorders
- Involved in GI motility and gastric acid secretions
- Inhibit gastric acid and gastrin production, mucus production, and bicarbonate secretion
- Prostaglandin analogue misoprostol (Cytotec) is most commonly used.

Objective 6: List four generic names and trade names for proton pump inhibitors.

- esomeprazole (Nexium)
- lansoprazole (Prevacid)
- omeprazole (Prilosec)
- pantoprazole (Protonix)

Objective 7: Explain the problems associated with laxative use.

- Nausea, vomiting, abdominal cramps, diarrhea, weakness, reduced appetite, lethargy, bitter taste, anorexia, gripping, constipation rebound, melanosis of the colon, discoloration of urine, hypokalemia, and electrolyte imbalance
- In severe cases, hypotension, bradycardia, mental depression, and coma
- Contraindicated in patients with renal impairment, atonic constipation, nausea, vomiting, abdominal pain, fecal impaction, esophageal obstruction, intestinal obstruction, intestinal perforation, GI bleeding, ulcerations, appendicitis, hypertension, and in patients younger than 2 years
- Cautious use in patients with a history of congestive heart failure, edema, rectal bleeding, and diabetes mellitus

Objective 8: Describe the drug treatment for diarrhea.

- Opioid and synthetic opioid drugs: most effective
- Absorbents: inexpensive and, to a certain extent, effective

Objective 9: Describe the mechanism of action for bulk-forming laxatives, osmotic laxatives, and laxative stimulants.

- Bulk-forming laxatives—absorb free water in the intestinal tract and oppose the dehydrating forces of the bowel by forming a gelatinous mass
- Osmotic laxatives—use the ions of sodium and magnesium to attract water (osmosis), which causes a more liquid stool to be formed. Hypertonic contents cause water to be retained and to be pulled from the bowel's capillaries back into the bowel lumen, resulting in an increase in pressure and volume in the colon and rectum, leading to the stimulation of the defecation reflex.
- Laxative stimulants—true purgatives that cause an increase in peristaltic movements and lead to defecation

Internet Sites of Interest

- The National Institute of Diabetes and Digestive and Kidney Diseases (NIDDK) at **http://digestive.niddk.nih.gov** presents information on how the digestive system works. The information is appropriate for patient teaching. Search for "digestive system."

- The same NIDDK site provides information on peptic ulcer disease. Search for "peptic ulcer."

- The Family Doctor website offers information on the use of OTC laxatives at **http://familydoctor.org**. Search for "laxatives."

- For information on the use of laxatives, see Medical News Today at **www.medicalnewstoday.com**. Search for "laxative use."

PEARSON
myhealthprofessionskit™

Go to www.myhealthprofessionskit.com to access the Companion Website created for this textbook. Simply select "Basic Health Science" from the choice of disciplines. Find this book and then log in using your username and password to access interactive learning games, assessment questions, animations, and more.

Chapter 28

Drugs Used to Treat Respiratory Conditions

Chapter Objectives

1. Describe the upper and lower respiratory tracts.
2. List the most commonly used medications for asthma.
3. Explain xanthine derivatives in the treatment of asthma.
4. Describe the mechanism of action of leukotriene inhibitors.
5. Explain the contraindications of mast cell stabilizers.
6. Describe the use of opioid cough suppressants.
7. Define expectorants and mucolytic agents.
8. Explain the mechanism of action for decongestants.

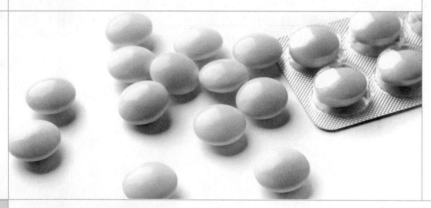

Key Terms

alveolar duct (al-vee-OH-lar DUKT) (page 497)

alveolar sacs (page 497)

alveoli (al-VEE-oh-lie) (page 497)

antitussives (an-tee-TUSS-ivz) (page 507)

asthma (page 497)

atelectasis (at-tuh-LEK-tuh-sis) (page 508)

bronchioles (BRONG-kee-ols) (page 497)

bronchitis (page 502)

bronchodilators (page 502)

bronchospasm (page 502)

cystic fibrosis (SIS-tik fy-BRO-sis) (page 508)

decongestants (page 509)

emphysema (em-fih-ZEE-muh) (page 503)

expectorants (page 508)

leukotriene inhibitors (loo-ko-TRY-een) (page 505)

mast cells (page 505)

mucolytics (myoo-ko-LIT-tiks) (page 508)

nebulizer (NEH-byoo-ly-zer) (page 502)

nonproductive cough (page 507)

productive cough (page 507)

xanthine derivatives (ZAN-theen) (page 503)

Introduction

All cells of the body require oxygen to break down nutrients and thereby release energy and produce energy (adenosine triphosphate [ATP]). The cells must also excrete the carbon dioxide that results from the process. Obtaining oxygen and removing carbon dioxide are the primary functions of the respiratory system, which includes tubes that filter incoming air and transport air into and out of the lungs as well as microscopic air sacs where gases are exchanged. The respiratory organs also entrap particles from incoming air, help control the temperature and water content of the air, produce vocal sounds, and participate in the sense of smell and the regulation of blood pH.

Organs of the Respiratory System

The organs of the respiratory system can be divided into two groups, or tracts. Those in the *upper respiratory tract* include the nose, nasal cavity, paranasal sinuses, and pharynx. Those in the *lower respiratory tract* include the larynx, trachea, bronchial tree, and lungs (Figure 28-1 ■).

The lower respiratory tract is essential for the exchange of oxygen and carbon dioxide. As the bronchi enter the lungs, they subdivide into bronchial tubes and small **bronchioles** (which are 1 mm or less in diameter and have abundant smooth muscle and elastic fibers). At the end of each bronchiole is an **alveolar duct**. These ducts lead to thin-walled outpouchings called **alveolar sacs**. Alveolar sacs lead to smaller microscopic air sacs called **alveoli**, which lie within capillary networks (Figure 28-2 ■).

Drug Effects on Asthma

Asthma is a chronic disease caused by the increased reactivity of the tracheobronchial tree to various stimuli. It is a leading cause of chronic illness and school absenteeism in children (Figure 28-3 ■). Asthma is also one of the most common chronic conditions in the United States, affecting about 23 million Americans, with 7 million of these being children.

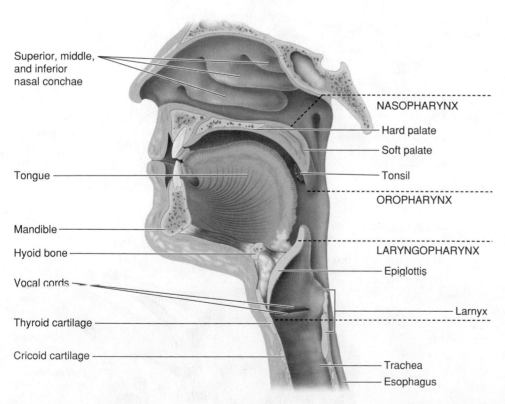

Superior, middle, and inferior nasal conchae

NASOPHARYNX

Hard palate

Soft palate

Tongue

Tonsil

OROPHARYNX

Mandible

Hyoid bone

LARYNGOPHARYNX

Vocal cords

Epiglottis

Larnyx

Thyroid cartilage

Cricoid cartilage

Trachea

Esophagus

A

Figure 28-1 ■ The upper (**A**) and lower (**B**) respiratory tracts.

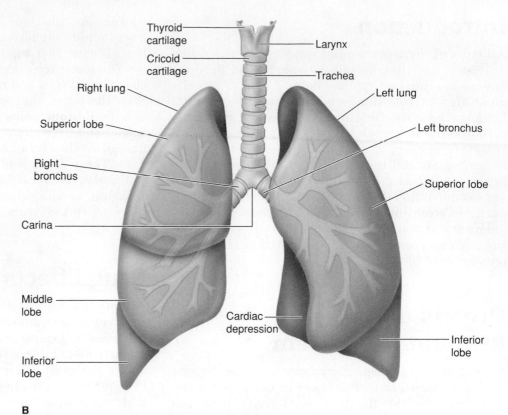

Figure 28-1 ■ (continued)

B

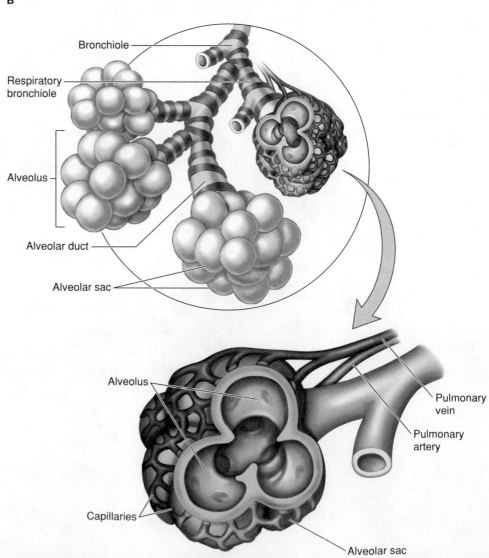

Figure 28-2 ■ Bronchioles and alveoli.

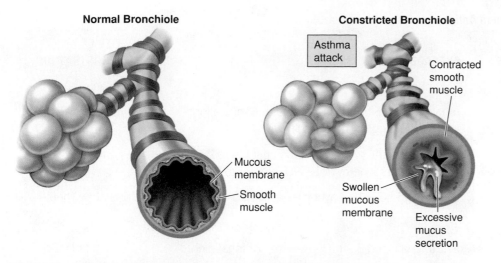

Figure 28-3 ■ The effects of asthma on the bronchioles.

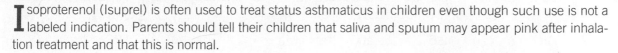

Focus on Pediatrics

Isoproterenol for Asthma

Isoproterenol (Isuprel) is often used to treat status asthmaticus in children even though such use is not a labeled indication. Parents should tell their children that saliva and sputum may appear pink after inhalation treatment and that this is normal.

Asthma is frequently classified according to its cause: allergy, exercise induced, or infections of the respiratory tract. Symptoms include breathlessness, cough, wheezing, and chest tightness. The airway becomes inflamed with edema (abnormal accumulation of fluid) and mucous plugs; hyperactivity of the bronchial tree adds to the symptoms. During asthmatic attacks, when bronchiole constriction and increased secretions are present, bronchodilators are used for relief. Classifications of the most common medications that are used for asthma are listed in Table 28-1 ■.

Table 28-1 ■ The Most Common Antiasthma Drugs

GENERIC NAME	TRADE NAME	AVERAGE ADULT DOSAGE	ROUTE OF ADMINISTRATION
Beta₂-Adrenergic Agonists			
albuterol	Proventil, Ventolin	2–4 mg tid	PO
		1–2 inhalations q4–6h; 2 inhalations before exercise	Inhalation
epinephrinc	EpiPen	Individualized: solution 1:1,000, 0.3–0.5 mL	Inhalation, subcutaneous, IM
formoterol	Foradil	One 12-mg capsule q12h	Inhalation (aerolizer inhaler)
ipratropium	Atrovent, Atrovent HFA	2 inhalations qid at 4-h intervals (maximum: 12 inhalations in 24 h)	Inhalation (MDI)
		500 mcg (1 unit-dose vial) q6–8h	Inhalation (nebulizer)
		Intranasal: 2 sprays of 0.06% in each nostril tid–qid up to 4 d	Nasal spray

(continued)

Table 28-1 ■ The Most Common Antiasthma Drugs (*continued*)

GENERIC NAME	TRADE NAME	AVERAGE ADULT DOSAGE	ROUTE OF ADMINISTRATION
isoetharine	Bronkosol	3–7 inhalations 1:3 dilution	Inhalation
isoproterenol	Isuprel	Inhalations 4–6 times/d (maximum: 6 inhalations in any hour during 24-h period)	Inhalation (MDI)
		Solution: 0.5 mL of 0.5% solution diluted to 2–2.5 mL with water or saline over 10–20 min, up to 5 times/d	IPPB
levalbuterol	Xopenex	0.63 mg tid q6–8 h; may increase to 1.25 mg tid PRN	Inhalation (nebulizer)
metaproterenol	Alupent	20 mg q6–8h	PO
		2–3 inhalations q3–4h (maximum: 12 inhalation/d)	Inhalation (MDI)
		5–10 inhalations of undiluted 5% solution	Inhalation (nebulizer)
		2.5 mL of 0.4–0.6% solution q4–6h	IPPB
pirbuterol	Maxair	2 inhalations (0.4 mg) q6h (maximum: 12 inhalations/d)	Inhalation
salmeterol	Serevent	2 inhalations of aerosol (42 mcg) or 1 powder diskus (50 mcg) bid, 12h apart	Inhalation (various)
terbutaline	Brethine	2.5–5 mg tid at 6-h intervals (maximum: 15 mg/d)	PO
		0.25 mg q15–30 min, up to 0.5 mg in 4 h	Subcutaneous
		2 inhalations separated by 60 sec q4–6h	Inhalation
Xanthine Derivatives			
aminophylline	Phyllocontin, Truphylline, etc.	Loading dose: 6 mg/kg over 30 min; maintenance dose: 0.25–0.75 mg/kg/h	IV
		0.6 mg/kg/h qid	PO
dyphylline	Dilor, Dyflex, etc.	200–800 mg q6h up to 15 mg/kg qid	PO
		250–500 mg q6h (maximum: 15 mg/kg qid)	IM
oxtriphylline	Choledyl	200–800 mg q6h up to 15 mg/kg	PO
theophylline	Somophyllin, Theo-Dur, etc.	Loading dose: 5 mg/kg	PO
		Maintenance dose: 0.5 mg q8–12h	PO (sustained release)
		Maintenance dose: 0.5 mg/kg/h	IV
Corticosteroids			
beclomethasone	Beclovent, Beconase*, QVAR, Vance-nase, Vanceril	2 inhalations tid–qid, up to 20 inhalations/d	Inhalation, nasal
budesonide	Pulmicort, Rhinocort, Turbuhaler	Maintenance: 1–2 inhalations (200 mcg/inhalation 1–2 times/d)	Inhalation
dexamethasone	Aeroseb-Dex, Decadron, Decaspray	Up to 3 inhalations tid–qid (maximum: 800 mcg bid)	Inhalation

GENERIC NAME	TRADE NAME	AVERAGE ADULT DOSAGE	ROUTE OF ADMINISTRATION
flunisolide	AeroBid, Nasalide, Nasarel	2 sprays orally or intranasally in each nostril bid; may increase to tid if needed	PO, nasal
fluticasone	Flonase, Flovent	100 mcg (1 inhalation in each nostril 1–2 times/d (maximum: 4 times/d)	Nasal
		1–2 inhalations bid	Inhalation
hydrocortisone	Cortaid, Dermacort	10–320 mg/d in 3–4 divided doses (maximum: 2 g/d)	PO
mometasone furoate monohydrate	Nasonex	2 sprays (50 mcg each) in each nostril/d	Nasal
prednisolone	Delta-Cortef, Prelone	5–60 mg/d in single or divided doses	PO
prednisone	Deltasone, Meticorten	40 mg q12h for 3–5 d	PO
triamcinolone	Azmacort, Tri-Nasal	2 puffs 3–4 times/d or 4 puffs bid	Inhalation
		2 spray/nostril once daily (maximum: 8 sprays/d)	Nasal
Leukotriene Inhibitors			
montelukast	Singulair	10 mg at bedtime	PO
zafirlukast	Accolate	20 mg bid	PO
zileuton	Zyflo	600 mg qid	PO
Mast Cell Stabilizers			
cromolyn	Intal, NasalCrom	1 spray or 1 capsule inhaled qid	MDI
		1 spray in each nostril 3–6 times/d at regular intervals	Nasal
nedocromil	Alocril, Tilade	2 inhalations qid at regular intervals (NOT for acute asthma attacks!)	Inhalation
Combination Drugs			
fluticasone with salmeterol	Advair Diskus, Advair HFA	1 puff bid approx, 12h apart	Inhalation
budesonide with formoterol	Symbicort	2 inhalations per dose, q12h	Inhalation

*Beconase AQ is a nasal spray; Beconase is also available as an inhalation aerosol.
bid, twice a day; IM, intramuscular; IPPB, intermittent positive-pressure breathing; IV, intravenous; MDI, metered-dose inhaler; PO, oral; PRN, as needed; qid, four times a day; tid, three times a day.

Focus Point

Severe Asthma

Severe forms of asthma are associated with frequent attacks of wheezing dyspnea, especially at night, and chronic limitation of activity. Asthma causes the contraction of the airway smooth muscle, mucosal thickening, and abnormally thick plugs of mucus.

✳ Apply Your Knowledge 28.1

The following questions focus on what you have just learned about organs of the respiratory system and the effects of drugs on asthma.

CRITICAL THINKING

1. What is the primary function of the respiratory system?
2. What organs are included in the lower respiratory tract?
3. What are the symptoms of asthma?
4. What are the classifications of antiasthma drugs?
5. What are the trade names of cromolyn, montelukast, aminophylline, and terbutaline?

BRONCHODILATORS

Bronchodilators are agents that widen the diameter of the bronchial tubes. They include beta$_2$-adrenergic agonists, such as salmeterol (Serevent), and xanthines, such as theophylline (Theo-Dur) and aminophylline (Truphylline, Somophyllin).

Focus On

Beta$_2$-Adrenergic Agonists

Beta$_2$-adrenergic agonists are the drugs of choice in the treatment of acute bronchoconstriction, and they have replaced some of the older agents, such as epinephrine, because they cause fewer cardiac adverse effects. Some of these drugs (isoproterenol [Isuprel]) produce therapeutic effects immediately but last for 2 to 3 hours, but other drugs, such as salmeterol (Serevent), provide 12 hours of therapy.

How do they work?

Beta$_2$-adrenergic agonists produce bronchodilation by relaxing smooth muscles of the bronchial tree. This effect decreases airway resistance, facilitates mucus drainage, and increases vital capacity.

How are they used?

Beta$_2$-adrenergic agonists are used to relieve **bronchospasm** (the contraction of smooth muscle in the walls of the bronchi and bronchioles) associated with acute or chronic asthma, **bronchitis** (inflammation of the mucous membrane of the bronchial tubes), or other reversible obstructive airway diseases. Some of them are also used to prevent exercise-induced bronchospasm. Many of these types of agents are inhaled by using a **nebulizer** (a device that disperses a fine-particle mist of medication into the deeper parts of the respiratory tract).

What are the adverse effects?

Adverse effects of such beta$_2$-adrenergic drugs as epinephrine (EpiPen) and isoproterenol (Isuprel) may cause restlessness, headache, dizziness, palpitations, tachycardia, insomnia, nausea, vomiting, and anorexia.

What are the contraindications and interactions?

Contraindications are hypersensitivity to sympathomimetic amines, narrow-angle glaucoma, and hemorrhagic and traumatic or cardiogenic shock. Safety during pregnancy or lactation is not established. Beta$_2$-adrenergic drugs should be used cautiously in older adults and debilitated patients and in those with prostatic hypertrophy, hypertension, diabetes mellitus, hyperthyroidism, Parkinson's disease, tuberculosis, and psychoneurosis. No significant drug interactions with beta$_2$-adrenergic agents have been reported.

What are the important points patients should know?

Instruct patients not to exceed the recommended dosage. They should use caution if driving or performing tasks that require alertness. Advise patients to eat small, frequent meals to avoid nausea, vomiting, and a change in taste. Instruct patients to immediately report chest pain, dizziness, insomnia, weakness, tremors, an irregular heartbeat, difficulty breathing, a productive cough, or a lack of therapeutic effects to their physicians.

Focus on Geriatrics

Cautious Use of Beta$_2$-Adrenergic Drugs in Elderly Patients

Care must be taken when using beta$_2$-adrenergic drugs, such as epinephrine, in older adults. These drugs are contraindicated in numerous conditions that affect elderly patients, including hypertension, Parkinson's disease, heart disease, glaucoma, and arteriosclerosis.

Focus On

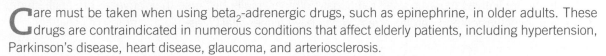

Xanthine Derivatives

Xanthine derivatives are a group of drugs chemically related to caffeine that dilate bronchioles in the lungs. Xanthines are most often used to treat asthma and are administered by the oral or intravenous route. Examples of xanthenes include aminophylline (Truphylline, Somophyllin) and theophylline (Theo-Dur).

How do they work?

Xanthine derivatives relax smooth muscle by direct action on the bronchi and pulmonary vessels. They stimulate the medullary respiratory center, resulting in an increase in the vital capacity of the lungs. Methylxanthines (such as caffeine) are bases of xanthine derivatives, which must be converted to theophylline. Theophylline (Theo-Dur) has a narrow therapeutic range and is not used as commonly today.

How are they used?

Xanthine derivatives are used for prophylaxis and the symptomatic relief of bronchial asthma as well as bronchospasm associated with chronic bronchitis and **emphysema** (a condition in which the walls between the alveoli lose their elasticity; the alveoli become weakened and break; air is trapped in the alveoli; and the exchange of oxygen and carbon dioxide is reduced).

What are the adverse effects?

The common adverse effects of xanthine derivatives include palpitations, tachycardia, flushing, hypotension, insomnia, nervousness, nausea, vomiting, diarrhea, tachypnea, and respiratory arrest.

What are the contraindications and interactions?

Xanthine derivatives are contraindicated in hypersensitivity to these agents. Xanthine preparations should not be given to patients who have coronary artery disease, a history of angina pectoris, or severe renal or liver impairment. Safety during pregnancy or lactation is not established. Xanthine derivatives should be used cautiously in children and older adults and in those with

(Continued)

Focus On (Continued)

hyperthyroidism, hypertension, peptic ulcer, prostatic hypertrophy, glaucoma, and diabetes mellitus.

The xanthine drugs may produce drug interactions with antibiotics, rifampin (Rifadin), phenobarbital (Bellatal), phenytoin (Dilantin), cimetidine (Tagamet), and caffeine.

What are the important points patients should know?

Advise patients to take these medications at the same time every day. They should avoid charbroiled food (or food cooked using charcoal), which may increase theophylline (Theo-Dur) elimination and reduce the half-life as much as 50%. Instruct patients to limit caffeine intake because it may increase the incidence of adverse effects. Instruct them to avoid cigarette smoking, which may significantly lower the plasma concentration of xanthine drugs. Women should not breastfeed while taking these drugs without consulting a physician.

Focus on Geriatrics

Cautious Use of Xanthines

Xanthine derivatives must be used cautiously in older adults because their adverse effects include severe hypotension and cardiac arrest, which have higher fatality rates in this group of patients.

Focus On

Corticosteroids

Corticosteroids, such as prednisone (Deltasone), are steroid hormones used to treat a wide variety of inflammatory diseases. Inhaled corticosteroids help prevent asthmatic attacks. Oral corticosteroids are used for the short-term management of acute severe asthma.

How do they work?

The precise mechanism of action of corticosteroids is not known. It is thought that they diminish the activation of inflammatory cells and increase the production of anti-inflammatory mediators, which in turn reduces mucus production and edema and decreases airway obstruction.

How are they used?

Corticosteroids are used to treat respiratory conditions, such as nasal congestion, and allergic conditions, such as rhinitis and asthma.

What are the adverse effects?

The adverse effects of corticosteroids include the irritation of mucous membranes, headache, pharyngitis, epistaxis, nausea, vomiting, asthma-like symptoms, and coughing. Less common adverse effects include blood in the nasal mucus, runny nose, abdominal pain, diarrhea, fever, flu-like symptoms, body aches, dizziness, and bronchitis.

What are the contraindications and interactions?

Corticosteroids are contraindicated in patients with known hypersensitivity to these types of drugs. They should not be used if symptoms of hypercorticism (such as Cushing's syndrome) are present. They must be used with caution in patients with immune system infections, tuberculosis, herpes simplex, ulcers, nasal surgery, and nasal trauma and in women who are pregnant or lactating. They should not be used in children younger than age 4 years. Corticosteroids may interact with ritonavir (Norvir), ketoconazole (Nizoral), other cytochrome P450 inhibitors, and other inhaled corticosteroids.

What are the important points patients should know?

Advise patients to avoid exposure to chicken pox or measles while taking corticosteroids and to contact their physicians if exposure occurs. Women who are pregnant or lactating should not use corticosteroids without their physician's approval.

Focus on Pediatrics

Growth Retardation and Corticosteroids

Growth retardation is of particular concern when corticosteroids are used in children. Guidelines for use of corticosteroids with certain age groups of children must be followed closely.

Focus On

Leukotriene Inhibitors

Leukotriene inhibitors, such as zafirlukast (Accolate), are bronchodilator and leukotriene-receptor antagonists. Leukotrienes are metabolized from arachidonic acid, which is also responsible for forming prostaglandins. Leukotrienes cause inflammation and allergic reactions. They increase edema, vascular permeability, and mucus in bronchioles.

How do they work?

A leukotriene inhibitor blocks either the synthesis of or the body's inflammatory responses to leukotrienes. Blocking the receptors also blocks the tissue's inflammatory response. Thus, leukotriene inhibitors control asthmatic attacks.

How are they used?

Leukotriene inhibitors are used in the prophylaxis and treatment of chronic asthma or allergic rhinitis.

What are the adverse effects?

Adverse effects of leukotriene inhibitors include arrhythmias, dizziness, lightheadedness, anxiety, headache, and euphoria. Common adverse effects are nausea, diarrhea, dry mouth, and abdominal discomfort.

What are the contraindications and interactions?

Leukotriene inhibitors are contraindicated in hypersensitive patients and in those with severe asthma attacks, bronchoconstriction caused by asthma or nonsteroidal anti-inflammatory drugs, and status asthmaticus. They should not be used by lactating women and should be used cautiously in patients with severe liver disease, pregnant patients, and children younger than 12 months. No significant drug interactions with leukotriene inhibitor agents have been reported.

What are the important points patients should know?

Instruct patients not to use these drugs for the reversal of an acute asthmatic attack and instead to inform their physicians if they need short-acting inhaled bronchodilators more often than leukotriene inhibitors.

Focus Point

Oral Administration Advantage

The principal advantage of leukotriene inhibitors is that they are taken orally. Some patients (especially children) do not comply well with inhaled medications.

Focus On

Mast Cell Stabilizers

Mast cells are large cells found in connective tissue that contain a wide variety of biochemicals, including histamine. Mast cells are involved in inflammation secondary to injuries and infections, and they are sometimes implicated in allergic reactions. A mast cell stabilizer is able to stabilize mast cell membranes against rupture caused by antigenic substances. As a result, less histamine and other inflammatory substances are released in airway tissue. Examples of mast cell stabilizers include cromolyn (Intal) and nedocromil (Tilade).

(Continued)

Focus On (*Continued*)

How do they work?

Mast cell stabilizers are synthetic asthma-prophylactic agents with unique action. They inhibit the release of bronchoconstrictors, such as histamine, from sensitized pulmonary mast cells, thereby suppressing an allergic response.

How are they used?

Cromolyn sodium (Intal) is used primarily for the prophylaxis of mild to moderate seasonal and perennial bronchial asthma and allergic rhinitis. It is also used for the prevention of exercise-related bronchospasm and the prevention of acute bronchospasm induced by known pollutants or antigens. Nedocromil sodium (Tilade) is used as maintenance therapy for patients with mild to moderate asthma.

What are the adverse effects?

Common adverse effects include nausea, vomiting, dry mouth, throat irritation, cough, hoarseness, slightly bitter aftertaste, headache, dizziness, urticaria, and rash.

What are the contraindications and interactions?

Mast cell stabilizers are contraindicated in patients with coronary artery disease or a history of arrhythmias, dyspnea, acute asthma, and status asthmaticus. These agents should not be used during pregnancy or in children younger than age 6 years. Cromolyn sodium (Intal) should be given cautiously in patients with renal or hepatic dysfunction. No clinically significant interactions with cromolyn sodium or nedocromil sodium have been established.

What are the important points patients should know?

Advise patients that throat irritation, cough, and hoarseness can be minimized by gargling with water, drinking a few swallows of water, or sucking on a lozenge after each treatment. Women should not breastfeed while taking these drugs.

Focus on Geriatrics

Contraindications of Mast Cell Stabilizers

Mast cell stabilizers, such as cromolyn, are contraindicated in patients with coronary artery disease, a history of arrhythmias, and renal or hepatic dysfunction—all conditions with higher rates of occurrence in elderly patients.

✳ Apply Your Knowledge 28.2

The following questions focus on what you have just learned about the various types of drugs used for respiratory disorders.

CRITICAL THINKING

1. What are the four examples of xanthine derivatives?
2. What are the three examples of leukotriene inhibitors?
3. What are the three examples of bronchodilators?
4. What are the mechanisms of action of beta$_2$-adrenergic agonists on asthma patients?
5. What are the indications of xanthine derivatives?
6. What are mast cells and their involvement in asthma?
7. What are the contraindications of cromolyn?
8. What are the indications of leukotriene inhibitors?
9. Why must xanthine derivatives be used cautiously in older adults?

Focus On

Antitussives

Antitussives are agents that reduce coughing. They are also called *cough suppressants.* The initial stimulus for a cough probably arises in the bronchial mucosa, where irritation results in bronchoconstriction. *Coughing* is a sudden expulsion of air from the lungs and through the mouth. A cough is often described as productive or nonproductive. A **productive cough** brings up fluid or mucus from the lungs. A **nonproductive cough** is a sudden ejection of air from the lungs and through the mouth that does not expel (produce) mucus or fluid from the throat or lungs. Antitussives are classified into two major groups: opioid and nonopioid. Various cough suppression agents are summarized in Table 28-2 ■.

How do they work?

The opioid cough suppressants cause respiratory depression similar to that of morphine. An antitussive action occurs at doses that are lower than those required for analgesia. Examples of opioid cough suppressants are codeine (generic only), hydrocodone (Histussin), and chlorpheniramine and hydrocodone (Tussionex).

Nonopioid cough suppressants, such as dextromethorphan (Robitussin DM, Vicks Formula 44 Cough), do not suppress respiration. These drugs reduce the activity of peripheral cough receptors and appear to increase the threshold of the central cough center.

How are they used?

The opioid cough suppressants are used to suppress nonproductive cough, but they have limited use because of unwanted side effects. Codeine and hydrocodone (Histussin) are not generally effective but are used because they elevate the cough threshold.

Nonopioid cough suppressants are indicated for temporary relief of cough spasms in nonproductive coughs caused by colds, pertussis, and influenza. The major nonopioid cough suppressants are over-the-counter (OTC) medications.

What are the adverse effects?

The adverse effects of antitussives may include difficulty breathing, drowsiness, skin rash, itching, dizziness, constipation, nausea, nervousness, and restlessness.

What are the contraindications and interactions?

Antitussives are contraindicated in patients with known hypersensitivity, asthma, emphysema, diabetes, heart disease, seizure conditions, thyroid conditions, chronic bronchitis, and liver disease. They should be used only if directed by a physician in women who are pregnant or lactating.

Antitussives interact with monoamine oxidase inhibitors (MAOIs), alcohol, sedatives and hypnotics, cold and allergy medications, muscle relaxants, and analgesics.

What are the important points patients should know?

Advise patients to call their physicians if their coughing does not improve or if it lasts longer than 1 week, worsens, or produces yellow-colored mucus. They should also contact their physicians if symptoms of fever, rash, sore throat, vomiting, or continuing headache occur.

Table 28-2 ■ Major Types of Cough Suppressants

GENERIC NAME	TRADE NAME	AVERAGE ADULT DOSAGE	ROUTE OF ADMINISTRATION
Opioids			
chlorpheniramine and hydrocodone	Tussionex	5 mL bid	PO
hydrocodone	Hycodan, Robidone A	5–10 mg q4–6h PRN (maximum: 15 mg/dose)	PO
codeine	(generic only)	10–20 mg q4–6h PRN (maximum: 120 mg/d)	PO
Nonopioids			
benzonatate	Tessalon Perles	100–200 mg tid (maximum, 600 mg/d)	PO
dextromethorphan	Robitussin DM, Romilar CF	10–20 mg q4h or 30 mg q6–8h (maximum: 120 mg/d) or 60 mg of sustained-action liquid bid	PO
diphenhydramine	Benadryl, Benahist	25 mg q4–6h (max: 100 mg/d)	PO

bid, twice a day; PRN, as needed; PO, oral; tid, three times a day.

Focus on Natural Products

Natural Expectorant

Wild cherry bark acts as an expectorant and as a mild sedative. It is available in syrup and tincture forms. It is good for coughs, colds, bronchitis, and asthma. However, wild cherry bark should not be used during pregnancy.

Focus Point

Opioids for Cough

Opioid analgesics are among the most effective drugs used as cough suppressants. Their effect is often achieved at doses below those required to produce analgesia. For example, 15 mg of codeine is usually sufficient to relieve coughing.

Focus On

Expectorants and Mucolytics

Expectorants and **mucolytics** are medications that are capable of dissolving or promoting liquefaction of mucus in the lungs. They also facilitate the elimination of mucus through coughing. These medications (Table 28-3 ■) are available OTC and by prescription. Expectorants and mucolytics include acetylcysteine (Mucomyst), guaifenesin (Fenesin), and dornase alfa (Pulmozyme).

How do they work?

Acetylcysteine (Mucomyst) lowers viscosity and facilitates the removal of secretions. Guaifenesin (Fenesin) enhances reflex outflow of respiratory tract fluids by the irritation of gastric mucosa.

How are they used?

These agents are used as adjuvant therapy in patients with abnormal, sticky, or thickened mucous secretions in acute and chronic bronchopulmonary disease and in pulmonary complications of **cystic fibrosis** (a disorder marked by abnormal secretions of the exocrine glands causing obstruction of bronchial

pathways), tracheostomy, and **atelectasis** (absence of gas from the lungs).

What are the adverse effects?

The adverse effects of these expectorants and mucolytics are not significant. A low incidence of nausea and drowsiness is reported.

What are the contraindications and interactions?

Expectorants and mucolytics are contraindicated in patients with hypersensitivity to these agents. They should be avoided in pregnancy and lactation. Guaifenesin may interact with heparin therapy by inhibiting platelet function and increasing the risk of hemorrhage.

What are the important points patients should know?

Instruct patients to increase fluid intake to help loosen mucus and drink at least 8 glasses of fluids daily. They should contact their physicians if cough persists beyond 1 week. Advise women to avoid breastfeeding while taking these drugs without their physicians' approval.

Table 28-3 ■ **Expectorants and Mucolytics**

GENERIC NAME	TRADE NAME	AVERAGE ADULT DOSAGE	ROUTE OF ADMINISTRATION
acetylcysteine	Mucomyst	10 mL of 20% solution or 2–20 mL of 10% solution q2–6 h	Inhalation
dornase alfa	Pulmozyme	2.5 mg/d inhaled through a nebulizer	Inhalation
guaifenesin	Fenesin, Humibid	100–400 mg q4h	PO
potassium iodide	Pima, SSKI	300–1,000 mg after meals, bid–tid up to 1.5 g tid	PO

bid, twice a day; PO, oral; tid, three times a day.

Focus On

Decongestants

Decongestants are a class of drugs that reverse excessive blood flow (congestion) into an area. These agents are available in oral and nasal preparations. Table 28-4 ■ shows the most commonly used decongestants, such as pseudoephedrine (Sudafed).

How do they work?

Decongestants are vasoconstricting agents that shrink the swollen mucous membranes of the nasal airway passage of the upper respiratory tract. Most oral agents are adrenergic medications or medications that mimic the effects of the sympathetic nervous system.

How are they used?

The most common uses for decongestants are for the relief of nasal congestion caused by the common cold, upper respiratory allergies, and sinusitis.

What are the adverse effects?

All patients may experience nervousness, insomnia, restlessness, dizziness, headaches, and irritability. Decongestants may also cause tachycardia, blurred vision, nausea, and vomiting.

What are the contraindications and interactions?

Decongestants should not be used by patients who are taking other sympathomimetic drugs. They also are contraindicated in patients with diabetes, heart disease, uncontrolled hypertension, hyperthyroidism, and prostatic hypertrophy.

Nasal decongestants may cause severe hypertension with certain MAOIs. They may also decrease the vasopressor response with reserpine (Serpalan), methyldopa (Aldomet), and urine acidifiers. Nasal decongestants increase the duration of action of urine alkalinizers (sodium citrate, lactate, and sodium bicarbonate). They decrease the antihypertensive effects of methyldopa (Aldomet).

What are the important points patients should know?

Instruct patients to avoid taking oral decongestants within 2 hours of bedtime because pseudoephedrine (Sudafed) may act as a stimulant. Advise patients to discontinue the medication and consult their physician if extreme restlessness or signs of sensitivity occur. Women should not breastfeed while taking decongestants without consulting their physicians.

Table 28-4 ■ The Most Commonly Used Decongestants

GENERIC NAME	TRADE NAME	AVERAGE ADULT DOSAGE	ROUTE OF ADMINISTRATION
Oral Decongestants			
Pseudoephedrine	Sudafed	60 mg q4–6h or 120 mg sustained release q12h	PO
Combination Decongestants/Antihistamines			
cetirizine-pseudoephedrine	Zyrtec-D	5–10 mg once daily	PO
clemastine fumarate	Tavist	1.34 mg bid; may increase to 8.04 mg/d	PO
fexofenadine-pseudoephedrine	Allegra D	60 mg tid	PO
loratadine-pseudoephedrine	Claritin-D and others	10 mg/d on empty stomach	PO
naproxen-pseudoephedrine	Aleve Cold & Sinus	275–1,100 mg/d	PO
Nasal Decongestants			
phenazoline 0.05%	Allerest	2 drops or sprays in each nostril q3–6h, up to 3–5 d	Nasal
oxymetazoline 0.05%	Afrin	2–3 drops in each nostril bid, up to 3–5 d	Nasal
phenylephrine 1%	Neo-Synephrine, Sinex	1–2 drops in each nostril q3–4h	Nasal
tetrahydrozoline 0.1%	Tyzine	2–4 drops in each nostril q3h PRN	Nasal

PO, oral; PRN, as needed.

✳ Apply Your Knowledge 28.3

The following questions focus on what you have just learned about antitussives and decongestants.

CRITICAL THINKING

1. What is another name for antitussives?
2. What are the classifications of antitussives?
3. Why are codeine and hydrocodone generally not effective on the central cough center?
4. What are the trade names of dornase alfa and acetylcysteine?
5. What are the conditions known as cystic fibrosis and atelectasis?
6. What are the adverse effects of decongestants?
7. What are the trade names of pseudoephedrine, fexofenadine-pseudoephedrine, and phenylephrine?
8. What is the mechanism of action for decongestants?

PRACTICAL SCENARIO 1

A 60-year-old man with a history of depression and hypertension visited his local pharmacy to buy a decongestant and cough suppressant for a bad chest cold. He asked the pharmacist to recommend a brand. The pharmacist recommended Sudafed (pseudoephedrine) for his congestion and Robitussin DM (dextromethorphan) for his cough. At home, the man took the recommended dose of each medicine. Within 1 hour, he began having palpitations, chest pains, and severe headache. He was sweating, and his heart rate was 120 beats per minute. His wife called the emergency medical services (EMS). The EMS team obtained an electrocardiogram and asked the man's medical history. The man reported taking phenelzine (Nardil) for depression and atenolol (Tenormin) for hypertension. His wife stated that he had just taken Sudafed and Robitussin for his cold and cough. The EMS team stabilized his heart rate and transferred him to the hospital for observation.

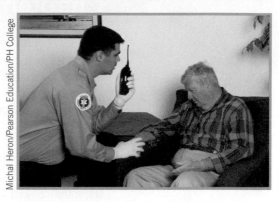

Critical Thinking Questions

1. What is the significance of the man's use of phenelzine, atenolol, and the OTC cold and cough medications?
2. What mistake did the pharmacist make in helping the man choose OTC cough and cold preparations?
3. What patient teaching would you provide this patient if he was seen in your office for a routine checkup and review of his prescriptions?

PRACTICAL SCENARIO 2

A 7-year-old girl was brought to the emergency department with a severe asthma attack.

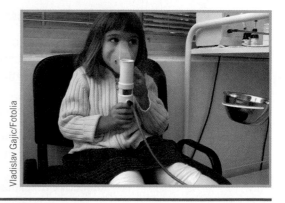

Critical Thinking Questions

1. What is the drug of choice in the treatment of acute bronchoconstriction?
2. List all medications used for asthma.

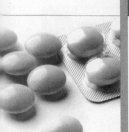

Chapter Capsule

This section repeats the objectives from the beginning of the chapter and then provides a summary of the most important concepts for that objective. Use this section as a quick review and to check your knowledge.

Objective 1: Describe the upper and lower respiratory tracts.

- Upper respiratory tract—nose, nasal cavity, paranasal sinuses, and pharynx
- Lower respiratory tract—larynx, trachea, bronchial tree, and lungs

Objective 2: List the most commonly used medications for asthma.

- Asthma—most commonly treated by bronchodilators, xanthine derivatives, leukotriene inhibitors, corticosteroids, and mast cell stabilizers

Objective 3: Explain xanthine derivatives in the treatment of asthma.

- Xanthine derivatives—treat asthma by relaxing smooth muscle via direct action on the bronchi and pulmonary vessels

Objective 4: Describe the mechanism of action for leukotriene inhibitors.

- Leukotriene inhibitors—block either the synthesis of leukotrienes or the body's inflammatory responses to leukotrienes

Objective 5: Explain the contraindications of mast cell stabilizers.

- Mast cell stabilizers—contraindicated in patients with coronary artery disease, history of arrhythmias, dyspnea, acute asthma, status asthmaticus, during pregnancy, and in children younger than the age of 6; cromolyn sodium (Intal) should be used cautiously in patients with renal or hepatic dysfunction.

Objective 6: Describe the use of opioid cough suppressants.

- Opioid cough suppressants—used to suppress nonproductive cough but have limited use because of unwanted side effects; codeine and hydrocodone (Histussin) are not as effective but are used to elevate the cough threshold.

Objective 7: Define expectorants and mucolytic agents.

- Expectorants and mucolytics—medications capable of dissolving or promoting the liquefying of mucus in the lungs and facilitating the elimination of mucus through coughing

Objective 8: Explain the mechanism of action of decongestants.

- Decongestants—vasoconstricting agents that shrink the swollen mucous membranes of the nasal airway passage of the upper respiratory tract; most oral agents—adrenergic medications or medications that mimic the effects of the sympathetic nervous system

Internet Sites of Interest

- Information on various asthma topics and guidelines are available on the National Heart Lung and Blood Institute website at **http://www.nhlbi.nih.gov**. Search for "asthma."

- The Family Doctor offers useful information on OTC decongestants at **http://familydoctor.org**. Search for "over the counter decongestants."

- Various lung disorders, including asthma and cough, are discussed in detail on the American Lung Association website at **http://www.lungusa.org**.

- The Asthma and Allergy Foundation of America provides information, advocacy, and research on asthma at **http://www.aafa.org**.

- A wealth of information about asthma and its treatments (including alternative therapies), screening tools, and prevention tips are found at MedlinePlus at **http://www.nlm.nih.gov/medlineplus/asthma.html**.

PEARSON myhealthprofessionskit™

Go to www.myhealthprofessionskit.com to access the Companion Website created for this textbook. Simply select "Basic Health Science" from the choice of disciplines. Find this book and then log in using your username and password to access interactive learning games, assessment questions, animations, and more.

Chapter 29

Drugs Used to Treat Musculoskeletal Conditions

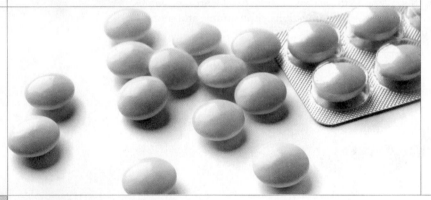

Key Terms

dysphagia (dis-FAY-jee-uh) (page 517)

flatulence (FLAT-yoo-lentz) (page 517)

hyperuricemia (hy-per-yoo-rih-SEE-mee-uh) (page 523)

nephrotic syndrome (neh-FROT-ik) (page 525)

oligospermia (ol-lih-go-SPER-mee-uh) (page 522)

osteopenia (os-tee-oh-PEE-nee-uh) (page 516)

osteoporosis (os-tee-oh-por-OH-sis) (page 516)

spasticity (spas-TIH-sih-tee) (page 526)

Introduction

Disorders of the musculoskeletal system are very common in people of all ages. Musculoskeletal conditions include osteoarthritis, muscle spasms, gout, bursitis, tendonitis, and rheumatoid arthritis (RA). Medications used to treat these conditions include skeletal muscle relaxants, nonsteroidal anti-inflammatory drugs (NSAIDs), aspirin, and gold salts.

Musculoskeletal System

The musculoskeletal system consists of two body systems: (1) the muscular system and (2) the skeletal system. The muscular system includes three types of muscle tissues: (1) skeletal, (2) cardiac, and (3) smooth.

Skeletal muscle, which is discussed in this chapter, contains connective tissues, nerves, and blood vessels. Skeletal muscles produce movement, maintain posture and body position, support soft tissue, and maintain body temperature.

The skeletal system includes the bones of the skeleton and the cartilages, ligaments, and other connective tissues that stabilize or connect the bones. The five primary functions of the skeletal system are (1) support, (2) storage of minerals and lipids, (3) blood cell production, (4) protection, and (5) leverage (Figure 29-1 ■).

Calcium is the most abundant mineral in the human body. Its proper balance and interaction with other minerals and hormones are essential to optimal functioning of several body systems, particularly the musculoskeletal system. A typical human body

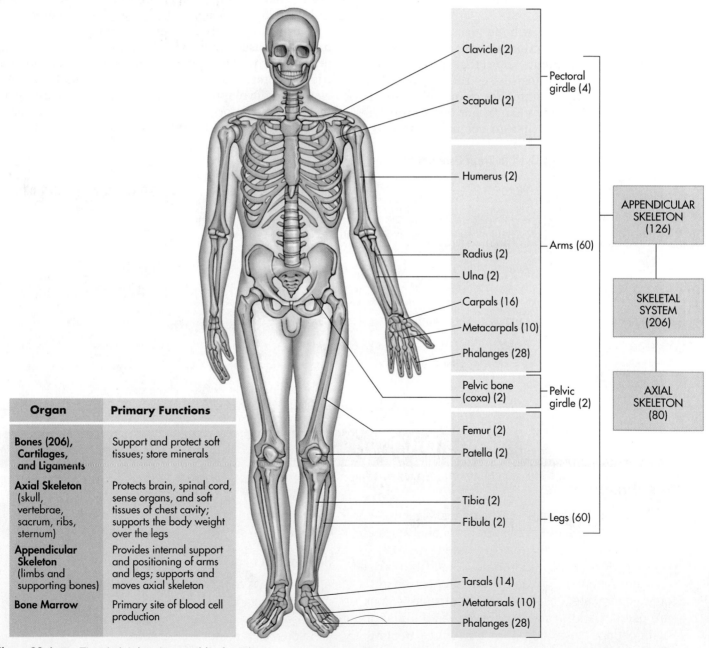

Organ	Primary Functions
Bones (206), Cartilages, and Ligaments	Support and protect soft tissues; store minerals
Axial Skeleton (skull, vertebrae, sacrum, ribs, sternum)	Protects brain, spinal cord, sense organs, and soft tissues of chest cavity; supports the body weight over the legs
Appendicular Skeleton (limbs and supporting bones)	Provides internal support and positioning of arms and legs; supports and moves axial skeleton
Bone Marrow	Primary site of blood cell production

Figure 29-1 ■ The skeletal system and its functions.

contains 1 to 2 kg of calcium, with roughly 99% of it deposited in the skeleton. Calcium ion homeostasis is maintained by a negative feedback system involving a pair of hormones with opposing effects. These hormones—parathyroid hormone and calcitonin—coordinate the storage, absorption, and excretion of calcium ions. Three target sites are involved: (1) bones (storage), (2) digestive tract (absorption), and (3) kidneys (excretion).

Osteoporosis

The bones of the skeleton become thinner and weaker as a normal part of the aging process. Inadequate ossification (the process of bone formation) is called **osteopenia**, and most people become slightly osteopenic as they age. This reduction in bone mass begins between the ages of 30 and 40.

When the reduction in bone mass is sufficient to compromise normal function, the condition is known as **osteoporosis**. The fragile bones that result are likely to break when exposed to stresses that younger individuals could easily tolerate. For example, a hip fracture can occur when a woman in her 90s simply tries to stand. Any fractures that do occur lead to loss of

independence and immobility that further weakens the skeleton.

With its loss of normal bone density, osteoporosis literally leads to porous bone that can be described as being compressible like a sponge rather than dense like a brick. It occurs more often in women than in men, especially in postmenopausal women, whose levels of the hormone estrogen are greatly decreased. Osteoporosis can cause permanent disability if not arrested, and the treatment varies depending on the cause.

AGENTS AFFECTING POSTMENOPAUSAL OSTEOPOROSIS

The treatment of postmenopausal osteoporosis is an important area of new drug development because estrogen replacement therapy (ERT) and hormone replacement therapy (HRT)—once popular forms of treatment for several postmenopausal conditions, including osteoporosis—have been associated with increased cardiovascular problems as well as a potential increased risk of endometrial and breast cancer in some patients (Table 29-1 ■). New drug developments include the selective estrogen-receptor modulators (SERMs). such as raloxifene (Evista), plus new-generation bisphosphonates.

Table 29-1 ■ Drugs Used to Treat Osteoporosis

GENERIC NAME	TRADE NAME	AVERAGE ADULT DOSAGE	ROUTE OF ADMINISTRATION
Bisphosphonates			
alendronate sodium	Fosamax; Fosamax-70	5–10 mg/d 70 mg once a wk	PO
risedronate sodium	Actonel	5 mg/d	PO
Hormonal Agents			
calcitonin salmon	Calcimar, Miacalcin	1 spray/d	Intranasal spray
raloxifene	Evista	60 mg/d	PO
sodium fluoride	Slow Fluoride	In cycles	PO
PO, oral.			

Focus On

Bisphosphonates

The first bisphosphonate available for clinical use was etidronate (Didronel), but several new analogues are now available, including pamidronate (Aredia), alendronate (Fosamax), tiludronate (Skelid), and risedronate (Actonel). For the treatment of osteoporosis, only alendronate (Fosamax) and risedronate (Actonel) are used. Alendronate (Fosamax) was the first oral bisphosphonate to be approved for the treatment

and prevention of osteoporosis in postmenopausal women.

How do they work?

Alendronate is a highly selective inhibitor of bone demineralization and resorption (breakdown). It appears to increase bone mineral density. The mechanism of action of risedronate is not fully understood.

How are they used?

Only alendronate and risedronate have been approved for the treatment of osteoporosis, but other bisphosphonates are used for other purposes. For example, etidronate, pamidronate, and tiludronate are used for Paget's disease, a disorder similar to osteoporosis in that bones become very weak and brittle but are characterized by constant bone resorption and formation, resulting in enlarged and abnormal bones. Pamidronate is also indicated for hypercalcemia of malignancy. Ibandronate sodium (Boniva) is a once-monthly medication for postmenopausal osteoarthritis used to build bone mass and maintain bone density.

What are the adverse effects?

Several gastrointestinal (GI) adverse effects may occur that include **flatulence** (presence of excess gas in the stomach and intestines), acid regurgitation, **dysphagia** (difficulty in swallowing), and gastritis. Other effects include headache, musculoskeletal pain, and rash.

What are the contraindications and interactions?

Alendronate and risedronate are contraindicated in hypersensitivity to these agents, severe renal impairment, hypocalcemia, lactation, and pregnancy. These agents should be used cautiously in patients with renal impairment, congestive heart failure, hyperphosphatemia, liver disease, fever or infection, and peptic ulcer. Calcium and food (especially dairy products) reduce alendronate absorption.

What are the important points patients should know?

Review with patients the correct administration of these medications and advise patients to report fever, especially when accompanied by arthralgia and myalgia. Instruct patients to take the drugs at least 30 minutes before food, beverages, or other medications. Women should not breastfeed while taking these drugs.

Hormonal Agents

For patients who are unable to take ERT or bisphosphonates, such hormonal agents as calcitonin (Calcimar, Miacalcin) and raloxifene (Evista) are often prescribed.

Focus On

Calcitonin

Calcitonin is secreted by the parafollicular cells of the thyroid glands of mammals. Calcitonin is a natural product obtained from salmon. Human calcitonin is also available (Cibacalcin) but is not as potent or long lasting.

How does it work?

The principal effects of calcitonin are to lower serum calcium and phosphate by action on the bones and kidneys. Calcitonin inhibits bone resorption and lowers serum calcium. Thus, calcitonin increases bone density and reduces the risk of vertebral fractures.

How is it used?

Calcitonin is approved for the treatment of osteoporosis in postmenopausal women, hypercalcemia, and symptomatic Paget's disease.

What are the adverse effects?

The adverse effects of calcitonin include headache, eye pain, hypersensitivity reactions, and anaphylaxis (reported for human calcitonin [Cibacalcin] only). Urination frequency, chills, chest pressure, weakness, dizziness, nasal congestion, and shortness of breath are other adverse effects of calcitonin.

What are the contraindications and interactions?

Calcitonin is contraindicated in patients with hypersensitivity to fish proteins or to synthetic calcitonin. It should be avoided in patients with a history of allergy. Safe use in children and during pregnancy and lactation is not established. Calcitonin should be used cautiously in patients with renal impairment and pernicious anemia. Calcitonin may interact with and may decrease serum lithium (Eskalith) levels.

(Continued)

Focus On (Continued)

. . . .

What are the important points patients should know?

Advise patients to watch for redness, warmth, or swelling at the injection site and to report any of these effects to their physicians because they may indicate an inflammatory reaction. Instruct patients to consult their physicians before using such over-the-counter (OTC) preparations as some supervitamins, hematinics (which improve the condition of the blood), and antacids containing calcium and vitamin D.

Focus on Natural Products

Dimethyl Sulfoxide

Dimethyl sulfoxide, also known as DMSO, has a long history as a topical agent that can help reduce pain and inflammation in various musculoskeletal disorders, such as tendonitis. DMSO should only be used under the guidance of a qualified health-care professional.

Focus On

Raloxifene Hydrochloride

Raloxifene (Evista) is one of the SERMs and is considered to be an estrogen antagonist.

How does it work?

Raloxifene acts by combining with estrogen receptors. It decreases bone resorption and increases bone mass and density by acting through the estrogen receptor. Raloxifene has not been associated with endometrial proliferation or the increased risk of uterine or breast cancers.

How is it used?

Raloxifene is used primarily to prevent and treat osteoporosis in postmenopausal women. It is also used to reduce the risk of breast cancer in postmenopausal women. This agent is able to reduce total serum cholesterol and low-density lipoprotein.

What are the adverse effects?

The adverse effects of raloxifene include hot flashes, migraines, headache, flu-like symptoms, uterine disorders, vaginal bleeding, urinary tract disorders, and breast pain. Other adverse effects are depression, insomnia, and dizziness.

What are the contraindications and interactions?

Raloxifene is contraindicated in women who are or who might become pregnant and in those with active (or a history of) venous thromboembolic events (for example, pulmonary embolism or retinal vein thrombosis). It is also contraindicated with the concurrent use of a systemic ERT. Raloxifene should be used cautiously with diazepam (Valium), lidocaine (Anestacon), and diazoxide (Proglycem). It can interact with cholestyramine (Questran) and warfarin (Coumadin).

What are the important points patients should know?

Advise patients to contact their physician immediately if unexplained calf pain or tenderness occurs. They should avoid prolonged restriction of movement during travel. Be sure patients are aware that raloxifene (Evista) can induce hot flashes. Patients should not breastfeed while taking this drug.

Focus Point

Raloxifene

Raloxifene is the first of the SERMs to be approved for the prevention of osteoporosis.

✳ Apply Your Knowledge 29.1

The following questions focus on what you have just learned about the musculoskeletal system, osteoporosis, and related medications.

CRITICAL THINKING

1. What is osteoporosis?
2. What are the primary functions of the skeletal system?
3. What hormones coordinate the storage, absorption, and excretion of calcium ions?
4. What drugs are used to treat or prevent osteoporosis?
5. What is the mechanism of action of calcitonin?
6. What are the indicators of raloxifene?

Rheumatoid Arthritis

Rheumatoid arthritis (RA) is a systemic autoimmune disease that involves the inflammation of the membranes lining the joints and often affects internal organs. Most patients exhibit a chronic fluctuating course of disease that can result in progressive joint destruction, deformity, and disability. It occurs two to three times more often in women, and the peak onset occurs between the fourth and sixth decades of life.

Most commonly, the joints first affected by RA include the metacarpophalangeal joints of the hands, metatarsophalangeal joints of the feet, and the wrists. Other areas affected by this disease include the spine, shoulders, ankles, and hips. RA involves not only joint capsules but also tendons, ligaments, and skeletal muscles. The goals in the management of RA are to:

✳ Prevent or control joint damage.
✳ Prevent loss of function.

✳ Decrease pain.
✳ Maintain the patient's quality of life.
✳ Avoid or minimize adverse effects of the treatment.

Antirheumatic Drugs

Drug therapy for RA involves the treatment of symptoms and the use of disease-modifying agents. Drugs with anti-inflammatory activity are the agents of choice for the symptomatic relief of RA. Salicylates, NSAIDs, and cyclooxygenase 2 (COX-2) inhibitors (as discussed in Chapter 15) reduce joint pain and swelling, but they do not alter the course of the disease or prevent joint destruction. Corticosteroids have excellent anti-inflammatory activity and are immunosuppressants. Disease-modifying antirheumatic drugs (DMARDs) reduce or prevent joint damage and preserve joint function. The DMARDs are listed in Table 29-2 ■.

Table 29-2 ■ Disease-Modifying Drugs for Rheumatoid Arthritis

GENERIC NAME	TRADE NAME	AVERAGE ADULT DOSAGE	ROUTE OF ADMINISTRATION
Gold Compounds			
Auranofin	Ridaura	3–6 mg/d; may increase up to 3 mg tid after 6 mo	PO
aurothioglucose	Solganal	10–50 mg; initially, 10 mg and then increased weekly until 1 g is reached	IM
gold sodium thiomalate	Myochrysine	Dose may be continued at 25–50 mg every other wk for 2–20 wk	IM
Miscellaneous Agents			
adalimumab	Humira	40 mg every other wk (may use 40 mg/wk if not on concomitant methotrexate)	Subcutaneous

(continued)

Table 29-2 ■ **Disease-Modifying Drugs for Rheumatoid Arthritis** (*continued*)

GENERIC NAME	TRADE NAME	AVERAGE ADULT DOSAGE	ROUTE OF ADMINISTRATION
etanercept	Enbrel	25 mg twice weekly or 0.08 mg/kg (or 50 mg) once weekly	Subcutaneous
hydroxychloroquine sulfate	Plaquenil	200–600 mg/d	PO
methotrexate	Folex, Mexate	2.5–5 mg bid for 3 doses/wk	PO
sulfasalazine	Azulfidine	250–500 mg/d (maximum: 8 g/d)	PO

bid, twice a day; IM, intramuscular; PO, oral; tid, three times a day.

Focus On

Gold Compounds

Gold compounds, such as auranofin (Ridaura), aurothioglucose (Solganal), and gold sodium thiomalate (Myochrysine), were first proved to be effective in a large group of patients in 1960. Because of their toxicity, they are used infrequently today.

How do they work?

The mechanism of anti-inflammatory action of gold compounds is not clearly understood. Gold uptake by macrophages with subsequent inhibition of migration and phagocytic action occurs, thereby suppressing immune responsiveness, which may be the principal mechanism of action.

How are they used?

Gold compounds are effective for active RA. They are generally used when adequate trials with salicylates or other NSAIDs have not been satisfactory.

What are the adverse effects?

The adverse effects of gold compounds include hypersensitivity, syncope, bradycardia, thickening of the tongue, and a metallic taste in the mouth. Hematologic abnormalities are thrombocytopenia, leukopenia, and aplastic anemia.

What are the contraindications and interactions?

These agents are contraindicated in patients with a gold allergy or a history of severe toxicity from previous therapy with gold or other heavy metals. Gold compounds should not be used in patients with uncontrolled diabetes mellitus, renal or hepatic insufficiency, or a history of hepatitis. Gold compounds may increase the risk of blood dyscrasias if they are used with antimalarials, immunosuppressants, and penicillamine (Cuprimine), another DMARD.

What are the important points patients should know?

Be sure that patients are aware of possible adverse effects and know to report them to their physicians. If therapy is interrupted at the onset of gold toxicity, serious reactions can be avoided. Advise patients to report any unusual color or odor of their urine and to avoid contact with anyone who has a cold, has had a recent vaccination, or has been recently exposed to a communicable disease.

Focus Point

Gold Compounds

Adverse reactions to gold compounds are most likely to occur during the second and third months of therapy. However, reactions may appear at any time during therapy or even several months after treatment has been discontinued.

Focus On

Hydroxychloroquine

Hydroxychloroquine sulfate (Plaquenil) is classified as an anti-infective and an antimalarial. This agent is used mainly to treat malaria.

How does it work?

The mechanism of the anti-inflammatory action of this drug in rheumatic diseases is unclear.

How is it used?

Hydroxychloroquine is approved for RA but is not considered one of the most efficacious DMARDs. Hydroxychloroquine is often used for the treatment of lupus erythematosus.

What are the adverse effects?

The adverse effects of hydroxychloroquine are fatigue, headache, mood or mental changes, anxiety, retinopathy, blurred vision, and difficulty focusing. Other adverse effects include anorexia, nausea, vomiting, diarrhea, and abdominal cramps.

What are the contraindications and interactions?

Hydroxychloroquine is contraindicated in patients with known hypersensitivity to this agent. Safe use in pregnancy and lactation is not established. Hydroxychloroquine must be used cautiously in patients with hepatic disease, alcoholism, and impaired renal function.

Aluminum- and magnesium-containing antacids and laxatives decrease hydroxychloroquine absorption. This agent may interfere with the response to rabies vaccine.

What are the important points patients should know?

Teach patients about the adverse effects and symptoms of prolonged therapy with this drug. Advise them to follow the drug regimen exactly as prescribed by their physicians and to make sure to keep this drug out of the reach of children. Because this drug may cause damage to the eyes, advise patients to get regular eye examinations. Instruct patients to avoid breastfeeding while taking this drug without consulting their physicians.

Focus on Pediatrics

Hydroxychloroquine

Hydroxychloroquine has not been established for safe use in juvenile arthritis. It should not be used during pregnancy (because it crosses the placental barrier) nor during lactation.

Focus On

Methotrexate

Formerly called amethopterin, methotrexate (Folex, Mexate) was once considered the DMARD of first choice in the treatment of patients with RA. However, newer DMARDs, such as adalimumab (Humira) and etanercept (Enbrel), are becoming first-choice agents (see Table 29-2 ■).

How does it work?

Methotrexate is a folic acid blocker and immunosuppressant that affects lymphocyte and macrophage function.

How is it used?

Methotrexate is principally used in combination regimens to maintain induced remissions in patients with neoplastic diseases. Methotrexate is also used to treat those with severe psoriasis, psoriatic arthritis, and RA.

What are the adverse effects?

The most common toxicity of methotrexate is dose-related bone marrow suppression. Infertility with azoospermia (absence of living spermatozoa in the semen) and amenorrhea also occur. GI upset and mouth sores are less serious common adverse effects.

What are the contraindications and interactions?

Methotrexate is contraindicated in pregnancy and lactation, in men and women of childbearing age, hepatic and renal insufficiency, and preexisting blood dyscrasias. Methotrexate should be used cautiously in patients with infections, peptic ulcer, ulcerative colitis, cancer patients with pre-existing bone marrow impairment, and poor nutritional status.

(Continued)

Focus On (*Continued*)

Alcohol, azathioprine (Azasan), and sulfasalazine (Azulfidine) increase the risk of hepatotoxicity if used with methotrexate. Chloramphenicol (Chlorofair), sulfonamides, salicylates, NSAIDs, phenytoin (Dilantin), tetracyclines, and probenecid (Benemid) may increase methotrexate levels with increased toxicity.

What are the important points patients should know?

Be sure patients are aware of the dangers of this drug and know to promptly report any abnormal symptoms to their physicians. They should know that the most common adverse affects are stomach upset, mouth sores, headache, and drowsiness. Alcohol ingestion increases the incidence and severity of methotrexate hepatotoxicity. Instruct patients that they should not self-medicate with vitamins or OTC compounds that include folic acid, which alters methotrexate response. They should avoid exposure to sunlight and ultraviolet light and wear sunglasses and sunscreen.

Focus Point

Methotrexate

P rolonged treatment with small frequent doses of methotrexate may lead to hepatotoxicity, which is best diagnosed by liver biopsy.

PENICILLAMINE

Penicillamine (Cuprimine) is a metabolite of penicillin and is rarely used today because of toxicity. Therefore, it is not discussed here for the treatment of RA.

Focus On

Sulfasalazine

Sulfasalazine (Azulfidine) is a GI and anti-inflammatory agent.

How does it work?

Sulfasalazine is a locally acting sulfonamide that is believed to be converted by intestinal microflora to sulfapyridine, providing antibacterial action, and to 5-aminosalicylic acid or mesalamine, which may exert an anti-inflammatory effect. It may also inhibit prostaglandins that are known to cause diarrhea and affect mucosal transport as well as interfere with the absorption of fluids and electrolytes from the colon.

How is it used?

Sulfasalazine is effective in RA and reduces the rate of appearance of new joint damage. It has been used in juvenile chronic arthritis and ankylosing spondylitis.

What are the adverse effects?

Approximately 30% of patients using sulfasalazine discontinue the drug because of toxicity. Common adverse effects include nausea, vomiting, headache, and rash. Other adverse effects include anemia, **oligospermia** (a subnormal concentration of spermatozoa in the ejaculate), blood dyscrasias, liver injury, and allergic reactions.

What are the contraindications and interactions?

Sulfasalazine is contraindicated in patients with sensitivity to this agent or other sulfonamides and salicylates. It should not be used in patients with agranulocytosis, intestinal and urinary tract obstruction, or porphyria. Sulfasalazine is contraindicated in pregnancy and in children younger than 2 years of age. It should be used cautiously in patients with severe allergy or bronchial asthma, hepatic or renal impairment, and in children younger than the age of 6 years. Antibiotics may alter the absorption of sulfasalazine.

What are the important points patients should know?

Instruct patients that this drug may color the urine and skin orange-yellow. Women should not breastfeed while taking sulfasalazine without consulting their physicians.

✳ Apply Your Knowledge 29.2

The following questions focus on what you have just learned about RA and antirheumatic drugs.

CRITICAL THINKING

1. What is the definition of RA?
2. What are the drugs of choice for the symptomatic relief of RA?
3. What are three generic names of gold compounds for RA?
4. What are the adverse effects of gold compounds?
5. What are DMARDs?
6. What is the mechanism of action of methotrexate?
7. What are the indications of sulfasalazine?
8. What are the contraindications of gold compounds?

Gout and Gouty Arthritis

Several distinct diseases are characterized by crystal deposition in and around joint spaces. This deposition can lead to acute inflammation of the joint. Gout is a metabolic disorder of sodium urate deposition (which involves uric acid crystals) in which uric acid accumulates in the bloodstream or joint cavities, causing inflammation and pain. Gout is classified as primary, secondary, or gouty arthritis. Primary gout is a disease primarily found in men, with a peak incidence in the fifth decade of life.

The cause of gout is either the overproduction or underexcretion of uric acid. Primary gout is generally caused by the overproduction of uric acid and may be caused by enzyme deficiencies in the metabolic pathway for purines or genetic dysfunction. Secondary gout, characterized by underexcretion of uric acid, may be caused by diminished renal function,

interaction with various medications, or unknown causes.

Primary gout has three manifestations: (1) asymptomatic **hyperuricemia** (elevated uric acid blood level), (2) acute gouty arthritis, and (3) chronic gouty arthritis. In acute gouty arthritis, the onset of the attack is abrupt and typically occurs at night or early in the morning as synovial fluid is reabsorbed. In acute gouty arthritis, immobilization of the affected joints—most often the big toes, heels, ankles, wrists, fingers, elbows, or knees—is very important.

DRUGS FOR GOUTY ARTHRITIS

Anti-inflammatory drug therapy should begin immediately, and urate-lowering drugs should not be given until the acute attack has been controlled. Specific drugs include colchicine, allopurinol, NSAIDs, and corticosteroids (Table 29-3 ■).

Table 29-3 ■ Anti-Gout Medications

GENERIC NAME	TRADE NAME	AVERAGE ADULT DOSAGE	ROUTE OF ADMINISTRATION
allopurinol	Aloprim, Zyloprim	200–800 mg/d	PO, IV
colchicine	colchicine (generic only)	0.5–0.6 mg/d prophylactically; 0.5–1.2 mg q1–2 h for acute attack	PO
probenecid	Benemid	250–500 mg bid	PO
sulfinpyrazone	Anturane	100–400 mg/d	PO

bid, twice a day; IV, intravenous; PO, oral.

Focus On

Colchicine

Colchicine is an anti-inflammatory agent specifically used for gout and is ineffective for any other disease. Colchicine is not an analgesic, so it does not relieve the symptoms of any condition but gout.

How does it work?

Colchicine acts by inhibiting the formation of white blood cells, which decreases joint inflammation.

How is it used?

Colchicine may be used to treat acute gouty attacks or to reduce the incidence of attacks in chronic gout.

What are the adverse effects?

The most common adverse effects are GI disturbances, such as nausea, vomiting, diarrhea, and abdominal pain. Colchicine may decrease the intestinal absorption of vitamin B_{12}.

What are the contraindications and interactions?

Colchicine is contraindicated in blood dyscrasias, severe GI conditions, severe renal conditions, severe hepatic conditions, and severe cardiac disease. The use of IV colchicine is contraindicated in patients with renal and hepatic dysfunction. Severe local irritation can result from subcutaneous or intramuscular use. It is also contraindicated during pregnancy, and its safe use in children has not been established.

What are the important points patients should know?

Instruct patients taking colchicine at home to withhold the drug and to report to their physicians any onset of GI symptoms or signs of bone marrow depression (nausea, sore throat, bleeding gums, sore mouth, fever, fatigue, malaise, and unusual bleeding or bruising). Advise patients to keep colchicine on hand at all times to start therapy or to increase dosage—if a physician directs—at the first suggestion of an acute attack. Advise patients to avoid beer, ale, and wine because they may precipitate gouty attack. Women taking colchicine should not breastfeed without consulting their physicians.

Focus on Geriatrics

Colchicine Use in Elderly Patients

Colchicine should be used with care in elderly patients because of the dangers of cardiac, renal, hepatic, and GI diseases.

Focus On

Allopurinol

Allopurinol (Aloprim, Zyloprim) is known as an anti-gout agent because it improves the solubility of uric acid. It is used for chronic gout and will not relieve an attack already started. The drug must be taken regularly for a few months to be effective.

How does it work?

Allopurinol reduces endogenous uric acid by selectively inhibiting the action of xanthine oxidase, the enzyme responsible for converting xanthine derivatives to uric acid (the end product of purine catabolism). Allopurinol has no analgesic, anti-inflammatory, or uricosuric (increasing excretion of uric acid) actions.

How is it used?

Allopurinol is used to control primary hyperuricemia that accompanies severe gout and to prevent possibilities of acute gouty attack.

What are the adverse effects?

Allopurinol may cause drowsiness, headache, dizziness, nausea, vomiting, diarrhea, and abdominal pain. In some cases, this agent may cause hepatotoxicity and renal insufficiency. Allopurinol can produce pruritus and skin rash.

What are the contraindications and interactions?

Allopurinol is contraindicated in patients with hypersensitivity to this agent. Allopurinol is also contraindicated as an initial treatment for acute gouty attacks. This medication should be avoided in children (except in those with hyperuricemia secondary to cancer and chemotherapy). Safety during pregnancy and lactation is not established. Allopurinol should be used cautiously in patients with impaired hepatic or renal function, a history of peptic ulcer, lower GI tract disease, and bone marrow depression.

Drug interaction of allopurinol with alcohol, caffeine, and thiazide diuretics may increase the uric acid level; it may also increase the risk of skin rash if used with ampicillin (Amcill) and amoxicillin (Amoxil). Allopurinol enhances the anticoagulant effect of warfarin (Coumadin).

What are the important points patients should know?

Advise patients to drink enough fluid (at least 3,000 mL, or 3 quarts, per day) to produce a urine output of at least 2,000 mL, or 2 quarts, per day. Instruct patients to report diminishing urine output, cloudy urine, an unusual color or odor of urine, pain or discomfort on urination, and the onset of itching or rash. Tell patients to stop taking allopurinol if a skin rash appears even after 5 or more weeks of therapy. Patients should minimize exposure to ultraviolet light or sunlight and not drive or engage in potentially hazardous activities until their response to this drug is known. This drug should only be taken under constant medical supervision, and women taking allopurinol should not breastfeed without consulting their physicians.

Uricosuric Agents

Probenecid (Benemid) and sulfinpyrazone (Anturane) are uricosuric drugs that are used to decrease the amount of urate in patients with increasingly frequent gouty attacks.

How do they work?

These agents work by competitively inhibiting the renal tubular reabsorption of uric acid, thereby promoting its excretion and reducing serum urate levels.

How are they used?

Uricosuric therapy should be initiated if several acute attacks of gouty arthritis have occurred or when plasma levels of uric acid in patients with gout are so high that tissue damage is almost inevitable.

What are the adverse effects?

Adverse effects of uricosuric agents do not provide a basis for preferring one or the other. Both of these organic acids cause GI irritation, but sulfinpyrazone is more active in this regard. Probenecid is more likely to cause allergic dermatitis, but a rash may appear after the use of either compound. Another adverse effect of using probenecid is **nephrotic syndrome** (a clinical state characterized by edema, various abnormal substances present in the urine, decreased plasma albumin, and usually increased blood cholesterol).

What are the contraindications and interactions?

Uricosuric therapy is contraindicated in patients with blood dyscrasias and uric acid kidney stones. Safety during pregnancy, lactation, and in children younger than 2 years of age is not established. These agents should be used cautiously in patients with a history of peptic ulcer.

Salicylates may decrease uricosuric activity and methotrexate (Folex, Mexate, Rheumatrex) elimination. There is an increased risk of nitrofurantoin (Furadantin) toxicity if used with probenecid or sulfinpyrazone.

What are the important points patients should know?

Advise patients to drink fluids liberally (approximately 3,000 mL per day) to maintain daily urine output of at least 2,000 mL or more. Physicians may advise the restriction of high-purine foods during early therapy until uric acid levels stabilize. Foods high in purine include organ meats (sweetbreads, liver, kidneys), meat extracts, meat soups, and gravy. Instruct patients to avoid alcohol because it may increase serum urate levels. They should be instructed not to stop taking these drugs or to take aspirin or other OTC medications without first consulting their physicians.

Focus Point

Uricosuric Therapy

Urate-lowering drugs should not be started until after the acute attack has completely resolved—a process that takes 2 to 3 weeks.

✳ Apply Your Knowledge 29.3

The following questions focus on what you have just learned about gouty arthritis and its drug therapy.

CRITICAL THINKING

1. What are the definitions of *gout* and *gouty arthritis*?
2. How many types of gout are known?
3. What are the trade names of probenecid, allopurinol, and sulfinpyrazone?
4. What drug is specifically used for gout and what are the most common adverse effects of this agent?
5. What is the mechanism of action of allopurinol?
6. What are examples of uricosuric agents?

Muscle Spasms and Pain

Muscular spasms and pain are often associated with traumatic injuries and **spasticity** (an inability of opposing muscle groups to move in a coordinated manner) from such chronic debilitating disorders as cerebral palsy, strokes, or head and spinal cord injuries. Muscle spasms can also be caused by an overmedication of antipsychotic drugs, epilepsy, and hypocalcemia. The transmission of impulses from motor nerves to muscle cells occurs across spaces known as *neuromuscular junctions*. These spaces are sensitive to chemical changes in their immediate environment. Therefore, somatic motor nerve impulses cannot be generated, which may also decrease the availability of calcium ions to the myofibrillar contractile system.

There are two types of muscle spasms: *tonic* and *clonic* spasms. Whereas a single, prolonged contraction is called a *tonic spasm*, multiple, rapidly repeated contractions are known as *clonic spasms*. Most muscle spasms and strains are self-limited and respond to rest, physical therapy, and the short-term use of aspirin and other analgesics.

SKELETAL MUSCLE RELAXANTS

The treatment of muscle spasms may be nonpharmacologic and pharmacologic (muscle relaxants). Nonpharmacologic treatments include the immobilization of the affected muscle, the application of heat or cold, ultrasonography, hydrotherapy, and massage. Local anesthesia may also effect the relaxation of limited muscle groups, and the local anesthetic block of efferent somatic motor outflow is sometimes used to relieve localized skeletal muscle spasms.

Spasticity results from increased muscle tone caused by hyperexcitable neurons or a lack of inhibition in the spinal cord (or at the skeletal muscles). Many neurologic disorders that cause spasticity require the long-term use of muscle relaxants. The skeletal muscles are voluntary muscles under control of the central nervous system (CNS). Skeletal muscle relaxants work by blocking somatic motor nerve impulses through the depression of specific neurons within the CNS.

Focus On

Centrally Acting Muscle Relaxants

These agents, such as baclofen (Lioresal), cyclobenzaprine (Flexeril), and lorazepam (Ativan), relieve symptoms of muscular stiffness and rigidity. Centrally acting muscle relaxants improve the mobility of the part of the body that is affected. Pharmacotherapy for muscle spasms can be a combination of analgesics, anti-inflammatory medications, and centrally acting skeletal muscle relaxants. The centrally acting muscle relaxants are listed in Table 29-4 ■.

How do they work?

The exact mechanism of action of these agents is unknown, but they may affect the brain or spinal cord to inhibit upper motor neuron activity.

How are they used?

Skeletal muscle relaxants are used to treat local spasms to reduce pain and increase range of motion. Baclofen (Lioresal) is often a drug of first choice because of its wide safety margin.

What are the adverse effects?

All the centrally acting agents can cause sedation. Common adverse effects include drowsiness, dizziness, weakness, and fatigue. Tizanidine (Zanaflex) and other centrally acting agents may cause hallucinations or *ataxia* (loss of coordination, such as that caused by benzodiazepines).

What are the contraindications and interactions?

Baclofen (Lioresal) is contraindicated in patients with bacteremia (the presence of viable bacteria in circulating blood) and clotting disorders. Carisoprodol (Soma) should be avoided in patients with acute intermittent porphyria and in children younger than age 5 years. Clonazepam (Klonopin) is contraindicated in patients with liver disease and glaucoma. None of the centrally acting muscle relaxants should be used during pregnancy and lactation.

Centrally acting muscle relaxants, such as baclofen, should not be used with alcohol and other CNS depressants, monamine oxidase inhibitors, and antihistamines. Baclofen may increase blood glucose levels, making it necessary to increase the dosages of sulfonylureas and insulin.

What are the important points patients should know?

Instruct patients to avoid consuming alcoholic beverages and other CNS depressants because this combination will potentiate CNS depression. Incidence of CNS symptoms are reportedly high in patients older than 40 years. Advise patients with diabetes to closely monitor their blood glucose for loss of glycemic control. Patients should avoid driving and using heavy machinery until the effect is stabilized because these drugs are prone to cause drowsiness and dizziness. Tell patients to report all adverse reactions to their physicians. Instruct patients not to self-dose with OTC drugs without their physicians' approval. These drugs should not be stopped abruptly, and the stopping of these drugs should be directed by a physician. Instruct female patients that these drugs should not be taken during pregnancy or while breastfeeding.

Table 29-4 ■ Centrally Acting Muscle Relaxants

GENERIC NAME	TRADE NAME	AVERAGE ADULT DOSAGE	ROUTE OF ADMINISTRATION
baclofen	Lioresal	15–80 mg/d in divided doses	PO
carisoprodol	Soma	350 mg tid–qid	PO
chlorphenesin carbamate	Maolate	400–800 mg/d in divided doses	PO
chlorzoxazone	Paraflex, Parafon	250–750 mg tid–qid	PO
clonazepam	Klonopin	0.5–20 mg tid	PO
cyclobenzaprine	Flexeril	10–60 mg/d in divided doses	PO

(continued)

Table 29-4 ■ Centrally Acting Muscle Relaxants (*continued*)

GENERIC NAME	TRADE NAME	AVERAGE ADULT DOSAGE	ROUTE OF ADMINISTRATION
dantrolene	Dantrium	Initially, 25 mg/d and then 50–400 mg/d in divided doses	PO
diazepam	Valium	2–10 mg bid–qid	PO
		2–10 mg	IM, IV
lorazepam	Ativan	1–10 mg bid–tid	PO
methocarbamol	Robaxin	1.5 g qid for 2–3 d and then 4–4.5 g/d in 3–6 divided doses	PO
		0.5–1 g q8h	IM
		1–3 g/d in div. doses (maximum: rate of 300 mg/min)	IV
orphenadrine citrate	Banflex, Norflex	100 mg bid	PO
		60 mg bid	IM, IV

bid, twice a day; IM, intramuscular; IV, intravenous; PO, oral; qid, four times a day; tid, three times a day.

Focus Point

Baclofen

Baclofen (Lioresal) is at least as effective as diazepam (Valium) in reducing spasticity and produces much less sedation.

✳ Apply Your Knowledge 29.4

The following questions focus on what you have just learned about skeletal muscle relaxants and centrally acting muscle relaxants.

CRITICAL THINKING

1. What are neuromuscular junctions?
2. How many types of muscle spasms are known?
3. What are the nonpharmacologic treatments for muscle relaxants?
4. What is the drug of first choice of the centrally acting muscle relaxants?
5. What are the trade names of lorazepam, baclofen, methocarbamol, and dantrolene?

PRACTICAL SCENARIO 1

Leonora, a slightly built 73-year-old woman, visits her long-time family physician complaining of low-grade but constant back pain. The nurse's examination finds that her weight has remained consistent over time but that she has lost almost 2 inches in height in the past 10 years. Reviewing her chart, the doctor notes that Leonora has been postmenopausal for more than 25 years, declined to take hormone replacement therapy, and broke her ankle 2 years ago after stepping off a curb into the street. Physical examination shows kyphosis (humpback). The physician orders a dual-emission X-ray absorptiometry scan to measure bone density but tells Leonora that even without the results of the scan, she is quite sure that the osteopenia most people experience as they get older has, in this case, degenerated into osteoporosis.

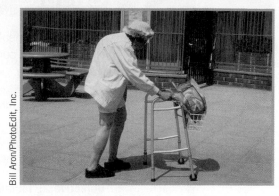

Bill Aron/PhotoEdit, Inc.

Critical Thinking Questions

1. What is the significance of the fact that Leonora has been postmenopausal for many years?
2. What is the difference between osteopenia and osteoporosis and why does one lead to a reduction in height in patients?
3. Would drug therapy or lifestyle changes work best for Leonora in managing her osteoporosis?

PRACTICAL SCENARIO 2

A 56-year-old postmenopausal woman was diagnosed with osteoporosis. Her physician prescribed bisphosphonates.

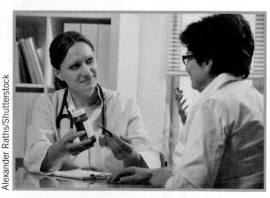

Alexander Raths/Shutterstock

Critical Thinking Questions

1. Explain several new bisphosphonates analogs that are now available.
2. Explain the common adverse effects of bisphosphonates.

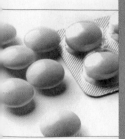

Chapter Capsule

This section repeats the objectives from the beginning of the chapter and then provides the most important concept for that objective. Use this section as a quick review and to check your knowledge.

Objective 1: Describe the major functions of the skeletal system.

- Support, storage of minerals and lipids, blood cell production, protection, and leverage

Objective 2: Identify the most common bisphosphonate agents used for osteoporosis.

- Alendronate (Fosamax)—first oral bisphosphonate approved for treatment and prevention of osteoporosis in postmenopausal women
- Risedronate (Actonel)

Objective 3: Define *rheumatoid arthritis*.

- Systemic autoimmune disease; involves inflammation of the membranes lining the joints; often affects internal organs
- A chronic fluctuating course of disease that can result in progressive joint destruction, deformity, and disability
- Occurs two to three times more often in women; peak onset is between the fourth and sixth decades of life

Objective 4: List the major drugs used for rheumatoid arthritis.

- Treatment of symptoms—drugs with anti-inflammatory activity, such as salicylates, nonsteroidal anti-inflammatory drugs (NSAIDs), and cyclooxygenase 2 (COX-2) inhibitors; corticosteroids have excellent anti-inflammatory activity and are immunosuppressants
- Treatment to prevent joint damage and preserve joint function—disease-modifying antirheumatic drugs (DMARDs), such as methotrexate (Folex, Mexate), sulfasalazine (Azulfidine), etanercept (Enbrel), and adalimumab (Humira)

Objective 5: Describe the major indications of methotrexate.

- Principally used in combination regimens to maintain induced remissions in neoplastic diseases; also used to treat severe psoriasis, psoriatic arthritis, and rheumatoid arthritis

Objective 6: Explain gouty arthritis and the cause of gout.

- Disorder of sodium urate deposition (which involves uric acid crystals) characterized by crystal deposition in and about joint spaces, which can lead to acute inflammation of the joint
- Primarily a disease found in men, with a peak incidence in the fifth decade of life
- Caused by either an overproduction or underexcretion of uric acid
- Primary gout has three manifestations: asymptomatic hyperuricemia, acute gouty arthritis, and chronic gouty arthritis
- The onset of *acute gouty arthritis* is abrupt, typically occurring at night or early in the morning as synovial fluid is reabsorbed

Objective 7: Describe the mechanism of action for colchicine.

■ Inhibits the formation of white blood cells to decrease joint inflammation

Objective 8: Explain the indications of allopurinol.

■ Used to control primary hyperuricemia (high levels of uric acid in the blood circulation) that accompanies severe gout and to prevent acute gouty attack

Objective 9: Name three disorders that may cause spasticity.

■ Cerebral palsy
■ Stroke
■ Head or spinal cord injuries

Objective 10: List commonly used central skeletal muscle relaxants.

■ baclofen (Lioresal)
■ carisoprodol (Soma)
■ chlorphenesin carbamate (Maolate)
■ chlorzoxazone (Paraflex, Parafon)
■ clonazepam (Klonopin)
■ cyclobenzaprine (Flexeril)
■ dantrolene (Dantrium)
■ diazepam (Valium)
■ lorazepam (Ativan)
■ methocarbamol (Robaxin)
■ orphenadrine citrate (Banflex, Norflex)

Internet Sites of Interest

■ The National Institute of Neurological Disorders and Stroke, a division of the NIH, provides information about spasticity and its treatments at **http://www.ninds.nih.gov**. Search for "spasticity."

■ MedicineNet.com provides an in-depth look at rheumatoid arthritis at **http://www.medicinenet.com**. Search for "rheumatoid arthritis."

■ Johns Hopkins University's, Division of Rheumatology offers a comprehensive discussion about treatments for rheumatoid arthritis at **http://www.hopkinsmedicine.org/patient_care_conditions_treatments.html**. Click on Rheumatology.

■ For more information about the rheumatoid arthritis drug methotrexate (Folex, Mexate, Rheumatrex) visit **http://www.rxlist.com/trexall-drug.htm**. Click "methotrexate."

myhealthprofessionskit™

Go to www.myhealthprofessionskit.com to access the Companion Website created for this textbook. Simply select "Basic Health Science" from the choice of disciplines. Find this book and then log in using your username and password to access interactive learning games, assessment questions, animations, and more.

Chapter 30

Drugs Used to Treat Eye Conditions

Chapter Objectives

After completing this chapter, you should be able to:

1. Describe the structure and function of the eye.
2. Explain glaucoma and the types of glaucoma.
3. State the rationale for the use and the mechanism of action for carbonic anhydrase inhibitors in the treatment of glaucoma.
4. Identify direct-acting miotics (cholinergic drugs) and list two generic and trade names.
5. Explain mydriatic agents and their indications.
6. State the mechanism of action of antimuscarinics.

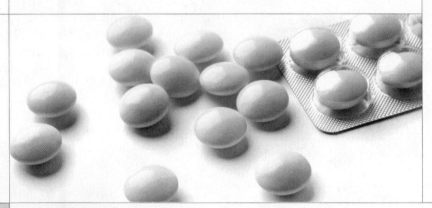

Key Terms

accommodation (page 533)

aqueous humor (AY–kwee–us) (page 533)

blepharitis (blef-fah-RY-tis) (page 541)

cataract (page 534)

choroid layer (KO-royd) (page 533)

ciliary body (SIL-ee-ayr-ee) (page 533)

ciliary muscle (page 533)

cornea (page 533)

glaucoma (glauw-KO-ma) (page 534)

iris (page 533)

lens (page 533)

optic nerve (page 533)

photoreceptors (page 534)

pupil (page 533)

retina (page 534)

retinal detachment (page 538)

retinopathy (ret-tin-NOP-pa-thee) (page 534)

sclera (page 533)

vitreous humor (VIT-ree-us) (page 534)

Introduction

A number of the key drug groups mentioned elsewhere in the text are used in ophthalmology. Such drug groups as antimicrobials, corticosteroids, adrenergic drugs, muscarinic drugs, and nonsteroidal anti-inflammatory drugs (NSAIDs) have ophthalmic indications. In this chapter, the effects of these drugs on the eye are emphasized.

Structure and Function of the Eye

The eye is a hollow, spherical structure about 2.5 cm in diameter. Its wall has three distinct layers. These layers consist of an outer layer (**sclera**), a middle layer (**choroid layer** or "coat"), and an inner layer (retina). The spaces within the eye are filled with fluids that support its wall and internal parts.

The anterior of the sclera bulges forward as the transparent **cornea**—the window of the eye—and helps to focus entering light rays. Along the circumference, the cornea is continuous with the sclera (the white portion of the eye). In the back of the eye, the **optic nerve** and certain blood vessels pierce the sclera.

The middle layer includes the choroid layer, ciliary body, and iris (Figure 30-1 ■). The choroid layer contains many pigment-producing melanocytes. The melanin that these cells produce absorbs excess light and helps to keep the inside of the eye dark.

The **ciliary body**, which is the thickest part of the middle layer, extends forward from the choroid layer and forms an internal ring around the front of the eye, which constitutes the **ciliary muscle**. Many strong but delicate fibers, called *suspensory ligaments*, extend inward from the ciliary processes and hold the transparent **lens** in position. The distal ends of these fibers attach along the margin of a thin capsule that surrounds the lens. The ciliary muscles and suspensory ligaments, along with the structure of the lens itself, enable the lens to adjust its shape to facilitate focusing—a phenomenon called **accommodation**. The functions of the ciliary body are controlled by the parasympathetic nervous system. The uveal tract of the eye consists of the iris, ciliary body, and choroid.

The **iris** is a thin diaphragm composed mostly of connective tissue and smooth muscle fibers. From the outside, the iris is the colored portion of the eye. The ciliary body secretes a watery fluid called **aqueous humor** into the posterior chamber. The iris extends forward from the periphery of the ciliary body and lies between the cornea and lens (see Figure 30-1 ■). The fluid circulates from this chamber through the **pupil**—a circular opening in the center of the iris—and into the anterior chamber. Aqueous humor fills the space between the cornea and lens, helps nourish these parts, and aids in maintaining the shape of the front of the eye. It subsequently leaves the anterior chamber through veins and a special drainage canal—the scleral venous sinus (Schlemm canal)—located in its wall at the junction of the cornea and the sclera. The iris consists of circular and radially arranged bands of smooth muscle, innervated by the autonomic nervous system, that control the size of the pupil. The autonomic nervous system plays an important part in the regulation

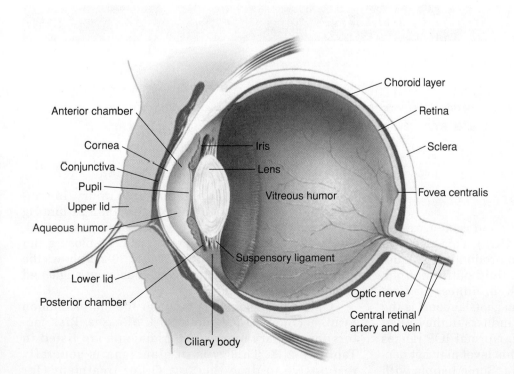

Figure 30-1 ■ Anatomy of the eye.

Table 30-1 ■ Effects of Autonomic Nervous System on the Eye

PARTS OF THE EYE	EFFECTS OF SYMPATHETIC STIMULATION	EFFECTS OF PARASYMPATHETIC STIMULATION
Ciliary muscle	Relaxation (for far vision)	Accommodation
Ciliary processes	Vasoconstriction of ciliary processes increases aqueous humor production	Increased outflow of aqueous humor and vasodilation
Iris	Contraction of the radial muscle: pupil dilation (mydriasis)	Contraction of the circular muscle: pupil constriction (miosis)
Conjunctival vasculature	Vasoconstriction	Vasodilation
Lacrimal apparatus	Vasoconstriction	Increased secretion and vasodilation

of eye functions. Such structures as the iris, ciliary body, lens, lacrimal glands, and ocular vasculature receive autonomic innervation. The effects of this stimulation are summarized in Table 30-1 ■.

The inner layer consists of the **retina**, which contains the visual receptor cells (**photoreceptors**). This layer is continuous with the optic nerve in the back of the eye and extends forward on the inner layer of the eyeball.

The space bounded by the lens, ciliary body, and retina is the largest compartment of the eye and is called the *posterior cavity*. It is filled with a transparent, jelly-like fluid called **vitreous humor**. The vitreous body supports the internal parts of the eye and helps maintain its shape.

Disorders of the Eye

The eyes are subject to various disorders—some of which are serious. These disorders may include inflammation, infections, injuries, glaucoma, **cataract** (an opacity of the lens of the eye), and diabetic **retinopathy** (degeneration of the blood vessels of the retina). One of the most common and serious disorders of the eye is glaucoma, for which treatment usually begins with medication. Therefore, in this chapter, most emphasis will be on drugs used in treatment of glaucoma. The other disorders or conditions of the eye that are initially treated with lasers or surgery are not discussed here. Anti-inflammatory drugs and antibiotics are explained in other chapters.

Focus on Pediatrics

Congenital Cataracts

Congenital cataracts may result from chromosomal abnormalities and maternal diseases during pregnancy. If the cataracts are dense and obscure the view of the optic disk, an ophthalmologist must determine the possible long-term effects on the infant's vision and surgery may be recommended.

Glaucoma

Glaucoma damages the optic nerve and is often caused by elevated intraocular pressure (IOP). This elevation of the IOP results from excessive production of aqueous humor or diminished ocular fluid outflow. When the pressure is persistently high, blindness may occur secondary to optic nerve damage. Glaucoma is the second-most common cause of blindness in the United States (cataract is number one). Normal IOP ranges from 11 to 21 mm Hg; however, this level may not necessarily be healthy for all people. Some people with

normal pressure develop optic nerve injury. In contrast, many patients have IOP of more than 21 mm Hg without any optic nerve injury (ocular hypertension). The two types of glaucoma are acute angle-closure and chronic open-angle glaucoma. Figure 30-2 ■ shows the normal condition of the eye as well as open-angle and angle-closure glaucoma.

Open-angle glaucoma is by far the more common form, accounting for about 90% of cases. Risk factors for primary open-angle glaucoma are listed in Table 30-2 ■. This type of glaucoma is generally responsive to drug therapy. Other treatments for

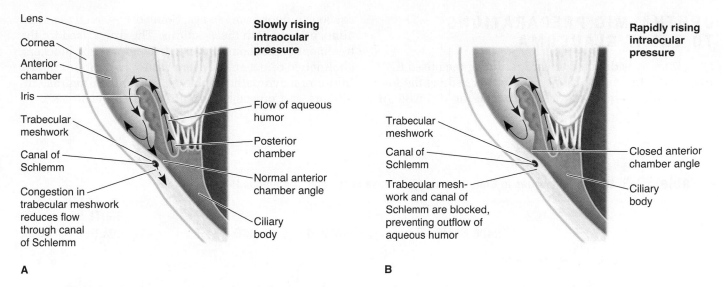

Figure 30-2 ■ The pathophysiology of glaucoma: slowing rising intraocular pressure (IOP) (**A**) and rapidly rising IOP (**B**).

Table 30-2 ■ Risk Factors for Primary Open-Angle Glaucoma

Elevated intraocular pressure	Diabetes
Older age	Hypertension
Family history	Myopia
Black race	Use of corticosteroids

open-angle glaucoma may include lasers or surgery. Most of the drugs used in the treatment of open-angle glaucoma are also used in the acute management of narrow-angle glaucoma before surgery.

Angle-closure glaucoma accounts for 10% of all glaucomas in the United States. Angle-closure glaucoma can be primary caused by pupillary block. It is most common among Eskimos and Asians. Primary angle closure is more common in women, elderly patients, and patients with a family history of angle-closure glaucoma.

Focus on Geriatrics

Glaucoma in Elderly Adults

Although glaucoma can occur in any age group, it is six times more common in persons older than 60 years of age.

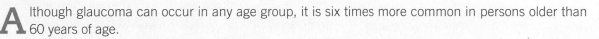

✳ Apply Your Knowledge 30.1

The following questions focus on what you have just learned about the structure and functions of the eye.

CRITICAL THINKING

1. What are the three layers of the eye?
2. Which layer of the eye contains the ciliary body?
3. What is the meaning of *accommodation*?
4. What are the iris and pupil?
5. Where is the location of the photoreceptors in the eye?
6. What is diabetic retinopathy?
7. How many types of glaucoma exist and which type is more common in women and elderly patients?
8. What are the risk factors for primary glaucoma?

OPHTHALMIC PREPARATIONS TO TREAT GLAUCOMA

Drug therapy is directed toward reducing the raised IOP. In general, the medications used either reduce the formation of aqueous humor or enhance the drainage of aqueous humor from the eye. Some drugs, such as adrenaline, possess both these actions. The drugs used for the treatment of glaucoma include beta-adrenergic blockers, cholinergic direct-acting agents (miotics), cholinesterase inhibitors, sympathomimetics, carbonic anhydrase inhibitors, and prostaglandin inhibitors (Table 30-3 ■).

Table 30-3 ■ Drug Therapies in Glaucoma that Decrease Formation of Aqueous Humor

GENERIC NAME	TRADE NAME	AVERAGE ADULT DOSAGE	ROUTE OF ADMINISTRATION
Beta-Adrenergic Blocking Agents			
betaxolol	Betoptic, Kerlone	1 drop 0.5% solution bid	Topical
carteolol	Ocupress	1 drop 1% solution bid	Topical
levobunolol	Betagan	1–2 drops 0.25–0.5% solution 1–2 times/d	Topical
metipranolol	OptiPranolol	1 drop 0.3% solution bid	Topical
timolol	Betimol, Timoptic	1–2 drops of 0.25–0.5% solution 1–2 times/d	Topical
Alpha$_2$–Adrenergic Blocking Agents			
apraclonidine	Lopidine	1 drop 0.5% solution bid	Topical
brimonidine tartrate	Alphagan P	1 drop 0.2% solution bid	Topical
Carbonic Anhydrase Inhibitors			
acetazolamide	Diamox	250 mg 1–4 times/d	PO
dichlorphenamide	Daranide, Oratrol	100–200 mg, followed by 100 mg bid	PO
dorzolamide hydrochloride	Trusopt	1 drop 2% solution tid	PO
methazolamide	Neptazane	50–100 mg bid–tid	PO
Osmotic Diuretics			
glycerine anhydrous	Ophthalgan	1–1.8 g/kg 1–1.5 h before ocular surgery; may repeat q5h	PO
isosorbide	Ismotic	1–3 g/kg bid–qid	PO
mannitol	Osmitrol	1.5–2 mg/kg as a 15–25% solution over 30–60 min	IV

bid, twice a day; IV, intravenous; PO, oral; qid, four times a day; tid, three times a day.

Focus On

Beta-Adrenergic Blockers

Beta-blocker agents are relatively safe, highly efficacious, act longer than the cholinergic agonists, and have no effects on pupil size or accommodation.

How do they work?

Beta-blockers lower the cyclic adenosine monophosphate (cAMP) levels within the ciliary body necessary for aqueous humor production. This reduces elevated IOP in chronic open-angle glaucoma by reducing the formation of aqueous humor.

How are they used?

The beta-blockers are considered the drugs of first choice in the treatment of intraocular hypertension and chronic open-angle glaucoma.

What are the adverse effects?

The most common adverse effects are local, mild ocular stinging; dry eyes; tearing; blurred vision; and eye irritation. Beta-adrenergic blockers may also have the adverse effects of systemic beta-blockers. These agents may mask symptoms of acute hypoglycemia in patients with diabetes (tachycardia and tremor but not sweating).

Beta-adrenergic blockers may precipitate thyrotoxic crisis in patients with hyperthyroidism.

What are the contraindications and interactions?

Beta-adrenergic blockers are contraindicated in patients with angle-closure glaucoma (unless used with a miotic), sinus bradycardia, and cardiogenic shock. Safety during pregnancy and in children younger than 18 years of age is not established. These drugs should be used cautiously in patients with heart failure or diabetes mellitus, in those who have evidence of airflow obstruction, and during lactation.

Reserpine (Serpalan) may interact with beta-blockers and cause addictive hypotensive effects or bradycardia. Verapamil (Calan) may cause addictive heart block.

What are the important points patients should know?

Advise patients to report unusual or significant changes in pulse rate to their physicians, according to the parameters provided. Instruct patients to follow their dosing regimen exactly as prescribed. They should not stop these drugs abruptly. Instruct patients to report difficulty in breathing promptly to their physicians because the drug may need to be withdrawn.

Carbonic Anhydrase Inhibitors

Carbonic anhydrase inhibitors are diuretic agents, but they are also available as eye preparations.

How do they work?

Carbonic anhydrase inhibitors act on the enzyme responsible for the conversion of carbon dioxide to bicarbonate and hydrogen ions. The mechanism of action of this group (in glaucoma) is different from that described for the kidneys in Chapter 24. In the eye, carbonic anhydrase plays a significant role in aqueous humor formation by the ciliary body cells. In the ciliary bodies, carbonic anhydrase facilitates the secretion of bicarbonate ions in the aqueous humor. Carbonic anhydrase inhibitors therefore decrease the formation of aqueous humor.

How are they used?

Glaucoma has become the main clinical indication for the carbonic anhydrase inhibitors. Most of these drugs must be administered systemically. Dorzolamide (Trusopt) is available in a topical preparation.

What are the adverse effects?

The carbonic anhydrase inhibitors are closely related to the sulfanilamide antibacterial agents. As such, they produce a similar profile of adverse effects, including skin rashes, kidney stones, and aplastic anemia. Other adverse effects associated with this group are depression, anorexia, and electrolyte imbalances (especially potassium).

What are the contraindications and interactions?

Carbonic anhydrase inhibitors are contraindicated in patients with chronic noncongestive angle-closure glaucoma. These drugs should be avoided in patients with hypersensitivity and marked renal or hepatic dysfunction. Safety during pregnancy or lactation is not established. Carbonic anhydrase inhibitors should be used cautiously in patients with a history of hypercalciuria, diabetes mellitus, gout, and asthma. These drugs may interact with amphetamines, ephedrine (Efedron), and procainamide (Procan) to decrease renal excretion.

(Continued)

Focus On (*Continued*)

What are the important points patients should know?

Instruct patients to avoid touching the eye with the tip of the drug dispenser. Tell them to discontinue the drug and report to their physicians if ocular irritations, infections, or systemic hypersensitivity occurs. Be sure to advise patients that some of these drugs may cause drowsiness and that they should avoid hazardous activities until the response to drugs is known. If patients are using oral medications (acetazolamide), they should report numbness, tingling, burning, drowsiness, visual problems, sore throat, fever, and renal problems. Advise them to eat potassium-rich foods and take potassium supplements while taking acetazolamide in high doses or for prolonged periods.

Focus on Natural Products

Bilberry for Eye Health

The berries, roots, and leaves of the bilberry plant have been used to improve night vision; to prevent cataracts, macular degeneration, and glaucoma; and to prevent and treat diabetic retinopathy and myopia. However, bilberry should be avoided during pregnancy and lactation and may cause constipation if large amounts of the dried fruit are consumed. Higher-than-recommended doses of this herb for extended periods will result in toxicity and may even result in death.

Osmotic Diuretics

Osmotic diuretic drugs are commonly used in patients needing eye surgery or for acute closed-angle glaucoma. These agents include glycerin anhydrous (Ophthalgan), isosorbide (Ismo), and mannitol (Osmitrol). The osmotic diuretics are discussed in Chapter 24.

Focus On

Direct-Acting Miotics (Cholinergic Agents)

Miotic muscarine agonists (Table 30-4 ■) are agents that constrict the pupils. Miotics are often used to treat glaucoma.

How do they work?

Miotic agents act primarily to increase the drainage of aqueous humor out of the anterior cavity through the canal of Schlemm. They achieve this effect through miosis (pupil constriction) and contraction of the ciliary muscles responsible for accommodation. These effects are mediated by the parasympathetic nervous system.

How are they used?

The muscarinic agonists are used in open-angle and angle-closure glaucoma. Examples of muscarinics include acetylcholine chloride, pilocarpine (Adsorbocarpine), and carbachol (Miostat).

What are the adverse effects?

Systemic adverse effects of topical muscarinic agonists are few, with headache being the most common. The most common adverse effect of the muscarinic agonists on the eye is pupil constriction.

What are the contraindications and interactions?

Cholinergic agents (miotics) are contraindicated in patients with hypersensitivity, contact allergy, cataract, **retinal detachment** (separation of the retina from the corneal layer), and depression. Cholinergic drugs may interact with monamine oxidase inhibitors (MAOIs) and cause an increased risk of hypertensive emergency. They may increase the effects of beta-blockers and other antihypertensives on blood pressure and heart rate.

What are the important points patients should know?

Advise patients to use caution during nighttime driving and in performing hazardous activities in poor light. Instruct them to report to their physicians if any sensitivity or severe adverse drug reactions occur.

Table 30-4 ■ Drug Therapy in Glaucoma that Increases the Outflow of Aqueous Humor

GENERIC NAME	TRADE NAME	AVERAGE ADULT DOSAGE	ROUTE OF ADMINISTRATION
Direct-Acting Miotics (Cholinergic Agents)			
carbachol	Isopto Carboptic, Miostat	1–2 drops 0.75%–3% solution q4h–tid	Topical
pilocarpine hydrochloride	Isopto Carpine Miocarpine	1 drop of 1% solution in affected eye	Topical
Indirect-Acting Miotics (Cholinesterase Inhibitors)			
demecarium bromide	Humorsol	1–2 drops of 0.125%–0.25% solution 2 times/wk	Topical
physostigmine salicylate	Antilirium	1 drop of 0.25%–0.5% solution 1–4 times/d	Topical
Sympathomimetics			
dipivefrin hydrochloride	Propine	1 drop in eye q12h	Topical
epinephrine borate	Epinal	1–2 drops as needed	Topical
phenylephrine hydrochloride	Neo-Synephrine	1 drop of 2.5% or 10% solution before examination	Topical
Prostaglandins and Prostamides			
bimatoprost	Lumigan	1 drop of 0.03% solution daily in the evening	Topical
latanoprost	Xalatan	1 drop of 1.5-mg solution daily in the evening	Topical
travoprost	Travatan	1 drop in affected eye(s) once daily in the evening	Topical
unoprostone	Rescula	1 drop of 0.15% solution bid	Topical

bid, twice a day; tid, three times a day.

Focus On

Indirect-Acting Miotics (Cholinesterase Inhibitors)

The cholinesterase inhibitors are more potent and longer acting than the direct-acting miotic agents.

How do they work?

The cholinesterase inhibitors produce severe miosis and muscle contractions. These actions cause a decreased resistance to aqueous outflow.

How are they used?

The cholinesterase inhibitors are used to treat open-angle glaucoma. Examples of this group include demecarium (Humorsol) and physostigmine (Antilirium).

What are the adverse effects?

Ophthalmic-related adverse effects of cholinesterase inhibitors include lacrimation, burning conjunctivitis, retinal detachment, and conjunctival thickening. Systematic adverse effects are nausea, vomiting, diarrhea, abdominal cramps, difficulty breathing, urinary incontinence, salivation, and fainting.

What are the contraindications and interactions?

Cholinesterase inhibitors are contraindicated in patients with hypersensitivity to these agents. The drugs are also contraindicated in patients with any acute inflammatory disorders

(Continued)

Focus On (Continued)

of the eye and during pregnancy and lactation. The cholinesterase inhibitors should be used cautiously in patients with chronic angle-closure glaucoma and in patients with myasthenia gravis. Drug interactions occur with carbachol (Miostat), beta-blockers, atropine (Atropisol), ipratropium (Atrovent), and echothiophate (Phospholine Iodide).

What are the important points patients should know?

Instruct patients that aching around the eyebrows or temporary burning or stinging may occur initially but usually disappears as the body adjusts to the medication. Vision may be temporarily blurred or unstable after applying eye drops. Advise patients to use caution if driving and performing duties requiring clear vision. Because the medication may cause sensitivity to bright light, instruct patients to wear sunglasses. Advise patients to inform their physicians about changes in vision, eye pain, sweating, nausea, vomiting, diarrhea, difficulty breathing, increased urination or salivation, or irregular heartbeat.

Focus Point

Eye Protection and Insecticides and Pesticides

Individuals working with insecticides or pesticides that contain organophosphate or carbonate and who are using cholinesterase inhibitors must wear respiratory masks, change their clothes frequently, and wash exposed clothes thoroughly.

Focus On

Sympathomimetic Agents

Sympathomimetics have both alpha- and beta-adrenergic activity (see Chapter 18). Apraclonidine (Iopidine) and brimonidine (Alphagan P) are relatively selective alpha$_2$ agonists. Dipivefrin (Propine) and phenylephrine (AK-Dilate Ophthalmic) are beta-adrenergic agonists.

How do they act?

The sympathomimetics can decrease the formation of aqueous humor and increase its outflow by activating adrenoreceptors associated with the ciliary body.

How are they used?

The sympathomimetic drugs we have listed can be used in the management of glaucoma.

What are the adverse effects?

Common adverse effects of dipivefrine and phenylephrine include headache, blurred vision, a stinging sensation during instillation, and increased sensitivity to light. *Rebound nasal congestion* (hyperemia and edema of mucosa), nasal burning, and sneezing may also occur. Other adverse effects of sympathomimetics include palpitation, tachycardia, bradycardia (overdosage), extrasytoles, hypertension, sweating, sleeplessness, anxiety, and dizziness.

What are the contraindications and interactions?

Sympathomimetic agents are contraindicated in patients with hypersensitivity to these drugs and in patients with severe coronary disease, severe hypertension, angle-closure glaucoma (ophthalmic preparations), pregnancy, and lactation. Ophthalmic solution (10%) of dipivefrin (Propine) and phenylephrine (AK-Dilate Ophthalmic) should be used cautiously in cardiovascular disease, diabetes mellitus, hyperthyroidism, hypertension, pregnancy, elderly patients, and infants. Epinephrine (Bronkaid Mist) should not be used while wearing soft lenses because discoloration of the lenses may occur. There are no known drug interactions with ophthalmic preparations. Dobutamine (Dobutrex) may increase the risk of hypertension when it is given along with beta-adrenergic blockers. The effects of dopamine (Dopastat) may be increased when given with a tricyclic antidepressant (TCA) or MAOI. Epinephrine may interact with a TCA and cause an increased risk of sympathomimetic effects. Excessive hypertension may occur when epinephrine is used with propranolol (Inderal).

What are the important points patients should know?

Patients should be aware that the instillation of 2.5% to 10% strength ophthalmic solution can cause burning and stinging. Instruct them to not exceed the recommended dosage regardless of formulation. Tell patients that systemic absorption from nasal and conjunctival membranes could occur. Instruct patients to discontinue the drug and report to their physicians if adverse effects occur and to wear sunglasses in bright light because the pupils will be large and the eyes may be more sensitive to light than usual. Advise patients that some ophthalmic solutions may stain contact lenses.

Focus Point

Eye Drops and Contact Lenses

Patients with contact lenses must remove them and leave them out for at least 15 minutes after the administration of eye drop preparations.

Focus On

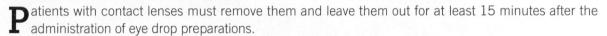

Prostaglandin Agonists

Research has shown that prostaglandins also have a role in the movement of aqueous humor through the eye.

How do they work?

Prostaglandin agonist agents increase aqueous humor outflow by reducing congestion in the trabecular meshwork, resulting in lowered IOP.

How are they used?

Prostaglandin agonists are used in the treatment of open-angle glaucoma and intraocular hypertension to lower IOP. Travoprost (Travatan) can be used as first-line monotherapy or in combination with timolol.

What are the adverse effects?

The ocular adverse effects of prostaglandin agonists include ocular dryness, visual disturbance, ocular burning, foreign body sensation, eye pain, pigmentation of the periocular skin, **blepharitis** (inflammation of one or both eyes), cataract, ocular irritation, eye discharge, tearing, increase pigmentation of the iris, and photophobia.

What are the contraindications and interactions?

Prostaglandin agonists should be avoided in patients with hypersensitivity and during pregnancy. These agents are to be used cautiously in patients with active intraocular inflammation, those wearing contact lenses, and in lactating women. These agents may interact with thimerosal (Mersol) and other topical ophthalmic drugs.

What are the important points patients should know?

Instruct patients, especially those with green eyes, of a possible change in iris pigmentation, which is an irreversible condition.

Focus Point

Allergic Blepharoconjunctivitis

Apraclonidine (Iopidine) should be used only for the short term for lowering IOP because with chronic use, it is associated with allergic blepharoconjunctivitis.

Apply Your Knowledge 30.2

The following questions focus on what you have just learned about the treatment of glaucoma.

CRITICAL THINKING

1. What are the trade names of acetazolamide, methazolamide, mannitol, cartelol, and apraclonidine?
2. Why are beta-blockers better than cholinergic agonists?
3. When are osmotic diuretics commonly used for eye disorders?
4. What are three examples of muscarinic agonists?
5. What is the mechanism of action of cholinesterase inhibitors?
6. What are three trade names of sympathomimetics used in glaucoma?
7. What are the indications of prostaglandin agonists?
8. What are the trade names of bimatoprost, pilocarpine, and phenylephrine?

DRUG THERAPY FOR MINOR EYE CONDITIONS

There is a broad range of agents indicated for eye examinations, minor irritations, and injury. These drugs include antimicrobials, local anesthetics, and anti-inflammatories. Antimicrobials and anti-inflammatory drugs are discussed in Chapters 12, 13, and 15. Some drugs, including mydriatic drugs and cycloplegic agents, are used for ophthalmic examinations.

Mydriatic Agents

Mydriatic drugs are agents that dilate the pupil of the eye. These drugs are commonly used during eye examinations to permit examination of the retina. Examples of mydriatics or sympathomimetics include hydroxy-amphetamine (Paredrine) and phenylephrine hydro-chloride (Mydfrin), which are used to dilate pupils in angle-closure glaucoma. These drugs were discussed previously in this chapter.

Focus On

Cycloplegics (Anticholinergic) Agents

Cycloplegic drugs (Table 30-5 ■) cause paralysis of ciliary muscles, resulting in pupillary dilation.

How do they work?

Such antimuscarinic agents as atropine (Atropisol), homatropine (AK-Homatropine), and cyclopentolate (Ak-Pentolate) act by blocking all muscarinic responses to acetylcholine. The mechanism of action for anticholinergic agents includes mydriasis (pupillary dilation) and cycloplegia (paralysis of ciliary muscles).

How are they used?

Anticholinergic drugs are used locally by inserting drops in the eyes for eye examinations and preoperatively for eye surgery; however, they can also aggravate glaucoma-producing mydriasis and cycloplegia.

What are the adverse effects?

Antimuscarinic drugs may cause mydriasis, blurred vision, photophobia, increased IOP, cycloplegia, eye dryness, and local redness.

What are the contraindications and interactions?

Contraindications include hypersensitivity to antimuscarinic drugs, angle-closure glaucoma, urinary bladder neck obstruction caused by prostatic hypertrophy, intestinal atony, severe ulcerative colitis, tachycardia secondary to cardiac insufficiency, acute bleeding, and myasthenia gravis. Safety during pregnancy or lactation is not established.

Antimuscarinic agents should be used cautiously in elderly patients and in patients with brain damage (in children), hyperthyroidism, asthma, and hepatic or renal disease. Antimuscarinic drugs may interact with the ocular antihypertensive effects of carbachol (Miostat), pilocarpine (Adsorbocarpine), and physostigmine (Antilirium).

What are the important points patients should know?

Instruct patients to use caution when driving or engaging in other potentially hazardous activities because these drugs may cause blurred vision. Patients should be advised to avoid touching the dropper to any skin or eye surface. Advise patients to not wear soft contact lenses when eye drops are being inserted and to immediately report difficulty breathing; swelling of the lips, tongue, or face; hives; palpitations; and unusual behavior.

Table 30-5 ■ Cycloplegics (Anticholinergic Drugs)

GENERIC NAME	TRADE NAME	AVERAGE ADULT DOSAGE	ROUTE OF ADMINISTRATION
atropine sulfate	Isopto Atropine Atropisol	1 drop of 0.5% solution daily	Topical
cyclopentolate	Cyclogyl, Pentolair	1 drop of 0.5%–2% solution 40–50 min before surgery	Topical
homatropine	Isopto Homatropine Isopto Hyoscine	1–2 drops of 2% or 5% solution before eye examination	Topical
scopolamine hydrobromide	Mydriacyl	1–2 drops of 0.25% solution 1 h before eye examination	Topical
tropicamide	Tropicacyl	1–2 drops of 0.5%–1% solution before eye examination	Topical

PRACTICAL SCENARIO 1

A 72-year-old African American man with a history of hypertension, coronary artery disease, and diabetes mellitus presents with the inability to clearly see objects at a distance and visual field loss. He also states that two days ago, he missed some stairs as he was walking up to the second floor of his home. The physician conducts an eye examination and determines that the patient's IOP is 25 mm Hg, there is no hemorrhage in the retina, and his right eye has a mild cataract. The physician diagnoses this patient as having glaucoma.

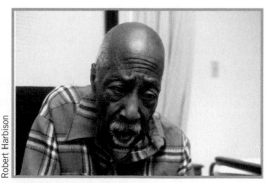

Robert Harbison

Critical Thinking Questions

1. After the physician leaves the room, the patient asks the medical assistant about this condition. How should the medical assistant explain the diagnosis to this patient, including its complications and possible relationship to his other disorders?
2. What treatment options would you tell the patient about that are available?
3. What would you tell the patient about his lifestyle that may be helpful with regard to this diagnosis?

PRACTICAL SCENARIO 2

A 72-year-old man went for an annual eye checkup. A medical assistant administered two different types of eye drops to dilate his pupils before the physician examined his eyes.

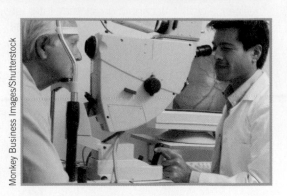

Monkey Business Images/Shutterstock

Critical Thinking Questions

1. What are the most common mydriatic drugs used to dilate the eyes?
2. If the patient has had a history of diabetes mellitus, what condition is likely to be present?

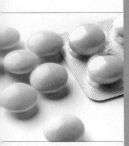

Chapter Capsule

This section repeats the objectives from the beginning of the chapter and then provides a summary of the most important concepts for that objective. Use this section as a quick review and to check your knowledge.

Objective 1: Describe the structure and function of the eye.

- A hollow, spherical structure about 2.5 cm in diameter with three distinct layers in its walls: an outer layer (sclera), a middle layer (choroid layer or "coat"), and an inner layer (retina)
- Spaces within the eye—filled with fluids that support its wall and internal parts
- Structures—the iris, ciliary body, lens, lacrimal glands, and ocular vasculature receive autonomic innervation

Objective 2: Explain glaucoma and the types of glaucoma.

- Damage to the optic nerve—often caused by elevated IOP
- Results from excessive production of aqueous humor or diminished ocular fluid outflow
- Can cause blindness secondary to optic nerve damage
- Two types of glaucoma: acute angle closure and chronic open angle

Objective 3: State the rationale for the use and the mechanism of action for carbonic anhydrase inhibitors in the treatment of glaucoma.

- Plays a significant role in aqueous humor formation by the ciliary body cells of the eye
- Facilitates the secretion of bicarbonate ions in the aqueous humor, decreasing the formation of aqueous humor
- Main clinical indication: glaucoma
- Most administered systemically

Objective 4: Identify direct-acting miotics (cholinergic drugs) and list two generic and trade names.

- Agents that constrict the pupil—often used to treat glaucoma
- Carbachol (Miostat, Isopto Carboptic)
- Pilocarpine hydrochloride (Miocarpine, Isopto Carpine)

Objective 5: Explain mydriatic agents and their indications.

- Agents that dilate the pupil of the eye; commonly used during eye examinations to permit examination of the retina
- Used locally by inserting drops in the eyes for eye examinations and preoperatively for eye surgery; however, can aggravate glaucoma-producing mydriasis and cycloplegia

Objective 6: State the mechanism of action of antimuscarinics.

- Act by blocking all muscarinic responses to acetylcholine
- Mechanism of action of antimuscarinic agents—mydriasis (pupillary dilation) and cycloplegia (paralysis of ciliary muscles)

 Internet Sites of Interest

- Learn more about glaucoma at the Glaucoma Research Foundation website at **http://www.glaucoma.org**.
- More information about carbonic anhydrase inhibitors can be found on the Mayo Clinic website at **http://www.mayoclinic.com**. Search for "carbonic anhydrase inhibitors."

myhealthprofessionskit

Go to www.myhealthprofessionskit.com to access the Companion Website created for this textbook. Simply select "Basic Health Science" from the choice of disciplines. Find this book and then log in using your username and password to access interactive learning games, assessment questions, animations, and more.

Checkpoint Review 4

MULTIPLE CHOICE

Select the best answer for the following questions.

1. Which of the following neurotransmitters is released by the preganglionic sympathetic neuron?
   a. Norepinephrine
   b. Acetylcholine
   c. Dopamine
   d. Serotonin

2. Which of the following neurotransmitters is released by the parasympathetic postganglionic neurons?
   a. Serotonin
   b. Norepinephrine
   c. Dopamine
   d. Acetylcholine

3. Sympathomimetics are also called:
   a. Cholinergic antagonists
   b. Cholinergic agonists
   c. Adrenergic agonists
   d. Adrenergic antagonists

4. The "pacemaker," or SA node, is located in which of the following chambers of the heart?
   a. Left atrium
   b. Right atrium
   c. Right ventricle
   d. Left ventricle

5. Which of the following are class I antidysrhythmic drugs?
   a. Beta-adrenergic blockers
   b. Drugs that bind to sodium channels
   c. Drugs that interfere with potassium outflow
   d. Calcium channel blockers

6. Which of the following drugs has antisympathetic class III action?
   a. Bretylium (Bretylol)
   b. Verapamil (Calan)
   c. Propranolol (Inderal)
   d. Lidocaine (Xylocaine)

7. Alpha$_2$-receptor agonists are used to treat:
   a. Hypertension
   b. Hypotension
   c. Hepatitis
   d. Impotence

8. Sublingual nitroglycerin is rapidly effective and lasts for about:
   a. 15 minutes
   b. 30 minutes
   c. 1 hour
   d. 3 hours

9. Which of the following describes stage 2 of anesthesia?
   a. Surgical
   b. Analgesia
   c. Medullary paralysis
   d. Excitement

10. Beta$_2$-receptor agonists are used in patients with:
    a. Cardiac arrhythmias associated with digitalis intoxication
    b. Chronic obstructive airway disease
    c. Hypertension
    d. Thyrotoxicosis

11. The most common adverse effects of phenytoin (Dilantin) include which of the following?
    a. Nosebleed
    b. Asthma
    c. Bloody urine
    d. Gingival hyperplasia

12. Specialized cells in the epidermis called *melanocytes* produce:
    a. Melatonin
    b. Melanin
    c. Melanogen
    d. Melanotropin

13. Beta-receptor antagonists are used in the management of:
    a. Hypertension and weight reduction
    b. Cardiac arrhythmias
    c. Angina pectoris
    d. All of the above

14. Which of the following stages of anesthesia is called an *anesthetic accident*?
    a. Medullary paralysis
    b. Excitement
    c. Surgical anesthesia
    d. Analgesia

15. Pilocarpine is used most commonly in which of the following?

    a. Gynecology
    b. Ophthalmology
    c. Dermatology
    d. Cardiology

16. Cholinergic blockers are also called:

    a. Sympatholytics
    b. Sympathomimetics
    c. Parasympatholytics
    d. Parasympathomimetics

17. Which of the following is the cause of primary (essential) hypertension?

    a. Obesity
    b. Chronic glomerulonephritis
    c. Excessive alcohol
    d. Unknown

18. Discontinuation of nitroglycerin should take place over time because the length of action of these drug preparations can cause:

    a. Hypertension
    b. Vasospasms
    c. Bradycardia
    d. Vomiting

19. Which of the following is/are the mechanism(s) of action for quinidine?

    a. Slowing of the heart rate
    b. Decreasing the contractile force of the heart
    c. Depressing the myocardium and the conduction system
    d. All of the above

20. General anesthetics are contraindicated in patients who have received monoamine oxidase inhibitors within how many days?

    a. 2
    b. 4
    c. 7
    d. 14

21. Which of the following must patients do when taking nitroglycerin?

    a. Avoid food or liquids.
    b. Avoid alcoholic beverages.
    c. Avoid coffee and tea.
    d. Discard unused tablets after 5 minutes.

22. Which of the following is the mainstay of treatment for acute or chronic inflammatory disorders of the skin and may be topical or oral?

    a. Emollients (skin-softening agents)
    b. Keratolytic agents
    c. Antibiotics
    d. Corticosteroids

23. Which of the following drugs are mainstays of hypertensive therapy?

    a. Diuretics
    b. Statin drugs
    c. Beta-adrenergic blockers
    d. Centrally acting adrenergic blockers

24. Rhabdomyolysis (degeneration of skeletal muscle tissue) is a rare but life-threatening adverse effect of:

    a. Diuretics
    b. Angiotensin II receptor blockers
    c. Statins
    d. Fat-soluble vitamins

25. Parasympathomimetics (or cholinergic agonists) produce symptoms of:

    a. Fight or flight
    b. Rest and digest
    c. Fight and rest
    d. Speed and rest

26. Acne vulgaris is an inflammatory disorder of which of the following glands?

    a. Sweat
    b. Sebaceous
    c. Bartholin
    d. Mammary

27. Dopamine is released from which of the following?

    a. Kidneys
    b. GI tract
    c. Brain
    d. All of the above

28. Which of the following is an example of a beta-adrenergic blocker?

    a. Verapamil
    b. Diltiazem
    c. Inderal
    d. Amiodarone

29. A chemical compound containing nitrogen that is derived from the amino acid tyrosine is called:

    a. Catecholamine
    b. Melanin
    c. Melatonin
    d. Cardiolipin

30. Which of the following agents are used in the treatment of corns, calluses, and plantar warts?

    a. Topical antibiotics
    b. Topical corticosteroids
    c. Keratolytics
    d. Emollients

31. Peripherally acting blockers are antihypertensive in that their effects depend on the inhibition of:

    a. Renin release
    b. Norepinephrine release
    c. Acetylcholine release
    d. Serotonin release

32. Beta$_1$-receptor agonists are used to treat which of the following?

    a. Cardiac arrest
    b. Circulatory shock
    c. Hypotension
    d. All of the above

33. Atropine acts by selectively blocking all muscarinic responses to:

    a. Dopamine
    b. Acetylcholine
    c. Norepinephrine
    d. Serotonin

34. Which of the following agents is a popular choice for infiltration anesthesia?

    a. Lidocaine
    b. Nitrous oxide
    c. Sevoflurane
    d. Cocaine

35. Which of the following is the trade name of lidocaine?

    a. Marcaine
    b. Carbocaine
    c. Novocain
    d. Xylocaine

36. The primary use of bethanechol (Urecholine), which is a cholinergic agonist used in the cardiovascular field, is in the diagnosis of:

    a. Prolapse of the mitral valve
    b. Atrial tachycardia

    c. Myocardial infarction
    d. Hypertensive crises

37. During spinal anesthesia, the anesthetic agent is injected into which of the following spaces or parts of the spinal column?

    a. Pia mater
    b. Arachnoid
    c. Subarachnoid
    d. Epidural

38. Which of the following is the most commonly used route to administer local anesthetics?

    a. Local infiltration
    b. Topical anesthesia
    c. Spinal anesthesia
    d. Epidural anesthesia

39. Which of the following is the most frequent adverse effect associated with barbiturates?

    a. Blurred vision
    b. Thrombocytopenia
    c. Sedation
    d. Aplastic anemia

40. Stage 3 (surgical anesthesia) is characterized by progressive:

    a. Muscular contraction
    b. Circulatory collapse
    c. Muscular relaxation
    d. Dysfunction of the respiratory system, which can cause sudden death

41. Valproic acid is classified as an:

    a. Antipyretic
    b. Anticonvulsant
    c. Anticoagulant
    d. Antineoplastic

42. The trade name of ethosuximide is:

    a. Celontin
    b. Dilantin
    c. Ativan
    d. Zarontin

43. Cholinergic drugs exhibit effects similar to which of the following substances?

    a. Monoamine oxidase inhibitors
    b. Methotrimeprazine
    c. Acetylcholine
    d. Amphetamines

44. Stimulation of beta₂ receptors results in which of the following?

a. Postural hypotension
b. Nasal congestion
c. Bronchoconstriction
d. Bronchodilation

45. Which of the following is a cholinergic drug?

a. Noradrenaline
b. Dopamine
c. Acetylcholine
d. Any calcium channel blocker

46. Which of the following properties of general anesthetics is essential for the drug to cross the blood–brain barrier?

a. Lipophilic
b. Hydrophilic
c. Proteinphilic
d. None of the above

47. All the following inhaled anesthetics are commonly used in the United States except:

a. Nitrous oxide
b. Sevoflurane
c. Diethyl ether
d. Isoflurane

48. Which of the following drugs is in the group of ester-type local anesthetics?

a. Bupivacaine
b. Etidocaine
c. Ropivacaine
d. Benzocaine

49. Which of the following drugs is used to treat ophthalmic disorders and in preoperative situations?

a. Niacin
b. Atropine
c. Alcohol
d. Amantadine

50. Beta₂-receptor agonists are used in patients with all the following except:

a. Premature labor
b. Circulatory shock
c. Anaphylactic shock
d. Chronic obstructive airway disease

51. An opacity of the eye's lens is called:

a. Glaucoma
b. Cataract
c. Retinopathy
d. Choroiditis

52. Gold sodium thiomalate (Myochrysine) is effective in which of the following disorders?

a. Bronchitis
b. Hepatitis
c. Acute glomerulonephritis
d. Active rheumatoid arthritis

53. All the following are adverse effects of estrogen replacement therapy in the treatment of postmenopausal osteoporosis except:

a. Breast cancer
b. Lung cancer
c. Endometrial cancer
d Cardiovascular problems

54. Carbonic anhydrase inhibitors act on the enzyme responsible for the conversion of carbon dioxide to which of the following?

a. Bicarbonate and calcium ions
b. Bicarbonate and sodium ions
c. Bicarbonate and hydrogen ions
d. None of the above

55. Colchicine is used for which of the following conditions or diseases?

a. Peptic ulcer
b. Gout
c. Severe hepatic conditions
d. Severe cardiac disease

56. Which of the following is an example of a new drug that is a selective estrogen-receptor modulator for the treatment of postmenopausal osteoporosis?

a. carisoprodol (Soma)
b. lorazepam (Ativan)
c. acetazolamide (Diamox)
d. raloxifene (Evista)

57. Baclofen is at least as effective as which of the following drugs?

a. lorazepam (Dantrium)
b. dorzolamide (Trusopt)
c. diazepam (Valium)
d. levobunolol (Betagan)

58. Even when applied directly to the eye, several drugs may have systemic effects. This is because the drug enters via which of the following routes?

a. The lungs
b. The nasolacrimal ducts
c. The mouth and nasopharyngeal ducts
d. All of the above

59. The anterior of the sclera of the eye that bulges forward is called the:
    a. Retina
    b. Pupil
    c. Iris
    d. Cornea

60. All the following are primary functions of the skeletal system except:
    a. Blood cell production
    b. Storage of minerals
    c. Production of heat and energy
    d. Protection of other organs

61. Which of the following is the generic name of Fosamax?
    a. risedronate sodium
    b. alendronate sodium
    c. raloxifene
    d. calcitonin salmon

62. The ciliary body is the thickest part of which layer of the eye?
    a. Inner
    b. Middle
    c. Outer
    d. Inner and middle

63. Pigment-producing melanocytes are located in which of the following organs?
    a. Mouth
    b. Liver
    c. Spleen
    d. Eye

64. Photoreceptors are located in which of the following portions of the eyes?
    a. Pupils
    b. Retina
    c. Aqueous humor
    d. Choroid

65. Which of the following is a systemic autoimmune disease?
    a. Osteoporosis
    b. Osteomyelitis
    c. Rheumatoid arthritis
    d. Rheumatoid fever

66. When the lenses of the eyes adjust shape and facilitate focusing, it is known as:
    a. Presbyopia
    b. Diplopia
    c. Amblyopia
    d. Accommodation

67. All the following are risk factors for primary open-angle glaucoma except:
    a. Myopia
    b. Diabetes
    c. Peptic ulcer
    d. Black race

68. When benzodiazepines are combined with other central nervous system depressants, which of the following adverse effects can occur?
    a. Coma and renal failure
    b. Coma and respiratory depression
    c. Hypertension
    d. Hyperthermia

69. Which of the following is one of the most common and serious disorders of the eye?
    a. Retinal detachment
    b. Conjunctivitis
    c. Glaucoma
    d. Cataract

70. Adverse effects of acetazolamide (Diamox) include:
    a. Blurred vision, urinary retention
    b. Dry mouth, thirst
    c. Paresthesias, drowsiness, nausea
    d. Congestive heart failure

71. Auranofin (Ridaura) is used in the treatment of:
    a. Rheumatoid arthritis
    b. Multiple sclerosis
    c. Ear infections
    d. Ulcerative colitis

72. Which of the following hormones is secreted by the kidneys?
    a. Vasopressin
    b. Oxytocin
    c. Luteinizing
    d. Erythropoietin

73. Following the proximal convoluted tubule is the:
    a. Distal convoluted tubule
    b. Loop of Henle
    c. Glomerular capsule
    d. Collecting duct

74. Which of the following is a major adverse effect of potassium-sparing diuretics?
    a. Hyperkalemia
    b. Hypercalcemia
    c. Hypokalemia
    d. Hypocalcemia

75. Antidiuretic hormone is also called:

 a. Oxytocin

 b. Adrenocorticotropic hormone

 c. Vasopressin

 d. Prolactin

76. Graves's disease is characterized by:

 a. Hypothyroidism

 b. Hyperthyroidism

 c. Myxedema

 d. Congenital hypothyroidism

77. Iodide is used alone for which of the following disorders or conditions?

 a. Hyperkalemia

 b. Hyperthyroidism

 c. Acute bronchitis

 d. Asthma

78. Propylthiouracil is classified as a(n):

 a. Diuretic drug

 b. Antihistamine

 c. Antithyroid agent

 d. Antihypertensive agent

79. Glucagon hormone is secreted by which of the following glands?

 a. Pancreas

 b. Thymus

 c. Thyroid

 d. Adrenal gland

80. The sulfonylureas are categorized as:

 a. Oral hypoglycemics

 b. Oral contraceptives

 c. Oral anticoagulants

 d. Loop diuretics

81. The alpha cells of the islets of the pancreas secrete:

 a. Insulin

 h. Thymosin

 c. Heparin

 d. Glucagon

82. Which of the following agents is used for nasal congestion and asthma?

 a. Furosemide

 b. Corticosteroids

 c. Potassium iodide

 d. Regular insulin

83. Loop diuretics are toxic to which of the following organs of the body?

 a. Ears

 b. Eyes

 c. Lungs

 d. Ovaries

84. Which of the following chronic conditions of the lungs is the most common in the United States?

 a. Nasal polyps

 b. Pneumonia

 c. Asthma

 d. Pulmonary edema

85. Bronchodilators that widen the diameter of the bronchial tubes include which of the following agents?

 a. Corticosteroids

 b. Narrow-spectrum antibiotics

 c. Beta$_2$-adrenergic agonists

 d. Alpha$_2$-adrenergic agonists

86. Gestational diabetes develops during:

 a. Childhood

 b. The neonatal period

 c. Lactation

 d. Pregnancy

87. The antacids are all:

 a. Weak acids

 b. Weak alkalines

 c. Strong acids

 d. Strong alkalines

88. Which of the following are among the most misused drugs?

 a. Opioid analgesics

 b. Antidiarrheals

 c. Laxatives

 d. Antacids

89. All the following are indications of androgens in women except:

 a. Postpartum breast engorgement

 b. Fibrocystic breast disorders

 c. Breast cancer

 d. Endometriosis

90. Which of the following portions of the body secretes gonadotropin-releasing hormone?

    a. The hypothalamus
    b. The anterior pituitary
    c. The posterior pituitary
    d. The ovaries

91. A patient who is receiving insulin should be taught to be cautious about which of the following adverse effects?

    a. Malignant hyperthermia
    b. Severe hypotension
    c. Hypoglycemic reaction
    d. Malignant hypertension

92. Which of the following are the most effective drugs for controlling diarrhea?

    a. Osmotics
    b. Electrolytes
    c. Adsorbents
    d. Opioid antidiarrheals

93. A 70/30 combination of insulin means:

    a. NPH 70% and regular insulin 30%
    b. NPH 30% and regular insulin 70%
    c. NPH 30% and Novolin 70%
    d. NPH 70% and Novolin 30%

94. Stool softeners are sometimes called:

    a. Laxatives
    b. Osmotics
    c. Adsorbents
    d. Emollients

95. Which of the following is the best-known synthetic estrogen?

    a. Norethindrone
    b. Diethylstilbestrol
    c. Megestrol
    d. Norgestrel

96. Which of the following is the trade name of insulin glargine (long acting)?

    a. Novolin
    b. Lantus
    c. Humalog
    d. Humulin U

97. Which of the following chemical substances increases sodium ion reabsorption in the distal convoluted tubules and collecting ducts of the nephrons?

    a. Erythropoietin
    b. Insulin
    c. Glucagon
    d. Aldosterone

98. Water balance is regulated by the secretion of which of the following hormones?

    a. Vasopressin
    b. Thyroxin
    c. Erythropoietin
    d. Growth hormone

99. Exophthalmos (protrusion of the eyeball) is seen in which of the following conditions or disorders?

    a. Hyperparathyroidism
    b. Hyperthyroidism
    c. Hypertension
    d. Myxedema

100. Laxative stimulants are contraindicated in all the following conditions except:

    a. Fecal impaction
    b. Abdominal pain
    c. Pregnancy
    d. Constipation

101. Which of the following diuretics are used primarily for cerebral edema?

    a. Osmotic agents
    b. Carbonic anhydrase inhibitors
    c. Thiazide agents
    d. Loop diuretics

102. Which of the following portions of the male reproductive system stores sperm cells?

    a. Vas deferens
    b. Prostate gland
    c. Scrotum
    d. Epididymis

103. Which of the following agents stimulates powerful uterine contractions?

    a. Prolactin
    b. Progesterone
    c. Oxytocin
    d. Estrogen

104. Which of the following is the trade name of spironolactone?

    a. Dyrenium
    b. Aldactone
    c. Midamor
    d. Lasix

105. Which of the following drugs is an antiemetic?

    a. Ipecac
    b. Chlorpromazine
    c. Magnesium hydroxide
    d. Senna

106. Uterine relaxants include which of the following agents?

    a. Beta$_2$-adrenergic agonists
    b. Alpha$_2$-adrenergic agonists
    c. Cholinergic agonists
    d. Oxytocin hormone

107. Estrogen therapy in older women is used to prevent or treat which of the following disorders or conditions?

    a. Breast cancer
    b. Pregnancy
    c. Endometriosis
    d. Osteoporosis

108. Stoppage of blood flow is known as:

    a. Hemopoiesis
    b. Hemostasis
    c. Hemosiderosis
    d. Hemolysis

109. Which of the following chemical substances is released from the platelets?

    a. Serotonin
    b. Heparin
    c. Histamine
    d. Fibrinogen

110. Tagamet and Zantac are known as which of the following?

    a. Histamine agonists
    b. Histamine antagonists
    c. Antispasmodics
    d. Antacids

111. Which of the following is an example of an oral anticoagulant?

    a. Heparin
    b. Urokinase
    c. Streptokinase
    d. Coumadin

112. Allergic rhinitis is also known as:

    a. Rhinovirus
    b. Coryza
    c. Hives
    d. Hay fever

113. Which of the following anticoagulants should not be used during pregnancy?

    a. Warfarin
    b. Heparin
    c. Enoxaparin
    d. Ardeparin

114. The adrenal medulla synthesizes, stores, and secretes which of the following?

    a. Epinephrine and norepinephrine
    b. Androgen and glucocorticoids
    c. Parathormone
    d. Thyroxine

115. All the following leafy green foods contain vitamin K except:

    a. Parsley
    b. Swiss chard
    c. Spinach
    d. Sweet potatoes

116. Patients should be instructed to avoid exposure to UV light while taking which of the following drugs?

    a. Coumarin derivatives
    b. Thrombolytics
    c. Xanthine derivatives
    d. Progestins

117. Xanthine derivatives are used for prophylaxis and the symptomatic relief of which of the following conditions or disorders?

    a. Bronchial asthma
    b. Osteoporosis
    c. Dementia
    d. Pancreatitis

118. The process of blood clotting occurs in a series of sequential steps that are referred to as a:

    a. Prothrombin activator
    b. Cascade
    c. Thrombus
    d. Low-molecular-weight heparin

119. Most of the circulating clotting proteins are synthesized by which of the following organs in the human body?

    a. Lungs
    b. Liver
    c. Bones
    d. Brain

120. Conjugated estrogens (during the first trimester) may increase the risk for which of the following?

 a. Dysrhythmia in the fetus
 b. Heart failure in the fetus and infant
 c. Malabsorption in the infant
 d. Malformations in the fetus and infant

121. Which of the following is an example of antiplatelet agents?

 a. Heparin
 b. Abciximab
 c. Abbokinase
 d. Warfarin

MATCHING 1

For questions 122–126, match the lettered drug class to the numbered description.

DESCRIPTION	DRUG CLASS
122. _____ Converted to theophylline	a. Leukotriene inhibitors
123. _____ Causes masculinization of the fetus	b. Oxytocic agents
124. _____ Used to treat gastrointestinal disorders	c. Prostaglandins
125. _____ Metabolized from arachidonic acid	d. Androgen derivatives
126. _____ Produces phasic contractions characteristic of normal delivery	e. Xanthine derivatives

MATCHING 2

For questions 127–131, match the lettered drug trade name to the numbered drug generic name.

GENERIC NAME	TRADE NAME
127. _____ dalteparin	a. Lovenox
128. _____ danaparoid	b. Innohep
129. _____ ardeparin	c. Orgaran
130. _____ enoxaparin	d. Fragmin
131. _____ tinzaparin	e. Normiflo

FILL IN THE BLANK

Select terms from your reading to fill in the blanks.

132. The space between each synapse is bridged by chemicals called _____.

133. Intraorbital block is often used for _____ surgery.

134. Atropine is a classic anticholinergic or _____ antagonist drug.

135. Neurons that release acetylcholine are termed _____.

136. Cryoanesthesia involves the reduction of nerve conduction by localized _____.

137. Alpha-receptor antagonists can be reversible or _____.

138. There are two types of cholinergic receptors: muscarinic and _____.

139. Beta-blockers competitively antagonize the responses to _____ that are mediated by beta receptors.

140. Cholinergic blockers are also called _____.

141. Volatile anesthetics are combined with intravenous agents in regimens of so-called _____ anesthesia.

142. Oral androgens should be taken with meals to reduce _____.

143. The testes secrete _____.

144. The best-known synthetic _____ is diethylstilbestrol (Stilbestrol).

145. The ovaries are the primary source of progesterones and _____.

146. Primary digestion occurs in the _____.

147. H$_2$-receptor antagonists are used for the short-term treatment of active _____.

148. The prostaglandins are involved in gastrointestinal _____ and gastric acid secretions.

149. Bronchodilators include _____ adrenergic agonists and _____.

150. Leukotriene inhibitors are bronchodilators and leukotriene receptor _____.

151. The pancreas is an accessory organ of the _____.

Unit 5

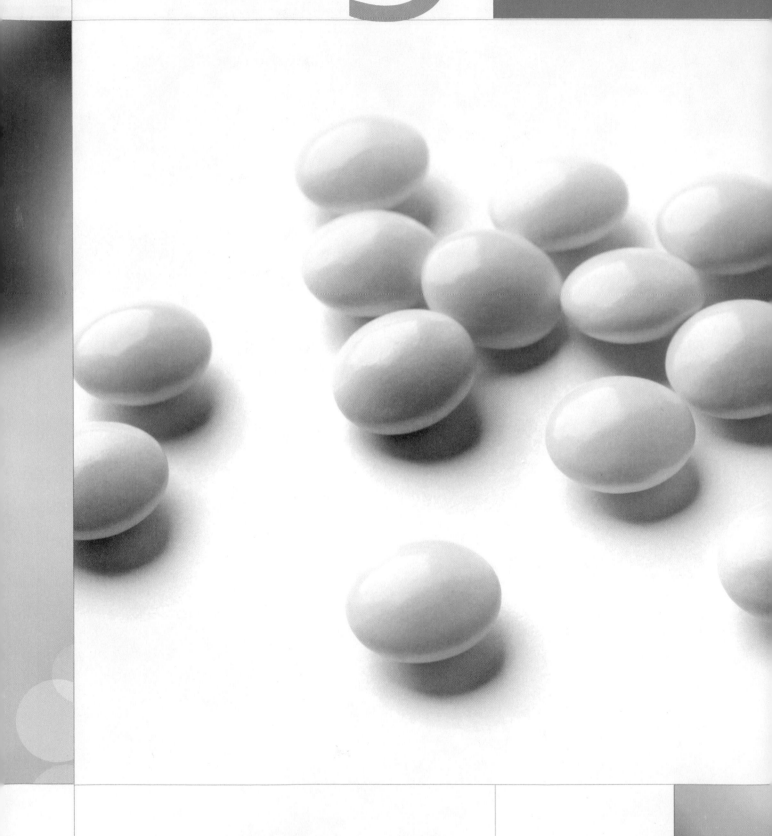

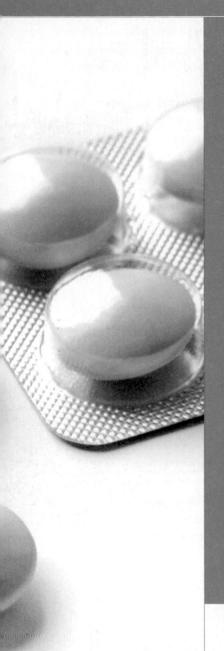

SPECIAL POPULATIONS

" Health professionals must ensure that drugs are administered safely and effectively to patients of all ages. "

Chapter 31

Drugs Used to Treat Geriatric Patients

Chapter Objectives

After completing this chapter, you should be able to:

1. Discuss the process of aging.
2. Explain the leading causes of diseases and death in elderly patients older than.
3. Identify the factors that influence drug absorption in older adults.
4. Discuss creatinine clearance in elderly patients and use the measurement formula.
5. Identify polypharmacy and its effects on elderly patients.
6. List common cardiovascular disorders in elderly individuals.
7. Discuss the effects of sedatives and hypnotics on elderly patients.
8. List six principles that are important in treating elderly patients.

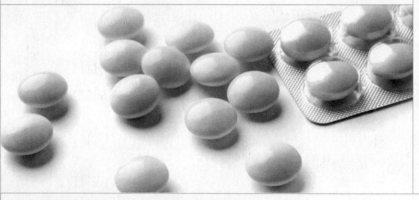

Key Terms

Alzheimer's disease (AL-zhy-merz) (page 564)

cognitive (page 559)

creatinine clearance (kree-AT-tih-neen) (page 560)

glycoprotein (page 560)

polypharmacy (page 561)

stroke (page 559)

thiazides (page 562)

Introduction

The process of aging is complex and includes biological, psychological, sociological, and behavioral changes. *Biologically*, the body gradually loses the ability to renew itself. Various body functions begin to slow down and the vital senses become less acute. *Psychologically*, aging persons experience changing sensory processes; perception, motor skills, problem-solving abilities, and emotions are frequently altered. *Sociologically*, they must cope with the changing roles and definitions of self that society imposes on elderly people. *Behaviorally*, aging individuals may move more slowly and have less dexterity.

Major changes that are not physiological also occur during the aging process and impact health, including **cognitive** (intellectual processes, such as thinking, reasoning, and remembering) changes, such as forgetting to take daily medications; economic changes caused by decreased income, increased health expenses, and other factors; and unforeseen changes, including the death of a spouse.

Geriatric Drug Therapy

The elderly population requires increased health-care attention. In the United States, the elderly population grew more than tenfold during the twentieth century. In 1900, there were just over 3 million Americans 65 or older. In 2009, the same group numbered nearly 40 million. Drug therapy for geriatric patients requires specific knowledge of their physiology, pathology, and other age-related factors. Drug dosages must be adjusted according to an elderly patient's weight, amount of body fat, laboratory results (e.g., blood urea nitrogen, creatinine, serum protein, liver enzymes, electrolytes), and current health conditions.

Significant changes in common responses to certain drugs can occur in older people. Other drugs may affect elderly patients in only slightly differing ways. As people age, their drug usage patterns change—generally increasing—because the incidence of disease or multiple diseases increases with age. In addition, many older adults experience problems with nutrition and finances that may decrease dosing compliance in prescribed drugs. Health-care practitioners who deal with elderly patients must be aware of these issues and understand how to deal with them. Equally important, it is essential for health-care personnel to be aware of the leading causes of death in elderly individuals.

Disease and Death in Elderly People

Heart disease and cancer have been the two leading causes of death among people 65 and older for the past two decades. More than one-third (35%) of all deaths are caused by heart disease, including heart attacks and chronic ischemic heart disease. Cancer accounts for about one-fifth (22%) of all deaths.

Other important chronic diseases among persons 65 and older include **stroke** (cerebrovascular disease), chronic obstructive pulmonary disease, diabetes, pneumonia, and influenza. Alzheimer's disease and several important renal diseases (such as chronic nephritis and nephrotic syndrome) have gained significance as causes of death among the elderly population during the past two decades. Alzheimer's disease is now among the 10 leading causes of death for older white people but not for other racial groups.

Physiologic Changes in Elderly Individuals

Most organ systems show a decline that begins during young adulthood and continues as people age. Individuals age differently, and elderly people accumulate physiologic deficiencies with the passage of time in varying amounts. The most important decline appears to be in renal function. The physiologic changes in older adults are shown in Table 31-1 ■.

Table 31-1 ■ Physiologic Changes in Geriatric Patients

ORGANS	PHYSIOLOGIC CHANGES
Heart	Cardiac output and blood flow decrease
Liver	Function of enzymes and blood flow decrease
Kidneys	Blood flow, glomerular filtration, and nephron function decrease
Stomach	Gastric secretions decrease
Intestines	Peristalsis and motility decrease; first-pass effect decrease

CHANGES IN PHARMACOKINETICS

Pharmacokinetics deal with the absorption, distribution, metabolism, and elimination of drugs as well as the amount of time each of these processes requires. In many cases, pharmacokinetics can explain why different people react differently to a drug.

Absorption

Although drug absorption is not altered in any major way with age, the rate at which some drugs are absorbed does change. Conditions that influence drug absorption in older adults include slower gastric emptying, altered nutritional habits, and greater use of over-the-counter (OTC) medications.

Distribution

Elderly people tend to have increased body fat but reduced lean body mass and reduced total body water (Table 31-2 ■).

Serum albumin, which binds to many drugs, especially weak acids, is usually decreased. There may be a concurrent increase in alpha-1 acid **glycoprotein**—a specific serum protein that binds to many basic drugs. Changes such as these may alter a drug's appropriate loading dose. Because of a decreased volume of distribution, the loading dose of a drug, such as digoxin (Lanoxin), should be reduced (if it is used at all) in an older person with heart failure. Because of reduced drug clearance, maintenance doses also may have to be reduced.

Table 31-2 ■ Pharmacokinetic Changes Due to Aging

TYPE OF CHANGE	YOUNG ADULTS (BEGINNING AT AGE 20 YEARS)	OLDER ADULTS (BEGINNING AT AGE 60 YEARS)
Body fat	18%–20% of body weight (men)	36%–38% of body weight (men)
	26%–33% of body weight (women)	38%–45% of body weight (women)
Body water	61% of body weight	53% of body weight
Hepatic blood flow	100% in a young adult	55%–60% in an older adult
Kidney weight	100% in a young adult	80% in an older adult
Lean body mass	19% of body weight	12% of body weight
Serum albumin	4.7 g/d	3.8 g/d

Focus Point

Age Affects Pharmacokinetic Process

The efficiency of pharmacokinetic processes varies across one's life span. In very young and very old people, the manner in which their bodies handle drugs can be significantly different from that of young or middle-aged adults.

Metabolism

The liver's capacity to metabolize drugs does not appear to consistently decline as age increases. This is true for all drugs. However, as we age, the liver's ability to heal from an injury (such as from viral hepatitis or alcohol use) declines. The health-care professional should realize that a history of recent liver disease in an elderly patient should lead to caution when administering drugs that are mostly cleared by the liver. This is true even after the patient has apparently completely recovered from hepatic damage. Also in elderly people, heart failure and other diseases that affect liver function (such as malnutrition) are more common. Heart failure may alter liver metabolism and reduce hepatic blood flow. Impaired hepatic function may also result from severe nutritional deficiencies.

Elimination

Because of decreased cardiac output and blood flow in the circulatory system, the liver and kidneys are affected. By age 65, nephron function may decline

by 35%, and after age 70, blood flow to the kidneys may be decreased 40%.

Creatinine clearance is an indicator of the glomerular filtration rate. Evaluating renal function based on serum creatinine alone may not be accurate for older adults because of the decrease in muscle mass. Creatinine is a by-product of the muscle breakdown of stored proteins. However, creatinine is primarily excreted by the kidneys. A decrease in muscle mass can cause a decrease in serum creatinine. In elderly patients, serum creatinine may be within normal values because of a lack of muscle mass, but there could still be a decrease in renal function. In young or middle-aged adults, serum creatinine would be increased with a decrease in renal function.

The serum creatinine level may be measured by the 24-hour creatinine clearance test to evaluate renal function. Creatinine clearance can also be calculated by this formula:

Creatine clearance in mL / min

$$= \frac{(140 - age) \times (weight\ in\ kg)}{72 \times serum\ creatinine\ in\ mg\ /\ dL}$$

The normal creatinine clearance value for an adult is 80 to 130 mL/min.

With liver and kidney dysfunction, the efficacy of a drug dose is usually decreased. If several drugs are being taken, drug effects may be intensified in elderly patients. If the efficiency of the hepatic and renal systems is decreased, the half-life of the drug is prolonged, resulting in drug toxicity. Special medications must be administered in reduced dosages in elderly patients (Table 31-3 ■).

Table 31-3 ■ Medications Administered in Elderly Patients That Require Reduced Dosages

DRUG OR CLASS OF DRUG	ADVERSE EFFECTS
aminoglycosides	Ototoxicity, nephrotoxicity
carbamazepine (Carbatrol)	Ataxia, drowsiness
cimetidine (Tagamet)	Confusion
digoxin (Lanoxin)	Overdose toxicity
levodopa (Dopar)	Hypotension
morphine (Avinza)	Respiratory depression
thioridazine (Mellaril)	Confusion
thyroxine	Myocardial infarction
vitamin D (Calcijex)	Renal toxicity
warfarin (Coumadin)	Bleeding

CHANGES IN PHARMACODYNAMICS

The term *pharmacodynamics* refers to how drugs interact at target organs or receptor sites. Pharmacodynamics examines the way drugs bind with receptors, the concentration required to elicit a response, and the time required for each of these events. Because there is a lack of affinity to receptor sites throughout an elderly person's body, the pharmacodynamic response may be changed.

Many changes in pharmacodynamics in elderly individuals result from altered pharmacokinetics or diminished homeostatic responses. There may be changes with age in the characteristics or numbers of some receptors. The elderly patient may be more or less sensitive to drug action because of age-related changes in the central nervous system (CNS), changes in the number of drug receptors, and changes in the affinity of receptors to drugs. If the patient is more sensitive to the drug's action, the dose may need to be lowered and vice versa. Changes in organ functions are important to consider in drug dosing. Most studies show that the elderly experience a decrease in responsiveness to beta-adrenoceptor stimulants.

In the cardiovascular system of older adults who do not have obvious cardiac disease, the increment of cardiac output required by mild to moderate exercise is successfully provided until at least age 75. However, the increased output results mostly from increased stroke volume in the elderly (in young adults, it results from tachycardia). Average blood pressure and symptomatic orthostatic hypotension increase with age. An elderly patient should be checked for orthostatic hypotension during every physician visit. Other physiologic changes in older adults include increased blood sugar, impaired temperature regulation, and poor tolerance to hypothermia.

Focus on Natural Products

Yohimbe

Yohimbe is a natural supplement widely taken to treat erectile dysfunction. However, in the absence of standardization in dietary supplement labeling in the United States, there is no reliable way to determine the amount of the drug *yohimbine* that is contained in the supplement. Yohimbe is not recommended for patients with hypertension or hepatic, renal, or peptic ulcer diseases—all common conditions affecting elderly individuals.

Polypharmacy

The practice of prescribing multiple medicines to a single patient simultaneously is called **polypharmacy**. In general, it is better to use as few medicines as possible. Polypharmacy increases the patient's costs for treatment as well as increases the chances for multiple adverse effects and drug interactions. Administration of many drugs together is more common in the elderly population because of their need for different medical specialists and the use of OTC drugs and herbal therapies.

Polypharmacy may cause liver dysfunction, malnutrition, confusion, and falls. Liver dysfunction contributes to delirium or an acute confusional state. Confusion and disturbances of perception (including misinterpretations of information) are commonly seen.

Herbal preparations must also be considered drugs, and their use with prescribed medications contributes to polypharmacy.

Focus on Geriatrics

Polypharmacy

Multiple drug therapies may cause confusion in elderly patients and lead to medication errors and further drug interactions.

✳ Apply Your Knowledge 31.1

The following questions focus on what you have just learned about disease, death, and physiologic changes in elderly people.

CRITICAL THINKING

1. What are the major changes during the aging process that impact health?
2. What are the two leading causes of death among elderly people?
3. What is the most important physiologic decline in elderly individuals?
4. What factors may influence medication absorption in older adults?
5. What is an indicator of the glomerular filtration rate?
6. What are the adverse effects of morphine, thyroxine, warfarin, and aminoglycosides?
7. What are the contraindications of yohimbe?
8. What is polypharmacy?

Changes in the Effects of Drugs on Elderly Patients

Antihypertensives, cardiac glycosides, antiarrhythmics, CNS drugs (sedative–hypnotics, opioid analgesics, antidepressants, and antipsychotics as well as medications used for Alzheimer's disease), antiinflammatory drugs, antimicrobial drugs, and gastrointestinal (GI) drugs (antiulcer drugs and laxatives) all have different effects on elderly patients. Drug selection for this group of patients is extremely important. Drugs with longer half-lives may accumulate and cause toxicity.

CARDIOVASCULAR DRUGS

Such cardiovascular disorders as hypertension, congestive heart failure, myocardial infarction, and stroke are very common in older adults. Almost one-third of all deaths in Western countries are attributed to heart disease. Many drugs can be used for these disorders, and some of them must be used cautiously in elderly individuals.

Antihypertensive Drugs

In the United States, blood pressure increases with age, especially in elderly women. It is clear that uncontrolled hypertension leads to serious health problems and, especially in elderly people, should be treated very seriously.

Weight reduction and salt restriction are indicated before drug therapy, which usually begins with **thiazides**, the most commonly prescribed class of diuretics. These agents often cause hyperglycemia, hyperuricemia, and hypokalemia in elderly patients because of their higher incidence of arrhythmias, type II diabetes, and gout. It is important that antihypertensives be used in lowered doses. If the patient also has atherosclerotic angina, calcium channel blockers are effective and safe when their use is controlled. Beta-blockers are prescribed less often because of their effects on patients with obstructive airway disease, although they are important if heart failure is present. Angiotensin-converting enzyme (ACE) inhibitors are less useful unless diabetes or heart failure is present.

Alpha$_1$-blockers, such as prazosin (Minipress) and terazosin (Hytrin) and centrally acting alpha$_2$-agonists, such as methyldopa (Aldomet), clonidine (Catapres), guanabenz (Wytensin), and guanfacine (Tenex), are infrequently used for elderly patients because of their adverse effects.

Focus on Geriatrics

Antihypertensives and Elderly Patients

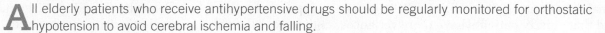

All elderly patients who receive antihypertensive drugs should be regularly monitored for orthostatic hypotension to avoid cerebral ischemia and falling.

Cardiac Glycosides

Physicians often overuse cardiac glycosides, partially because of their fear of heart failure in elderly patients. Because older patients are more susceptible to arrhythmias, the toxic effects of cardiac glycosides are particularly dangerous and the long-term use of these drugs should be carefully monitored because of their narrow therapeutic range. The half-life of digoxin (Lanoxin) may be increased by 50% or more in elderly patients, and renal function must be considered when a dosing regimen is being contemplated. In geriatric patients, coronary atherosclerosis, hypokalemia, hypomagnesemia, and hypoxemia all contribute to a high incidence of digitalis-induced arrhythmias. Other less common digitalis toxicities, including delirium, endocrine abnormalities, and visual changes, are also seen in elderly patients. With close monitoring of serum digoxin levels, creatinine clearance tests, and vital signs (the pulse should not be less than 60 beats/min), digoxin is considered safe for older adults.

Antiarrhythmic Drugs

Treating elderly patients who have dysrhythmias (also called *arrhythmias*) is challenging. Whereas clearances of quinidine and procainamide decrease, their half-lives increase in aging patients. Older people exhibit changes in hemodynamic reserve, an incidence of severe coronary disease, and different frequencies of electrolyte disturbances—all of which contribute to arrhythmias. Disopyramide (Norpace) should be avoided because of its major toxicities. The half-life of lidocaine (Anestacon) is increased in elderly patients, and its loading dose should be reduced in geriatric patients to avoid toxicity.

However, patients with atrial fibrillation do as well with simple control of their ventricular rate as they do with conversion to normal sinus rhythm. For safety, measures should still be taken to reduce possible thromboembolism in chronic atrial fibrillation (such as with anticoagulant drugs or aspirin therapy).

Anticoagulants

Bleeding may occur with the chronic use of anticoagulants in elderly patients. Warfarin (Coumadin) is 99% protein-bound, and with a decrease in serum albumin, which is common among older adults, there is an increase in free, unbound circulating warfarin. There is a significant risk for bleeding as a result. Regular testing to determine the level of warfarin in the blood and to regulate anticoagulant drug therapy is essential for everyone taking the drug, particularly elderly individuals.

Focus Point

Prothrombin Time

Elderly patients who are taking anticoagulants must undergo periodic monitoring of prothrombin time or international normalized ratio to determine the level of anticoagulant in the blood and to regulate anticoagulant drug therapy.

CENTRAL NERVOUS SYSTEM DRUGS

Numerous drugs influence the action of chemical mediators and affect neurotransmitter release and reception. These drugs may act by blocking receptors and prevent the transmitters from binding them. CNS drugs for geriatric patients—sedative–hypnotics, narcotic analgesics, antidepressants, antipsychotics, and drugs used for Alzheimer's disease—are discussed in this section.

Sedatives and Hypnotics

Insomnia is a common problem for elderly patients. Sedatives and hypnotics are the second-most common group of drugs prescribed for or taken OTC by elderly patients. In those who are 60 to 70 years old, the half-lives of many barbiturates and benzodiazepines show their greatest age-related increase. These agents are eliminated more slowly if the patient has reduced renal function or a liver disease. It is generally believed that elderly patients have more variances in their sensitivity to sedative and hypnotic drugs on a pharmacodynamic basis. To avoid injuries and accidents, ataxia and other motor impairments should be especially watched for in older individuals taking these drugs.

Narcotic Analgesics

Narcotics may cause dose-related adverse effects when taken by elderly patients. Geriatric patients are often more sensitive to the respiratory effects of narcotic analgesics because of the way respiratory function changes with increased age. Patients should be evaluated regarding their sensitivity to these agents before administration, and caution should be continually used. Hypotension may also result from narcotic use. However, for conditions requiring strong analgesia (such as cancer), opioids are frequently underutilized for this group of patients. Good pain management plans are easily obtained, and the underutilization of narcotic analgesics is generally unjustified.

Antidepressants and Antipsychotics

Phenothiazines, such as promazine (Prozine-50) and perphenazine (Phenazine), and phenothiazine-like drugs, such as haloperidol (Haldol), have sometimes been overused in managing psychiatric diseases in elderly patients. These agents are effective in treating schizophrenia, delirium, dementia, aggressiveness, and paranoia but are not fully satisfactory for geriatric patients. These drugs do not appear to be effective in dementia caused by Alzheimer's disease. When an antipsychotic drug that has sedative effects is required in elderly patients, a phenothiazine, such as thioridazine (Mellaril), is adequate except in patients with a pre-existing extrapyramidal disease. Older drugs, such as chlorpromazine (Thorazine), should be avoided in elderly patients because of their orthostatic hypotension-inducing effects. Drug doses should be gradually increased according to the patient's tolerance and the desired therapeutic effect. There should be close monitoring for possible adverse effects.

The half-lives of some phenothiazines are increased in the geriatric population, and dosages should be started at just a fraction of the amounts used for young adults. Lithium (Eskalith) must be dosage-adjusted because of its clearance by the kidneys, and thiazide diuretics should not be used with lithium because it further reduces renal clearance.

Older adults are more likely to experience toxic effects of antidepressants, but they are just as responsive to them as other adults. Senile dementia and major depression must be carefully diagnosed because they may resemble each other. If a tricyclic antidepressant is to be used, nortriptyline (Aventyl) and desipramine (Norpramin) are good choices because of their reduced antimuscarinic effects.

Focus Point

Depression and Suicide

The suicide rate among people older than age 65 is more than twice the national average, and psychiatric depression—a leading cause of suicide—is often undertreated in elderly patients.

Medications Used for Alzheimer's Disease

Alzheimer's disease is characterized by progressive memory and cognitive function impairment, which may lead to a completely vegetative state and, ultimately, death. The biochemical defects responsible for Alzheimer's disease have not been identified. It is believed that abnormal neuronal lipoprotein processing, together with changes in choline acetyltransferase, brain glutamate, dopamine, norepinephrine, serotonin, and somatostatin, are causative factors.

Cholinomimetic drugs are usually the focus of treatment for Alzheimer's patients. Cerebral vasodilators have been deemed ineffective. A cholinesterase inhibitor called tacrine (Cognex) enters the CNS quickly and has a duration of 6 to 8 hours. This drug apparently increases the release of acetylcholine from cholinergic nerve endings and may inhibit monoamine oxidase; decreases the release of gamma-aminobutyric acid; and increases the release of norepinephrine, dopamine, and serotonin from nerve endings. However, it has significant toxic effects, including nausea, vomiting, and liver toxicity.

Donepezil (Aricept), rivastigmine (Exelon), and galantamine (Reminyl) have been shown to improve cognitive activity in some patients with Alzheimer's disease. They may even reduce morbidity from other diseases and slightly prolong the life of the patient. These agents should be used with caution in patients receiving other cytochrome P450 enzyme inhibitors, such as ketoconazole (Nizoral) and quinidine (Quinora).

Focus on Geriatrics

Central Nervous System Drug Toxicities

Alzheimer's patients are often very sensitive to CNS toxicities of drugs that have antimuscarinic effects.

ANTI-INFLAMMATORY DRUGS

For osteoarthritis and rheumatoid arthritis, nonsteroidal anti-inflammatory drugs (NSAIDs), such as naproxen (Naprosyn) and ibuprofen (Advil, Motrin), must be used with special care because of toxicity. Although aspirin causes GI irritation and bleeding, newer NSAIDs may cause irreversible kidney damage. They accumulate more rapidly in geriatric patients, especially in those with renal disease. Elderly patients receiving large doses of NSAIDs must be carefully monitored for changes in renal function.

For those who cannot tolerate full NSAID doses, corticosteroids, such as hydrocortisone (Cortef, Hydrocortone) and prednisone (Deltasone, Meticorten), are very useful. However, these agents can cause osteoporosis that is related to the dose and duration of corticosteroid therapy. Increased calcium and vitamin D intake may reduce these effects. Frequent exercise should also be encouraged during corticosteroid therapy.

GASTROINTESTINAL AGENTS

Histamine-2 (H_2) receptor blockers are safer drugs than other antiulcer agents for the treatment of peptic ulcers. Ranitidine (Zantac), famotidine (Pepcid), and nizatidine (Axid) may be used for elderly patients. Cimetidine (Tagamet) is not suggested for older adults because of its side effects and multiple potential drug interactions.

Laxatives are commonly taken by elderly patients. In long-term facilities, such as nursing homes, 75% of older adult patients use laxatives on a daily basis. Fluid and electrolyte imbalances may occur with excessive use. Increased GI motility with laxative use may decrease the absorption of other drugs.

ANTIMICROBIAL DRUGS

Elderly patients appear to have reduced host defenses due to alterations in their T-lymphocyte function. As a result, they are more susceptible to serious infections and diseases, such as cancer. Antimicrobial drugs have been used since 1940 to compensate for this deterioration of natural body defenses. Important changes in the half-lives of antimicrobial drugs may be expected because of decreased renal function. This is very important in the case of aminoglycosides owing to their toxicities to the kidneys and other organs. For example, the half-lives of gentamicin (Garamycin), kanamycin (Kantrex), and netilmicin (Netromycin) are more than doubled in elderly patients.

Penicillins, such as amoxicillin (Amoxil); cephalosporins, such as cefotaxime (Claforan); sulfonamides, such as sulfadiazine (Gantanol[3]); and tetracyclines, such as tetracycline HCl (Achromycin), are considered safe for elderly patients. If the patient has a decrease in renal drug clearance and the drug has a prolonged half-life, the drug dose should be reduced.

✱ Apply Your Knowledge 31.2

The following questions focus on what you have just learned about changes in the effects of drugs on the elderly population.

CRITICAL THINKING

1. Why should all elderly patients who receive antihypertensive drugs be regularly monitored?
2. Which psychiatric disorder is a leading cause of suicide in elderly patients?
3. Why is cimetidine (Tagamet) not suggested for older adults?
4. What are two factors that indicate drug doses for elderly patients should be reduced?
5. What group of patients are often very sensitive to CNS toxicities of drugs with antimuscarinic effects?

Special Considerations

Inadequate health-care and prescription coverage often force older patients to avoid taking required medications that are important for their quality of life. For example, newer NSAID therapies for arthritis treatment may cost more than $100 a month.

Noncompliance because of forgetfulness may result in patients not staying on a regular drug regimen, thereby greatly reducing effectiveness. Deliberate noncompliance may also occur based on prior poor experience with a drug. Other noncompliance in taking drugs may be caused by physical disabilities or difficulty in using spoons, syringes, and other equipment. Enlisting the elderly patient as an educated, willing participant in drug therapies is vital. Labels should be large enough for patients to read, and any other impediments to sticking to a drug regimen should be noted and efforts should be made to overcome them.

Health-care practitioners should adhere to the following principles when treating elderly patients:

* Take drug histories carefully.
* Prescribe drugs only for specific, rational indications.
* Define the goal of drug therapy.
* Start with small doses, adjust slowly, and check blood levels when necessary.
* Maintain suspicion regarding drug reactions and interactions by knowing what other drugs the patient is taking.
* Keep the drug regimen as simple as possible. Try to use drugs that may be taken at the same time every day and use the smallest number of drugs possible.

Focus Point

More Drugs Prescribed for the Elderly Population

People older than 65 account for more than 32% of the drugs prescribed in the United States, even though they represent only about 12% of the total population.

PRACTICAL SCENARIO 1

An 82-year-old man arrives at the hospital complaining of chest pains. An electrocardiogram reveals congestive heart failure, and he is treated with various drugs, including a diuretic and an ACE inhibitor. His condition stabilizes, and he is discharged. Seven days later, he experiences nausea and confusion. His doctor treats the nausea but does not treat the confusion, assuming it is related to senility. The patient develops a tremor in his hands, which is an adverse effect of the drug prescribed for his nausea. He is given benztropine, which then causes constipation. The doctor gives him docusate tablets for the constipation, but the patient's confusion increases until he is extremely anxious. Next, the doctor prescribes an antipsychotic, which calms the patient down but results in depression. The doctor prescribes an antidepressant, but the patient soon dies from ventricular tachycardia.

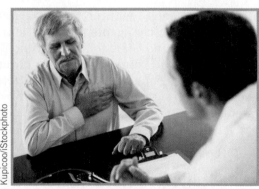
Kupicoo/iStockphoto

Critical Thinking Questions

1. What action by the physician may have led to this patient's death?
2. What are the principles that might have helped the physician make different drug therapy decisions for the patient?
3. What assumptions did the physician make early in the course of therapy that may have been unwarranted or incorrect?

PRACTICAL SCENARIO 2

A 73-year-old woman has insomnia. Her physician prescribes a benzodiazepine. This patient also has cirrhosis of the liver.

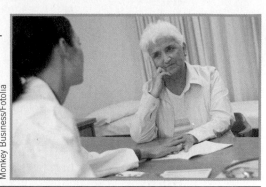

Monkey Business/Fotolia

Critical Thinking Questions

1. What is the most important caution that her physician should consider when prescribing a benzodiazepine for this patient?
2. What is the half-life of a benzodiazepine in an elderly patient?

Chapter Capsule

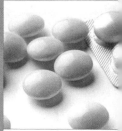

This section repeats the objectives from the beginning of the chapter and then provides a summary of the most important concepts for that objective. Use this section as a quick review and to check your knowledge.

Objective 1: Discuss the process of aging.

- Physiologic changes—decreased cardiac output and blood flow, function of liver enzymes and blood flow, kidney blood flow, glomerular filtration, nephron function, gastric secretions, peristalsis and motility, first-pass effect, body water, hepatic blood flow, kidney weight, lean body mass, serum albumin, and increased body fat

- Biological, psychological, sociological, and behavioral changes; changes in sensory processes and in roles and self-definitions; slowdown of physical movement; decreased dexterity

Objective 2: Explain the leading causes of diseases and death in elderly patients older than 65.

- Heart disease, including heart attacks and chronic ischemic heart disease—35% of deaths among elderly individuals

- Cancer—about 22% percent of deaths in the elderly population

- Chronic diseases—stroke, chronic obstructive pulmonary disease, diabetes, pneumonia, and influenza

- Alzheimer's disease and several serious renal diseases—have increased over the past two decades as causes of death in elderly individuals

Objective 3: Identify the factors that influence drug absorption in older adults.

- Slower gastric emptying
- Altered nutritional habits
- Greater use of OTC medications

Objective 4: Discuss creatinine clearance in elderly patients and use the measurement formula.

- Creatinine clearance is an indicator of the glomerular filtration rate; creatinine is a by-product of the muscle breakdown of stored proteins but is excreted primarily by the kidneys; serum creatinine level can be measured by the 24-hour creatinine clearance test to evaluate renal function

■ Creatinine clearance can also be calculated by this formula:

$$\text{Creatinine clearance in mL / min} = \frac{(140 - \text{age}) \times (\text{weight in kg})}{72 \times \text{serum creatinine in mg / dL}}$$

Objective 5: Identify polypharmacy and its effects on elderly patients.

■ Polypharmacy   prescribing multiple medicines to a single patient simultaneously by one or more physicians; taking herbal drugs in addition to prescribed drugs

■ Effects—increased costs of treatment; increased chances for side effects and drug interactions; possible liver dysfunction, malnutrition, confusion, and falls

Objective 6: List common cardiovascular disorders in elderly individuals.

■ Hypertension

■ Congestive heart failure

■ Myocardial infarction

■ Stroke

Objective 7: Discuss the effects of sedatives and hypnotics on elderly patients.

■ The half-lives of many sedatives and hypnotics increase in patients ages 60 to 70.

■ The reduced elimination of the drugs occurs if the patient has impaired renal function or a liver disease.

■ Elderly patients often have more variances in their sensitivity to these drugs.

■ Ataxia and other motor impairments can occur.

Objective 8: List six principles that are important in treating elderly patients.

■ Take drug histories carefully.

■ Prescribe drugs only for specific, rational indications.

■ Define the goal of drug therapy.

■ Start with small doses, adjust slowly, and check blood levels.

■ Know what other drugs the patient is taking.

■ Keep the drug regimen as simple as possible.

 ## Internet Sites of Interest

■ For a review of renally excreted drug dosing, visit **http://www.rxkinetics.com/renal.html**.

■ WebMD presents an article on the prescribing of sedatives for elderly people with insomnia based on material from the *British Medical Journal* at **http://www.webmd.com**. Search for "sedatives elderly."

■ PharmacyTimes.com offers "Understanding and Managing Polypharmacy in the Elderly" at **http://www.pharmacytimes.com**. Search for "polypharmacy in the elderly."

PEARSON
myhealthprofessionskit™

Go to www.myhealthprofessionskit.com to access the Companion Website created for this textbook. Simply select "Basic Health Science" from the choice of disciplines. Find this book and then log in using your username and password to access interactive learning games, assessment questions, animations, and more.

Chapter Objectives

After completing this chapter, you should be able to:

1. List drugs that may result in toxicity in newborns or infants.

2. Describe drug toxicities in neonates from percutaneous absorption.

3. List three example drugs that should not be used in neonates because of their lowered protein binding.

4. Explain the factors that affect pharmacokinetics in children.

5. Describe the means by which adult doses must be adjusted for pediatric drug administration.

6. Discuss pharmacodynamics in newborns, infants, and children.

7. List five drugs that produce pharmacological effects in nursing infants.

8. Explain the effects of radioactive substances in breast milk.

Chapter 32

Drugs Used to Treat Pediatric Patients

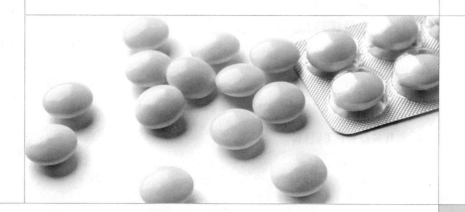

Key Terms

elixirs (ee-LICKS-ers) (page 571)
gestation (jes-STAY-shun) (page 571)
infants (page 570)
kernicterus (ker-NIK-ter-rus) (page 571)

neonates (NEE-oh-nayts) (page 570)
peripheral blood circulation (page 570)
peristalsis (payr-iss-STALL-sis) (page 570)

suspensions (page 571)
toddlers (page 570)

Introduction

Lack of knowledge and understanding of the clinical pharmacology of specific drugs in pediatric patients, particularly in newborns, can result in many problems in drug therapy. The problem of establishing efficacy and dosing guidelines for infants is further complicated by the fact that the pharmacokinetics of many drugs change greatly as an infant ages from birth to several months after birth. The dose-response relationships of some drugs may change markedly during the first few weeks after birth. Then, during the first few months of life, physiologic processes and their resulting pharmacokinetic variables change significantly. This is why it is vital to pay special attention to the pharmacokinetics of pediatric patients. The differences between younger patients and other groups have not been greatly researched.

The term **neonates** refers to newborns from birth to 28 days old, **infants** are from 29 days old to walking age (typically 1 year), and **toddlers** are children from approximately 1 year to 3 years.

Pharmacokinetics

The basic pharmacologic principles that apply to adults (see Chapter 1) also apply to neonates, infants, and younger children. Only the ways in which they differ in neonates and infants are discussed in this chapter.

DRUG ABSORPTION

In infants and children, the drug absorption process is similar to that of adults. Factors such as blood flow at the site of administration and gastrointestinal (GI) function influence drug absorption. These factors change rapidly soon after birth.

Physiologic conditions that can reduce the rate of blood flow to the site of administration include heart failure, cardiovascular shock, and vasoconstriction. For example, there is very little muscle mass in a preterm infant who is sick. Drugs may remain in the muscles and be absorbed more slowly than anticipated. If **peripheral blood circulation** (the circulation in the body's extremities) improves, a sudden increase of circulating drugs may result in potentially toxic drug concentrations. Drugs that can be especially dangerous

in these situations include aminoglycoside antibiotics, anticonvulsants, and cardiac glycosides.

Because of rapidly changing biochemical and physiologic changes that occur in the GI tract of infants, drugs that are inactivated by the low pH of gastric contents should not be given orally. **Peristalsis** (the rhythmic movement of the intestines) in neonates is irregular and may be slower than anticipated. Great care must be taken in administering drugs to neonates because of the unpredictability of their rates of absorption.

The rate of gastric emptying is an important determinant of the overall rate and extent of drug absorption. It is variable during the neonatal period and is affected by gestational maturity, postnatal age, and type of feeding. Gastroesophageal reflux, respiratory distress syndrome, and congenital heart disease in neonates can delay gastric emptying.

Chemical agents applied to the skin of a premature infant may result in inadvertent poisoning. For example, drug toxicities in neonates are reported for percutaneous absorption of such agents as hexachlorophene (Phisohex), laundry detergents with pentachlorophenol, hydrocortisone (Alphaderm), and disinfectant solutions with aniline.

DRUG DISTRIBUTION

Neonates have higher percentages of water than adults. Extracellular water makes up 40% of body weight in neonates, compared with 20% in adults. Most neonates experience diuresis in the first two days of life. It is important, especially for water-soluble drugs, to determine the concentration of a drug at receptor sites.

The amount of body fat in full-term neonates is about 15%. Organs that accumulate high concentrations of lipid-soluble drugs in older children may accumulate smaller amounts of these types of agents in younger infants. Another important factor is drug binding to plasma proteins. Albumin's affinity for acidic drugs and the total plasma protein concentration increase during the time from birth into early infancy. These do not reach normal adult values until 10 to 12 months of age. Usually, protein binding of drugs is lowered in neonates. This has been seen with local anesthetic drugs, diazepam (Valium), phenobarbital (Barbital), ampicillin (Amcill), and phenytoin (Dilantin). Therefore, the concentration of free (unbound) drug in plasma is increased. This results in greater drug effect or toxicity.

Focus on Pediatrics

Physiologic Impacts on Pharmacokinetics

The physiologic processes that influence pharmacokinetics in children include GI function, tissue blood flow, body fluid levels, plasma protein concentrations, liver function, and renal function.

Certain drugs compete with serum bilirubin in binding to albumin. Drugs given to a neonate with jaundice can displace bilirubin from albumin, and because of the greater permeability of a neonate's blood–brain barrier, large amounts of bilirubin may enter the brain and cause **kernicterus**, which is a serious form of jaundice in newborns.

DRUG METABOLISM

Most drugs are metabolized in the liver. Drug-metabolizing oxidases and conjugating enzymes exhibit substantially lower activity in neonates. Because of these lower metabolic activities, many drugs have slow clearance rates and longer half-life elimination times. Drug doses and dosing schedules must be altered appropriately. If not, the neonate may experience adverse effects from drugs that are metabolized in the liver.

The limited knowledge and understanding of the clinical pharmacology of specific drugs in pediatric patients predispose this population to problems in the course of drug treatment, particularly in newborns and infants. There are no FDA requirements for pediatric studies, which means that determining appropriate efficacy and dosage guidelines for the therapeutic use of drugs in children must rely extensively on pharmacologic data derived primarily from adults. The problem of establishing efficacy and dosage guidelines for infants is further complicated by the fact that the pharmacokinetics of many drugs change appreciably as an infant ages from birth (which is sometimes premature) to several months after birth. The dose-response relationships of some drugs may change markedly during the first few weeks after birth.

Pharmacokinetics and organ responsiveness also change dramatically during development from the embryonic and fetal periods to adulthood. Prematurely born neonates at gestations as short as 24 weeks are now surviving (a full-term **gestation**, or the period of fetal development from conception until birth, is 40 weeks).

DRUG EXCRETION

The glomerular filtration rate (GFR) is much lower in newborns than in older children and adults. Based on body surface area, a neonate's GFR is only 30% to 40% that of an adult. Premature babies show an even lower GFR. However, GFRs do improve greatly during the first week after birth. By the end of the third week, glomerular filtration is 50% to 60% of an adult's. Adult values are reached by the time an infant is 6 to 12 months old. Drugs that require renal function for elimination are removed from the body very slowly during the first weeks of life.

Toddlers may have shorter elimination half-lives of drugs than older children and adults—probably as a result of higher renal elimination and metabolism. One example concerns the drug digoxin. The dose per kilogram of this drug is much higher for toddlers than for adults, which is a fact that is still not fully understood.

* Apply Your Knowledge 32.1

The following questions focus on what you have just learned about pediatric pharmacokinetics.

CRITICAL THINKING

1. What physiologic processes may influence pharmacokinetics in children?
2. What are the definitions of the terms *neonate*, *infant*, and *toddler*?
3. What is the cause of kernicterus?
4. What is the result of lower metabolic activities in neonates?
5. Why is the GFR in newborns much lower than in older children?

Pediatric Dosage Forms and Compliance

Actual pediatric dosages are determined by taking into account the form of the drug and how a parent or caregiver will dispense it to the child. Elixirs and suspensions are popular forms for pediatric administration. **Elixirs** are alcoholic solutions that offer consistent dissolution and distribution of the drugs they contain. **Suspensions** are dosage forms that contain undissolved drug particles and must be shaken to evenly distribute them. This is essential because if a suspension drug form is not adequately shaken, it will cause dangerous variations in dosages. For example, an uneven distribution of drug is a potential cause of inefficacy or toxicity in children taking phenytoin (Dilantin) suspensions. The prescriber must provide proper instructions to the pharmacist and the child's parents or caregivers.

Major dosing errors may result from incorrect calculations because many pediatric doses are calculated by using body weight. A common but potentially fatal mistake is that 10 times the amount of medication is administered because a decimal point was placed incorrectly. A good rule to use in avoiding decimal point errors is to always use a zero to the left of a decimal point for doses that are less than 1 (Figure 32-1 ■). Also, zeros should not be used after decimal points if they are not needed.

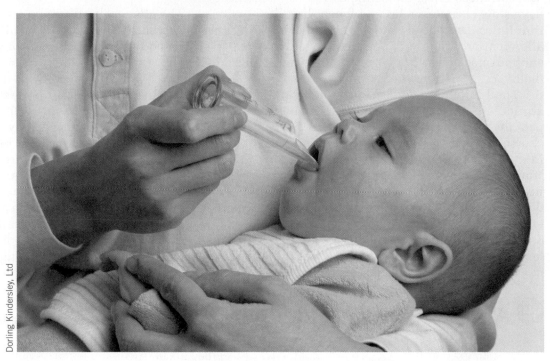

Figure 32-1 ■ Using the measuring device provided by the pharmacy or physician is important for giving the correct dose to children. © Dorling Kindersley.

Dorling Kindersley, Ltd

Pharmacodynamics

The mechanisms of action of drugs in newborns, infants, and children involve a complex sequence of events. An inadequate response to an effective concentration of a drug may result from the presence or absence of receptors, inadequate drug–receptor binding, or the inability of the organ or tissue to respond to the postreceptor signal. One particular drug may have a specific affinity for a special cell. Some drugs may act by affecting the enzyme functions of the body.

Each of these events progresses at different rates during development—beginning with growth to biochemical maturation and eventually to structural maturation, at which point the organ can respond fully to the events initiated by a drug.

Certain drugs pose particular difficulties when used in neonates because of the unique character of their distribution or elimination in patients in this age group or because of the unusual side effects they may cause. These drugs include antibiotics, digoxin (Lanoxin), indomethacin (Indameth), and methylxanthines.

Drug Administration During Lactation

Many women avoid breastfeeding because they incorrectly believe that drugs they may be taking are in sufficient quantities to cause great risk to their infants. In actuality, more babies die because of problems from baby formula than from the milk of their mothers.

Still, it is important to realize that most drugs taken by lactating women do pass through to the breast milk. Drug concentration in breast milk is usually low. In a one-day period, the amount of drug an infant receives from nursing is much less than what would be considered a "therapeutic dose." If a drug is prescribed as safe for a mother to take while she is breastfeeding, she should take it 1 to 2 hours before breastfeeding or 3 to 4 hours after breastfeeding to minimize the effect on the infant. Most over-the-counter (OTC) medications provide information on the label about their safety during lactation. Nursing mothers should avoid OTC products that contain multiple ingredients, such as cold remedies, as well as those containing more than 20% alcohol. Nursing mothers should not take more than the dosage listed on the product label.

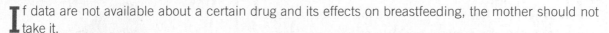

Focus on Pediatrics

Drug Safety During Lactation

If data are not available about a certain drug and its effects on breastfeeding, the mother should not take it.

Many antibiotics are highly detectable in breast milk. Tetracyclines appear at about 70% of maternal serum concentrations and can stain the developing teeth of an infant. Isoniazid (Laniazid) can quickly reach equilibrium between maternal blood and breast milk. Its concentrations in breast milk can cause signs of pyridoxine deficiency in the infant if the mother does not take pyridoxine supplements (Beesix).

Sedatives and hypnotics can produce pharmacologic effects in nursing infants. Barbiturates can produce sedation and poor sucking reflexes; sedation can also be caused by chloral hydrate. Diazepam (Valium) can also sedate a nursing infant but, more importantly, can result in significant drug accumulation.

Heroin, methadone (Dolophine), and morphine (Avinza) can cause narcotic dependence in infants, and these infants may have to be tapered off, as would their mothers. Excessive amounts of alcohol can produce alcoholic effects in infants. Lithium (Eskalith) enters breast milk in concentrations equal to those in maternal serum, and the baby may be exposed to relatively large amounts of this drug as a result. Radioactive substances can increase the risk of thyroid cancer in infants, and chemotherapeutic, cytotoxic, or immune-modulating agents are also potentially dangerous to the pediatric population. No matter what medication the breastfeeding mother is taking, she should monitor her infant for any signs of drug effect and report this to the infant's health-care provider.

Focus on Natural Products

Lobelia Dangers

Lobelia is found in dietary supplements that are marketed for use by children and infants as well as pregnant women. Lobelia may be very dangerous to use because it contains alkaloids with pharmacologic actions that are similar to nicotine. It can cause autonomic nervous system depression or stimulation, bronchial dilation, increased respiratory rate, respiratory depression, sweating, rapid heart rate, hypotension, and even coma or death.

Pediatric Drug Dosages

It is not always safe to proportionally reduce adult doses to determine safe pediatric doses. Patients or their parents should always follow their physician's instructions about pediatric dosages and double-check them with the drug manufacturer's product inserts and labels. The FDA is moving toward more stringent demands on the testing and thorough labeling of new drug products for children. The recommended pediatric dose—usually stated as milligrams per kilogram or milligrams per pound—should always be followed.

✳ Apply Your Knowledge 32.2

The following questions focus on what you have just learned about pediatric dosage forms.

CRITICAL THINKING

1. What pediatric dosage forms are more popular for drug administration?
2. Which pediatric dosage form must be shaken before administration to an infant?
3. What factor is the major cause of dosing errors?
4. What is the effect of heroin in nursing infants?
5. What is the result of the difference in pharmacokinetics in children compared with those in young adults?

PRACTICAL SCENARIO 1

Alice, age 32, is breastfeeding her newborn. Alice has developed a cold and says she is not sleeping at night because of her symptoms. She wants to take an over-the-counter (OTC) decongestant and cough suppressant. But Alice's health-care provider instructed her that she cannot take any medication while breastfeeding without first checking with her physician. Alice is confused and questions you about this.

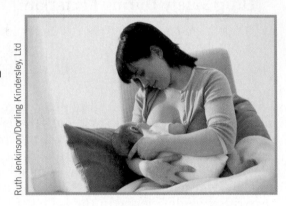
Ruth Jenkinson/Dorling Kindersley, Ltd

Critical Thinking Questions

1. How would you address Alice's concerns?
2. Is it safe for Alice to take an OTC product for her cold symptoms while she is breastfeeding?
3. How can Alice help to minimize any effect on her infant from taking a medication?

PRACTICAL SCENARIO 2

A newborn baby was in the neonatal care ward with seizures. Her pediatrician prescribed a barbiturate medication for intramuscular injection.

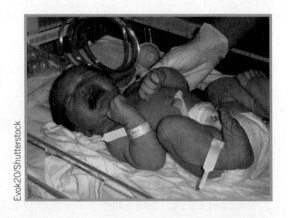
Evok20/Shutterstock

Critical Thinking Questions

1. Describe the four stages of pharmacokinetics.
2. Because an infant's kidneys do not develop fully until 6 months of age, what important consideration should the pediatrician remember before administering any medications?

Chapter Capsule

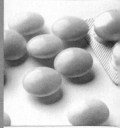

This section repeats the objectives from the beginning of the chapter and then provides a summary of the most important concepts for that objective. Use this section as a quick review and to check your knowledge.

Objective 1: List drugs that may result in toxicity in newborns or infants.

■ Drugs that can be especially dangerous to newborns or infants include aminoglycoside antibiotics, anticonvulsants, and cardiac glycosides.

Objective 2: Describe drug toxicities in neonates from percutaneous absorption.

■ Agents that may result in inadvertent poisoning in neonates include hexachlorophene, pentachlorophenol-containing laundry detergents, hydrocortisone, and aniline-containing disinfectant solutions.

Objective 3: List three example drugs that should not be used in neonates because of their lowered protein binding.

■ Local anesthetic drugs
■ Diazepam
■ Phenobarbital

Objective 4: Explain the factors that affect pharmacokinetics in children.

■ Drug absorption—physiologic conditions that can reduce the rate of blood flow to the site of administration include heart failure, cardiovascular shock, and vasoconstriction; if peripheral blood circulation improves, a sudden increase of circulating drugs may result in potentially toxic drug concentrations; rate of gastric emptying.

■ Drug distribution—neonates have higher percentages of water than do adults; their amount of body fat is about 15%; another important factor is drug binding to plasma proteins; protein binding of drugs is lowered in neonates.

■ Drug metabolism—neonates exhibit substantially lower drug-metabolizing activities of oxidases and conjugating enzymes; the dose-response relationships of some drugs may change markedly during the first few weeks after birth.

■ Drug excretion—in newborns, the glomerular filtration rate is much lower than in older children or adults; drugs that require renal function for elimination are removed from the body very slowly during the first weeks of life.

Objective 5: Describe the means by which adult doses must be adjusted for pediatric drug administration.

■ Pediatric drug dosages are based on proportionally reduced adult doses.
■ They can be based on body surface area, age, and body weight.

Objective 6: Discuss pharmacodynamics in newborns, infants, and children.

■ An inadequate response to an effective concentration of a drug may result from the presence or absence of receptors or inadequate drug–receptor binding.
■ A particular drug has a specific affinity for a special cell.
■ Some drugs may act by affecting the enzyme functions of the body.

■ Certain drugs pose particular difficulties when used in neonates because of the unique character of their distribution or elimination in patients in this age group or because of the unusual side effects they may cause.

Objective 7: List five drugs that produce pharmacological effects in nursing infants.

■ Antibiotics
■ Sedatives and hypnotics
■ Heroin
■ Alcohol
■ Lithium

Objective 8: Explain the effects of radioactive substances in breast milk.

■ These substances can increase the risk of thyroid cancer in infants, and chemotherapeutic, cytotoxic, and immune-modulating agents are also potentially dangerous to babies.

 Internet Sites of Interest

■ Search **http://www.medscape.com** for "pediatric pharmacotherapy."
■ The site **http://www.mapharm.com/med_calc_pedi.htm** provides information about medical assisting pharmacology with calculation examples.
■ Search for "drugs and other substances in breast milk" at **http://www.kidsgrowth.com**.

PEARSON
myhealthprofessionskit™

Go to www.myhealthprofessionskit.com to access the Companion Website created for this textbook. Simply select "Basic Health Science" from the choice of disciplines. Find this book and then log in using your username and password to access interactive learning games, assessment questions, animations, and more.

Chapter Objectives

After reading this chapter, you should be able to:

1. Describe various stages of reproduction that may potentially be affected by drug toxicity.

2. Define the terms *reproductive toxicology, developmental toxicity,* and *embryo toxicity* and *fetotoxicity.*

3. Explain the four principles concerning a drug's potential to induce developmental disorders.

4. Define *pharmacokinetics* in pregnant women.

5. Discuss the possible outcomes if toxic agents contact a developing embryo or fetus during embryogenesis or organogenesis.

6. Describe which drugs used during lactation can cause disruption to the infant's normal sleeping patterns.

7. Define the term *teratology.*

8. Discuss immunizations during pregnancy.

9. Identify which vaccine may be administered during pregnancy without any harm to the mother or baby.

Chapter 33

Drugs Used to Treat Pregnant Patients

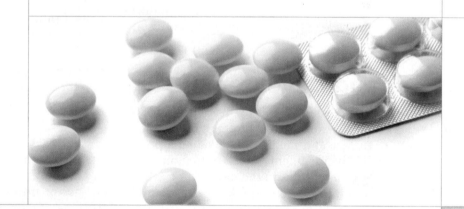

Key Terms

cohort (KO-hort) (page 582)

developmental toxicity (dee-vel-op-MEN-tul tok-SIS-ih-tee) (page 583)

dysmorphology (dis-mor-FAH-lo-jee) (page 583)

embryotoxicity or fetotoxicity (em-bree-oh-tok-SIS-ih-tee or fee-toh-tok-SIS-ih-tee) (page 583)

epidemiological (ep-ih-dee-mee-oh-LAH-jih-kul) (page 582)

fetal (FEE-tul) (page 578)

fetotoxic (fee-toh-TOK-sik) (page 582)

metabolites (meh-TAB-oh-lahyts) (page 581)

oogonia (ooh-ooh-GO-nee-uh) (page 578)

perinatal (peh-ree-NAY-tul) (page 578)

phenylketonuria (feh-nul-kee-toh-NOOR-ee-uh) (page 583)

reproductive toxicology (ree-pro-DUK-tiv tok-sih-KAH-lo-jee) (page 583)

teratogenicity (teh-rat-oh-jeh-NIH-sih-tee) (page 583)

teratogens (teh-RAT-oh-jens) (page 581)

teratology (teh-rah-TAH-lo-jee) (page 583)

tidal volume (TY-dul VAHL-yoom) (page 579)

transplacental (trans-plah-SEN-tul) (page 578)

Introduction

Pregnancy begins with conception and ends with the delivery of the baby. During the life span, organs and body systems undergo physiological changes that affect the absorption, metabolism, distribution, and elimination of medications. Health professionals must understand these changes to ensure that drugs are administered safely and effectively to patients of all ages. It is important to understand the effects of medications before becoming pregnant, during the entire time a fetus is carried, and throughout early life.

Drugs can affect all stages of pre- and postnatal development. During embryonic life, the majority of organs and systems are forming. Drugs and other substances, including radiation, may be particularly harmful during the first trimester of pregnancy. Pregnant women must be educated about the use of medications when attempting to become pregnant because the effects of medications on an embryo may be severe. The study of drug effects on pregnant patients is not as advanced as the study of other areas of pharmacology, although advances are being made. Drugs used during pregnancy have the potential to cause **fetal** malformations, restricted growth, functional defects, and death.

Health and Development

Although most normal pregnancies require only minimal medical intervention, high-risk pregnancies may require intensive care and medications. When a pregnant woman is ill, the treatment or lack of treatment of her condition may be harmful to the developing fetus. It is widely known that cigarette smoking and alcohol use are damaging to fetuses, but many prescription and over-the-counter (OTC) drugs also have harmful effects. Herbal supplements must also be carefully used, and proper nutrition during pregnancy is essential. The effects of improper nutrition and the use of certain medications have been linked to diseases later in the life of the fetus, including fertility disorders, metabolic imbalances, diabetes, cardiovascular conditions, and even schizophrenia.

STAGES OF REPRODUCTION

Each developmental stage has its own sensitivities to toxic agents. The following list details specific potential outcomes of use of toxic agents and poor nutrition at each stage of development.

* Germ cell formation: sterility, damage to sperm or egg cells, chromosomal defects, menstrual and menopausal defects, hormone imbalances
* Fertilization: impotence, sterility, chromosomal defects, reduced sperm function
* Implantation: spontaneous abortion, low birth weight, stillbirth
* Embryogenesis: spontaneous abortion, birth defects, chromosomal defects, low birth weight, stillbirth
* Organogenesis: spontaneous abortion, birth defects, retarded development, functional disorders (such as autism), **transplacental** carcinogenesis
* **Perinatal** period: premature birth, birth defects (usually nervous system related), stillbirth, neonatal death, toxicity, withdrawal symptoms
* Postnatal period: mental retardation, infant death, retarded development, metabolic and functional disorders, developmental disabilities (such as epilepsy or cerebral palsy)

About one month after the first day of the last menstruation, primordial germ cells are present in an embryo. These cells differentiate into **oogonia** and oocytes or into spermatogonia. During a female's life span, nearly 400 oocytes undergo ovulation. In males, the onset of meiosis begins at puberty, and spermatogenesis continues throughout the reproductive life. Therefore, prenatal and postnatal drug exposure may be toxic during any stage of development. Each sex reacts differently to various toxic agents.

✳ Apply Your Knowledge 33.1

The following questions focus on what you have just learned about health and development.

CRITICAL THINKING QUESTIONS

1. Why are many medications prohibited during the first trimester of pregnancy?
2. What are the potential outcomes when toxic agents are used during organogenesis?
3. How can fetal toxicity from drugs be best prevented?

DRUG ADMINISTRATION DURING PREGNANCY AND LACTATION

Great caution should be taken when administering drugs during pregnancy and lactation. When possible, it should be avoided completely or nonpharmacologic methods should be undertaken. However, for specific, serious conditions, pharmacotherapy is required. If epilepsy, hypertension, or psychiatric disorders exist before pregnancy, drug therapy should not be discontinued during pregnancy or lactation. Conditions that occur during pregnancy, such as gestational diabetes and hypertension, must be treated to maintain the health of the growing fetus. Because such infections as acute urinary tract infections and sexually transmitted diseases may harm fetuses, antibiotics may be indicated. Regardless of the condition, health-care practitioners must determine whether the therapeutic benefits of drug administration outweigh potential adverse effects.

PHARMACOTHERAPY IN THE PREGNANT PATIENT

The effects of a drug on the mother and the fetus must be considered before it can be administered. Certain substances easily pass from the mother to the fetus through the semipermeable placenta. Other substances are blocked from this passage. The membranes of the fetus detoxify some substances, such as insulin, as they cross the membrane. Drugs that are bound to plasma proteins, ionized, or water-soluble are not as likely to cross the placenta.

Major physiological and anatomic changes occur in pregnant women. Some of these changes alter drug pharmacokinetics and pharmacodynamics. Changes in hormone levels as well as pressure exerted on the blood supply by the expanding uterus may affect the absorption of drugs. Progesterone slows the transit time for food and drugs in the gastrointestinal (GI) tract. This allows for a longer time for absorption of drugs taken orally. Gastric emptying also slows, and gastric acidity is decreased. Inhaled drugs may be absorbed more readily because increased **tidal volume** and pulmonary vasodilation occur in pregnancy women.

Cardiac output, plasma volume, and regional blood flow may be increased, causing dilution of drugs and decreased plasma protein concentration. Lipid level alterations may affect drug transport and distribution (primarily during the third trimester). Drug metabolism increases may cause higher doses of certain drugs to be used (primarily anticonvulsants). Because fat-soluble drugs are distributed into breast milk (which is rich in lipids), they may be passed to the lactating infant.

Blood flow through the mother's kidneys increases between 40% and 50% by the third trimester. This affects glomerular filtration rate, renal plasma flow, and renal tubular absorption. Drug excretion is then affected, including the onset of action and dosage timing.

PREGNANCY DRUG CATEGORIES AND REGISTRIES

Only a small number of prescription drugs have been verified as being teratogenic or are strongly suspected as teratogens. Alternative drugs can be safely used instead. Newer or infrequently used drugs should be avoided in pregnant women until their outcomes are better understood. The FDA has created drug pregnancy categories, as shown in Table 33-1 ■.

Illicit drugs, such as cocaine, also affect fetuses. Although testing drugs in human subjects for teratogenicity is unethical and legally prohibited, animal testing is regularly undertaken. However, these studies do not provide identical outcomes because human placentas (and other components) are structurally different from those of animals. The following rule must be remembered: No prescription drug, OTC medication, herbal product, or dietary supplement should be taken during pregnancy unless a physician verifies that the therapeutic benefits to the mother clearly outweigh the potential risks for the unborn.

Unfortunately, the current pregnancy drug labeling system does not give specific clinical information to help understand the true safety of medications. It does not indicate how doses should be adjusted during pregnancy. Most drugs are ranked as Category C for pregnancy because high doses produce teratogenicity in animals. All drugs in Category D or Category X must be avoided during pregnancy because of potentially severe birth defects. Women of childbearing age must be checked about their intentions of becoming pregnant before being prescribed any drugs that are potentially harmful to the fetus.

PREGNANCY REGISTRIES

Pregnancy registries gather information from women who have taken certain medications during pregnancy to determine those that are safe for use by others when they become pregnant. By comparing women who did not take a specific medication while pregnant with those who did, data are compiled on fetal outcomes. Pregnancy registries are maintained by drug companies, governmental agencies, and special interest groups. Here is a list of pregnancy registries:

✳ http://otispregnancy.org lists asthma medications.

✳ http://www.apregistry.com/who.htm lists antiretroviral medications.

Table 33-1 ■ **Food and Drug Administration Pregnancy Drug Categories**

RISK CATEGORY	DESCRIPTION	EXAMPLES
A	Well-controlled studies of pregnant women with no demonstrated increased risk of fetal abnormalities in any trimester	Folic acid, insulin, prenatal multivitamins, thyroxine
B	Either animal reproduction studies have not demonstrated a fetal risk but there are no controlled studies in pregnant women, or animal reproduction studies have shown an adverse effect that was not confirmed in controlled studies in women in the first trimester.	Acetaminophen, azithromycin, cephalosporins, penicillins, ibuprofen in the first and second trimesters
C	Either studies in animals have revealed adverse effects on the fetus and there are no controlled studies in women, or studies in women and animals are not available. Drugs should be given only if the potential benefit justifies the potential risk to the fetus.	Most prescription medications, most antihypertensives, antimicrobials (such as clarithromycin, co-trimoxazole [Bactrim], and fluoroquinolones), corticosteroids, SSRIs
D	Well-controlled studies of pregnant women have demonstrated fetal risk, but benefits of therapy may outweigh the risk, especially in life-threatening situations or serious diseases that cannot be effectively treated with safer drugs.	ACE inhibitors and ARBs in the second and third trimesters; alcohol, gentamicin, ibuprofen in the third trimester; nicotine; conjugated estrogens (Premarin); tetracyclines
X	Well-controlled or observational animal studies have shown positive risk of fetal abnormalities; use of these products is contraindicated in pregnant women and those who may become pregnant. THERE IS NO INDICATION FOR USE IN PREGNANCY.	Isotretinoin (Accutane), misoprostol, thalidomide

ACE, angiotensin-converting enzyme; ARB, angiotensin receptor blocker; SSRI, selective serotonin reuptake inhibitor.

✳ http://www.motherisk.org/women/index.jsp lists antipsychotic medications.

✳ http://www2.massgeneral.org/aed lists epilepsy medications.

Also, the FDA's list of pregnancy registries is located at http://www.fda.gov/ScienceResearch/SpecialTopics/WomensHealthResearch/ucm134848.htm.

✳ Apply Your Knowledge 33.2

The following questions focus on what you have just learned about drug administration during pregnancy and lactation.

CRITICAL THINKING QUESTIONS

1. Why must drug therapy be continued during pregnancy when the patient has hypertension?
2. Why may physiological and anatomic changes in pregnant women alter drug pharmacokinetics and pharmacodynamics?
3. Why may increases in metabolism require higher doses of anticonvulsants?
4. Which federal agency has created drug pregnancy categories and why?
5. Which category of pregnancy drugs is contraindicated in pregnant women? List three examples.

TOXIC EFFECTS AND RESPONSES

Developmental toxicity may cause many different conditions, including chromosomal and genetic disorders, infertility, intrauterine death, spontaneous abortion, low birth weight, prematurity, functional disorders, and birth defects. Toxic effects may occur at different times and be highly unpredictable. Many structural malformations occur during the period of organogenesis (between 20 and 70 days after the first day of last menstruation). They can also occur from 1 week before the missed menstruation until the woman is 44 days past due. Exposure to radiographs may also have unpredictable timed effects. Also, teratogens may be **metabolites** and not the actual administered compounds.

During fetal development, common responses to toxic agents include restricted growth, structural malformations, functional impairment, fetal death, and transplacental carcinogenesis. Because organ and system maturation occurs beyond organogenesis and the prenatal period, responses may occur over a much longer period of time. This may lead to behavioral, reproductive, immunologic, and other responses, including those related to endocrine, metabolic, and intelligence functions. Also, carcinogenic effects of certain agents are increased because fetal tissues are more vulnerable to their effects.

Focus Point

Radiographs

The primary manifestations of intrauterine radiation effects on humans are growth retardation and central nervous system defects.

PHARMACOKINETICS

During pregnancy, metabolism and kinetics of drugs are more complicated. Influences include uptake, distribution, metabolism, and excretion by the mother. Other factors involve the passage and metabolism of agents through the yolk sac and placenta. Embryos and fetuses distribute, metabolize, and excrete agents differently than in the postnatal period, with reabsorption and swallowing of substances from the amniotic fluid being unique to fetal development.

During pregnancy, GI motility and distribution to plasma proteins is decreased compared with other times during life. However, nearly all other resorptive, distributive, metabolic, and excretive processes are increased. These include lung function, skin–blood circulation, distribution to plasma volume, distribution to body water, distribution to fat deposition, and the glomerular filtration rate. However, the metabolic liver activity in developing fetuses may be increased or decreased depending on many factors.

Because total body water may be increased up to 81% during pregnancy, drugs can be distributed in a greatly increased volume. Because albumin is decreased in concentration, the binding of acidic drugs, such as aspirin or phenytoin, is likewise decreased. Increased female hormones due to pregnancy may inactivate certain medications and environmental agents. During the last trimester, greatly increased renal plasma flow causes a more rapid elimination of drugs without being changed by the kidneys.

✳ Apply Your Knowledge 33.3

The following questions focus on what you have just learned about toxic effects and responses.

CRITICAL THINKING QUESTIONS

1. What are the common responses to toxic agents during fetal development?
2. Why are drugs with shorter half-lives preferable during lactation?
3. Why do many structural malformations occur during the first trimester?
4. Why is distribution of plasma protein decreased during pregnancy?
5. Why does more rapid elimination of drugs occur during the last trimester?
6. Why should radiographs not be used during the first trimester of pregnancy?

Drug Effects on the Newborn

The passage of drugs to fetuses and the way that fetal kinetics work are of most concern with long-term drug therapy. The placenta allows oral medications to pass between the maternal and fetal circulation. Drugs cross the placenta by passive diffusion. It should be understood that basically any drug will reach the fetus. The only drugs that are not able to cross the placenta are conjugated steroid and peptide hormones, such as growth hormone and insulin. Others, such as modified immunoglobulins (such as abciximab), are instead metabolized by the placenta itself.

By the third month of pregnancy, the liver of the fetus can activate or inactivate chemical substances by the process of *oxidation*. Accumulation of biologically active substances can take place in the fetal compartment. At this stage, fetuses have not yet developed the blood–brain barrier, making many chemicals **fetotoxic**. Penicillins, cephalosporins, and antiretrovirals concentrate in the fetal compartment. Fetuses can also swallow excreted substances in the amniotic fluid.

RISKS OF TOXICITY

Risks of toxicity concerning embryos and fetuses are assessed in a variety of methods. These include animal experimentation, **epidemiological** studies, case studies, and other methods. Drugs that have been proven to have significant toxicity to embryos and fetuses include:

✳ Angiotensin-converting enzyme inhibitors and angiotensin II receptor antagonists

✳ Alcohol

✳ Androgens

✳ Antimetabolites

✳ Benzodiazepines

✳ Carbamazepine

✳ Cocaine

✳ Coumarin anticoagulants

✳ Diethylstilbestrol

✳ Ionizing radiation

✳ Iodine overdose

✳ Lead

✳ Lithium

✳ Methyl mercury

✳ Misoprostol

✳ Penicillamine

✳ Phenobarbital and primidone in anticonvulsive doses

✳ Phenytoin

✳ Polychlorinated biphenyls

✳ Retinoids

✳ Tetracycline after week 15

✳ Thalidomide

✳ Trimethadione

✳ Valproic acid

✳ Vitamin A (over 25,000 international units per day)

Ideally, every pregnancy should be studied and all outcomes assessed. Many analytical studies use the **cohort** approach, in which a specific adverse outcome is studied in women who were exposed to the same toxic agent. Sometimes, case-control studies within cohort groups of women are conducted. These lead to the identification of possible statistical associations between the exposure and outcome.

Prolonged use of certain medicines during pregnancy is likely to cause fetal harm. Women who have epilepsy, diabetes, or thyroid dysfunction often regularly use long-term medications, making pregnancy especially dangerous. Also, women with psychiatric illnesses may require fetotoxic medications on a long-term basis.

✳ Apply Your Knowledge 33.4

The following questions focus on what you have just learned about drug effects on fetuses.

CRITICAL THINKING QUESTIONS

1. What is the reason that the placenta allows oral medications to pass to the fetus?

2. In which month of pregnancy does the liver of the fetus begin to activate or inactivate chemical substances by the process of oxidation?

3. What methods may be used to assess the risks of toxicity concerning embryos or fetuses?

4. What term is used to study a specific adverse outcome in women who were exposed to the same toxic agent?

5. What may be the long-term effects on the fetus of drugs used to treat psychiatric illnesses in the mother?

Drugs Used During Pregnancy

Nearly 80% of pregnant women use prescription or OTC drugs. Exposures to occupational and environmental agents while pregnant are also very common. It is best to avoid taking any medications unless absolutely necessary when pregnant. Illegal drugs, tobacco, and alcohol must be avoided. Classifications of drugs in relation to pregnancy are primarily based on human toxicity testing.

RISKS OF MEDICATIONS DURING PREGNANCY

Most pregnant women take between three and eight different medications during their pregnancies. The risks of each medication should be discussed between pregnant patients and their physicians before beginning use or before patients even become pregnant. If a patient has already taken any medication and is pregnant, the physician should continue to communicate with her about potential outcomes. This communication should include whether diagnostic procedures may be required to assess any fetal harm and consideration of termination of pregnancy if the harm is severe. It is not enough to rely on safety warnings printed on package inserts, reference books, and other sources to inform patients about the potential toxicities of medications.

TOXIC STATES

Reproductive toxicology is the study of the effects of toxic agents during the entire reproductive process. **Developmental toxicity** involves adverse effects that occur before adulthood. **Teratology** is the study of structural birth defects in general, although it also relates to certain functional defects. **Embryotoxicity or fetotoxicity** involves toxic effects resulting from prenatal exposure as well as structural or functional abnormalities of the postnatal manifestations of these effects. **Teratogenicity** is defined as a manifestation of developmental toxicity by induction or an increase of frequency of structural disorders in the embryo or fetus.

Poor nutrition has been linked to many birth defects, as have such disease states as German measles (rubella) and toxoplasmosis. Perhaps the most famous case of severe birth defects occurred in the thalidomide disaster, wherein the mild sedative thalidomide taken by pregnant women caused fetal limb deformities. Although the prevalence of birth defects, which affect between 3% and 4% percent of babies, is not increasing, the potential for them as caused by the use of toxic agents is real. Another area of concern is exposure to environmental toxicity—often in the workplace.

The best prevention of toxic states on fetuses is achieved through public education. Curbing such habits as smoking and alcohol use is essential. Proper vaccination with all recommended vaccines is also critical. Drugs are classified into categories based on their potential to cause harm to developing fetuses, but these categories must be understood so they can be used properly. Also, when a metabolic disorder, such as **phenylketonuria**, is detected early enough, the diet may be adjusted so phenylalanine is present in only very low levels to prevent mental retardation. The removal of toxic agents from the market is the best way to avoid future harm.

In general, pregnant women must be educated so that no drugs of any kind are taken during pregnancy unless they are essential for proper health and development. When a drug is required, the potential risks must be discussed and understood. There are four established principles concerning a drug's potential to induce developmental disorders:

✳ **Principle 1:** Dose-effect relationship. The dose response is important in determining the level of toxicity. Most drugs have a threshold or "no effect" level. The daily dose is important to consider as well as the route of exposure.

✳ **Principle 2:** Species susceptibility. Not every drug has the same effects on humans as it does on other animals. Environmental factors may also be related.

✳ **Principle 3:** Period of development. Depending on the stage of development, drugs may have differing effects. This explains how during early development, **dysmorphology** (the study of birth defects, especially those that affect the anatomy) more likely occurs as a result of a specific drug that later in development causes functional disorders instead.

✳ **Principle 4:** Mode of action. To understand potential toxicity, a drug's molecular targets should be identified. The transport and metabolism of toxic agents play significant roles in this area.

✳ Apply Your Knowledge 33.5

The following questions focus on what you have just learned about drugs used during pregnancy.

CRITICAL THINKING QUESTIONS

1. Why is the education of pregnant women important to inform them not to take any medications unless they are absolutely necessary?
2. What term is used to study the effects of toxic agents during the entire reproductive process?
3. What is the definition of *teratogenicity*?
4. What is phenylketonuria?
5. What is the definition of the term *dysmorphology*?
6. What was the result when pregnant women took the drug thalidomide?

PHARMACOTHERAPY DURING LACTATION

Breast milk receives secretions that carry a large number of drugs, although this has only been documented as causing a few infant injuries. Safer alternative drugs are usually available for use during lactation. Studies of drugs used during lactation must continue to fully understand their effects. Drugs that are highly lipid-soluble are most likely to enter the breast milk. These include central nervous system medications. Usually, these agents exist in the breast milk at lower than clinically significant levels. Drugs that exist in the maternal plasma (such as warfarin) and are bound to albumin are not able to penetrate the mother's breast milk.

Drugs that should be avoided during breastfeeding are listed by the American Academy of Pediatrics' Committee on Drugs. Health-care professionals working with pregnant and breastfeeding women should pay attention to drug guides and the information they contain about the risks of using specific drugs during these times. Table 33-2 ■ lists specific drugs associated with adverse effects during breastfeeding.

Table 33-2 ■ Specific Drugs Associated with Adverse Effects During Breastfeeding

GENERIC NAME	TRADE NAME	EFFECTS
acebutolol	Sectral	Bradycardia, hypotension, tachypnea
amiodarone	Cordarone	Hypothyroidism
atenolol	Tenormin	Bradycardia, cyanosis
bromocriptine	Parlodel	Suppression of lactation and potential hazards to the mother
ergotamine	Ergostat	Diarrhea, vomiting, and convulsions (when used in the recommended doses for migraine medications)
fluoxetine	Prozac	Colic, feeding and sleeping disorders, reduced weight gain
haloperidol	Haldol	Decline in developmental scores
lithium	Eskalith	One-third to one-half therapeutic blood concentration in infants
phenobarbital	Luminal	Methemoglobinemia, sedation, infantile spasms after weaning from milk containing phenobarbital
primidone	Mysoline	Feeding problems, sedation
sulfasalazine	Azulfidine	Bloody diarrhea

Other drugs that may have adverse effects during breastfeeding include various amphetamines, which can cause irritability and poor sleeping patterns. Aspirin and other salicylates can cause metabolic acidosis. Cocaine can cause cocaine intoxication, diarrhea, irritability, tremulousness, seizures, and vomiting.

If possible, the use of a potentially risky drug during lactation should be postponed until the baby is weaned. Alternatively, a safer medicine should be used instead. If a drug must be used that has potentially risky effects, it should be administered immediately after breastfeeding so time will lapse between administration and the next breastfeeding. New mothers should be educated about the effects of alcohol, illicit drugs, and tobacco products during lactation.

Some drugs do not affect the nursing infant because they are destroyed in the infant's GI system or cannot be absorbed across the GI tract. Therefore, although a drug may be present in the breast milk, it is usually in such small amounts that no noticeable harm will be caused. However, premature, neonatal, and extremely ill infants may be at a greater risk for adverse drug effects because they lack drug-metabolizing enzymes. In general, drugs with shorter half-lives are preferable because those with longer half-lives (or active metabolites) can accumulate in the plasma of the infant. If possible, drugs with a high protein-binding ability should be selected because they are not secreted into the milk as readily. Because of a lack of testing, all OTC herbal products and dietary supplements should be avoided during lactation.

Recreational Drugs

Recreational drugs may also be harmful to developing embryos and fetuses and to nursing infants. They include alcohol, nicotine, opiates, caffeine, cannabis, cocaine, and other drugs.

ALCOHOL

Nursing infants receive about 10% of the alcohol consumed by their mothers. Alcohol can change the taste of breast milk and result in feeding problems.

Milk levels of alcohol decrease along with plasma levels of alcohol. The faster alcohol is consumed, the faster its levels change in breast milk. Sipping an alcohol drink slowly does not cause levels of alcohol in breast milk to rise sufficiently because the body has time to metabolize it. Studies show that one to two servings of alcoholic beverages per week have no effect on nursing infants, but amounts higher than that have been shown to pose more significant risks to infant health. When an alcoholic beverage is consumed, the mother should avoid breastfeeding for 2 hours so the alcohol can be fully metabolized. If alcohol use is chronic or excessive, the baby should be weaned from breastfeeding and given baby formula instead.

NICOTINE

Smoking tobacco products has been linked to poor milk supply as well as poor nursing, restlessness, and vomiting by the infant. Secondhand smoke causes a higher rate of infant respiratory illnesses. Mothers who continue smoking tend to breastfeed their infants less than those who do not. It is important to realize that infants who are bottle-fed instead of breastfed also have nicotine in their urine. Secondhand smoke is dangerous for infants regardless of the manner of their feeding. Nicotine and its major metabolite—cotinine—pass into breast milk quickly. Levels increase with the number of cigarettes smoked. Many other chemicals are also present in the breast milk of smoking mothers.

OPIATES

All opiates penetrate breast milk, including heroin, morphine, methadone, and others. There have been documented cases of infant death caused by extremely high levels opiates in breast milk. Infants may also become addicted to opiates if used in sufficient quantities. Methadone is safer than other opiates, but in general, all these agents should not be used by mothers when they are nursing their babies. Each case should be individually reviewed, and abrupt weaning should be avoided so withdrawal from opiates does not occur in the infant.

Focus Point

Codeine

Codeine is a morphine derivative with a more restricted analgesic and sedative effect during pregnancy than morphine.

CAFFEINE

Caffeine is quickly absorbed and readily enters breast milk. Because the livers of infants are immature, the elimination of caffeine takes much longer than in adults. Normal amounts of coffee are usually well tolerated by infants, but continued use of higher than normal amounts causes infants to become irritable, jittery, and not satisfied by breastfeeding. Often, it takes weeks for the infant to clear the caffeine level. Babies consuming caffeine often cannot sleep normally and may not be receiving normal amounts of iron from breast milk.

CANNABIS

Cannabis (marijuana or hashish) can be detected in breast milk and is stored in the brain and fat. The main effects of cannabis are related to the motor development of exposed infants, which is delayed. If cannabis is used regularly, the infant must be weaned from breast milk consumption.

COCAINE

Cocaine can be detected in breast milk but is cleared much more quickly than substances such as cannabis. However, the metabolites of cocaine are cleared much more slowly. Effects of cocaine on infants include hypertonia, tachycardia, excitation, and trembling. Habitual users of cocaine should avoid breastfeeding entirely.

Focus Point

Alcohols

Alcohols may be used topically as disinfectants during pregnancy. However, the consumption of alcohol during pregnancy causes a specific complex of congenital organic and functional developmental defects known as *fetal alcohol syndrome*.

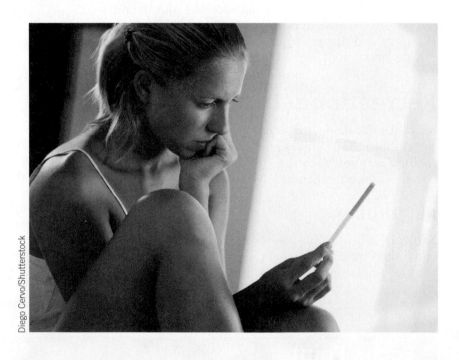

The consumption of alcohol during pregnancy can cause fetal alcohol syndrome.

Diego Cervo/Shutterstock

✳ Apply Your Knowledge 33.6

The following questions focus on what you have just learned about recreational drugs.

CRITICAL THINKING QUESTIONS

1. Why are fat-soluble drugs passed more quickly than other drugs to lactating infants?
2. What are the signs and symptoms of cocaine intoxication in lactating infants?
3. What are the adverse effects on infants whose mothers drink too much coffee?
4. If a mother consumes an alcoholic beverage, how long should she wait before breastfeeding her infant?
5. Why is smoking tobacco prohibited during lactation and breastfeeding?

Vaccinations During Pregnancy and Lactation

Protective and booster immunizations should be given before pregnancy for safety. Although no vaccines have proven embryotoxic or teratogenic effects, it is wise that excessive medication use be limited during the first trimester. Routine immunization should be avoided during pregnancy. However, when there is a high risk of infection because the mother has not received a common vaccine, she should be vaccinated regardless.

One of the concerns of vaccinations during pregnancy is that ethyl mercury is used as a preservative in vaccines, which may be a risk for fetuses' brains. Measles and mumps vaccines are contraindicated because fetuses may contract either disease. Most vaccines in general, should be avoided during pregnancy unless there is an actual high risk of contracting a specific disease without the vaccination.

Most of the normally administered vaccinations are not contraindicated during lactation. However, the live oral polio vaccine should not be given to the mother until the infant has been immunized at 6 weeks or older. The killed-virus injectable form of the smallpox vaccine is recommended during lactation.

Focus Point

Tetanus Vaccine

There are no indications of embryotoxic properties in the tetanus vaccine and it is safe to administer to pregnant women.

PRACTICAL SCENARIO 1

A 32-year-old woman who is 7 months pregnant has consumed four to five glasses of wine per week and has been unable to quit smoking. She also consumes three to four cups of coffee per day. She is admitted to her local hospital and delivers her baby prematurely.

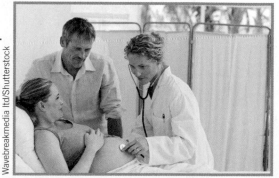
Wavebreakmedia ltd/Shutterstock

Critical Thinking Questions

1. What would be the best way to prevent premature delivery of the baby in this scenario?
2. What are the effects of nicotine, alcohol, and coffee on fetuses?
3. Which of these three substances is most dangerous to premature babies?

PRACTICAL SCENARIO 2

A 21-year-old woman went to the emergency room with a high fever, dyspnea, and chest pain. Her radiographs showed bilateral pneumonia, and her blood tests indicated a bacterial infection. She received antibiotics for 10 days (orally and intravenously). After discharge from the hospital, she took a pregnancy test and brought the results to her gynecologist, who determined she was 6 weeks pregnant.

Auremar/Shutterstock

Critical Thinking Questions

1. What are the adverse effects of any medications during the early stages of pregnancy?
2. What is the possibility of adverse effects on her baby?

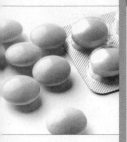

Chapter Capsule

This section repeats the objectives from the beginning of the chapter and then provides a summary of the most important concepts for that objective. Use this section as a quick review and to check your knowledge.

Objective 1: Describe various stages of reproduction that may potentially be affected by drug toxicity.

■ Drug toxicity may occur at different times and be highly unpredictable. Many structural malformations occur during the period of organogenesis. They can also occur from 1 week before the missed menstruation until the woman is 44 days past due. Because organ and system maturation occurs beyond organogenesis and the prenatal period, responses may occur over a much longer period of time.

Objective 2: Define the terms *reproductive toxicology*, *developmental toxicity*, and *embryotoxicity* and *fetotoxicity*.

■ Reproductive toxicology—the study of the effects of toxic agents during the entire reproductive process

■ Developmental toxicity—involves adverse effects that occur before adulthood

■ Embryotoxicity and fetotoxicity—involve toxic effects resulting from prenatal exposure as well as structural or functional abnormalities of the postnatal manifestations of these effects

Objective 3: Explain the four principles concerning a drug's potential to induce developmental disorders.

■ **Principle 1:** Dose-effect relationship. The dose response is important in determining the level of toxicity. Most drugs have a threshold or "no effect" level. The daily dose is important to consider as well as the route of exposure.

■ **Principle 2:** Species susceptibility. Not every drug has the same effects on humans as it does on other animals. Environmental factors may also be related.

■ **Principle 3:** Period of development. Depending on the stage of development, drugs may have differing effects. This explains how during early development, dysmorphology more likely occurs as a result of a specific drug that later in development causes functional disorders instead.

- **Principle 4:** Mode of action. To understand potential toxicity, a drug's molecular targets should be identified. The transport and metabolism of toxic agents plays a significant role in this area.

Objective 4: Define *pharmacokinetics* in pregnant women.

- During pregnancy, metabolism and kinetics of drugs are more complicated; gastrointestinal motility and distribution to plasma proteins are decreased compared to other times during life; however, nearly all other resorptive, distributive, metabolic, and excretive processes are increased.

- Pregnant woman experience increased lung function, skin-blood circulation, distribution to plasma volume, distribution to body water, distribution to fat deposition, and the glomerular filtration rate.

- Because total body water may be increased up to 81% during pregnancy, drugs can be distributed in a greatly increased volume.

- Increased female hormones because of pregnancy may inactivate certain medications and environmental agents.

Objective 5: Discuss the possible outcomes if toxic agents contact a developing embryo or fetus during embryogenesis or organogenesis.

- Embryogenesis— spontaneous abortion, birth defects, chromosomal defects, low birth weight, stillbirth

- Organogenesis—spontaneous abortion, birth defects, retarded development, functional disorders (such as autism), transplacental carcinogenesis

Objective 6: Describe which drugs used during lactation can cause disruption to the infant's normal sleeping patterns.

- Fluoxetine, various amphetamines, and caffeine

Objective 7: Define the term *teratology*.

- Teratology is the study of structural birth defects in general, although it also relates to certain functional defects

Objective 8: Discuss immunizations during pregnancy.

- Protective and booster immunizations should be given before pregnancy for safety. Although no vaccines have proven embryotoxic or teratogenic effects, it is wise that excessive medication use be limited during the first trimester. Routine immunization should be avoided during pregnancy. However, when there is a high risk of infection because the mother has not received a common vaccine, she should be vaccinated regardless. One of the concerns of vaccinations during pregnancy is that ethyl mercury is used as a preservative in vaccines, which may be a risk for fetuses' brains. Measles and mumps vaccines are contraindicated because fetuses may contract the disease. Most vaccines, in general, should be avoided during pregnancy unless there is an actual high risk of contracting a specific disease without the vaccination.

Objective 9: Identify which vaccine may be administered during pregnancy without any harm to the mother or baby.

■ The tetanus vaccine is safe for pregnant women, with no indications of embryotoxic properties.

 Internet Sites of Interest

■ The stages of human reproduction are discussed at **http://www.nature.com/scitable/topicpage/meiosis-genetic-recombination-and-sexual-reproduction-210**.

■ For information about drugs during pregnancy, see **http://www.pharmainfo.net/reviews/drugs-pregnancy**.

■ Drug use during pregnancy is discussed at **http://www.merck.com/mmhe/sec22/ch259/ch259a.html**.

■ Developmental disorders are explained at **http://www.firstsigns.org/delays_disorders/other_disorders.htm**.

■ Information about medications and diet during pregnancy is listed at **http://www.pregnancy-info.net/meds_during_pregnancy.html**.

■ The Teratology Society's website is located at **https://www.teratology.org**.

PEARSON myhealthprofessionskit™

Go to www.myhealthprofessionskit.com to access the Companion Website created for this textbook. Simply select "Basic Health Science" from the choice of disciplines. Find this book and then log in using your username and password to access interactive learning games, assessment questions, animations, and more.

Checkpoint Review 5

Select the best answer for the following questions.

1. Which of the following over-the-counter medications should be avoided by nursing mothers?

   a. iodine
   b. ascorbic acid
   c. nicotinamide
   d. cold remedies

2. Elderly patients appear to have reduced host defenses caused by alterations in the function of which of the following leukocytes?

   a. B lymphocytes
   b. T lymphocytes
   c. Macrophages
   d. Monocytes

3. Which of the following experiences the most age-related pharmacokinetic changes?

   a. Lean body mass
   b. Heart weight
   c. Kidney weight
   d. Body water

4. Which of the following age groups have higher percentages of water?

   a. Neonates
   b. Infants
   c. Teenagers
   d. Elderly adults

5. Prescribing multiple medications to a single patient simultaneously is called:

   a. Polydactylism
   b. Polypharmacy
   c. Pharmacology
   d. Polypharmacology

6. Pharmacokinetics deal with all the following except:

   a. Distribution
   b. Elimination
   c. Metabolism
   d. Mechanisms of action

7. Most of the common disorders seen in elderly people concern which of the following systems?

   a. Respiratory
   b. Cardiovascular
   c. Urinary
   d. Integumentary

8. All elderly patients who receive antihypertensive drugs should be regularly monitored for:

   a. Orthostatic hypotension
   b. Hyperglycemia
   c. Hypouricemia
   d. Hypernatremia

9. Suicides are more than twice as common in which of the following age groups?

   a. Young children
   b. Teenagers
   c. Young adults
   d. Elderly adults

10. Which of the following is present in higher percentages in neonates compared with adults?

    a. Water
    b. Fat
    c. Plasma protein
    d. Lean mass

11. Which of the following drug forms is most popular for pediatric administration?

    a. Powders and pills
    b. Intramuscular injections
    c. Elixirs and suspensions
    d. Suppositories

12. Tetracyclines show up as about 70% of maternal serum concentrations, and breastfeeding may cause which of the following adverse effects in infants?

    a. Staining of incoming teeth
    b. Staining of urine and tears
    c. Staining of skin and hair
    d. Renal failure

13. Exposure to radioactivity during pregnancy may increase the risk of cancer in infants. Which of the following organs is at most risk?

    a. Pancreas
    b. Thyroid
    c. Spleen
    d. Liver

14. All the following drugs may produce pharmacologic effects in nursing infants except:

    a. Lithium and alcohol
    b. Antacids and vitamins
    c. Sedatives and hypnotics
    d. Heroin and antibiotics

For questions 15 to 19, match the lettered trade name to the numbered generic name.

GENERIC NAME	TRADE NAME
15. _____ fluoxetine	a. Tenormin
16. _____ lithium	b. Luminal
17. _____ primidone	c. Mysoline
18. _____ phenobarbital	d. Eskalith
19. _____ atenolol	e. Prozac

Select terms from your reading to fill in the blanks.

20. In newborns, the glomerular filtration rate is much _____ than in older children or adults.

21. Creatinine clearance is an indicator of glomerular _____.

22. The administration of many drugs together is more common in the _____ because of the use of different physicians and specialties.

23. Pregnancy registries are maintained by special interest groups, governmental agencies, and _____ _____.

24. The pregnancy drug category that indicates a drug should never be used during pregnancy is drug category _____.

25. The study of birth defects is referred to as _____.

26. Precursor cells from which oocytes develop are called _____.

27. Agents that cause congenital malformations and developmental abnormalities are called _____.

28. Prenatal and postnatal drug exposure may be toxic during _____ _____ of development.

29. During pregnancy, cardiac output and regional blood flow may be increased, causing the dilution of drugs and _____ plasma protein concentration.

30. Many structural malformations occur during the period of _____.

31. Drugs can be distributed in a greatly increased volume because total _____ _____ may be increased up to 81% during pregnancy.

32. Drugs cross the placenta by _____ diffusion.

Glossary

absence seizures   Brief seizures characterized by the arrest of activity and occasional muscle contractions and relaxations

absorption   The process of drug movement into the systemic circulation

abuse potential   The potential for a drug to cause dependence, abuse, or both

accommodation   Focusing of the lens of the eye

acetaminophen   An analgesic used to relieve mild to moderate pain; it also has antipyretic properties

acids   Substances that react with bases; aqueous acids have a pH of less than 7

acromegaly (ak-roh-MEHG-uh-lee)   A disorder in which the extremities, such as the hands, feet, and head, are greatly enlarged

activated charcoal   Charcoal that has been treated with oxygen; used to reduce absorption of poisons in the body

active immunity (ih-MYOO-nih-tee)   A form of acquired immunity that develops in an individual in response to an immunogen

acute   (a) Characterized by sharpness or severity (acute pain; an acute infection); (b) having a sudden onset, sharp rise, and short course (an acute disease; an acute inflammation)

Addison's disease (ADD-iss-uns)   Adrenocortical insufficiency caused by an autoimmune response to the adrenal gland

additive effect   When two substances or actions used in combination produce a total effect the same as the sum of the individual effects

additives   Chemicals that are added to foods to facilitate their processing and preservation, enhance their restorative or stimulating properties, and control natural contaminants

adenocarcinoma (ah-deh-no-kar-sih-NO-muh)   A malignant tumor arising from a glandular origin

adenohypophysis (add-eh-no-hy-PO-fih-sis)   Anterior lobe of the pituitary gland

adjuvant (AJ-eh-vant)   Aiding or contributing to

adrenergic (add-ruh-NUR-jik)   Referring to neurons that release norepinephrine, epinephrine, or dopamine

adverse effects   Harmful effects

affinity   Attractive force

agonist (AH-go-nist)   A drug that binds to a receptor and produces an appropriate physiologic response that is similar to what an endogenous substance would do

akathisia (ak-kuh-THIS-zee-uh)   Difficulty in initiating muscle movement

alimentary canal   Part of digestive system that includes the mouth, pharynx, esophagus, stomach, small intestine, large intestine, rectum, and anus

alkalies   Basic, ionic salts that dissolve in water; soluble bases have a pH of more than 7

alkaloids (AL-kuh-loyds)   Organic nitrogen-containing compounds that are alkaline and usually bitter tasting; combine with acids to make a salt

alkylating agents (AL-kih-lay-ting)   Agents that cause the replacement of hydrogen by an alkyl group, specifically one that inhibits cell division and growth

alopecia (al-o-PEE-shuh)   Hair loss

alpha tocopherol (AL-fa toh-KAW-fer-rol)   Vitamin E; a substance that protects fragile red blood cell walls (mainly in premature infants) from breaking down

alpha-adrenergic receptors (AL-fuh add-ruh-NUR-jik ree-SEP-ters)   Parts of cells that respond to adrenaline

aluminum hydroxide   Base element used as an antacid

alveolar duct (al-vee-OH-lar dukt)   End of each bronchiole

alveolar sacs   Thin-walled air sacs in the bronchioles

alveoli (al-VEE-oh-lie)   Microscopic air sacs in the capillary networks of bronchioles

Alzheimer's disease (AL-zhymerz)   A disease characterized by progressive memory and cognitive function impairment, which may lead to a completely vegetative state and, ultimately, death

amylase (AM-mil-lace)   Digestive enzyme

anabolic steroids (AN-uh-bol-lik STER-oidz)   Hormonal substances related to estrogen, progestins, testosterone, and corticosteroids, which promote muscle growth

analgesia (ah-nul-JEE-zee-ah)   Insensibility to pain without loss of consciousness

analgesic (ah-nul-JEE-zik)   Relating to, characterized by, or producing pain relief with or without antipyretic or anti-inflammatory action

anaphylactic shock (an-nuh-fih-LAK-tik)   A sudden and severe allergic reaction that may be life threatening

androgens   Male sex hormones

anemia (uh-NEE-mee-uh)   A deficiency of hemoglobin, red blood cell number, or red blood cell volume

anesthesia (an-ess-THEE-zee-ah)   Loss of sensation or consciousness

anesthetics (an-ess-THET-iks)   Substances that produce anesthesia

angina pectoris (an-JY-nuh pek-TOR-iss)   A common form of ischemic heart disease that often precedes and accompanies myocardial infarction; described as chest pain and squeezing pressure that can radiate to the jaw and arm

anions (AN-eye-ons)   Negatively charged ions

antagonist (an-TAH-go-nist)   An agent that acts in physiologic opposition; in pharmacology, it is an agent that prevents an agonist from binding to a receptor, thereby blocking its effects

antibacterial spectrum (an-tie-BAK-tee-ree-ul SPEK-trum)   The range of bacteria against which an agent is effective

antibiotics (an-tie-by-AW-tik)   Substances produced by microorganisms that in low concentrations are able to inhibit or kill other microorganisms

antibodies (an-tih-BAH-deez)   Special proteins manufactured by the lymphocytes when a foreign substance invades the body

anticholinergics (AN-tee-kol-in-UR-jiks)   Drugs that inhibit the actions of acetylcholine by occupying the acetylcholine receptors

antidiuretic hormone (ADH)   A hormone (also called *vasopressin*) that is released from the posterior lobe of the pituitary gland; exerts an antidiuretic effect; its absence can cause diabetes insipidus

antigens (AN-tih-jenz)   Specific chemical targets, usually pathogens, parts, or products of pathogens, or other foreign compounds against which antibodies react

antihistamine   A drug that inhibits the action of histamine by blocking it from attaching to histamine receptors

antimetabolites (an-tee-meh-TAH-bo-lytz)   Substances that prevent cancer cell growth by affecting DNA production; effective only against cells that are actively participating in cell metabolism

antimicrobial (an-tie-my-KRO-bee-ul)   Referring to an agent that destroys or inhibits the growth of microorganisms, especially pathogenic microorganisms

antioxidant   An agent that prevents cellular structure from being broken down by oxygen

antipsychotics   Any of the powerful tranquilizers (for example, phenothiazines or butyrophenones) used especially to treat psychosis and believed to act by blocking dopamine nervous receptors; also *neuroleptics*

antipyretics (an-tih-pye-REH-tiks)   Drugs that reduce elevated body temperature (fever) to normal levels

antitumor antibiotics   Agents made from natural products produced by species of the soil fungus *Streptomyces*; very effective in the treatment of certain tumors

antitussives (an-tee-TUSS-ivz)   Agents that reduce coughing

antivenom   Purified antibody against venoms or venom components

apothecary system (ah-PAW-thuh-keh-ree)   A very old English system of measurement that has been replaced by the metric system

approved name   A drug's nonproprietary (or generic) name

aqueous humor (AY-kwee-us)   Watery fluid that fills the space between the cornea and lens, helps nourish these parts, and aids in maintaining the shape of the front of the eye; secreted from the ciliary body

arabic number   A number commonly used in expressing quantity and value, such as 0, 1, 2, 3, 4, 5, 6, 7, 8, and 9

ascorbic acid (as-SCOR-bik)   Vitamin C; a substance required for building and maintaining strong tissues for wound healing, resistance to infection, and enhanced iron absorption

aseptic (ay-SEP-tik)   Hand washing and other precautions to reduce the risk of infection

asplenia (as-PLEN-ee-yuh)   Loss of the spleen

asthma   A chronic disease caused by increased reactivity of the tracheobronchial tree to various stimuli

ataxia   An inability to coordinate muscle activity

atelectasis (at-tuh-LEK-tuh-sis)   Absence of gas in the lungs, causing collapse

atrioventricular node (AY-tree-oh-ven-TRI-kyoo-ler)   Node that provides the only normal conduction pathway between the atrial and ventricular syncytia; its fibers delay impulse transmission; located in the inferior portion of the septum, which separates the atria, and just beneath the endocardium

atrium (AY-tree-um)   Smaller upper-receiving chamber of the heart

atropine   An alkaloid extracted from various plants that has competitive antagonist actions for muscarinic acetylcholine receptors

attenuated (ah-TEN-yoo-ay-ted) Reduced severity of (a disease) or virulence or vitality of a pathogenic agent

automaticity (aw-toe-muh-TIH-sih-tee) The heart impulse's automatic, spontaneous initiation

bacteria Single-celled organisms with a cell wall and cellular organelles that allow them to live independently in the environment

bactericidal (bak-tee-ree-uh-SY-dul) Capable of killing microbes

bacteriostatic (bak-tee-ree-oh-STAH-tik) Capable of inhibiting microbial growth

basal ganglia A group of cell bodies in the medulla involved in the regulation of motor activity

benign (be-NYN) Of a mild type or character that does not threaten health or life; related to cancer; slow growing

benzene An organic chemical compound with carcinogenic properties that is used as an industrial solvent as well as an ingredient in many industrial chemicals

benzodiazepines Psychotropic agents used as antianxiety agents, muscle relaxants, sedatives, and hypnotics

beri-beri (BEH-ree BEH-ree) A disease caused by a deficiency of thiamine and characterized by edema, cardiovascular abnormalities, and neurologic symptoms

beta-adrenergic receptors (BAY-tuh add-ruh-NUR-jik) Receptors that respond to norepinephrine or epinephrine

bevel The slanted part at the needle's tip

bioavailability The degree and rate at which a substance (as a drug) is absorbed into a living system or is made available at the site of physiologic activity

biotransformation The process of conversion of drugs within the body

blepharitis (blef-fah-RY-tis) Inflammation of one or both eyes

blood pressure Commonly means *arterial pressure*; pressure created in the vessels by the pumping action of the heart; varies from one vessel to another within the systemic circuit

blood volume Total amount of blood in vascular system

booster A substance that increases the effectiveness of a medication

bradycardia (bray-dee-KAR-dee-uh) An abnormally slow heartbeat

bradykinesia (bray-dee-kuh-NEE-shuh) Extremely slow movement

bradykinin (brah-dee-KYE-nin) A polypeptide that mediates inflammation, increases vasodilation, and contracts smooth muscle

broad spectrum Referring to agents that are effective against a wide range of organisms

bronchioles (BRONG-kee-ols) The portion of the bronchial tubes that are less than 1 mm in diameter and have abundant smooth muscle and elastic fibers

bronchitis Inflammation of the mucous membrane of the bronchial tubes

bronchodilators Agents that widen the diameter of the bronchial tubes

bronchospasm Contraction of smooth muscle in the walls of the bronchi and bronchioles

bundle of His A large group of fibers that enter the upper part of the intraventricular septum and are divided into right and left bundle branches lying just beneath the endocardium—between the atrioventricular node and the Purkinje fibers; also known as the *atrioventricular bundle*

calciferol (kal-SIH-fuh-rol) Vitamin D_3

calcitonin (kal-sih-TOE-nin) A thyroid hormone that lowers blood levels of calcium and phosphate and promotes bone formation

calcitriol (kal-SIH-tree-ol) The active vitamin D hormone

calibrated Marked with graduated measurements

candidiasis (kan-dih-dy-AY-sis) An infection or disease caused by *Candida spp.*, especially *Candida albicans,* usually resulting from debilitation, physiologic change, prolonged administration of antibiotics, and barrier breakage

cannabinoids Organic substances, such as tetrahydrocannabinol (THC), found in cannabis

cannula (KAN-yoo-luh) The actual metal length that makes up the majority of the needle; it is attached to the hub

capsule A solid dosage form featuring a drug contained inside an external shell

carbohydrates Any of a large group of compounds that contain carbon, hydrogen, and oxygen and can be broken down to release energy in the body

carbon monoxide A gas that is highly toxic in large quantities; it forms when there is not enough oxygen to produce carbon dioxide

carcinogenic (kars-ih-no-JEN-ik) Cancer causing

cardiac output Volume of blood pumped per minute

carotene (KAH-roh-teen) Substance found in dark green and yellow vegetables and fruits and converted to vitamin A in the human body

cataract A clouding of the lens of the eye or its surrounding transparent membrane that obstructs the passage of light

catecholamines (kah-teh-KOH-luh-meenz) Any of various amines (epinephrine, norepinephrine, and dopamine) that contain a dihydroxybenzene ring; are derived from tyrosine; and function as hormones, neurotransmitters, or both

cations (KAT-eye-ons) Positively charged ions

cell-mediated immunity Immunity obtained when cells attack the antigens directly rather than producing antibodies; lymphocytes are the primary cells that provide this immunity

central nervous system The brain and spinal cord

cerebrum (seh-REE-brum) The largest part of the brain that includes nerve centers associated with sensory and motor functions and provides higher mental functions, including memory and reasoning

chelating (kee-LAY-ting) agents Organic compounds capable of forming coordinate bonds with metals

chemical name The name describing the chemical makeup of a drug

child-resistant packaging Blister packs and special lids requiring the user to press downward and turn simultaneously

cholecalciferol (koh-luh-kal-SIH-feh-rol) Vitamin D_3; a substance that controls calcium metabolism in bone building

cholesterol (koh-LES-teh-rol) A natural lipid found in cell membranes, particularly in animal muscle and organ cells

cholinergic (kol-i-NUR-jik) Referring to neurons that release acetylcholine

cholinergic blockers Drugs that inhibit the actions of acetylcholine by occupying the acetylcholine receptors

choroid layer (KO-royd) The middle layer of the eye

chronic Lasting a long time or marked by frequent recurrence

ciliary body (SIL-ee-ayr-ee) The thickest part of the middle layer of the eye; extends forward from the choroid layer and forms an internal ring around the front of the eye

ciliary muscle Muscle in the eye that enables the lens to adjust shape to facilitate focusing

coagulation (koh-ag-yew-LAY-shun) Blood clotting

cobalamin (koh-BAL-luh-min) Vitamin B_{12}; a substance that promotes the normal function of all cells, especially normal blood formation, and is necessary for proper nervous system function

cognitive Relating to intellectual processes, such as thinking, reasoning, and remembering

cohort A group of people who share a common characteristic or experience within a defined period

common fraction A fraction that represents equal parts of a whole; subclassified as proper, improper, mixed, and complex

congenital hypothyroidism A disorder of deficiency of thyroid hormones (hypothyroidism) during infancy that results in dwarfism and severe mental retardation

congestive heart failure A condition in which the heart pumps blood at an insufficient rate, the kidneys retain salt and water, and fluid accumulates in interstitial spaces

connective tissue Tissue that consists of fibroblasts, macrophages, and interlacing protein fibers (collagen) that supports, ensheathes, and binds together other tissues and includes adipose tissue, tendons, ligaments, aponeuroses, cartilage, and bone

controlled substances Drugs whose possession and use are controlled by the comprehensive Drug Abuse Prevention and Control Act

conversion The changing of units

convulsion An abnormal violent and involuntary contraction or series of contractions of the muscles; violent spasms

cornea The window of the eye that helps to focus entering light rays

creatinine (kree-AT-tih-neen) A chemical waste molecule produced in skeletal muscle tissue by the breakdown of creatine phosphate

creatinine clearance An indicator of the glomerular filtration rate; creatinine, a by-product of the muscle breakdown of stored proteins, is excreted by the kidneys

cryoanesthesia (KRY-o-an-ess-THEE-zee-ah) Reduction of nerve conduction by localized cooling

Cushing's disease (KUSH-ings) A disease in which Cushing's syndrome is caused by a tumor in the pituitary gland

Cushing's syndrome A condition that affects the trunk of the body in which a pad of fat develops between the shoulders, producing a buffalo hump, and the face becomes round and moon shaped

cutaneous flush, (kew-TAY-nee-us)   Skin reddening

cyanide   A highly toxic chemical compound that is found in many plants; it is produced by certain bacteria, fungi, and algae

cyclooxygenase (SYE-klo-OKS-ih-jeh-nase)   The name for a group of enzymes required to produce prostaglandins from arachidonic acid

cystic fibrosis (SIS-tik fy-BRO-sis)   A disorder marked by abnormal secretions of the exocrine glands, causing obstruction of bronchial pathways

decimals   Any real numbers expressed as a fraction of 10

decongestants   A class of drugs that reverse excessive blood flow (congestion) into an area

dehydration (dee-hy-DRAY-shun)   Excessive loss of body water

delirium tremens (DT)   An acute, sometimes fatal episode usually caused by withdrawal or abstinence from alcohol after habitual excessive drinking; symptoms include sweating, trembling, anxiety, confusion, and hallucinations

denominator (dee-NAW-mih-nay-ter)   The part of a fraction that is below the line and that functions as the divisor of the numerator (number above the line)

dermatitis (dur-mah-TY-tiss)   Inflammation of the skin

designer drugs   Drugs produced by a minor modification in the chemical structure of an existing drug, resulting in a new substance with similar pharmacologic effects

desired dose   The amount of drug to be administered at one time (must be in the same unit of measurement as the dosage unit)

detergent   A surfactant or mixture of surfactants having cleaning properties in dilute solutions

detoxification   The physiological or medicinal removal of toxic substances from a living organism, including the period of withdrawal

developmental toxicity   Adverse effects induced during pregnancy or as a result of parental exposure that can be manifested at any point in the life span of the organism

diabetes insipidus (dy-uh-BEE-tees in-SIP-uh-dus)   A disorder that is caused by the insufficient secretion of vasopressin by the pituitary gland or by a failure of the kidneys to respond to circulating vasopressin;

characterized by intense thirst and the excretion of large amounts of urine

diabetes mellitus (dy-uh-BEE-tees MEL-uh-tiss)   A serious endocrine disorder characterized by hyperglycemia (high blood glucose levels), resulting from deficient insulin secretion or decreased sensitivity of insulin receptors on target cells

diastole   Ventricles contract and eject blood

dilutions (dye-LOO-shuns)   Less concentrated mixtures

dissolution (dis-oh-LOO-shun)   The process of dissolving

distribution   The passage of an agent through blood or lymph to various body sites

diuretics (dy-yoo-REH-tiks)   Drugs that promote water loss from the body into the urine

dose   The amount of a drug that a patient takes for an intended therapeutic effect

dose-effect relationship   The relationship between the dose of a drug (or other agent) that produces harmful effects and the severity of the effects on the patient

drams   Fluidrams; apothecary unit of weight (equivalent to 1/8 oz)

dwarfism (DWARF-izm)   A condition in which the body is abnormally undersized

dysmorphology   The study of human congenital malformations (birth defects), particularly those affecting the morphology (anatomy) of the individual

dysphagia (dis-FAY-jee-uh)   Difficulty swallowing

dysrhythmia (dis-RITH-mee-uh)   Disturbance of the heart rhythm; also called *arrhythmia*

eczema (ECK-zih-mah)   The most common inflammatory skin condition, caused by endogenous and exogenous agents

edema (eh-DEE-muh)   An abnormal fluid accumulation in the body

efflux (EE-flucks)   The process of flowing out; something that is given off

electrocardiogram (ECG or EKG) (ee-lek-tro-KAR-dee-oh-gram)   A test that records the electrical activity of the heart; an electrograph is the tracing made on paper

elixirs (ee-LICKS-ers)   Alcoholic solutions that offer consistent dissolution and distribution of the drugs they contain; they are sweetened and contain alcohol and water

embolus (EM-bo-lus)   An abnormal particle circulating in blood, such as an air bubble or blood clot

embryo toxicity   The degree to which a substance can damage an embryo or fetus

emesis (EH-meh-sis) Vomiting

emollients (ee-MOLE-ee-ents) Skin-softening agents

emphysema (em-fih-ZEE-muh) Condition of the lung that is marked by distension and eventual rupture of the alveoli with progressive loss of pulmonary elasticity that is accompanied by shortness of breath with or without cough and that may lead to impaired heart action

endocardium (en-do-kar-dee-um) The thin membrane lining the inside of the cardiac muscle

endogenous (en-dah-jeh-nus) Caused by factors within the body or mind or arising from internal structural or functional causes (*endogenous* malnutrition or *endogenous* psychic depression); relating to or produced by metabolic synthesis in the body

endorphins (en-DOR-finz) Any of a group of endogenous peptides (such as enkephalin and dynorphin) found especially in the brain that bind chiefly to opiate receptors and produce some of the same pharmacologic effects (such as pain relief) as do opiates

enkephalins (en-KEH-fuh-linz) Peptides with opiate and analgesic activity that occur naturally in the brain and have a marked affinity for opiate receptors

epicardium (ep-ih-Kar-dee-um) Membrane lining the outside of the myocardium

epidemiological Related to epidemiology; the study of patterns of health and illness and associated factors at the population level

epidural anesthesia (ep-eh-DUR-al) Anesthesia produced by injection of a local anesthetic into the epidural (lumbar or caudal) space via a catheter that allows repeated infusions

epilepsy (EH-pih-lep-see) Various disorders marked by abnormal electrical discharges in the brain and typically manifested by sudden brief episodes of altered or diminished consciousness, involuntary movements, or convulsions

erythema (ear-ih-thee-mah) Skin redness caused by capillary dilation

essential amino acids Components of proteins that cannot be synthesized by the body and must be provided by the diet; there are nine essential amino acids

estrogens One of two major groups of female sex hormones; stimulate enlargement of the vagina, uterus, uterine tubes, ovaries, and external reproductive structures

ethanol (EH-the-nol) A flammable, colorless chemical compound produced by fermentation of grain

ethics Standards of behavior, including concepts of right and wrong, beyond what legal considerations are in any given situation

ethylene glycol A toxic organic compound used commercially in automotive antifreeze and as an ingredient in various plastics

excretion The last stage of pharmacokinetics that removes drugs from the system via the kidneys

expectorants Medications capable of dissolving or promoting liquefaction of mucus in the lungs

extremes The two outside terms in a proportion

fatty acids A group of acids that must be provided by the diet and can be either saturated or unsaturated

fetal Related to a fetus, a developing mammal or other vertebrate after the embryonic stage and before birth

fetotoxicity The state of being toxic to a fetus

fiber A type of complex carbohydrate that does not supply energy or heat to the body

fibrillation (fib-rih-LAY-shun) Very rapid, irregular contractions or twitching of the individual muscular fibers of the atria or ventricles

fight-or-flight response Reaction in the body when faced by a sudden threat or source of stress

first-pass effect Immediate exposure of orally administrated drugs to metabolism by liver enzymes before they reach the systemic circulation

flatulence (FLAT-yoo-lentz) The presence of excess gas in the stomach and intestines

fluoride A form of fluorine that has beneficial properties in low quantities but may be highly toxic in larger quantities

flutter Rapid, regular atrial contractions that often produce sawtooth waves in an electrocardiogram (ECG); rapid ventricular tachycardia that appears as a regular, undulating pattern in an ECG without QRS and T waves, as would normally be found

formaldehyde An organic compound that is a precursor to many other chemical compounds; it is used in many industrial applications but has toxic, allergenic, and carcinogenic properties

fraction A number usually expressed in the form a/b; expresses one or more equal parts of a whole

fungi (FUNG-guy) Nonphotosynthetic, eukaryotic single or multicellular organisms that are found throughout the environment; fungi have a cell wall containing *sterol*

fungicidal (FUN-jih-sy-dul) Having a killing action on fungi

gastric lavage (luh-VAAZH) Washing out the stomach with sterile water or a saltwater solution

gastrostomy tube (gah-straw-sto-mee) A surgically placed tube into the stomach that provides a route for feeding and administering medication

gauge Diameter of the needle shaft that varies from #18 to #28; the larger the gauge, the smaller the shaft's diameter

generic name A drug's approved nonproprietary or official name

gestation (jes-STAY-shun) The period of fetal development from conception until birth; about 40 weeks

gestational diabetes mellitus (jeh-STAY-shuh-nul) Disorder that may develop during pregnancy; symptoms may be similar to type 2 diabetes

gigantism (jy-GANT-izm) A condition in which the entire body or any of its parts is abnormally large

gingival hyperplasia (JIN-jih-vul hi-per-PLAY-zhuh) An increase in the number of cells in the gums of the mouth, causing them to have a swollen appearance

glaucoma (glauw-KO-muh) A disorder that damages the optic nerve and is often caused by elevated intraocular pressure

globulins (GLOB-yoo-linz) Proteins present in blood that contain antibodies

glomerular capsule (gloh-MAYR-yoo-lar KAP-sool) A thin-walled, sac-like structure of the renal corpuscle that surrounds the glomerulus

glomerular filtration Separation of wastes from body water to produce urine; occurs in the glomerulus

glomerulus (gloh-MAYR-yoo-lus) A filtering unit of the nephron composed of a cluster of blood capillaries

glucagon (GLOO-kuh-gon) Hormone secreted when blood glucose levels are low

glycoprotein A specific serum protein that binds to many basic drugs

glycoside (GLY-ko-side) An organic compound that yields sugar and nonsugar substances when hydrolyzed; an important cardiac glycoside is digoxin

goiter (GOY-ter) A swelling of the thyroid gland resulting from a shortage of iodine in the diet

grain Basic unit of weight of the apothecary system

gram The unit of weight of the metric system (equivalent to 15.432358 grains)

gram negative Refers to bacteria that cannot resist decolorization with alcohol after being treated with Gram's crystal violet; among these bacteria are *Escherichia coli*, *Salmonella spp.,* and other *Enterobacteriaceae*, *Pseudomonas*, *Moraxella*, *Helicobacter*, and *Legionella spp.*

gram positive Refers to bacteria that have the ability to resist decolorization with alcohol after being treated with Gram's crystal violet stain, imparting a violet color to the bacterium when viewed by a microscope; includes *Bacillus*, *Listeria*, *Staphylococcus*, *Streptococcus*, *Enterococcus*, and *Clostridium spp.*

Graves's disease A disorder in which the thyroid gland is overactive; characterized by numerous eye problems

half-life (t1/2) The time taken for the blood or plasma concentration of the drug to decrease from full to one-half

hallucinogens Psychedelics, dissociatives, and deliriants—all of which are psychoactive drugs that can cause subjective changes in perception, thought, emotion, and consciousness

hemodialysis (hee-mo-dy-AL-uh-sis) A method in which the patient's blood is passed through a tube to a semipermeable membrane (dialyzer) that filters out waste products

hemoperfusion (hee-mo-per-FU-zhun) The removal of poisons from blood by passing it through a tube containing treated charcoal or ion-exchange resins

hemostasis (hee-mo-STAY-sis) A physiologic progression of several steps that stops bleeding

heparin (HEH-puh-rin) An anticoagulant commonly administered subcutaneously

household system System of measurement used in most American homes that is not precisely accurate

hub Part of the needle that fits onto the syringe

humoral (HYOO-moh-rul) immunity Immunity based on the antigen–antibody response; obtained when B cells produce circulating antibodies to act against an antigen

hybridomas (hy-brih-DO-muhz) Fusion of a single immune cell to tumor cells that are grown in cultures

hypercholesterolemia (hi-per-koh-les-ter-raw-LEE-mee-uh) Higher-than-normal levels of cholesterol in the blood

hyperglycemia High blood sugar; a condition in which an excessive amount of glucose circulates in the blood plasma

hyperkalemia (hy-per-kah-LEE-mee-uh) An abnormally high amount of potassium ions in blood

hyperplasia (hy-per-PLAY-shuh) Abnormal cell growth

hypertension (hy-per-ten-shun) Blood pressure that is elevated above the normal limits

hypertensive crisis Severely elevated blood pressure

hyperthermia (hy-per-THER-mee-uh) A condition of increased body heat; body temperatures above 104°F (40°C) are life threatening; brain death begins at 106°F (41°C)

hyperthyroidism (hy-per-THY-royd-izm) Overactivity of the thyroid gland

hyperuricemia (hy-per-yoo-rih-SEE-mee-uh) Elevated blood level of uric acid

hypervitaminosis (hy-per-vy-tuh-mih-NOH-sis) Excess intake of vitamins

hypodermic (hy-po-DUR-mik) Refers to the administration of drugs under the skin; of or relating to the needles used

hypoglycemia (hy-po-gly-SEE-mee-uh) An abnormally low blood glucose level

hypokalemia (hy-po-kah-LEE-mee-uh) An abnormally low concentration of potassium ions in blood

hyponatremia (hy-po-nuh-TREE-mee-uh) An abnormally low concentration of sodium ions in blood

hypoparathyroidism (hy-po-par-uh-THY-royd-izm) A rare disorder in which the body produces little or no parathyroid hormone, resulting in an abnormally low level of blood calcium (hypocalcemia)

hypopituitarism (hy-po-pih-TOO-ih-tayr-izm) Underactivity of the pituitary gland

hypotension (hy-po-TEN-shun) An abnormal condition in which blood pressure is not adequate for full oxygenation of the tissues

hypothyroidism (hy-po-THY-royd-izm) Underactivity of the thyroid gland

hypoxia (hy-POK-see-uh) Lack of oxygen

iatrogenic (eye-ah-troh-JEH-nik) Produced inadvertently by medication or other treatment

immune response A specific defense of the body in response to a foreign substance

immunity The ability to resist infection and disease through the activation of specific defenses

immunocompromised (im-myoo-no-KOM-pro-miezd) A weakened immune system

immunogen (ih-MYOO-no-jen) Antigen

immunoglobulins (ih-myoon-o-GLOB-yoo-linz) Antibodies, derived from human plasma, formed by the body to specific antigens

improper fraction A fraction with a numerator that is greater than or the same as the denominator

infant A child aged 29 days old to walking age (typically 1 year)

injectable Medication that can be administered by intradermal (within the skin), subcutaneous (into fatty tissue under the skin), intramuscular (IM, into the muscle), and intravenous (IV, into the vein) injection

insomnia (in-SOM-nee-uh) Inability to sleep normally

insulin (IN-suh-lin) A pancreatic hormone that stimulates glucose metabolism

international units Units standardized by an international agreement; used to show the amount of drug required to produce a certain effect

interstate commerce The commerce, traffic, transportation, and exchange among states of the United States

intoxication (in-tok-sih-KAY-shun) An abnormal state induced by a chemical agent, such as a drug, serum, or toxin; essentially, a poisoning

invasive Pertaining to a route of medication administration that requires insertion of an instrument or device through the skin or a body orifice

iodine A chemical element with nutritive properties; in excessive quantities, it can be cytotoxic

iris Thin diaphragm in the eye that is composed mostly of connective tissue and smooth muscle fibers; the colored portion of an eye

ischemia (is-KEE-mee-uh) Insufficient blood flow to the myocardium

islets of Langerhans (EYE-lits of LANG-ur-hans) Small clusters of cells within the pancreas

isopropyl alcohol A chemical compound commonly used for cleaning and disinfecting; it is highly toxic if ingested

isotypes (EYE-so-typz) Species of atoms of a chemical element with the same atomic number and position in the periodic table and nearly identical chemical behavior but with differing atomic mass or mass number and different physical properties

keratinization (keh-rat-in-eh-ZAY-shun) Formation of keratin (a horny layer of skin)

keratinocytes (keh-RAH-tin-oh-syts) Epidermal cells that produce keratin

keratolytic (keh-rat-oh-LIH-tik) Referring to agents that separate or loosen the horny layer of the epidermis

kernicterus (ker-NIK-ter-rus) A serious form of jaundice in newborns

lead An element that exists as a soft, malleable metal; used in many construction applications; if ingested, it is toxic to the nervous system

legend drugs Prescription drugs

lens Transparent part of an eye; adjusts to facilitate focusing

leukotriene inhibitors (loo-ko-TRY-een) Drugs that inhibit the production of leukotrienes, which are the cause of the inflammatory response in asthma

lipophilic (lie-poh-FIL-lik) Related to the ability to dissolve more easily in lipids than in water

liter (LEE-ter) The unit of volume of the metric system (equivalent to 1.056688 quarts)

lithium (LITH-ee-um) A drug that reduces the activity of certain neurotransmitters and is used in the treatment of bipolar disorder

loading dose A comparatively large dose given at the beginning of treatment to quickly obtain therapeutic effects

loop of Henle (HEN-lee) A long, U-shaped part of the renal tubule extending through the medulla from the end of the proximal convoluted tubule to the beginning of the distal convoluted tubule

lymph (limf) The fluid that flows through the lymphatic vessels

lymphatic (lim-FAH-tik) vessels Network of vessels of the lymphatic system that begins in peripheral tissues and ends at connections to the venous system

lymphocytes (LIM-foh-sites) White blood cells that manufacture antibodies to overcome infection and disease

lymphoid (LIM-foyd) organs Organs connected to the lymphatic vessels that contain large numbers of lymphocytes

macrominerals (mak-ro-MIH-neh-ruls) Dietary minerals needed by the human body in high quantities

macrophages (MAK-ro-fah-jez) Immune cells derived from monocytes

magnesium carbonate Base element used as an antacid

magnesium sulfate A chemical compound containing magnesium, sulfur, and oxygen; its salt form is used for mineral baths

major minerals Elements that occur in large amounts in the body (i.e., calcium) and have a daily requirement of more than 100 mg/d

maintenance dose a dose that keeps the plasma drug concentration of a drug continuously in the therapeutic range

malignant (mah-LIG-nent) In terms of cells, rapidly proliferating with an atypical appearance

mast cells Large white blood cells found in connective tissue that contain a wide variety of biochemicals, including histamine; involved in inflammation secondary to injuries and infections and are sometimes implicated in allergic reactions

means The two inside terms in a proportion

medical emergency An injury or illness that poses an immediate threat to a person's health or life and requires help from a doctor or hospital

medication error The inappropriate or incorrect administration of a drug that should be preventable through effective system controls

medication reconciliation Keeping track of a patient's medications as they change health-care providers

melanosis Abnormal dark pigmentation

menorrhagia (men-no-RAH-jee-uh) Abnormally heavy or prolonged menstruation

mercury A chemical element that is a liquid metal at room temperature; it has many industrial applications but is highly toxic upon contact

metabolism The sum of chemical and physical changes in the tissues, consisting of anabolism and catabolism

metabolites Intermediates and products of metabolism

metastasis (meh-TAS-tuh-sis) The spreading of cancer cells from the primary site to secondary sites

meter a unit of length of the metric system (equivalent to 39.37007874 inches)

methyl alcohol Methanol; it has many applications in solvents and fuels but is highly toxic and can cause permanent blindness and death

metric system   The most common, most accurate, and safest system of measurement; based on the decimal system

metrorrhagia (mee-tro-RAH-jee-uh)   Uterine bleeding that occurs independent of the normal menstrual period

milliequivalents (mil-lee-ee-KWIH-vuh-lentz)   Measurements used to indicate the strength of certain drugs; more specifically, an expression of the number of grams of equivalent weight of a drug contained in 1 mL of a normal solution

minim (MIH-num)   The basic unit of volume of the apothecary system

minuend (min-YOO-end)   In subtraction, the number from which another number (subtrahend) is subtracted

mitosis (my-TOH-sis)   The splitting of one cell into two new cells

mixed fraction   A fraction that has a whole number and a proper fraction combined and whose value is always greater than one

monoclonal antibodies (maw-noh-KLO-nul)   Types of human proteins that are produced by fusing a single immune cell to tumor cells that are grown in cultures

mucolytics (myoo-ko-LIT-tiks)   Medications capable of dissolving or promoting liquefaction of mucus in the lungs

multiplicand (mul-tih-plih-KAND)   The number that is to be multiplied by another number

multiplier (MUL-tih-ply-er)   The number that multiplies another number (multiplicand)

muscarinic receptors (mus-kah-RIN-ik)   Receptors that innervate smooth muscle and slow the heart rate

mycoses (my-KOH-seez)   Fungal infections

myocardial infarction (my-oh-KAR-dee-ull in-FARK-shun)   MI; heart attack; occurs when a portion of the heart is deprived of blood supply, causing cells to die

myocardium (my-oh-KAR-dee-um)   The middle layer and most important structure of the heart; contains the heart muscles that regulate cardiac output

myxedema (mix-uh-DEE-muh)   The most severe form of hypothyroidism; often develops in older children and adults and is characterized by swelling of the hands, feet, and face (especially around the eyes); can lead to coma and death

narcotic   a medication that induces sleep or stupor and alters mood and behavior

nasogastric (NG) tube (nay-zo-GAS-trik)   Tube that is inserted through the nose for feeding or removing gastric secretions

nebulizer (NEH-byoo-ly-zer)   A device that disperses a fine-particle mist of medication into the deeper parts of the respiratory tract

neonates (NEE-oh-nayts)   Newborns from birth to 28 days old

nephrons (NEH-fronz)   The functional units of kidneys

nephrotic syndrome (neh-FROT-ik)   a clinical state characterized by edema, various abnormal substances present in the urine, decreased plasma albumin, and increased blood cholesterol

neurohypophysis (noor-oh-hy-PO-fih-sis)   Posterior lobe of pituitary gland

neuroleptic   Referring to psychotropic drugs used to treat psychosis

neurons   Nerve cells

neurotransmitters (noo-roh-TRANZ-mih-ters)   Certain chemical substances, concentrated in various parts of the central nervous system, that are released by neurons and allow communication from one nerve cell to another

nicotinic receptors (nik-oh-TIN-ik)   Receptors that respond to acetylcholine and nicotine and affect skeletal muscles

nomogram (NAW-mo-gram)   A numerical chart that shows relationships between two values

nonproductive cough   A sudden ejection of air from the lungs and through the mouth that does not expel (produce) mucus or fluid from the throat or lungs

nuclear pharmacy   A specialty area of pharmacy practice dedicated to the compounding and dispensing of radioactive materials for use in nuclear medicine procedures

nucleoside (NOO-klee-oh-sied)   Derived from a nucleic acid

nucleotides (NOO-klee-oh-tiedz)   The basic structural subunits of DNA

numerator (NOO-meh-ray-ter)   The top number in a fraction

nutrition   The process of how the body takes in and uses food and other sources of nutrients for growth and repair of tissues

nystagmus (nis-TAG-mus)   A constant, involuntary movement of the eye

oligospermia (ol-lih-go-SPER-mee-uh)   A subnormal concentration of spermatozoa in ejaculate

oncogenes (ON-koh-jeenz)   Cancer genes that develop from normal genes

oocytes (OO-oh-sites)   Female sex cells

oogonia   Immature reproductive cells of a female

opiate (OH-pee-ut)   A drug (such as morphine, heroin, and codeine) containing or derived from opium and tending to induce sleep and to alleviate pain

opioid (OH-pee-oyd)   Possessing some properties characteristic of opiate narcotics but not derived from opium

optic nerve   Nerve that runs through the back of the eye; transmits electrical pulses from the retina to the brain, providing vision

orphan drugs   Drugs developed under the Orphan Drug Act, which provides federal financial incentives to nonprofit and commercial organizations for the development and marketing of drugs used to treat rare diseases (those that affect fewer than 200,000 people in the United States)

osmolality (oz-moh-LAL-ih-tee)   The concentration of particles in plasma

osmosis (oz-MOH-sis)   The process in which sodium and magnesium ions attract water into the bowel, causing a more liquid stool to be formed

osteopenia (os-tee-oh-PEE-nee-uh)   Reduced bone mass

osteoporosis (os-tee-oh-por-OH-sis)   Reduced bone mass that compromises normal function and often leads to fractures

ounces   Household unit of measurement of weight equivalent to 480 grains or 31.10349 g

overdose   A toxic dose of a drug or another substance

oxytocin (awk-see-TOH-sin)   A hormone that stimulates powerful uterine contractions; aids labor in its later stages

palliative (PAH-lee-uh-tiv)   Able to ease a disease's effects but not able to cure

parasites (PAH-rah-syts)   Protozoans, roundworms, flatworms, and arthropods

parafollicular cells (par-uh-fo-LIK-u-lur)   Cells in the thyroid gland that release calcitonin

paralytic ileus (par-uh-LIT-ik ILL-ee-us)   Absence of peristaltic movements in the intestines

parasympathetic nervous system (pahr-ah-sim-pah-THET-ik)   The part of the nervous system that slows the heart rate, increases intestinal and glandular activity, and relaxes muscles

parasympatholytics (pahr-ah-sim-pah-tho-LIT-iks)   Drugs that inhibit the actions of acetylcholine by occupying the acetylcholine receptors

parenteral (puh-REN-teh-rul)   Introduction of a drug outside of the gastrointestinal tract; generally in injectable form

parkinsonism   Any of several neurological conditions that resemble Parkinson's disease and that result from a deficiency or blockage of dopamine caused by degenerative disease, drugs, or toxins

partial response   Relating to chemotherapy, a 50% or greater decrease in the tumor size or other objective disease markers and no evidence of any new disease for at least one month

passive immunity   The transfer of the effectors of immunity, which are called *immunoglobulins*, from an immune individual to another

pathogenic (pah-thoh-JEH-nik)   Disease causing

pathogens (PAH-tho-jenz)   Bacteria or viruses that invade the body

pediculicides (puh-DIK-yoo-lih-sydz)   Pharmacologic agents that kill lice

pellagra (peh-LEH-gruh)   A condition caused by a deficiency of vitamin B_3 and marked by dementia, dermatitis, diarrhea, and death

percent   A term meaning *hundredths* that can be expressed as a fraction, decimal, or ratio

perinatal   Related to the period around childbirth, especially five months before and one month after birth

peripheral blood circulation   Circulation in the body's extremities

peripheral nervous system   Part of the nervous system that is outside the brain and spinal cord

peripheral resistance   Friction in the arteries as blood flows through the vessels

peristalsis (payr-ih-STALL-sis)   The rhythmic movement of the intestine

petroleum distillates   Compounds extracted by distillation during the refining of crude oil; they are found in many products, including cosmetics, fertilizers, solvents, and fuels

pharmacodynamics (far-muh-koh-dy-NAH-mix)   The biochemical and physiologic effects of drugs and mechanisms of drug action

pharmacognosy (far-muh-KOG-nuh-see)   The study of drugs derived from herbal and other natural sources

pharmacokinetics (far-muh-koh-kih-NEH-tix)
The study of the absorption, distribution, biotransformation, metabolism, and excretion of drugs

pharmacology The study of drugs, including their actions and effects in living body systems

pharmacotherapeutics (far-muh-koh-thayr-ruh-PYOO-tix) The study of how drugs may be best used in the treatment of illnesses and which drug is most or least appropriate to use for a specific disease

phenol Carbolic acid; an organic compound produced as a precursor to many materials, primarily plastics and related materials

phenylketonuria A genetic disorder in which the body lacks the enzyme necessary to metabolize phenylalanine to tyrosine

phosphorus A highly reactive chemical element used in many products, including explosives, pesticides, toothpaste, and detergents

photoreceptors Visual receptor cells of the eye

phylloquinone (fil-loh-KWIH-nohn) Dietary form of vitamin K_1, which aids in blood clotting and bone development; treatment for warfarin (Coumadin) overdose

plant alkaloids Physiologically active organic bases containing nitrogen (and usually oxygen) that are found in seed plants; prevent cell division (or meiosis); also called *mitotic inhibitors*

platelet plug (PLATE-let) Plug formed by platelets that become sticky and adhere to the inner lining of the injured vessel and to each other

platelets (PLATE-lets) Megakaryocyte fragments important in the clotting of blood

pneumonitis (new-moh-NY-tis) Inflammation of the lungs

polypharmacy The practice of simultaneously prescribing multiple medicines to a single patient

porphyria (por-FEE-ree-uh) A genetic disorder caused by a deficiency of enzymes of the heme biosynthetic pathway

polysubstance abuse The overusage of a minimum of three psychoactive substances within a 12-month period

preanesthetics (pree-an-ess-THEH-tiks) Agents used to partially sedate patients before surgery

priapism (PRY-uh-pizm) A painful and prolonged erection

primary hypertension Hypertension that has no known cause; accounts for 90% of cases

productive cough A cough that brings up fluid or mucus from the lungs

progesterones One of the major groups of female sex hormones; promote changes in the uterus during the reproductive cycle

prophylactic dose A dose that is given in order to prevent a disease

prophylaxis (pro-fih-LAK-sis) Prevention, as in drug treatment or other therapy that is given to prevent a disease

proprietary name A drug's name assigned by the manufacturer and protected by copyright; brand or trade name

prostaglandins (prah-stuh-GLAN-dinz) Hormone-like substances that control blood pressure, contract smooth muscle, and modulate inflammation

protozoan (pro-toh-ZOH-un) A single-celled highly mobile microorganism

pruritus (proo-RYE-tus) Itching

psoriasis (soh-RY-uh-sis) A chronic, relapsing inflammatory skin disorder

psychological treatment Psychotherapy, involving an intentional, interpersonal relationship used by a trained psychotherapist to aid a client or patient in the problems of living

ptosis (TOE-sis) Drooping eyelid

puberty The phase in development when an individual becomes reproductively functional

pupil Circular opening in the iris of the eye

Purkinje fibers (pur-KIN-jee) Specialized conductive fibers located within the walls of the ventricles that conduct an electrical stimulus or impulse that enables the heart to contract in a coordinated fashion

radical cure A treatment that eliminates a microorganism from blood and tissue

ratio A mathematical expression that compares the relationship of one number with another number or expresses a part of a whole number

receptor A specific protein in cell membranes that specific drugs bind to, producing a pharmacologic effect

recommended dietary allowances (RDAs) Guidelines released every five years by the Food and Nutrition Board that are computed to meet the needs of all healthy individuals

refractory (ree-FRAK-toh-ree) The period during repolarization when cells cannot respond normally to a second stimulus

regional anesthesia   Affects a large but limited part of the body and is often used in obstetrics (labor and delivery)

reimportation   Importation of a drug into the United States that was originally manufactured in the United States

renal corpuscle (REE-nul KOR-pus-sul)   A filtering unit of the nephron composed of a cluster of blood capillaries called a *glomerulus*

renal tubule (REE-nul TOO-byool)   The part of the nephron that leads away from the glomerular capsule and becomes highly coiled

renin (REE-nin)   A hormone secreted by the kidneys that converts angiotensinogen to angiotensin I

reproductive toxicology   Adverse effects on the reproductive system caused by exposure to a toxic chemical

retina   The inner layer of eye that contains the visual receptor cells

retinal detachment   Separation of the retina from the corneal layer of the eye

retinopathy (ret-tih-NOP-ah-thee)   Degeneration of the blood vessels of the retina

rickets   A deficiency of calcitriol that is characterized by the malformation of skeletal tissue in growing children

risk management department   The division of an organization that focuses on the identification and management of potential risks in order to minimize them

Roman numeral   A number represented by a letter (for example, I = 1, V = 5, X = 10)

root cause analysis (RNA)   A method used in many health care facilities to identify causes of mistakes, reduce risks, and prevent future occurrences

salicylism   Aspirin overdose; it can be acute or chronic, with symptoms including nausea, vomiting, abdominal pain, seizures, and cerebral edema

salpingitis (sal-pin-JY-tis)   Inflammation or infection of a fallopian tube

sarcomas (sar-KO-muhs)   Malignant growths of muscle or connective tissue

scabicides (SKAY-bih-sydz)   Pharmacologic drugs that kill mites

scabies (SKAY-beez)   A group of dermatologic conditions caused by mites that burrow into the skin, causing intense itching

sclera   The outer layer of eye

scored   Notched

sedative   Tranquilizer; a substance that induces sedation by reducing irritability or excitement

seizures   Abnormal electrical activity in the brain

sentinel event   Unexpected occurrences involving death or serious physical or psychological injury or risk thereof

serotonin (sayr-uh-TO-nin)   A neurotransmitter that causes the blood vessel to go into spasms

serum sickness   A reaction to a foreign serum

side effects   Results of drug (or other) therapy in addition to or in extension of the desired therapeutic effects, which are usually (but not always) undesirable

sinoatrial node (syn-oh-AY-tree-ull)   The pacemaker; specialized cardiac muscle tissue that initiates one impulse after another; located just beneath the epicardium in the right atrium near the opening of the superior vena cava

soap   A salt of a fatty acid mainly used for washing, bathing, and cleaning and as a component in lubricants

somnolence (SAHM-no-lents)   A state of near sleep, a strong desire for sleep, or sleeping for unusually long periods

spasticity (spas-TIH-sih-tee)   Inability of opposing muscle groups to move in a coordinated manner

sperm   male sex cells

spina bifida (SPY-nuh BIFF-ih-duh)   A condition wherein the spinal column is imperfectly closed, resulting in the protrusion of the meninges or spinal cord

spinal anesthesia   Injection of anesthetic agent into the subarachnoid space through a spinal needle

spirit   An alcohol-containing liquid that may be used pharmaceutically as a solvent; also known as an *essence*

stable disease   In terms of cancer, a tumor that neither grows nor shrinks in size

STAT   Immediately

steatorrhea (stee-at-oh-REE-ah)   Elimination of large amounts of fat in the stool

stroke   Cerebrovascular accident

stroke volume   Amount of blood pumped by a ventricle in one minute

subarachnoid (sub-uh-RAK-noyd)   Area of spinal cord beneath the arachnoid membrane or between the arachnoid and pia mater and filled with cerebrospinal fluid

substance abuse   Drug abuse; a maladaptive pattern of use of a substance that is not considered dependent but does not exclude dependency

substance dependent   The state of needing a drug or another substance regardless of problems that occur, which are related to the use of the substance

substantia nigra (sub-STAN-shee-uh NY-gra)   A large cell mass involved in metabolic disturbances associated with Parkinson's disease

subtherapeutic doses   Drug doses that are below the level used to treat diseases

subtrahend (SUB-truh-hend)   In subtraction, the number that is to be deducted from another

suspensions   Dosage forms that contain undissolved drug particles and must be shaken to evenly distribute them

sustained release   Tablets and capsules that are specially coated and contain several doses so they dissolve at specific times; also called *delayed release* or *timed release*

sympathetic (sim-puh-THEH-tik)   Relating to the sympathetic part of the autonomic nervous system or the fight-or-flight response

sympathetic nervous system   The part of the nervous system that accelerates heart rate, constricts blood vessels, and raises blood pressure

sympathomimetics (sim-path-oh-mi-MET-iks)   Adrenergic agonists

synapses (SIN-aps-eez)   The point of contact between nerve cells and each other or other types of cells

syndrome (SIN-drohm)   A collection of signs and symptoms that together signify a specific disease

syrup   An aqueous solution containing a high concentration of sugars; also known as a *linctus*

systole   Ventricles relax and heart stops ejecting blood

tablet   A solid dosage form that is made by compressing the powdered form of a drug and bulk filling material under high pressure

tachycardia (tak-ee-KAR-dee-uh)   An abnormally fast heartbeat

tardive dyskinesia (TAR-div dis-kih-NEE-zhah)   Slowed ability to make voluntary movements

teratogenic (teh-rah-toh-JEN-ik)   Able to cause birth defects in fetuses

teratogenicity   Related to the development of malformations of an embryo or fetus

teratogens   Agents that can cause birth defects

teratology   The study of birth defects

testosterone   The most abundant androgen

tetrahydrocannabinol (THC)   The main psychoactive substance found in the cannabis plant

therapeutic   Meant to treat a disease or disorder

thiazides   The most commonly prescribed class of diuretics

thrombi (THROM-by)   Blood clots that form within a blood vessel and attach to the site of formation

thromboembolism (throm-bo-EM-bo-lizm)   The blocking of a blood vessel by a particle that has broken away from a blood clot at its site of formation

thrush   A yeast infection in the mouth caused by *Candida albicans,* a normal resident of the gastrointestinal tract and vagina

thyrotoxicosis (thy-ro-toks-ih-KOH-sis)   Graves's disease; a disorder in which the thyroid gland is overactive; characterized by numerous eye problems

tidal volume   The lung volume representing the normal volume of air displaced between normal inspiration and expiration when extra effort is not applied

tobacco dependence   The need for tobacco regardless of problems it may be causing to the health of the user

toddler   A child from approximately 1 to 3 years old

tolerance   The body's slow adaptation to a drug; increasingly higher doses are required to achieve the same effect; reduced responsiveness to a drug

toluene   A clear, water-insoluble liquid that is an important organic solvent; if inhaled, it can cause severe neurological harm

tonic–clonic   Contraction–relaxation

total body water   Amount of water in the body

total parenteral nutrition (TPN)   Intravenously administered fluids that supply all of a patient's daily nutritional requirements

toxic agent   Poisonous or harmful substance

toxicity (tok-SIH-sih-tee)   The state of being noxious; refers to a drug's ability to poison the body

toxicologists (tok-sih-KAW-loh-jistz)   Those who study poisons and toxics agents and their treatments

toxicology (tok-sih-KAW-luh-jee)   The study of poisons and poisonings, including adverse drug reactions

toxin (TOKS-in)   A chemical produced by a microorganism that can be harmful

toxoids (TOKS-oyds)   Protein toxins that have been modified to reduce their hazardous properties without significantly altering their antigenic properties

trade name A drug's proprietary or brand name

transplacental Related to the ability of a toxin or pathogen to cross the physical and biological barriers of the placenta separating the mother and fetus, to whom such substances may be dangerous

tubular reabsorption The method by which the kidneys selectively reclaim just the right amounts of substances that the body requires, such as water, electrolytes, and glucose

tubular secretion The method by which the cells of the tubules remove certain substances from the blood and deposit them into the fluid in the tubules

tumor suppressor genes A category of genes involved in carcinogenesis; they regulate and inhibit inappropriate cellular growth and proliferation

ulcers A break in skin or mucous membrane with loss of surface tissue, disintegration and necrosis of epithelial tissue, and often pus

unit A standard of measure, weight, or any other similar quality

universal antidote (AN-tih-doht) One agent that will counteract all poisons

urea (yoo-REE-uh) The most abundant organic waste that results in the breakdown of amino acids

uric acid (YOO-rik) A type of waste molecule formed by the recycling of nitrogenous base from RNA molecules

urticaria (er-tih-KAY-ree-uh) Vascular reaction of the skin characterized by a rash and severe itching

vaccination (vak-sih-NAY-shun) Active immunization

vaccine (vak-SEEN) A preparation of killed microorganisms, living attenuated organisms, or living virulent organisms that are administered to produce or artificially increase immunity to a particular disease

vasodilation (vass-oh-dy-LAY-shun) Dilation of blood vessels; this action relaxes the smooth muscle of the peripheral arterioles

vasopressin (vaz-oh-PRESS-in) A peptide hormone of the posterior pituitary gland; also called *antidiuretic hormone (ADH)*

vasospasms (VAY-soh-spah-zims) Spasms of the blood vessels

ventricles (VEN-trih-kuls) The lower heart chambers that pump blood out of the heart

vertigo (VER-tih-go) A sensation of revolving—either of the patient themselves or of their environment

viruses Tiny genetic parasites that require the host cell to replicate and spread

vitreous humor (VIT-ree-us) Transparent, jelly-like fluid in the posterior cavity of the eye; supports the internal parts of the eye and helps maintain the eye's shape

volatile liquids Inhalation anesthetic agents that are easily vaporized liquids

water deficit Low levels of body water; dehydration

water of metabolism The volume of body water that is a by-product of the oxidative metabolism of nutrients (about 10%)

wheal A slightly reddened, raised lesion

whole bowel irrigation Rapid administration of large volumes of an osmotically balanced polyethylene glycol solution given orally or via a nasogastric tube to flush out the entire gastrointestinal tract

withdrawal The effects felt by a person when discontinuing or reducing the use of a substance

xanthine derivatives (ZAN-theen) A group of drugs chemically related to caffeine that dilate bronchioles in the lungs

Appendices

Appendix A

Poisons and Antidotes

Drug	Antidote
Acetaminophen	Acetylcysteine
Anticholinesterases (cholinergics)	Atropine, pralidoxime
Antidepressants (monoamine oxidase inhibitors and tyramine-containing foods)	Phentolamine
Benzodiazepines	Flumazenil
Cyanide	Amyl nitrite, sodium nitrite, sodium thiosulfate
Digoxin (digitoxin)	Digoxin immune Fab (Digibind)
Fluorouracil (5-FU)	Leucovorin calcium
Heparin	Protamine sulfate
Ifosfamide	Mesna
Iron	Deferoxamine
Lead	Edentate calcium disodium, dimercaprol, succimer
Methotrexate	Leucovorin calcium
Opioid analgesics, heroin	Nalmefene, naloxone
Thrombolytic agents	Aminocaproic acid (Amicar)
Tricyclic antidepressants	Physostigmine
Warfarin (Coumadin)	Phytonadione (vitamin K)

Appendix B

Common Sound-Alike Drug Names

The following is a list of common sound-alike drug names. Trade names are capitalized, and generic names are in lowercase. In parentheses next to each drug name is the pharmacological classification or use of the drug. Source: www.pharmacytimes.com.

Accupril (ACE inhibitor)	Accutane (anti-acne drug)
acetazolamide (anti-glaucoma drug)	acetohexamide (oral antidiabetic drug)
Aciphex (proton pump inhibitor)	Accupril (ACE inhibitor)
Aciphex (proton pump inhibitor)	Aricept (anti–Alzheimer's disease drug)
Actos (oral hypoglycemic)	Actonel (diphosphonate—bone-growth regulator)
Adriamycin (antineoplastic)	Aredia (bone-growth regulator)
albuterol (sympathomimetic)	atenolol (beta-blocker)
Aldomet (antihypertensive)	Aldoril (antihypertensive)
Alkeran (antineoplastic)	Leukeran (antineoplastic)
Alkeran (antineoplastic)	Myleran (antineoplastic)
allopurinol (anti-gout drug)	Apresoline (antihypertensive)
alprazolam (anti-anxiety agent)	lorazepam (anti-anxiety agent)
Amaryl (oral hypoglycemic)	Reminyl (anti–Alzheimer's disease drug)
Ambien (sedative-hypnotic)	Amen (progestin)
amiloride (diuretic)	amlodipine (calcium channel blocker)
amiodarone (antiarrhythmic)	amrinone (inotropic agent)
amitriptyline (antidepressant)	nortriptyline (antidepressant)
Apresazide (antihypertensive)	Apresoline (antihypertensive)
Aripiprazole (antipsychotic)	Lansoprazole (proton pump inhibitor)
Arlidin (peripheral vasodilator)	Aralen (antimalarial)
Artane (cholinergic blocking agent)	Altace (ACE inhibitor)
Asacol (anti-inflammatory drug)	Avelox (fluoroquinolone antibiotic)
asparaginase (antineoplastic agent)	pegaspargase (antineoplastic agent)
Atarax (anti-anxiety agent)	Ativan (anti-anxiety agent)
atenolol (beta-blocker)	timolol (beta-blocker)
Atrovent (cholinergic blocking agent)	Alupent (sympathomimetic)
Avandia (oral hypoglycemic)	Coumadin (anticoagulant)
Avandia (oral hypoglycemic)	Prandin (oral hypoglycemic)
Bacitracin (antibacterial)	Bactroban (anti-infective, topical)
Benylin (expectorant)	Ventolin (sympathomimetic)

Brevital (barbiturate)	Brevibloc (beta-adrenergic blocker)
Bumex (diuretic)	Buprenex (narcotic analgesic)
bupropion (antidepressant; smoking deterrent)	buspirone (anti-anxiety agent)
Cafergot (analgesic)	Carafate (anti-ulcer drug)
calciferol (vitamin D)	calcitriol (vitamin D)
carboplatin (antineoplastic agent)	cisplatin (antineoplastic agent)
Cardene (calcium channel blocker)	Cardizem (calcium channel blocker)
Cardura (antihypertensive)	Ridaura (gold-containing anti-inflammatory)
Cataflam (NSAID)	Catapres (antihypertensive)
Catapres (antihypertensive)	Combipres (antihypertensive)
cefotaxime (cephalosporin)	cefoxitin (cephalosporin)
cefuroxime (cephalosporin)	deferoxamine (iron chelator)
Celebrex (NSAID)	Cerebyx (anticonvulsant)
Celebrex (NSAID)	Celera (antidepressant)
Cerebyx (anticonvulsant)	Celera (antidepressant)
chlorpromazine (antipsychotic)	chlorpropamide (oral antidiabetic)
chlorpromazine (antipsychotic)	prochlorperazine (antipsychotic)
chlorpromazine (antipsychotic)	promethazine (antihistamine)
Clinoril (NSAID)	Clozaril (antipsychotic)
clomipramine (antidepressant)	clomiphene (ovarian stimulant)
clonidine (antihypertensive)	Klonopin (anticonvulsant)
Combivir (AIDS drug combination)	Combivent (combination for COPD)
Cozaar (antihypertensive)	Zocor (antihyperlipidemic)
cyclobenzaprine (skeletal muscle relaxant)	cyproheptadine (antihistamine)
cyclophosphamide (antineoplastic)	cyclosporine (immunosuppressant)
cyclosporine (immunosuppressant)	cycloserine (antineoplastic)
Cytovene (antiviral drug)	Cytosar (antineoplastic)
Cytoxan (antineoplastic)	Cytotec (prostaglandin derivative)
Cytoxan (antineoplastic)	Cytosar (antineoplastic)
Dantrium (skeletal muscle relaxant)	danazol (gonadotropin inhibitor)
daunorubicin (antineoplastic)	doxorubicin (antineoplastic)
desipramine (antidepressant)	diphenhydramine (antihistamine)
dexamethasone (corticosteroid)	dextromethorphan (antitussive)
DiaBeta (oral hypoglycemic)	Zebeta (beta-adrenergic blocker)
digitoxin (cardiac glycoside)	digoxin (cardiac glycoside)
diphenhydramine (antihistamine)	dimenhydrinate (antihistamine)
dopamine (sympathomimetic)	dobutamine (sympathomimetic)
Doribax (antibiotic)	Zovirax (antiviral)
DTaP (diphtheria, tetanus toxoids, and acellular pertussis)	Tdap (tetanus toxoid, reduced diphtheria toxoid, and acellular pertussis)

(*continued*)

Durasal (salicylate)	Durezol (corticosteroid)
Edecrin (diuretic)	Eulexin (antineoplastic)
enalapril (ACE inhibitor)	Anafranil (antidepressant)
enalapril (ACE inhibitor)	Eldepryl (anti-parkinsonism agent)
Eryc (erythromycin base)	Ery-Tab (erythromycin base)
etidronate (bone-growth regulator)	etretinate (antipsoriatic)
etomidate (general anesthetic)	etidronate (bone-growth regulator)
E-Vista (antihistamine)	Evista (estrogen receptor modulator)
Femara (antineoplastic)	Femhrt (estrogen-progestin combination)
Fioricet (analgesic)	Fiorinal (analgesic)
Flomax (alpha-adrenergic blocker)	Volmax (sympathomimetic)
flurbiprofen (NSAID)	fenoprofen (NSAID)
folinic acid (leucovorin calcium)	folic acid (vitamin B complex)
Gantrisin (sulfonamide)	Gantanol (sulfonamide)
glipizide (oral hypoglycemic)	glyburide (oral hypoglycemic)
glyburide (oral hypoglycemic)	Glucotrol (oral hypoglycemic)
Hycodan (cough preparation)	Hycomine (cough preparation)
hydralazine (antihypertensive)	hydroxyzine (anti-anxiety agent)
hydrocodone (narcotic analgesic)	hydrocortisone (corticosteroid)
Hydrogesic (analgesic combination)	hydroxyzine (antihistamine)
hydromorphone (narcotic analgesic)	morphine (narcotic analgesic)
Hydropres (antihypertensive)	Diupres (antihypertensive)
Hytone (topical corticosteroid)	Vytone (topical corticosteroid)
imipramine (antidepressant)	Norpramin (antidepressant)
Inderal (beta-adrenergic blocker)	Inderide (antihypertensive)
Inderal (beta-adrenergic blocker)	Isordil (coronary vasodilator)
Indocin (NSAID)	Minocin (antibiotic)
K-Phos Neutral (phosphorus–potassium replenishment)	Neutra-Phos-K (phosphorus–potassium replenishment)
Lamictal (anticonvulsant)	Lamisil (antifungal)
Lamictal (anticonvulsant)	Ludiomil (alpha- and beta-adrenergic blocker)
Lamisil (antiviral)	Ludiomil (alpha- and beta-adrenergic blocker)
Lanoxin (cardiac glycoside)	Lasix (diuretic)
Lantus (insulin glargine)	Lente insulin (insulin zinc suspension)
Lioresal (muscle relaxant)	lisinopril (ACE inhibitor)
Lithostat (lithium carbonate)	Lithobid (lithium carbonate)
Lithotabs (lithium carbonate)	Lithobid (lithium carbonate)
Lodine (NSAID)	codeine (narcotic analgesic)
Lopid (antihyperlipidemic)	Lorabid (beta-lactam antibiotic)
lovastatin (antihyperlipidemic)	Lotensin (ACE inhibitor)

Ludiomil (alpha- and beta-adrenergic blocker)	Lomotil (antidiarrheal)
Medrol (corticosteroid)	Haldol (antipsychotic)
metolazone (thiazide diuretic)	methotrexate (antineoplastic)
metolazone (thiazide diuretic)	metoclopramide (GI stimulant)
metoprolol tartrate (beta- adrenergic blocker)	metoclopramide hydrochloride (GI stimulant)
metoprolol (beta-adrenergic blocker)	misoprostol (prostaglandin derivative)
Monopril (ACE inhibitor)	minoxidil (antihypertensive)
morphine sulfate (analgesic)	morphine sulfate extended release (analgesic)
nelfinavir (antiviral)	nevirapine (antiviral)
nicardipine (calcium channel blocker)	nifedipine (calcium channel blocker)
Norlutate (progestin)	Norlutin (progestin)
Noroxin (fluoroquinolone antibiotic)	Neurontin (anticonvulsant)
Norvasc (calcium channel blocker)	Navane (antipsychotic)
Norvir (antiviral)	Retrovir (antiviral)
Ocufen (NSAID)	Ocuflox (fluoroquinolone antibiotic)
Orinase (oral hypoglycemic)	Ornade (upper respiratory product)
paroxetine (antidepressant)	paclitaxel (antineoplastic)
Paxil (antidepressant)	paclitaxel (antineoplastic)
Paxil (antidepressant)	Taxol (antineoplastic)
penicillamine (heavy metal antagonist)	penicillin (antibiotic)
Percocet (narcotic analgesic)	Percodan (narcotic analgesic)
pindolol (beta-adrenergic blocker)	Parlodel (inhibitor of prolactin secretion)
pitavastatin (anti-cholesterol agent)	pravastatin (anti-cholesterol agent)
Pitocin (neuromodulator that induces childbirth)	Pitressin (antidiuretic hormone)
Plaquenil (antimalarial drug)	Provigil (analeptic drug for sleep disorders)
Platinol (antineoplastic)	Paraplatin (antineoplastic)
Pletal (antiplatelet drug)	Plavix (antiplatelet drug)
Pravachol (antihyperlipidemic)	Prevacid (GI drug)
Pravachol (antihyperlipidemic)	propranolol (beta-adrenergic blocker)
prednisolone (corticosteroid)	prednisone (corticosteroid)
Prilosec (inhibitor of gastric acid secretion)	Prozac (antidepressant)
Prinivil (ACE inhibitor)	Prilosec (GI drug)
Prinivil (ACE inhibitor)	Proventil (sympathomimetic)
Procanbid (antiarrhythmic)	Procan SR (antiarrhythmic)
propranolol (beta-adrenergic blocker)	Propulsid (GI drug)
Provera (progestin)	Premarin (estrogen)
Prozac (antidepressant)	Proscar (androgen hormone inhibitor)
quinidine (antiarrhythmic)	clonidine (antihypertensive)
quinidine (antiarrhythmic)	Quinamm (antimalarial)

(continued)

quinine (antimalarial)	quinidine (antiarrhythmic)
Regroton (antihypertensive)	Hygroton (diuretic)
risperidone (antipsychotic)	ropinirole (anti-parkinsonism agent)
sulfadiazine (antibiotic)	sulfasalazine (anti-inflammatory agent)
tramadol (analgesic)	trazodone (antidepressant)
zolmitriptan (anti-migraine serotonin agonist)	zolpidem (hypnotic)

ACE, angiotensin-converting enzyme; GI, gastrointestinal; NSAID, nonsteroidal anti-inflammatory drug.

Appendix C

Recommended Immunization Schedule for Persons Aged 0 Through 6 Years—United States • 2011
For those who fall behind or start late, see the catch-up schedule

Vaccine ▼ Age ►	Birth	1 month	2 months	4 months	6 months	12 months	15 months	18 months	19–23 months	2–3 years	4–6 years
Hepatitis B[1]	HepB	HepB			HepB						
Rotavirus[2]			RV	RV	RV[2]						
Diphtheria, Tetanus, Pertussis[3]			DTaP	DTaP	DTaP	*see footnote[3]*	DTaP				DTaP
Haemophilus influenzae type b[4]			Hib	Hib	Hib[4]	Hib					
Pneumococcal[5]			PCV	PCV	PCV	PCV					PPSV
Inactivated Poliovirus[6]			IPV	IPV		IPV					IPV
Influenza[7]						Influenza (Yearly)					
Measles, Mumps, Rubella[8]						MMR		see footnote[8]			MMR
Varicella[9]						Varicella		see footnote[9]			Varicella
Hepatitis A[10]						HepA (2 doses)				HepA Series	
Meningococcal[11]										MCV4	

This schedule includes recommendations in effect as of December 21, 2010. Any dose not administered at the recommended age should be administered at a subsequent visit, when indicated and feasible. The use of a combination vaccine generally is preferred over separate injections of its equivalent component vaccines. Considerations should include provider assessment, patient preference, and the potential for adverse events. Providers should consult the relevant Advisory

Committee on Immunization Practices statement for detailed recommendations: **http://www.cdc.gov/vaccines/pubs/acip-list.htm**. Clinically signifcant adverse events that follow immunization should be reported to the Vaccine Adverse Event Reporting System (VAERS) at **http://www.vaers.hhs.gov** or by telephone, **800-822-7967**. Use of trade names and commercial sources is for identifcation only and does not imply endorsement by the U.S. Department of Health and Human Services.

 Range of recommended ages for all children

 Range of recommended ages for certain high-risk groups

1. **Hepatitis B vaccine (HepB).** (Minimum age: birth)

   At birth:

   - Administer monovalent HepB to all newborns before hospital discharge.
   - If mother is hepatitis B surface antigen (HBsAg)-positive, administer HepB and 0.5 mL of hepatitis B immune globulin (HBIG) within 12 hours of birth.
   - If mother's HBsAg status is unknown, administer HepB within 12 hours of birth. Determine mother's HBsAg status as soon as possible and, if HBsAg-positive, administer HBIG (no later than age 1 week).

   Doses following the birth dose:

   - The second dose should be administered at age 1 or 2 months. Monovalent HepB should be used for doses administered before age 6 weeks.
   - Infants born to HBsAg-positive mothers should be tested for HBsAg and antibody to HBsAg 1 to 2 months after the completion of at least 3 doses of the HepB series, at age 9 through 18 months (generally at the next well-child visit).
   - The administration of 4 doses of HepB to infants is permissible when a combination vaccine containing HepB is administered after the birth dose.
   - Infants who did not receive a birth dose should receive 3 doses of HepB on a schedule of 0, 1, and 6 months.

   - The final (3rd or 4th) dose in the HepB series should be administered no earlier than age 24 weeks.

2. **Rotavirus vaccine (RV).** (Minimum age: 6 weeks)

   - Administer the first dose at age 6 through 14 weeks (maximum age: 14 weeks 6 days). Vaccination should not be initiated for infants aged 15 weeks 0 days or older.
   - The maximum age for the final dose in the series is 8 months 0 days.
   - If Rotarix is administered at ages 2 and 4 months, a dose at 6 months is not indicated.

3. **Diphtheria and tetanus toxoids and acellular pertussis vaccine (DTaP).** (Minimum age: 6 weeks)

   - The fourth dose may be administered as early as age 12 months, provided at least 6 months have elapsed since the third dose.

4. ***Haemophilus influenzae* type b conjugate vaccine (Hib).** (Minimum age: 6 weeks)

   - If PRP-OMP (PedvaxHIB or Comvax [HepB-Hib]) is administered at ages 2 and 4 months, a dose at age 6 months is not indicated.
   - Hiberix should not be used for doses at ages 2, 4, or 6 months for the primary series but can be used as the final dose in children aged 12 months through 4 years.

5. **Pneumococcal vaccine.** (Minimum age: 6 weeks for pneumococcal conjugate vaccine [PCV]; 2 years for pneumococcal polysaccharide vaccine [PPSV])

   - PCV is recommended for all children aged younger than 5 years. Administer 1 dose of PCV to all healthy children aged 24 through 59 months who are not completely vaccinated for their age.

   - A PCV series begun with 7-valent PCV (PCV7) should be completed with 13-valent PCV (PCV13).

   - A single supplemental dose of PCV13 is recommended for all children aged 14 through 59 months who have received an age-appropriate series of PCV7.

   - A single supplemental dose of PCV13 is recommended for all children aged 60 through 71 months with underlying medical conditions who have received an age-appropriate series of PCV7.

   - The supplemental dose of PCV13 should be administered at least 8 weeks after the previous dose of PCV7. See *MMWR* 2010:59(No. RR-11).

   - Administer PPSV at least 8 weeks after the last dose of PCV to children aged 2 years or older with certain underlying medical conditions, including a cochlear implant.

6. **Inactivated poliovirus vaccine (IPV).** (Minimum age: 6 weeks)

   - If 4 or more doses are administered prior to age 4 years, an additional dose should be administered at age 4 through 6 years.

   - The final dose in the series should be administered on or after the fourth birthday and at least 6 months following the previous dose.

7. **Influenza vaccine (seasonal).** (Minimum age: 6 months for trivalent inactivated influenza vaccine [TIV]; 2 years for live, attenuated influenza vaccine [LAIV])

   - For healthy children aged 2 years and older (i.e., those who do not have underlying medical conditions that predispose them to influenza complications), either LAIV or TIV may be used, except LAIV should not be given to children aged 2 through 4 years who have had wheezing in the past 12 months.

   - Administer 2 doses (separated by at least 4 weeks) to children aged 6 months through 8 years who are receiving seasonal influenza vaccine for the first time or who were vaccinated for the first time during the previous influenza season but only received 1 dose.

   - Children aged 6 months through 8 years who received no doses of monovalent 2009 H1N1 vaccine should receive 2 doses of 2010–2011 seasonal influenza vaccine. See *MMWR* 2010;59(No. RR-8):33–34.

8. **Measles, mumps, and rubella vaccine (MMR).** (Minimum age: 12 months)

   - The second dose may be administered before age 4 years, provided at least 4 weeks have elapsed since the first dose.

9. **Varicella vaccine.** (Minimum age: 12 months)

   - The second dose may be administered before age 4 years, provided at least 3 months have elapsed since the first dose.

   - For children aged 12 months through 12 years, the recommended minimum interval between doses is 3 months. However, if the second dose was administered at least 4 weeks after the first dose, it can be accepted as valid.

10. **Hepatitis A vaccine (HepA).** (Minimum age: 12 months)

    - Administer 2 doses at least 6 months apart.

    - HepA is recommended for children aged older than 23 months who live in areas where vaccination programs target older children, who are at increased risk for infection, or for whom immunity against hepatitis A is desired.

11. **Meningococcal conjugate vaccine, quadrivalent (MCV4).** (Minimum age: 2 years)

    - Administer 2 doses of MCV4 at least 8 weeks apart to children aged 2 through 10 years with persistent complement component deficiency and anatomic or functional asplenia and 1 dose every 5 years thereafter.

    - Persons with human immunodeficiency virus (HIV) infection who are vaccinated with MCV4 should receive 2 doses at least 8 weeks apart.

    - Administer 1 dose of MCV4 to children aged 2 through 10 years who travel to countries with highly endemic or epidemic disease and during outbreaks caused by a vaccine serogroup.

    - Administer MCV4 to children at continued risk for meningococcal disease who were previously vaccinated with MCV4 or meningococcal polysaccharide vaccine after 3 years if the first dose was administered at age 2 through 6 years.

The Recommended Immunization Schedules for Persons Aged 0 Through 18 Years are approved by the Advisory Committee on Immunization Practices (**http://www.cdc.gov/vaccines/recs/acip**), the American Academy of Pediatrics (**http://www.aap.org**), and the American Academy of Family Physicians (**http://www.aafp.org**).
Department of Health and Human Services • Centers for Disease Control and Prevention

Appendix D

Answer Key to Checkpoint Review Questions

Checkpoint Review 1

MULTIPLE CHOICE

1. d
2. b
3. c
4. a
5. d
6. c
7. a
8. b
9. c
10. c
11. b
12. a
13. a
14. b
15. b
16. d
17. d
18. c
19. b
20. c
21. d
22. c
23. c
24. b
25. b
26. d
27. a
28. c
29. a
30. c
31. b
32. c
33. b
34. d
35. d
36. b
37. d
38. a
39. b
40. b
41. d
42. c
43. b
44. b
45. b

MATCHING 1

46. e
47. c
48. a
49. d
50. b

MATCHING 2

51. e
52. d
53. b
54. c
55. a

CASE STUDIES

56. No, the father would not be allowed by law (the Privacy Act) to have access to the medical records because the child is a minor and the father does not have custody.

57. The pharmacy technician should look for the Comprehensive Drug Abuse Prevention and Control Act of 1970.

Checkpoint Review 2

IDENTIFYING FRACTIONS

1. 2-5/8, 4/4, 9/7
2. 1/100, 1/160
3. 1/3, 1/12
4. 1-1/16, 1-2/9, 7-7/9
5. ¾
6. 1
7. 3-1/3
8. 2-3/4
9. 1-1/3
10. 13/2
11. 47/6
12. 6/5
13. 32/3
14. 411/4
15. 1/1,000
16. 1/10
17. 3/10
18. 5/9
19. 1-5/12
20. 1-1/24
21. 1-1/3
22. 53/132
23. 5-50/119
24. 8-7/15
25. 1/4
26. 3/100
27. ½
28. 35/48
29. 3/32
30. 254-1/6
31. 1/30
32. 3/14
33. 3-1/3
34. 1/3

FILL IN THE BLANK

35. volume
36. 1/1,000
37. 1,000
38. 1
39. 1,000
40. milligram
41. kilogram
42. weight

CIRCLE

43. 4 kg
44. 0.6 g
45. 2.5 mm
46. 20 mg

WRITE OUT TERMS

47. gram(s)
48. millimeter(s)
49. centimeter(s)
50. kilogram(s)
51. microgram(s)
52. milliliter(s)

WRITE OUT TERMS

53. quart(s)
54. grain(s)
55. minim(s)
56. dram(s)

WRITE OUT TERMS

57. 1
58. 32

APOTHECARY QUANTITIES

59. gr x
60. 2 pt
61. ½ oz

62. 16 pt
63. 4 oz
64. gr iii

MEASUREMENTS

65. 3 T
66. 10 t
67. 6 gtt
68. 25 mEq

CONVERSIONS

69. 2
70. 1
71. 2
72. 3

TERMS

73. 20 milliequivalents
74. 15 pounds
75. 50 drops
76. 8 tablespoons

CALCULATIONS

77. ½
78. 2
79. 2
80. 1
81. 4
82. 2.5
83. 2
84. 5
85. 1
86. 2
87. 15
88. 1-1/2
89. 7.5
90. 3
91. 2
92. 7.5
93. ½

94. ½
95. 3
96. 1
97. 1
98. 1.5
99. 2.5
100. 0.7
101. 6

FORMULAS

102. desired dose
103. dosage unit
104. dose on hand
105. amount to administer

FILL IN THE BLANK

106. tuberculin syringe
107. 3
108. 70/30
109. USP
110. Continuous
111. Nomogram
112. Young's; Fried's
113. weight
114. Young's
115. Fried's
116. dosage calculations
117. medication errors
118. FDA
119. Quality
120. evaluation

Checkpoint Review 3

MULTIPLE CHOICE

1. d
2. c
3. b
4. c
5. d

6. c
7. b
8. a
9. b
10. c
11. a
12. d
13. b
14. a
15. c
16. d
17. c
18. b
19. a
20. d
21. a
22. c
23. d
24. b
25. a
26. c
27. a
28. c
29. c
30. d
31. c
32. b
33. c
34. d
35. b
36. a
37. a
38. c
39. b
40. c
41. c
42. d
43. d
44. d
45. b
46. a
47. b
48. b

MATCHING 1

49. e
50. d
51. a
52. c
53. b

MATCHING 2

54. e
55. c
56. d
57. a
58. b

FILL IN THE BLANK

59. Metronidazole
60. antiprotozoal
61. antibiotics
62. bacteria
63. bactericidal
64. SMZ/TMP
65. penicillins
66. gram-positive
67. nephrotoxicity
68. large amounts
69. 50; 60
70. beri-beri
71. nausea
72. Immunity
73. antigen
74. B-lymphocytes
75. antitoxin

Checkpoint Review 4

MULTIPLE CHOICE

1. b
2. d
3. c
4. b

5. b
6. a
7. a
8. c
9. d
10. b
11. d
12. b
13. d
14. a
15. b
16. c
17. d
18. b
19. d
20. d
21. b
22. d
23. a
24. c
25. b
26. d
27. d
28. c
29. a
30. c
31. b
32. d
33. b
34. a
35. d
36. b
37. c
38. a
39. c
40. c
41. b
42. d
43. c
44. d
45. c
46. a
47. c

48. d
49. b
50. c
51. b
52. d
53. b
54. c
55. b
56. d
57. c
58. b
59. d
60. c
61. b
62. b
63. d
64. b
65. c
66. d
67. c
68. b
69. c
70. c
71. a
72. d
73. b
74. a
75. c
76. b
77. b
78. c
79. a
80. a
81. d
82. b
83. a
84. c
85. c
86. d
87. b
88. c
89. c
90. a

91. c
92. d
93. a
94. d
95. b
96. b
97. d
98. a
99. b
100. d
101. a
102. d
103. c
104. b
105. b
106. a
107. d
108. b
109. a
110. b
111. d
112. d
113. a
114. a
115. d
116. d
117. a
118. b
119. b
120. d
121. b

MATCHING 1

122. e
123. d
124. c
125. a
126. b

MATCHING 2

127. d
128. c

129. e
130. a
131. b

FILL IN THE BLANK

132. neurotransmitters
133. ocular
134. muscarinic
135. cholinergic
136. cooling
137. irreversible
138. nicotinic
139. catecholamines
140. parasympatholytics
141. balanced
142. gastric upsets
143. testosterone
144. estrogen
145. estrogens
146. mouth
147. duodenal ulcer
148. motility
149. $beta_2$; xanthenes
150. antagonists
151. digestive system

Checkpoint Review 5

MULTIPLE CHOICE

1. d
2. b
3. c
4. a
5. b
6. d
7. b
8. a
9. d
10. a
11. c
12. a

13. b
14. b

MATCHING

15. e
16. d
17. c
18. b
19. a

FILL IN THE BLANK

20. lower
21. filtration rate

22. elderly
23. drug companies
24. X
25. dysmorphology
26. oogonia
27. teratogens
28. any stage
29. decreased
30. organogenesis
31. body water
32. passive

Appendix E

Answer Key to Apply Your Knowledge Sections

Apply Your Knowledge 1.1

CRITICAL THINKING

1. The dose-effect relationship is the relationship between the dose of a drug (or other agent) that produces therapeutic effects and the potency of the effects on a person. It is determined by pharmacokinetics and pharmacodynamics.

2. Biotransformation is also known as metabolism, the sum of chemical and physical changes in the tissues, consisting of anabolism and catabolism.

3. *Pharmacodynamics* refers to the biochemical and physiologic effects of drugs and mechanisms of drug action (the effects of a drug on the body or organism), and *pharmacokinetics* is the study of the absorption, distribution, biotransformation, and excretion of drugs.

4. A drug's half-life is defined as the time taken for the blood or plasma concentration of the drug to decrease from full to one-half (50%). The longer the half-life of the drug, the longer the drug remains in the body.

5. Pharmacognosy is the study of drugs derived from herbal and other natural sources.

6. The various factors that affect drug action include age, sex, body weight, diurnal body rhythms, diseases, allergies, psychological factors, drug half-life, tolerance, drug toxicity, and drug interactions.

7. An agonist is a drug that binds to a receptor and produces a stimulatory response that is similar to what an endogenous substance (such as a hormone) would have done if it were bound to the receptor. For example, adrenaline is an agonist at beta (β)-adrenoceptors. An antagonist is a drug that prevents an agonist from binding to a receptor and thus blocks its effects. For example, propranolol (Inderal) is a β-adrenoceptor antagonist.

8. *Affinity* is defined as a drug's attractive force for a target receptor. A receptor is the cell recipient—usually a specific protein—situated in either in cell membranes on cell surfaces or within the cellular cytoplasm.

9. Toxicity is the state of being noxious and refers to a drug's ability to poison the body. Drug tolerance is the development of resistance to the effects of a drug such that the drug's doses must be continually raised to elicit the desired response.

Apply Your Knowledge 1.2

CRITICAL THINKING

1. The main route of drug excretion—the last stage of pharmacokinetics that removes drugs from the system—is via the kidneys. Diseases of the kidneys can significantly prolong the duration of drug action.

2. The four main stages of biotransformation are:
   a. oxidation—combination with oxygen
   b. reduction—a reaction with a substance that involves the gaining of electrons
   c. hydrolysis—the cleaving of a compound into simpler compounds with the uptake of the hydrogen and hydroxide parts of a water molecule
   d. conjugation—the combination of substances with glucuronic or sulfuric acid, terminating biologic activity and making them ready for excretion

3. Factors that affect the rate of drug absorption include the acidity of the stomach, physiochemical properties, presence of food in the stomach or intestine, and routes of administration.

4. The four stages of pharmacokinetics are drug absorption, drug distribution, drug metabolism, and drug excretion.

5. Side effects are also called adverse effects. They are defined as results of drug (or other) therapy that are beyond the desired therapeutic effects. Side effects are usually (but not always) undesirable.

6. The microsomal enzymes are found in the liver. They play different roles in metabolism. For example, one enzyme (called cytochrome P-450) has an essential role in drug metabolism.

7. The blood–brain barrier consists of tightly packed cells in capillary walls of the brain. This barrier prevents substances (such as most drugs) from migrating from the bloodstream into the cells of the brain. Bioavailability is the effect of presystemic metabolism on a drug, controlling how much of the drug reaches the systemic circulation intact and the speed at which this happens.

8. Anything absorbed through the wall of the small intestine must go to the liver to be metabolized. Substances, including drugs, must enter the liver through the hepatic portal vein. It is the only port of entry into the liver for these substances.

Apply Your Knowledge 1.3

CRITICAL THINKING

1. Of the various types of allergic drug reactions, type I reactions involve immediate hypersensitivity, type II reactions are antibody dependent or cytotoxic reactions, type III reactions are complex mediated, and type IV reactions are cell mediated or delayed hypersensitivity.

2. A drug interaction occurs when the effects of one drug are altered by the effects of another drug (with either increased or decreased effects). Examples include amiodarone inhibiting the cytochrome P-450 isoenzyme, leading to reduced metabolism of warfarin and increased anticoagulant effects; carbamazepine reducing the anticoagulant effect of warfarin; phenytoin having a complex interaction with phenobarbital; and the pharmacodynamic synergy between diuretics and angiotensin-converting enzyme (ACE) inhibitors.

3. Anaphylactic shock is an idiosyncratic, sudden, severe allergic reaction that may be life threatening. Examples of causes of anaphylactic shock include certain drugs, vaccines, serum, or blood transfusions.

4. Synergism is the combined action for two or more agents that produce an effect greater than that which would have been expected from the two agents acting separately. For example, the combination of the antibacterial drug trimethoprim with sulfamethoxazole is more effective for treating infections than either drug acting alone. Potentiation is an interaction between two drugs that causes an effect greater than that which would have been expected from the additive properties of the drugs involved. For example, alcohol potentiates the sedating effects of the tranquilizer diazepam when the two drugs are ingested at the same time.

5. Idiosyncratic reactions are defined as unique, strange, or unpredicted reactions to drugs. They may be caused by underlying enzyme deficiencies, resulting from genetic or hormonal variation.

6. Drug tolerance may be produced by such drugs as opiates, nitrates, barbiturates, alcohol, and tobacco.

Apply Your Knowledge 2.1

CRITICAL THINKING

1. To combat the lack of drug regulation in the United States, Congress passed the first Pure Food and Drug Act in 1906.

2. The 1938 Food, Drug, and Cosmetic Act gave the Food and Drug Administration (FDA) the authority to approve or deny new drug

applications. The sulfanilamide disaster of 1937 caused Congress to pass this act.

3. The thalidomide disaster of 1962 involved the use of thalidomide (both a sleeping pill and antinausea agent during pregnancy) abroad. Before U.S. approval for use, its adverse effects on developing fetuses were discovered. Women who took thalidomide during the first trimester of pregnancy delivered babies with severe deformities, including malformed or missing limbs.

4. Whereas legend drugs are those requiring a prescription in order to be dispensed, non-legend drugs are available over the counter (OTC).

5. The Drug Enforcement Administration (DEA) is part of the Federal Bureau of Investigation (FBI). The Controlled Substances Act (CSA) is administered and enforced by the DEA under the authority of the Department of Justice (DOJ) and the Attorney General. The DEA is required to obtain the expert scientific advice of the FDA when seeking to add a substance to the list of controlled substances.

Apply Your Knowledge 2.2

CRITICAL THINKING

1. Orphan drugs are those that treat rare diseases affecting fewer than 200,000 people in the United States. Examples of orphan drugs include those used to treat AIDS, cystic fibrosis, blepharospasm, and snake bites.

2. The purpose of the Controlled Substances Act is to encompass all federal laws dealing with narcotic drugs, stimulants, depressants, and abused designer drugs that did not fit the historical classifications. It also served to consolidate the government's enforcement activities that had previously been handled by various competing agencies.

3. Schedule I drugs—high abuse potential, no accepted medical use, no prescription permitted; examples include heroin, lysergic acid diethylamide (LSD), and marijuana

    Schedule II drugs—high abuse potential, accepted medical use, prescription required,

no refills permitted without a new written prescription; examples include cocaine, codeine, and methamphetamine

Schedule III drugs—low to moderate abuse potential, accepted medical use, prescription required, 5 refills permitted in 6 months; examples include certain drugs compounded with small quantities of narcotics, other drugs with high potential for abuse, and certain barbiturates

Schedule IV drugs—low abuse potential, accepted medical use, prescription required, 5 refills permitted in 6 months; examples include barbital, chloral hydrate, and diazepam

Schedule V drugs—low abuse potential, accepted medical use, no prescription required for patients 18 years or older (though there are a few exceptions); examples include cough syrups with codeine, diphenoxylate hydrochloride with atropine sulfate, and kaolin–pectin–opium

4. The abuse of anabolic steroids is dangerous because without medical supervision, their use may lead to heart damage, liver damage, depression, hostility, aggression, stunted height, excessive hair growth, acne, and a risk of human immunodeficiency virus (HIV).

5. The Omnibus Budget Reconciliation Act (OBRA) of 1990 requires that pharmacists offer to counsel Medicaid and Medicare patients about drug information and potential adverse effects for all new and refilled prescriptions.

Apply Your Knowledge 2.3

CRITICAL THINKING

1. All health professionals must obey Occupational Safety and Health Administration (OSHA) guidelines because they ensure workplace safety and a healthy workplace environment. These guidelines help to protect against the transmission of such infectious diseases as HIV, AIDS, and hepatitis B. Violations can result in fines and other penalties, which may be severe based on the level and amount of infractions.

2. The Health Insurance Portability and Accountability Act (HIPAA) of 1996 generated various standards and rules designed to protect insured individuals. The four parts are:

- The Electronic Health Transaction Standards—standard code sets must be adopted by health organizations and used in all health transactions
- Unique Identifiers—designed to reduce multiple identification numbers when organizations deal with each other
- Security and Electronic Signature Standards—improve physical storage and maintenance, transmission, and individual health information access standards
- Privacy and Confidentiality Standards—limit nonconsensual use and release of private health information (now called *protected health information*)

3. The Food and Drug Administration (FDA) controls all drugs for legal use. All drug administration laws are initiated, implemented, and enforced by the FDA. The Drug Enforcement Administration (DEA) enforces controlled substance laws and regulations and prosecutes individuals and organizations who grow, manufacture, or distribute illegal substances. It also targets people who use violence in the coercion of others to help them in their illegal activities and distributes information about illegal substances to educate the public. The Centers for Disease Control and Prevention (CDC) provides statistics and information to health professionals about the treatment of common and rare diseases worldwide.

4. The four parts of Medicare are:

- Part A—hospital insurance that also covers hospice, home health-care services, and religious nonmedical health-care institutions; usually does not require the payment of a premium
- Part B—medical insurance for doctors' services, outpatient care, home health services, other medical services, and some preventive services; it requires the payment of a monthly premium
- Part C—"Medicare Advantage" offered by private companies approved by Medicare, covering emergency and urgent care; may offer extra coverage such as vision care, hearing care, dental care, or other wellness programs; usually requires an additional monthly premium
- Part D—only covers drugs that are approved by the FDA and does not cover people who already have Medicare Part A or B coverage; Part D may be obtained either by joining a prescription drug plan or a Medicare Advantage plan; it is voluntary, operating on an annual renewal basis, with varied plans and copayment amounts

5. The Combat Methamphetamine Epidemic Act of 2005 is focused on the provisions of the Patriot Act extension that deals with methamphetamine provisions. It was designed to stop illegal use of methamphetamine and regulated trafficking of this drug (and others such as crack cocaine) when these activities are used to finance terrorism. Drugs that fall under this act's jurisdiction must be kept behind a counter or in a locked case, which helps to limit sales of ingredients used to manufacture methamphetamine. These ingredients include ephedrine and pseudoephedrine.

Apply Your Knowledge 3.1

CRITICAL THINKING

1. The most common combining vowels are "o" and "i," with "o" being most common.

2. A prefix is a structure at the beginning of a word that modifies the meaning of the root. A root is the main part of a word that gives the word its central meaning. A suffix is a word ending that modifies the meaning of the root.

3. Cryptorchidism is the absence of one or both testes from the scrotum. *Hemopathy* is a term that means any disease of the blood. Photophobia is a symptom of excessive sensitivity to light and the aversion to sunlight or well-lit places. Colostomy is a surgical procedure that brings one end of the large intestine out through the abdominal wall so feces can be drained into a collection bag.

4. The following prefixes are listed beside their meanings:

ante-	meaning: before
alb-	meaning: white
semi-	meaning: half
epi-	meaning: upon, above
ecto-	meaning: outside

Apply Your Knowledge 3.2

ABBREVIATIONS

1. The following abbreviations are listed beside their meanings:

ad	meaning: to, up to
aq	meaning: water
liq	meaning: liquid
per	meaning: through or by
QN	meaning: every night
supp	meaning: suppository
x	meaning: multiplied by

2. The following abbreviations are listed beside their meanings:

gtt	meaning: drops
fl	meaning: fluid
mcg	meaning: microgram
kg	meaning: kilogram
Bx	meaning: biopsy
CVA	meaning: cerebrovascular accident
Dx	meaning: diagnosis
HBV	meaning: hepatitis B virus

3. The following terms are listed beside their abbreviations:

potassium	abbreviation: K
nitrogen	abbreviation: N
sodium	abbreviation: Na
iodine	abbreviation: I
iron	abbreviation: Fe

4. The following terms are listed beside their abbreviations:

catheter	abbreviation: cath.
electrocardiogram	abbreviation: ECG
genitourinary	abbreviation: GU
hemoglobin	abbreviation: Hgb

5. The following terms are listed beside their abbreviations:

intrauterine device	abbreviation: IUD
weight	abbreviation: wt
chest x-ray	abbreviation: CXR
microgram	abbreviation: mcg

Apply Your Knowledge 3.3

CRITICAL THINKING

1. Ten examples of solid drugs include pills, tablets, capsules, sustained-release tablets, sustained-release capsules, enteric-coated tablets, enteric-coated capsules, caplets, gelcaps, powders, granules, and troches (lozenges).

2. Caplets are shaped like capsules but have the form of tablets. Gelcaps are oil-based medications enclosed in soft gelatin capsules. Capsules contain drugs in external shells—usually made of hard cylindrical gelatin.

3. Syrups and linctuses are aqueous solutions containing high concentrations of sugars with or without medical substances added. A syrup is defined as a saturated solution of sucrose in water, into which herbal or other constituents may be incorporated. A linctus is defined as a form of elixir designed for the treatment of respiratory complaints. They should be mucilaginous in their action.

4. Emulsions are pharmaceutical preparations containing two agents that cannot ordinarily be combined or mixed. Usually, they feature an oil dispersed inside water, although they may be the reverse. Most creams and lotions are emulsions. Liniments are liquid suspensions for external application to the skin to relieve pain and swelling.

5. Creams are usually emulsions that are most often thicker than lotions. Because of more oily components, creams are usually greasier in nature than lotions. They are designed to be rubbed into the skin. Lotions are suspensions of drugs in a water base that are patted onto the skin rather than rubbed in. Lotions tend to settle in their containers and must be shaken before use.

Apply Your Knowledge 3.4

CRITICAL THINKING

1. Sustained-release drug forms contain several doses of a drug. The doses have special coatings that dissolve at different rates; therefore, the drug is gradually released into the digestive system. Sustained-released drugs are referred to as delayed release or timed release.

2. Tablets are pharmaceutical preparations made by compressing the powdered form of a drug and bulk-filling material under high pressure. A pill is a single-dose unit of medication made by mixing the powdered drug with a liquid, such as syrup, and rolling it into a round or oval shape.

3. Enteric-coated tablets and capsules feature special coatings that keep them from dissolving in the stomach, which contains hydrochloric acid. They do not dissolve until they reach the intestine, providing a delayed action that is desirable.

4. Troches are also called lozenges. Examples include cough suppressants and treatments for sore throat, commonly called cough drops.

5. Fluidextracts are concentrated solutions of drugs removed from plant sources by mixing ground plant parts with solvents, such as alcohol, and then separating the plant residue from the solvent. Tinctures are alcoholic preparations of soluble drugs—usually from plant sources—that may also contain water. Magmas contain particles suspended in liquids, exhibiting a more pasty quality in their consistencies than other suspensions.

6. Whereas emulsions contain two agents that cannot ordinarily be combined or mixed, lotions are suspensions of drugs in a water base.

7. Three examples of drugs administered by transdermal patch are nicotine, estrogen, and nitroglycerine.

Apply Your Knowledge 3.5

CRITICAL THINKING

1. The components of prescriptions include the name and address of the patient, address of the prescriber's office, date, inscription, superscription, subscription, signa, refill and special labeling, and the prescriber's signature and license or Drug Enforcement Administration (DEA) number.

2. The *inscription* describes the medication being prescribed in a prescription. The *superscription* is the Rx symbol, which designates the medication as one requiring a prescription to be dispensed. The *subscription* contains the dispensing directions to the pharmacist.

3. Standing orders are written orders sometimes left by physicians as ongoing prescriptions in a hospital, nursing home, or residential care setting. They are not legally valid unless properly written, dated, and signed.

4. The Rx symbol designates that the medication requires a prescription in order to be dispensed. The term *signa* means the directions for the patient regarding how to administer the medication.

5. The abbreviation MAR stands for medication administration record. Prescriptions in hospitals are usually written on drug charts or physician order sheets and then transcribed onto a MAR, which may be many pages in length.

Apply Your Knowledge 4.1

CRITICAL THINKING

1. The principles of drug administration include the patient's health status, medication history, illness or current condition, intended drug, and route of administration.

Also, any problems the patient may have in self-administering a medication must also be identified. Obtaining information about how and where the patient stores medications is important. Socioeconomic factors need to be considered for all patients but especially for elderly people.

2. The seven rights of drug administration are the *right* patient, drug, dose, route, time, technique, and documentation.

3. Problems seen in elderly patients when self-administering medications include poor eyesight, unsteady hands, and difficulty opening certain containers.

4. Medication history is important because it includes information about the drugs the patient is taking currently or has taken recently. This includes prescription drugs; such over-the-counter drugs as antacids, alcohol, and tobacco; and illegal drugs, such as marijuana. Sometimes, an incompatibility with one or more drugs affects choices of new medications.

5. The most important factors to keep in mind concerning drug administration are following all physician orders exactly as written, asking for clarification if needed, administering medications only after the order is written in the patient's chart, always implementing the seven rights of drug administration, and performing three drug order and label checks.

Apply Your Knowledge 4.2

CRITICAL THINKING

1. The safest method of medication administration is, in general, the enteral routes (especially the oral route). However, enteral routes do include the oral, nasogastric or gastrostomy tube, sublingual, and buccal routes.

2. The nasogastric route involves a tube inserted into the nasopharynx down to the patient's stomach for the purpose of feeding or for removing gastric secretions. A gastrostomy tube is surgically placed directly into the patient's stomach and provides another route for administering medications and nutrition.

3. The buccal route involves medications being placed between the gum and cheek and left there until they dissolve. It is a type of percutaneous route. It should be used when slower absorption is required.

4. Three drugs administered sublingually are nitroglycerin, ergotamine tartrate, and buprenorphine with naloxone.

5. The enteral route is the route of drug administration through the gastrointestinal tract.

Apply Your Knowledge 4.3

CRITICAL THINKING

1. A Z-track injection avoids irritation to the skin and subcutaneous tissues. It prevents any leakage back from the deep muscle into the upper subcutaneous layers by displacing the upper tissue laterally before the needle is inserted.

2. The vastus lateralis site is recommended for injecting infants because it has no major blood vessels or nerves nearby, making it very safe to use.

3. Prefilled cartridge syringes and needles are available that must be attached to a reusable holder (injection) system before use. The advantages of cartridge syringes are that the medications they contain are ready for use in emergency situations; they prevent medication errors because they are already calculated.

4. One method of tuberculin screening is the tine test, which is administered with individually packaged disposable sterile stamps with four prongs on the end that have been treated with tuberculin solution. However, the tine test is not as accurate as the Mantoux (purified protein derivative [PPD]) intradermal screening test.

5. Ampules are made of clear glass and usually contain a single dose of a drug. A vial consists of a small glass bottle that is sealed with a rubber cap and may range from single dose to multidose. They are pierced with

needles to access the medication. Air is injected into the vial before the medication can be withdrawn from it to prevent a vacuum from building up within the vial.

6. The parts of a needle are the bevel (the slanted part at the needle's tip), the cannula or shaft (the actual metal length that makes up the majority of the needle and is attached to the hub), and the hub (the part of the needle that fits onto the syringe.

7. Hypodermic means "subcutaneous" or "under the skin." Hypodermic syringes are available in sizes between 2 and 3 mL and are marked in either milliliters or minims.

8. The three parts of a syringe are the barrel (the outside part), which has printed scales used to measure medication amounts; the plunger (which fits inside the barrel); and the tip (which connects with the needle).

Apply Your Knowledge 4.4

CRITICAL THINKING

1. Oxygen toxicity may develop when 100% oxygen is breathed for a prolonged period.

2. In children younger than 3 years old, the use of the otic route requires that the earlobe be gently pulled down and back. In adults, the earlobe is gently pulled up and out. For both types of patients, they should remain lying on their opposite side for 5 minutes to allow the medication to run into and coat the surface of the inner ear canal.

3. *Transdermal* is defined as "through or by way of the skin." *Topical* is defined as "applied to the surface of the skin."

4. Nasal medications should be held over one nostril at a time and then administered drop by drop. Nasal sprays are usually used with the patient in the supine position with the head tilted back.

5. Nasal decongestants are the most common nasal instillations. Many of these medications are over-the-counter drugs.

6. The rectal route is useful if the patient is nauseated, vomiting, or unconscious.

Apply Your Knowledge 5.1

DO THE MATH

1. 8   2. 25   3. 15   4. 6   5. 21   6. 14
7. 15   8. 16   9. 27   10. 12   11. 11   12. 6
13. 10

MATCHING

1. b   2. b   3. a   4. a   5. b

Apply Your Knowledge 5.2

FILL IN THE BLANK

1. less   2. top number   3. combined
4. smaller; larger
5. invert; multiply the numerators and divisors (remember to reduce to lowest terms)
6. 35   7. 100   8. 88
9. 60   10. numerator

MULTIPLE CHOICE

1. b   2. a   3. d

Apply Your Knowledge 5.3

DO THE MATH

1. 32.95	2. 57.96	3. 13.506
4. 7.269	5. 28.212	6. 7.15
7. 15.59	8. 9.569	9. 21.6
10. 324.03	11. 0.1501	12. 403.144
13. 75,100.751	14. 348.58	15. 0.01596
16. 300	17. 5.4477611	18. 3.7426035
19. 4,120	20. 400	

Apply Your Knowledge 5.4

FILL IN THE BLANK

1. colon (:)   2. solution   3. 100 units:1 mL
4. unit

DO THE MATH

1. 1/3   2. 3/4   3. 1/50   4. 3/5
5. 4/7   6. 1/2

Apply Your Knowledge 5.5

DO THE MATH

1. 16   2. 9   3. 65   4. 8
5. 4   6. 35   7. 20   8. 100

Apply Your Knowledge 5.6

FILL IN THE BLANK

1. whole number   2. hundredths
3. fraction   4. denominator
5. percent; decimal

DO THE MATH

1. 0.02   2. 0.18   3. 0.4
4. 1.06   5. 0.008   6. 0.245
7. 1.5075   8. 0.045   9. 8%
10. 3,200%   11. 44%   12. 50%
13. 1.9%   14. 570%   15. 1,300%
16. 99%

Apply Your Knowledge 6.1

FILL IN THE BLANK

1. 25 g   2. 8 mL   3. 0.55 mg
4. 100 mcg   5. 7.2 mcg   6. 16 L
7. 2,000 mL   8. 4 m   9. 19 mm
10. 3.5 cm

MULTIPLE CHOICE

1. c   2. b   3. b   4. c   5. b

Apply Your Knowledge 6.2

FILL IN THE BLANK

1. ʒ
2. gr
3. dr or ʒ
4. qt
5. pt
6. M or ♍

Apply Your Knowledge 6.3

FILL IN THE BLANK

1. 4 cups   2. 15 tablespoons
3. 1 cup   4. 6 teaspoons
5. 450 drops   6. 2 tablespoons
7. 4 pints   8. 2 ounces
9. length   10. volume
11. weight   12. 24
13. 2.9 (can be rounded to 3 teaspoons)

Apply Your Knowledge 6.4

FILL IN THE BLANK

1. 169   2. 8.3   3. 0.6   4. 0.4
5. 120   6. 255   7. 15   8. 2
9. 5   10. 0.5   11. 75   12. 7.5
13. 1.5   14. 0.2   15. 0.1   16. 240
17. 90   18. 450   19. 2.5   20. 0.5
21. 0.25

Apply Your Knowledge 6.5

FILL IN THE BLANK

1. 55.4°F   2. 69.8°F   3. 93.2°F
4. 113°F   5. 152.6°F   6. 206.6°F
7. 211.8°F   8. 222.8°F   9. 3.33°C
10. 11.11°C   11. 24.44°C   12. 36.67°C
13. 40°C   14. −26.67°C

Apply Your Knowledge 7.1

MATCHING

1. d   2. e   3. a   4. f   5. c   6. b

DRUG DOSAGE CALCULATIONS

1. 1/2 tablet   2. 3 mL   3. 2 tablets   4. 4 mL

Apply Your Knowledge 7.2

LABELING

1. 6.125   2. 2   3. 3   4. 4   5. 4

DRUG DOSAGE CALCULATIONS

1. 2 capsules   2. 2 tablets   3. 10 mL
4. 12.5 mL or 2-1/2 teaspoons   5. 1 tablet

Apply Your Knowledge 7.3

LABELING

1. 900 mg   2. 1 to 4 tsp, 3 to 4 times daily
3. 19,200   4. 12.5   5. 15   6. 118.5

DRUG DOSAGE CALCULATIONS

1. 0.16 mL   2. 1.5 mL   3. 0.5 mL   4. 2 mL
5. 0.5 mL   6. 1.2 mL   7. 2 mL

Apply Your Knowledge 7.4

MULTIPLE CHOICE

1. c   2. b   3. a   4. d   5. a

DO THE MATH

1. 25 kg   2. 5 kg   3. 71.2 kg   4. 8 kg
5. 95 kg   6. 12.2 kg   7. 42.2 kg   8. 61.3 kg

Apply Your Knowledge 8.1

CRITICAL THINKING

1. A medication error is the inappropriate or incorrect administration of a drug that should be preventable through effective system controls.

2. The most common medication errors involve dosages.

3. The Internet may cause medication errors because there is increased availability of drugs through the Internet.

4. The risk factors for medication errors include the use of incorrect abbreviations, miscommunication, missing information, the lack of appropriate labeling, environmental factors, and poor management.

5. Medication errors can occur in three stages: during prescribing or ordering, when the medication is dispensed, and when it is administered and monitored for side effects.

Apply Your Knowledge 8.2

CRITICAL THINKING

1. Medication errors should be investigated and documented so the causes of the error can be determined and eradicated in the future. All patient records should be updated with the information.

2. At the federal level, the Food and Drug Administration (FDA) coordinates the reporting of medication errors, using its "MedWatch" program.

3. The MedWatch program provides timely information that is clinically important regarding medical products. This includes information about safety issues for drugs, biologics, medical devices, radiation-emitting devices, and special nutritional products. Health-care professionals are encouraged to use MedWatch to report errors and situations that may lead to errors. Reporting may be done anonymously.

4. The National Coordinating Council for Medication Error Reporting and Prevention (NCC MERP) provides assistance with medication errors. It has helped to standardize the medication error reporting system and coordinates medication error information while providing preventive education.

5. The advantages of documenting medication errors include quality improvement and assurance, assisting in legal cases, and for the improvement of medication administration processes.

Apply Your Knowledge 8.3

CRITICAL THINKING

1. Steps that can help in avoiding medication errors include:

   Assessment—asking patients about allergies, health condition, use of medications and herbal supplements, knowledge of their medications, and whether pharmacotherapy impairments exist

   Planning—avoiding abbreviations that may be misunderstood, questioning unclear orders, refusing verbal orders, following policies and procedures, having patients restate all directions, and having patients explain the goals of the medication therapy

   Implementation—eliminating distractions, following the seven "rights," verifying the identification, following correct procedures and techniques, performing exact dosage calculations, ensuring correct opening of medications, documenting procedures, confirming that an oral dose has been completely swallowed, and double-checking for long-acting oral dosage forms

   Evaluation—assessing the patient for correct outcomes and determining any adverse effects

2. Nearly half of those who experience fatal medication errors are older than age 60.

3. *Polypharmacy* is defined as receiving multiple medications—sometimes for the same condition—that have conflicting pharmacologic actions.

4. *Medication reconciliation* is defined as keeping track of a patient's medications as he or she changes health-care providers.

5. Older adults often need many different medications because they often have multiple health problems related to the aging process. Their medications may include prescription and over-the-counter medications, herbal supplements, and even vitamins. Also, older adults may see numerous physicians—all of whom may prescribe various medications.

Apply Your Knowledge 9.1

CRITICAL THINKING

1. Some nutrients are called essential because they are needed by the body for normal functioning. Essential nutrients cannot be synthesized by the body, so they must be derived from the diet. Essential nutrients include vitamins, minerals, amino acids, fatty acids, and some carbohydrates.

2. Two essential fatty acids are linoleic acid and linolenic acid. Omega-3 fatty acids are indicated to decrease the risk of coronary artery disease, decrease triglyceride levels and the growth rate of atherosclerotic plaque, slightly lower blood pressure, and decrease the risk of arrhythmias.

3. Cholesterol is a natural lipid found in cell membranes in highest concentrations in animal muscles and organ cells. Cholesterol does not exist in plants. It is essential for certain cell structures, but excess cholesterol can deposit in blood vessels, form atherosclerotic plaque, and lead to cardiovascular disease.

4. Water-soluble fiber helps to lower blood cholesterol levels and may also stabilize blood sugar levels in the body by slowing the absorption of carbohydrates.

5. Carbohydrates are converted to glucose and other monosaccharides. There are two basic types: simple sugars (found in fruits, some vegetables, milk, and table sugar) and complex carbohydrates (found in such grain foods as pastas, breads, and rice and fruits and vegetables such as potatoes, broccoli, corn, apples, and pears).

6. Macronutrients are needed by the body in relatively large amounts and constitute the bulk of the diet. They include carbohydrates, fats, proteins, macrominerals, and water.

7. Macrominerals include sodium, chloride, potassium, calcium, phosphorus, and magnesium.

8. Insoluble fiber primarily promotes regular bowel movements by contributing to stool bulk, which stimulates peristalsis. It also helps to prevent colon cancer and seems to

reduce the risk of heart attack. It increases and softens the bulk of the stool, promoting normal defecation. It can help treat and prevent constipation, diverticular disease, and irritable bowel syndrome. It is linked to the reduction in gallstone formation and the risks of certain types of cancer and other diseases.

Apply Your Knowledge 9.2

CRITICAL THINKING

1. Fat-soluble vitamins:
   Retinol (vitamin A)—affects the retina of the eye
   Calciferol (vitamin D)—controls calcium metabolism in bone building
   Tocopherol (vitamin E)—antioxidant effects
   Phylloquinone (vitamin K1)—blood clotting and bone development

2. Scurvy occurs because of a deficiency of ascorbic acid (vitamin C). It is marked by anemia, edema of the gums, and bleeding into the skin and mucous membranes.

3. Deficiency of thiamine leads to the disease beri-beri, which is characterized by edema, cardiovascular abnormalities, and neurologic symptoms.

4. The generic forms of the B vitamins are:
   Vitamin B_1 or thiamine—functions as a coenzyme in some important carbohydrate metabolic processes
   Vitamin B_3 or nicotinamide (niacin)—lowers cholesterol, triglycerides, and free fatty acids
   Vitamin B_5 or pantothenic acid—needed for formation of coenzyme A, which is required for numerous biochemical processes
   Vitamin B_6 or pyridoxine—a collection of substances that prevent neuritis, treat nausea during pregnancy, and suppress lactation when given orally
   Vitamin B_{12} or cobalamin—promotes normal function of all cells, especially normal blood formation, and is necessary for proper nervous system function

5. Pellagra is marked by dementia, dermatitis, diarrhea, and death. It is caused by the deficiency of nicotinamide. Spina bifida is an imperfect closure of the spinal column and resulting protrusion of the meninges or spinal cord as well as anencephaly. It is caused by a deficiency of folate (folic acid). Pernicious anemia is a type of megaloblastic anemia that causes fatigue, blood pressure changes, rapid heart rate, pallor, depression, muscle weakness, and shortness of breath. It is caused by a deficiency of cobalamin (vitamin B_{12}).

6. Rickets is caused by a deficiency of calcitriol and is characterized by the malformation of skeletal tissue in growing children. Children with rickets have soft long bones that bend under their own weight.

7. Antioxidants are agents that prevent the cellular structure from being broken down by oxygen. Tocopherol (vitamin E) and ascorbic acid (vitamin C) are antioxidants.

Apply Your Knowledge 9.3

CRITICAL THINKING

1. A lack of iodine in the diet contributes to goiter, congenital hypothyroidism, and myxedema. Goiter is a swelling of the thyroid gland. Congenital hypothyroidism is a condition of extreme hypothyroidism characterized by physical deformity, dwarfism, and mental retardation. Myxedema is a life-threatening complication of hypothyroidism marked by coma, hypothermia, and respiratory depression.

2. Essential trace elements are also called microminerals. They are defined as those having a required intake of less than 100 mg per day. They include iron, iodine, fluoride, zinc, chromium, selenium, manganese, molybdenum, and copper.

3. The major minerals that exist in the highest quantities in the human body are:
   Calcium—bone formation, impulse conduction, myocardial and skeletal muscle contractions, and blood clotting

Phosphorus—bone formation, tooth formation, energy, fat storage, metabolism of other nutrients

Sodium—helps body fluid balance and acid-base balance; regulates nerve transmission and cell membrane irritability

Potassium—necessary for normal cardiac and muscle function

Magnesium—required to form proteins, stimulates muscle contraction and nerve transmission, activates enzymes, and aids in bone formation

Chlorine—is a component of gastric hydrochloric acid

4. Zinc is especially important during such growth periods as pregnancy, lactation, infancy, childhood, and adolescence. Fluoride prevents dental caries, strengthening the ability of teeth to withstand erosive effects of bacterial acids.

5. Iron deficiency is caused by inadequate supply or dietary iron, excessive blood loss, an inability to form hemoglobin because of a lack of various factors, such as vitamins, and a lack of gastric hydrochloric acid necessary to help liberate iron for absorption.

6. Sodium is the major electrolyte in the extracellular fluid. It helps body fluid balance and acid–base balance and regulates nerve transmission and cell membrane irritability. The primary source of sodium is table salt. Potassium is a major electrolyte of intracellular fluid. It is found in blood, nerve tissue, and muscle fibers. Potassium is necessary for normal cardiac and muscle function. The best sources of potassium are oranges, bananas, red meats, vegetables, yams, milk products, and coffee.

7. Wilson's disease is a genetic disorder that causes an excess storage of copper in the body. Without treatment, it can result in liver and nerve damage.

Apply Your Knowledge 9.4

CRITICAL THINKING

1. Cachexia is a specific profound syndrome caused by malnutrition and a disturbance in glucose and fat metabolism. It is usually seen in patients with terminal cancer or AIDS and in patients who are in generally poor health. It is indicated by an emaciated appearance.

2. Breast milk and commercially prepared formula contain the balance of nutrients that infants' bodies need during the first year of life. Cow's milk does not meet these standards.

3. Total parenteral nutrition (TPN) supplies all the patient's daily nutritional requirements. TPN is used in the hospital or at home, allowing patients who have lost small intestine function to lead useful lives.

4. For TPN, a peripheral vein may be used for short periods, but when concentrated solutions are used for prolonged periods, thrombosis can occur. Therefore, central venous access is usually required.

5. Pregnant women should be advised to gain about 25 to 35 pounds during pregnancy. The rate of weight gain should be 2 to 5 pounds in the first trimester and about 1 pound per week thereafter. Gaining too little weight contributes to the risk of having a small baby. Gaining too much weight may cause an early delivery or a very large baby as well as such health issues as gestational diabetes, high blood pressure, and varicose veins.

Apply Your Knowledge 9.5

CRITICAL THINKING

1. The benefits of food additives include reducing waste, providing a greater variety of attractive foods, and improving flavor.

2. Potassium depletion may occur because of the effects of drugs on mineral metabolism. These drugs include diuretics (especially thiazide diuretics), corticosteroids, and purgatives (agents that promote bowel movements).

3. Foods that contain the highest amounts of tyramine include aged cheeses, certain alcoholic beverages, pickled fish, concentrated yeast extracts, and broad-bean pods.

4. The concept of drug interaction is often extended to include situations in which food

or certain dietary items influence the activity of a drug. For example, drug interactions with foods, herbs, or other natural substances may alter the activity of a drug.

5. The adverse health effects of approved food additives in the long term have not been established. Reported health problems suspected to be caused by some food additives have been trivial and largely anecdotal. For example, nitrite is used in cured meats to inhibit the growth of *Clostridium botulinum* and to impart a desired flavor. However, evidence indicates that nitrite is converted in the body to nitrosamines, which are known carcinogens in animals.

Apply Your Knowledge 9.6

CRITICAL THINKING

1. Herbal supplements are mixtures of ingredients based on plant sources designed for the improvement of health or the treatment of certain conditions. They are considered by the Food and Drug Administration (FDA) to be food products, not drugs.

2. Herbal supplements are regulated by the Dietary Supplement Health and Education Act (DSHEA) and the Dietary Supplement and Nonprescription Drug Consumer Protection Act.

3. Specialty supplements include chondroitin, glucosamine, amino acids, flaxseed, and fish oils with omega fatty acids.

4. The Dietary Supplement and Nonprescription Drug Consumer Protection Act was passed because of a lack of standardization in the dietary supplement industry. Manufacturers must now include contact information on product labels, must alert the FDA if a consumer contacts them about adverse effects of their products, must keep records of these events for at least 6 years, and must provide accurate labeling assessing what their products consist of.

5. The seven top-selling herbal supplements in the United States are cranberry, soy, garlic, saw palmetto, ginkgo, echinacea, and milk thistle.

6. The growth of the herbal and dietary supplement industry in the United States has been prompted by increased efforts to achieve good health, the lack of belief in traditional medicines, costs and dangerous side effects of traditional medicines, and the general belief that these supplements are more natural and "pure."

Apply Your Knowledge 10.1

CRITICAL THINKING

1. Accidental poisonings occur far more often at home than through industrial exposure, and the effects are usually acute. They usually result from the ingestion of toxic substances, with the majority of occurrences involving children. In most instances, accidental poisonings should be preventable.

2. Pharmacists can play a key role in preventing accidental poisonings, especially those caused by drugs. They can educate consumers about potentially poisonous substances in the home as well as about the drugs they dispense.

3. Cyanide has an unmistakable odor that is similar to bitter almonds and causes a cherry-red discoloration of the skin. Other symptoms include rapid breathing, changes in behavior and consciousness, headache, dizziness, seizures, and more.

4. Influential factors of poisoning risks include age, location, access to poisons, containers used to hold potential poisons, and lack of supervision.

5. Poisons can be detected by certain clinical features, chemical analysis of body fluids, and simple or complex toxicologic tests.

6. The actual amount of people in the United States who are poisoned each year varies widely. However, a good website that tracks statistics is http://www.poison.org/stats. For example, in 2009, in the Washington, D.C., area alone, there were more than 42,000 reported exposures to poisons.

7. Child-resistant packaging uses safety caps to make containers hard to open by children. These caps have been tested and confirmed that the majority of young children are

unable to open them, but the majority of adults can open them easily.

8. In every poisoning case, identification of the toxic agent should be attempted. This is because specific antidotal therapy is obviously impossible without the poison being correctly identified.

Apply Your Knowledge 10.2

CRITICAL THINKING

1. Patients with acetaminophen poisoning should be treated with the induction of emesis or gastric lavage followed by the administration of activated charcoal. Treatment with acetylcysteine is most effective if started within 10 hours after ingestion.

2. Corrosive acids cause irritation, bleeding, severe pain, and severe burns. Profound shock often develops, which may be fatal. The toxic effects of alkalies are attributable to the irritation and the destruction of local tissues. They cause severe pain in the mouth, pharynx, chest, and abdomen. Vomiting of blood and diarrhea are common, and the esophagus or stomach may become perforated either immediately or after several days.

3. Treatment for carbon monoxide poisoning requires effective ventilation in the presence of high oxygen concentrations and the absence of carbon monoxide. If necessary, ventilation should be supported artificially. Pure oxygen should be administered. Patients with cerebral edema should be treated with diuretics and steroids.

4. Ethylene glycol is a solvent found in products ranging from antifreeze and deicing solutions to carpet and fabric cleaners. Intravenous or oral ethanol is used as an antidote for ethylene glycol poisoning.

5. Formalin is a 40% solution of formaldehyde. Poisoning may be diagnosed by the characteristic odor of formaldehyde. Cellular functions are depressed, and after ingestion, immediate, severe abdominal pain, nausea, vomiting, and diarrhea occur. This may be followed by collapse, coma, severe metabolic acidosis, and anuria. Death is usually caused by circulatory failure.

6. Lugol's solution is a strong iodine solution that contains 5% iodine and 10% potassium iodide.

7. Lead poisoning causes severe damage to the brain, nerves, red blood cells, and digestive system. Symptoms of acute poisoning include a metallic taste in the mouth, abdominal pain, vomiting, diarrhea, collapse, and coma. Large amounts affect the nervous system, causing headache, convulsions, and death.

8. Systemic poisoning from magnesium sulfate can cause paralysis, hypotension, hypothermia, coma, and respiratory failure.

9. Methods used to remove ingested substances include chelating agents, gastric lavage, activated charcoal, emesis, sodium bicarbonate and other chemical therapies, enzyme therapies, water, milk, bread, soup, cathartics, gastrotomy, hemodialysis, blood transfusions, oxygen, fluid replacement, and advanced life support.

10. The most common poisonings seen today involve nonprescription drugs, household products, solvents, pesticides, and poisonous plants.

11. Alcohol profoundly affects the central nervous system (CNS), causing impairment to memory, reasoning, and judgment. It also affects reaction time and motor coordination, vision, hearing and causes neuropathy, a specific form of dementia, psychotic symptoms, insomnia, depression, encephalopathy, and severe depletion of vitamins.

12. Methyl alcohol (wood alcohol or methanol) has caused permanent blindness by producing severe optic nerve and CNS toxicity.

13. Digoxin is a component of digitalis, which is used to treat heart failure. Signs of poisoning by digoxin include cardiac arrhythmias, tachycardia, nausea, vomiting, seizures, visual abnormalities, dizziness, altered serum potassium levels, and more. It may result in multiple-organ failure and recurrence of toxicity after treatment has ended.

14. Treatment for ingested bleach consists of dilution with water or milk.

Apply Your Knowledge 10.3

CRITICAL THINKING

1. Methanol poisoning is treated with ethanol, opiate overdose is treated with naloxone, and benzodiazepine overdose is treated with activated charcoal.
2. Nitrite is preferred to treat cyanide poisoning because its administration produces methemoglobin in the body.
3. Poison control centers are available 24 hours a day in the United States because poisonings can occur at any time. The network of poison control centers coordinate activities across the country to collect and standardize product toxicology data. This wealth of information may be accessed at any time when poisoning is suspected, and many lives have been saved by this process.

Apply Your Knowledge 11.1

CRITICAL THINKING

1. Substance abuse may affect every level of a person's life. It may cause failure to fulfill parenting, school, or work obligations; hazardous behavior (such as driving under the influence); and recurrent related legal problems, such as driving under the influence (DUI). It results in continuing social and interpersonal problems. If a person is addicted to a substance, health problems may also occur.
2. Polysubstance abuse is the use of two or more different substances of abuse.
3. Central nervous system depressants include barbiturates, nonbarbiturate sedative–hypnotics, benzodiazepines, opioids, alcohol, and antihistamines.
4. Benzodiazepines are usually used to treat anxiety but also for muscle relaxation and the prevention of seizures.
5. Opioids (narcotic analgesics) are used for severe pain, diarrhea, and persistent cough.

Apply Your Knowledge 11.2

CRITICAL THINKING

1. Marijuana is a natural substance that is the most commonly used illicit drug in the United States.
2. Repeated use of lysergic acid diethylamide (LSD) can lead to impaired memory and reasoning ability as well as psychoses. Flashbacks may occur in some users, wherein the drug's effects reoccur without further administration.
3. The most commonly used central nervous system stimulants include amphetamines, methylphenidate, cocaine, and caffeine.
4. Cocaine overdose may lead to convulsions, dysrhythmias, stroke, and death from respiratory arrest.
5. Withdrawal from caffeine produces fatigue, headaches, depression, and impaired physical and mental performance.

Apply Your Knowledge 11.3

CRITICAL THINKING

1. Risk factors for drug abuse include absent or problem parents, substance-abusing peers or parents, permissive parents, poor parental discipline, access to prescriptions, student absenteeism, aggressive behavior in adolescents, poor social skills, poor academic performance, transition periods in adolescent life, early drug use, and the method of drug administration.
2. For heroin addiction, methadone is often used because it does not produce the same degree of euphoria, has longer-lasting effects, and helps addicts to withdraw without unpleasant withdrawal symptoms.
3. Schools can receive grants for drug testing and the education of parents, students, and teachers through the Office of National Drug Policy (ONDCP). More than 4,000

schools across the United States use random student drug testing programs to provide early intervention for those students labeled "at risk."

Apply Your Knowledge 11.4

CRITICAL THINKING

1. The physical adverse effects of smoking are usually serious later in life and include cancer, emphysema, and heart attacks. Half of all Americans who continue to smoke will die from a smoking-related disease. Those who do not die from smoking-related illnesses experience pneumonia, being chronically short of breath, and sometimes having to be on a respirator for much of their lives. On average, smoking reduces life expectancy by 14 years.

2. Nicotine directly stimulates the central nervous system, accelerates the heart rate, increases blood pressure, and may result in muscular tremors in certain people. The adverse effects of nicotine are caused through carbon monoxide levels, its addictive properties, irritants in the tar found in tobacco, and through passive smoke inhalation.

3. Withdrawal from nicotine causes anxiety, cravings, impaired attention, insomnia, continual thoughts about smoking, gastrointestinal disturbances, and headaches. Nicotine has been proven to be a psychoactive substance.

4. Smoking cessation techniques include smoking cessation clinics, literature about quitting techniques, nicotine replacements, bupropion, varenicline, drug counseling, hypnotherapy, acupuncture, progressive filters, and employer-offered financial incentives.

5. The benefits of stopping cigarette smoking include better overall health, longer life expectancy, saving money, lower insurance premiums, reduced risk of cancer, reduced risk of heart disease, reduced risk of chronic lung disease, relief of lower back pain, better interpersonal relationships,

and slowed wrinkling and other signs of aging.

Apply Your Knowledge 11.5

CRITICAL THINKING

1. In small quantities, alcohol has been shown to reduce the risk of heart attack and stroke.

2. Acute overdoses of alcohol cause vomiting, severe hypotension, respiratory failure, coma, and possibly death. High rates of alcohol consumption produce increased depressant effects on the brain.

3. Alcohol should never be combined with other central nervous system depressants because the effects are cumulative, resulting in profound sedation or coma.

4. The liver is the most affected organ when chronic alcohol abuse occurs.

5. Acute alcohol withdrawal is treated with such benzodiazepines as Valium or Librium as well as antiseizure medications. Additional treatments include behavioral counseling, self-help groups, and a drug called *disulfiram*.

Apply Your Knowledge 12.1

CRITICAL THINKING

1. Infectious disease can be controlled by breaking the chain of transmission in one or more places. Destroying nonhuman reservoirs and vectors of the pathogen can also break the chain of transmission.

2. Weapons of mass destruction may be nuclear, chemical, or biological (such as anthrax or smallpox) in nature.

3. Transmission of disease requires a chain of events that must occur unbroken to allow one human to infect another. The pathogenic organism must live and reproduce in a reservoir. The reservoir may be a human

being, as with the influenza virus; an animal, as in bats with rabies; or soil, as in enterobiasis. The pathogen must have a portal of exit, with a mode of transmission from the reservoir to a susceptible victim.

4. Pathogens are disease-causing microorganisms. Four classes of pathogens are bacteria, viruses, fungi, and parasites.

5. Subtherapeutic doses are those that are below the level used to treat diseases.

Apply Your Knowledge 12.2

CRITICAL THINKING

1. *Bacteriostatic* is defined as capable of inhibiting microbial growth. *Bactericidal* is defined as capable of killing microbes.

2. The mechanism of action for sulfonamides is the blocking of a specific step in the biosynthetic pathway of folic acid. They are primarily bacteriostatic, meaning that they slow the multiplication of bacteria. Sulfonamides interfere with PABA and folic acid formation, thereby destroying the bacteria.

3. Gram-positive bacteria are those that have the ability to resist decolorization with alcohol after being treated with Gram's crystal violet stain, which imparts a violet color to the bacterium when viewed by microscope. Penicillins are used to treat gram-positive bacterial infections.

4. The four generations of cephalosporins are classified as:

First-generation—exhibit highest activity against gram-positive bacteria and lowest activity against gram-negative bacteria

Second-generation—are more active against gram-negative bacteria and less active against gram-positive bacteria than the first-generation cephalosporins

Third-generation—are considerably less active than first-generation agents against gram-positive bacteria, have a much expanded spectrum of activity against gram-negative organisms, and are more resistant to gram-negative beta-lactamases

Fourth-generation—have improved gram-positive spectrum and expanded gram-negative activity of third-generation cephalosporins

Apply Your Knowledge 12.3

CRITICAL THINKING

1. Aminoglycosides combine with bacterial (not human) ribosomes to arrest protein synthesis. This interference prevents cell reproduction, resulting in death of the bacteria.

2.
Generic name:	Trade name:
gentamicin	Garamycin
Generic name:	Trade name:
kanamycin	Kantrex
Generic name:	Trade name:
netilmicin	Netromycin
Generic name:	Trade name:
tobramycin	Nebcin

3. The mechanism of action for the macrolides is inhibition of bacterial protein synthesis by binding to the bacterial ribosome, which stops bacterial growth. Macrolides bind equally to ribosomes from gram-positive and gram-negative bacteria.

4.
Trade name:	Generic name:
Biaxin	clarithromycin
Trade name:	Generic name:
Ilosone	erythromycin estolate
Trade name:	Generic name:
Zithromax	azithromycin

5. Regarding oral macrolides, patients should be instructed to take them with a full glass of water on an empty stomach (1 hour before or 2 hours after meals) to get the maximum effect. Enteric-coated, sustained-release preparations can be administered with food and are often prescribed for patients with a gastrointestinal tolerance.

Apply Your Knowledge 12.4

CRITICAL THINKING

1. The fluoroquinolones exert their bactericidal effect by interfering with an enzyme (DNA gyrase) that is required by bacteria for the synthesis of DNA. This action inhibits cell reproduction, resulting in the death of the bacteria.

2. Fluoroquinolones should be avoided in children younger than 18 years and in pregnant or lactating women.

3. The tetracyclines are used in the treatment of Rocky Mountain spotted fever, typhus fever, chlamydial infections, cholera, brucellosis, tularemia, and amebiasis. They are also prescribed as an alternative to penicillin for gonorrhea, syphilis, Lyme disease, anthrax, and *Haemophilus influenzae*. Doxycycline is highly effective in the prophylaxis of "traveler's diarrhea."

4. Tetracyclines should be avoided in pregnant women and in children younger than age 8 years because they can cause permanent staining of developing teeth and can possibly affect the growth of teeth and bones.

5.
Generic name:	Trade name:
minocycline	Minocin
Generic name:	Trade name:
doxycycline	Vibramycin
Generic name:	Trade name:
chlortetracycline	Aureomycin

Apply Your Knowledge 12.5

CRITICAL THINKING

1. The drug of choice for typhoid fever is chloramphenicol.

2. Spectinomycin suppresses protein synthesis in gram-negative bacteria, especially *Neisseria gonorrhoeae*.

3. Vancomycin suppresses cell wall synthesis and is bactericidal.

4. Clindamycin is the drug of choice for the treatment of gastrointestinal infections caused by *Bacteroides fragilis*.

5. The most serious side effects of vancomycin are ototoxicity and nephrotoxicity.

Apply Your Knowledge 12.6

CRITICAL THINKING

1. *Mycobacterium tuberculosis* is an acid-fast aerobic bacillus that causes tuberculosis. The disease can affect any organ system, but the most common sites are the lungs and lymph nodes.

2. The first-line antituberculotics include ethambutol, isoniazid, rifampin, and pyrazinamide.

3. Isoniazid is the most potent and selective of the known tuberculostatic antibacterial agents. It is tuberculocidal to growing bacteria and the most effective agent in the therapy of tuberculosis.

4. The adverse effects of rifampin include fatigue, drowsiness, headache, confusion, dizziness, nausea, vomiting, heartburn, skin rashes, and renal insufficiency. It may also cause a reddish-orange discoloration of such body fluids as tears, urine, sweat, and saliva.

5. Pyrazinamide is used for the short-term therapy of advanced tuberculosis before surgery and to treat patients unresponsive to such primary agents as isoniazid and streptomycin.

Apply Your Knowledge 12.7

CRITICAL THINKING

1. Human immunodeficiency virus (HIV) results in acquired immunodeficiency syndrome (AIDS). Not all individuals infected with HIV develop AIDS, but they continue to be carriers of the virus.

2. Generic name: Trade name:
   acyclovir   Zoviraxl

   Generic name: Trade name:
   ganciclovir   Cytovene

   Generic name: Trade name:
   oseltamivir   Tamiflu

   Generic name: Trade names:
   zidovudine   AZT, Retravir

3. Amantadine is used to treat a wide variety of patients of all ages who have symptoms of influenza, but it may also be used to treat some patients with Parkinsonism.

4. Acyclovir interferes with DNA synthesis and inhibits viral multiplication.

5. The AIDS virus infects a group of helper T lymphocytes, which are called CD4 cells. This results in the patient becoming more susceptible to other infections, such as bacteria, fungi, protozoans, and other viruses. Most AIDS patients die from these secondary infections.

Apply Your Knowledge 13.1

CRITICAL THINKING

1. Fungi enter the body mainly via respiratory, mucous, and cutaneous routes. In general, the agents of primary mycoses have a respiratory portal (spores inhaled from the air). Subcutaneous agents enter through compromised skin, and cutaneous and superficial agents enter through contamination of the skin surface.

2. Molds are fungi that grow in the form of multicellular filaments called *hyphae*. Microscopic fungi that grow as single cells are called *yeasts*. Some yeasts can become multicellular through the formation of a string of connected budding cells known as *false hyphae* (*pseudohyphae*).

3. Mycoses are fungal infections. Most normal, healthy people are resistant to them and are infected only when faced with overwhelming numbers of fungi. In other cases, opportunistic pathogens may invade a person whose natural resistance is low because of other illnesses or even some medications.

4. A common opportunistic infection is candidiasis (also called *moniliasis* or *thrush*). Thrush can occur during the use of broad-spectrum antibiotics or by the alteration of the environmental conditions in the female reproductive system because of pregnancy or oral contraceptive use. It usually results from debilitation (immunosuppression, especially AIDS).

5. Antifungal agents are classified into three categories: drugs for systemic mycoses, oral drugs for mucocutaneous infections, and topical drugs for mucocutaneous infections.

6. Generic name: Trade name:
   amphotericin B   Amphocin

   Generic name: Trade name:
   fluconazole   Diflucan

   Generic name: Trade name:
   ketoconazole   Nizoral

   Generic name: Trade name:
   clotrimazole   Lotrimin

7. Amphotericin B, administered by the intravenous route, is extremely useful for therapy of systemic fungus diseases. It is also used by nasal spray in the prophylaxis of aspergillosis in immunocompromised patients and orally for the treatment of oral candidiasis.

8. Griseofulvin is fungistatic and not fungicidal. Its action involves deposition in newly formed skin and nail beds, where it binds to keratin, protecting these sites from new infection.

Apply Your Knowledge 13.2

CRITICAL THINKING

1. Malaria is caused by several species of the protozoan *Plasmodium*, of which *Plasmodium vivax* and *Plasmodium falciparum* are the most common. It is transmitted by the anopheles mosquito when the insect bites a human host.

2. Generic names of antimalarial drugs include chloroquine, doxycycline (tetracycline),

hydroxychloroquine, mefloquine, prima-quine, pyrimethamine, and quinine.

3. Primaquine is indicated for the cure of relapsing vivax malaria. It eliminates symptoms and the infection as well as prevents relapse.

4. Quinine is an agent that is destructive to gametes (germ cells) and acts rapidly against all *Plasmodium* malaria except *Plasmodium falciparum*. The actual mechanism of action for quinine is unknown.

5. Children who will be traveling to countries that require antimalarial vaccinations should be vaccinated 4 to 6 weeks before embarking to ensure full protection. Also, for antimalarial prescription drugs, infants' and children's dosages usually must be specially prepared; thus, adequate time also needs to be allowed for this. Guidelines must be followed exactly because overdosage can be fatal. For adults, anyone traveling to a country requiring antimalarial vaccinations should receive them.

Apply Your Knowledge 13.3

CRITICAL THINKING

1. *Entamoeba histolytica* and *Giardia lamblia* are two protozoal organisms frequently responsible for causing dysentery in humans. Infection caused by *E. histolytica* is also called *amebic dysentery* or *amebiasis* and is relatively rare in the United States. Amebic infections generally remain confined to the intestines, where they may give rise to dysentery, or they may locate elsewhere, especially in the liver. The most commonly reported intestinal protozoal infection in the United States is giardiasis caused by *G. lamblia*. Most patients are asymptomatic. However, these organisms cause a diarrhea that can be transient or persistent. Infection results from the ingestion of *G. lamblia* cysts, which may exist in water that is contaminated with fecal matter.

2. Generic matter: metronidazole — Trade name: Flagyl

   Generic matter: paromomycin — Trade name: Humatin

   Generic matter: Iodoquinol — Trade name: Yodoxin

3. Metronidazole should not be used in patients with diseases of the central nervous system. It is also advisable to withhold it during pregnancy.

4. Iodoquinol is an anti-infective, antiamebicide, and antiprotozoal agent.

5. Iodoquinol causes infrequent adverse effects, including diarrhea, nausea, vomiting, abdominal pain, anorexia, headache, rash, and pruritus. Other adverse effects may include blurred vision, optic atrophy, permanent loss of vision, and thyroid hypertrophy.

Apply Your Knowledge 14.1

CRITICAL THINKING

1. Natural killer cells make up 5% to 10% of circulating lymphocytes. They attack foreign cells, normal cells infected with viruses, and cancer cells that appear in normal tissues.

2. Humoral immunity is based on the antigen–antibody response. B cells, which are responsible for humoral immunity, produce circulating antibodies to act against an antigen.

3. Cell-mediated immunity depends on the functions of the T cells, which are responsible for a delayed type of immune response. The T lymphocyte becomes sensitized by the first contact with a specific antigen. T cells and macrophages work together in cell-mediated immunity to destroy the antigen. T cells attack the antigens directly rather than producing antibodies. Cell-mediated immunity may also occur without macrophages.

4. Antigens are specific chemical targets that antibodies react with. They are usually

pathogens, parts or products of pathogens, or other foreign compounds. Antibodies are special proteins manufactured by lymphocytes to fight invaders. Macrophages are immune cells derived from monocytes that work with T cells in cell-mediated immunity to destroy antigens.

5. Cytotoxic T cells directly attack foreign cells or body cells infected by viruses. These lymphocytes are the primary cells that provide cell-mediated immunity.

Apply Your Knowledge 14.2

CRITICAL THINKING

1. Inactivated vaccines are killed. Most bacterial vaccines contain killed bacteria or their components. Examples of inactivated vaccines include anthrax, cholera, *Haemophilus influenzae* type b, Lyme disease, meningococcal polysaccharide, pertussis, pneumococcal conjugate, and tetanus. Attenuated vaccines are live. One way to attenuate a virus is through laboratory manipulation, in which a bacterium is developed that lacks a toxin, an enzyme, or some other normal constituent that causes symptoms of disease. The bacterium's virulence is thereby lessened. Examples of attenuated vaccines include Bacillus Calmette-Guérin and typhoid vaccines.

2. Active immunity is a form of acquired immunity that develops in an individual in response to an immunogen (antigen). It may be naturally acquired by exposure to an infectious disease or artificially acquired by receiving active immunizing agents (vaccines). Passive immunity involves the transfer of the effectors of immunity (immunoglobulins or antibodies) from an immune individual to another. This occurs naturally by the active transport across the placental barrier of immunoglobulin G (IgG) antibodies from mother to fetus and to a lesser extent by the

transfer of IgA antibodies in the mother's milk to the nursing infant.

3. Immunity is the state or condition of being resistant to invading microorganisms.

4. Toxoids are types of vaccines in which protein toxins have been modified to reduce their hazardous properties without significantly altering their antigenic properties. Examples include diphtheria and tetanus toxoids.

5. Subcutaneous vaccines include anthrax, cholera, meningococcal polysaccharide, pneumococcal conjugate, and poliovirus vaccines.

Apply Your Knowledge 14.3

CRITICAL THINKING

1. Viral vaccines include hepatitis A, hepatitis B, influenza virus (types A and B), poliovirus, and rabies vaccines.

2. Bacterial vaccines include Bacillus Calmette-Guérin, typhoid, anthrax, cholera, *Haemophilus influenzae* type b, Lyme disease, meningococcal polysaccharide, pertussis, pneumococcal conjugate, and tetanus vaccines.

3. Toddlers should receive yearly flu (influenza) vaccines.

4. Hepatitis B vaccination should be given at birth because it protects babies from the virus, which can cause liver damage and death.

5. Varicella (chicken pox) is a highly communicable disease that is generally benign but that also causes herpes and sometimes may be accompanied by serious complications, such as encephalitis and bacterial superinfection. The varicella vaccine is called Varivax.

6. The best time for girls to receive the HPV vaccine is ages 10 to 11. Girls should receive three intramuscular injections over a 6-month period, with the second dose given 2 months after the first dose and the third dose given 6 months after the first dose.

Apply Your Knowledge 14.4

CRITICAL THINKING

1. Between the ages of 20 and 70 years, adults should receive a booster dose of diphtheria every 10 years.
2. Bacillus Calmette Guérin (BCG) vaccine is recommended only in extremely high-risk individuals in whom other controls are impractical.
3. The "cancer vaccine" for women is called human papillomavirus (HPV) vaccine.
4. Neonates born to mothers who are positive for hepatitis B should be immunized immediately with the vaccine and hepatitis B immunoglobulin.
5. German measles is also called *rubella*.

Apply Your Knowledge 14.5

CRITICAL THINKING

1. Immunoglobulins are divided into two types: one that should be administered intramuscularly and one that should be administered intravenously.
2. The dosage and site for injection of immunoglobulins vary according to the amount required and the size of the patient. Typically, the site is in the buttocks for adults and the leg or arm in children. This route is intramuscular, but they may also be administered intravenously.
3. The immunoglobulins are given to provide passive immunity to one or more infectious diseases.
4. Immunoglobulin intramuscular (IGIM) must not be injected intravenously because it can cause serious anaphylactic reactions.
5. The shingles vaccine is recommended more commonly after age 65 because the virus lies dormant in the dorsal root ganglia and is reactivated usually after this age.

Apply Your Knowledge 15.1

CRITICAL THINKING

1. Neurotransmitters are chemical substances with actions related to the transmission of pain. They are concentrated in various parts of the central nervous system and allow communication from nerve cell to nerve cell.
2. The process of inflammation includes vasodilation (resulting in redness and heat), vascular permeability (endothelial cells leak fluid), exudation (fluids, proteins, red blood cells, and white blood cells escape from intravascular spaces), and vascular stasis (slowing of blood with vasodilation and fluid exudation to allow the body to respond to the stimulus).
3. Prostaglandins are hormone-like substances that control blood pressure, contract smooth muscle, and modulate inflammation.
4. Endorphins and enkephalins are neurotransmitters that play a role in the transmission of pain impulses. They are capable of binding with opiate receptors in the central nervous system (CNS) and thereby inhibit the transmission of pain impulses, providing an analgesic effect. They are released when painful stimuli affect the body.
5. Analgesics relieve pain with or without antipyretic or anti-inflammatory action. Antipyretics reduce an elevated body temperature (fever) to normal levels. They may also possess anti-inflammatory properties.
6. Nonsteroidal anti-inflammatory drugs (NSAIDs) are used to relieve some symptoms caused by arthritis, such as inflammation, swelling, stiffness, and joint pain. They are also used to relieve other kinds of pain or painful conditions, such as menstrual cramps, gout attacks, bursitis, tendonitis, sprains, and muscle strains.
7. Reye's syndrome is defined as a potentially fatal disease that damages many organs, especially the brain and liver. It also causes hypoglycemia. It is associated with aspirin consumption by children who have a viral illness, such as chicken pox.

8. Aspirin's mechanism of action is unknown. It may produce analgesia and block pain impulses by inhibiting synthesis of prostaglandin in the CNS. It is thought to relieve fever by central action in the hypothalamic heat-regulating center.

9. Ibuprofen is used for rheumatoid arthritis, osteoarthritis, and arthritis. It is also indicated for mild to moderate pain, dysmenorrhea, and fever.

10. Indomethacin produces anti-inflammatory, analgesic, and antipyretic effects by inhibiting prostaglandin synthesis.

Apply Your Knowledge 15.2

CRITICAL THINKING

1. Cyclooxygenase-2 (COX-2) inhibitors affect the synthesis of prostaglandins by selectively targeting only the COX-2 enzyme, which is required to produce prostaglandins from arachidonic acid. COX-2 inhibitors have similar anti-inflammatory activity without the adverse gastrointestinal effects associated with COX-1 inhibition. The isoenzyme COX-2 is primarily associated with inflammation.

2. With COX-2 inhibitors, there is an increased risk of serious cardiovascular thrombotic events, even myocardial infarction and stroke, which can be fatal. This risk may increase with a longer duration of use. These inhibitors have been linked to cardiovascular problems, especially in elderly patients. Many believe that various COX-2 inhibitors should be used cautiously in patients with a history of heart disease.

3. COX-1 is available in all cells, especially in the platelets, gastrointestinal tract, and kidneys. It helps to maintain homeostasis in these cells. COX-2 appears to be made in macrophages in response to damage to local tissues.

4. Aspirin (acetylsalicylic acid) is the most commonly used salicylate drug, with analgesic, antipyretic, anti-inflammatory, and anticoagulant effects. It should not be used by any patient who has a condition involving bleeding. Acetaminophen, such as aspirin, has analgesic and antipyretic actions but is not anti-inflammatory. It should not be used by patients who consume three or more alcoholic drinks per day because it can cause acute liver damage or failure.

5. Over long-term use of acetaminophen, adverse effects include skin eruptions, urticaria, hypotension, and hepatotoxicity. Overdose can cause hepatotoxicity, coma, and internal bleeding.

Apply Your Knowledge 15.3

CRITICAL THINKING

1. *Opioid* is a general term referring to natural, synthetic, or endogenous morphine-related substances. Examples of opioids include oxycodone and methadone. Opiates are drugs derived from opium poppies and include morphine and codeine.

2. Examples of synthetic opioids include buprenorphine (Buprenex, Subutex), butorphanol (Stadol, Stadol NS), fentanyl (Duragesic, Sublimaze), meperidine (Demerol), methadone (Dolophine, Methadone), and pentazocine (Talwin, Talwin NX).

3. The three major types of opioid receptors are delta, kappa, and mu. Delta receptors have functions that include analgesia, antidepressant effects, and physical dependence. Kappa receptors have functions that include analgesia, sedation, miosis, inhibition of antidiuretic hormone release, and dysphoria. Mu receptors have functions that include analgesia, physical dependence, respiratory depression, miosis, euphoria, and reduced gastrointestinal motility.

4. Classes of opioid analgesics include natural opioid analgesics, semisynthetic opioid analgesics, synthetic opioid antagonists, and synthetic opioid agonist antagonists.

5. Major adverse effects of opioid analgesics include respiratory depression, cortical depression, tolerance, dependence, and addiction.

Apply Your Knowledge 15.4

CRITICAL THINKING

1. Synthetic opioid antagonists have little or no agonist actions. They are effective in the management of severe respiratory depression induced by opioid drugs and of respiratory distress in newborns caused by administration of these drugs to women during pregnancy. They are also used for the diagnosis or treatment of opioid addiction. Naloxone and naltrexone are examples of synthetic opioid antagonists.

2. Semisynthetic opioid analgesics include hydrocodone, hydrocodone with acetaminophen, levorphanol, oxycodone, oxycodone with acetaminophen, oxycodone with aspirin, and oxymorphone.

3. The most prominent actions for oxycodone affect the central nervous system (CNS) and organs composed of smooth muscle. It binds with specific receptors in various sites of the CNS to alter the perception of pain and the emotional response to pain. Its precise mechanism of action is not clear.

4. Naloxone may cause reversal of analgesia, tremors, slight drowsiness, hyperventilation, sweating, nausea, vomiting, hypertension, and tachycardia.

5. Generic name: naltrexone   Trade names: Trexan, ReVia

   Generic name: oxycodone   Trade name: OxyContin

   Generic name: hydrocodone   Trade name: Hycodan

   Generic name: naloxone   Trade name: Narcan

Apply Your Knowledge 15.5

CRITICAL THINKING

1. Buprenorphine is a centrally acting synthetic and narcotic analgesic. This opiate agonist–antagonist has agonist activity approximately 30 times that of morphine and antagonist activity equal to or up to three times greater than that of naloxone.

2. The principal mechanism of action for fentanyl is analgesia and sedation, but its action is more prompt and less prolonged than that of morphine or meperidine.

3. The most prominent actions for meperidine are on the central nervous system and on organs composed of smooth muscle. It acts principally to induce analgesia and sedation.

4. Large doses of pentazocine may increase blood pressure and heart rate.

5. Generic name: meperidine   Trade name: Demerol

   Generic name: pentazocine   Trade name: Talwin

   Generic name: methadone   Trade names: Dolophine

   Generic name: fentanyl   Trade names: Duragesic, Sublimaze

Apply Your Knowledge 16.1

CRITICAL THINKING

1. Oncogenes develop from normal genes, termed *protooncogenes*, which are present in all cells. They are essential regulators of normal cellular functions, including the cell cycle. Genetic alteration of the protooncogenes may activate the oncogenes, which, along with tumor suppressor genes, are involved in the development of cancer.

2. There are usually four steps in the cell cycle, after the resting (G_0) stage:

   G_1—the first gap phase, in which the cell starts making proteins to prepare for division

   S—DNA synthesis occurs, and the chromosomes containing the genetic code are copies so both of the new cells formed have the right amount of DNA

   G_2—the second gap phase; it occurs just before the cell starts splitting into two cells

M—mitosis, when one cell splits into two new calls

3. The warning signs of cancer in children include unexplained or persistent lumps or limping, unexplained normocytic anemia, unexplained thrombocytopenic bruising, unexplained weight loss, abdominal mass, and unexplained persistent headache or vomiting on awakening.

4. Carcinomas are malignant growths arising from epithelial cells. An adenocarcinoma is a malignant tumor arising from glandular origin. Malignant growths of muscle or connective tissue are called *sarcomas*.

5. DNA synthesis occurs in the S stage of the cell cycle.

6. Mitosis is when one cell splits into two new cells. It is the final stage of the cell cycle, and it lasts only 30 to 60 minutes.

Apply Your Knowledge 16.2

CRITICAL THINKING

1. The five primary methods used to treat cancer include surgery, radiation therapy, chemotherapy, immunotherapy, and hormonal therapy.

2. Intravenous administration is the most common method of administration for chemotherapy, but oral chemotherapy is becoming more popular than ever because of its ease of use.

3. Generic name: nitrogen mustard Trade names: Leukeran, Mustargen

Generic name:	Trade name:
melphalan	Alkeran

Generic name:	Trade name:
busulfan	Busulfex

Generic name:	Trade name:
bleomycin	Blenoxane

4. Depression of bone marrow is usually the most serious limiting toxicity of cancer chemotherapy.

5. The five major types of alkylating agents are nitrogen mustards, ethyleneimines, alkyl sulfonates, nitrosoureas, and temozolomide.

6. Examples of antimetabolites include purine antagonists (Mercaptopurine), adenosine antagonists (fludarabine), pyrimidines antagonists (fluorouracil), and folic acid antagonists (methotrexate).

7. Green tea contains high levels of polyphenols, which exhibit antioxidant and chemopreventive properties. Studies suggest that it may reduce the incidence of colon, pancreas, and stomach cancers.

8. The majority of antitumor antibiotics inhibit DNA and RNA synthesis, causing cell death.

Apply Your Knowledge 16.3

CRITICAL THINKING

1. Interferons are a group of blood proteins that have antiviral effects. They are naturally produced in response to viral infections or tumors and are also commercially produced by means of genetic engineering.

2. Interleukin-2 is a type of cytokine immune system signaling molecule, a hormone that is important in the body's response to microbial infection and in discriminating between "foreign" (non-self) and "self."

3. Tumor necrosis factor (TNF) actually describes a group of cytokines that can cause cell death. The "alpha" type is the most well known of the various TNFs.

4. Monoclonal antibodies are monospecific antibodies that are the same because they are made by identical immune cells that are all clones of a unique parent cell.

5. The advantage of monoclonal antibodies is that with almost any substance, they can be created to specifically bind to the substance, detecting or purifying it.

Apply Your Knowledge 17.1

CRITICAL THINKING

1. The four major portions of the brain are the cerebrum, diencephalon, brain stem, and cerebellum.

2. Degeneration of certain neurons within the basal ganglia is responsible for Parkinson's disease.

3. The two major functions of the brain are regulation of bodily function and self-preservation.

4. The exact mechanism of action for central nervous system (CNS) stimulants is not clear, but they stimulate the cerebral cortex and increase the activity of norepinephrine, dopamine, and other catecholamines at CNS synapses. This increased activity can lead to euphoria, reduced appetite, insomnia, wakefulness, etc.

5. A sedative (anxiolytic) diminishes the activity of the CNS, which usually relieves anxiety. *Hypnotic* is the term used to describe a substance that induces sleep. The difference between most hypnotics and anxiolytics is the dosage, not the drug.

6. With benzodiazepines, overdosage may result in CNS and respiratory depression as well as hypotension and coma.

7. Generic name: Trade name:
   oxazepam   Serax

   Generic name: Trade name:
   midazolam   Versed

   Generic name: Trade name:
   diazepam   Valium

   Generic name: Trade name:
   alprazolam   Xanax

8. Barbiturates, such as phenobarbital, are contraindicated in anyone with a familial history of porphyria and in cases of severe respiratory or kidney disease. They should be avoided in patients with a history of previous addiction to sedative–hypnotics or uncontrolled pain and in women who are pregnant or lactating.

Apply Your Knowledge 17.2

CRITICAL THINKING

1. Seizures may be classified as: generalized tonic–clonic seizures, generalized absence seizures, generalized myoclonic seizures, and partial seizures. Status epilepticus is an emergency condition that may result in brain injury or death if not treated immediately.

2. Epilepsy is a permanent, recurrent seizure disorder. Examples of the known causes of epilepsy include brain injury at birth, head injuries, and inborn errors of metabolism. In some patients, the cause of epilepsy is never determined.

3. The most common prescribed antiseizure drugs include the hydantoins, benzodiazepines, barbiturates, and miscellaneous antiseizure drugs.

4. Generic name: Trade name:
   ethosuximide   Zarontin

   Generic name: Trade name:
   phenytoin   Dilantin

   Generic name: Trade name:
   valproic acid   Depakene

   Generic name: Trade name:
   carbamazepine   Tegretol

5. Phenytoin is approved by the Food and Drug Administration (FDA) for partial seizures with complex symptomatology and tonic–clonic seizures, psychomotor, and nonepileptic seizures, such as those caused by head trauma. It is also used to prevent or treat seizures occurring during or after neurosurgery. Phenytoin is prescribed as an antiarrhythmic agent, especially in the treatment of digitalis-induced arrhythmias.

6. Valproic acid is used alone or with other anticonvulsants in the management of absence and mixed seizures and mania and in migraine headache prophylaxis. It is the drug of choice for symptomatic and idiopathic generalized seizures, juvenile myoclonic epilepsy, and childhood absence seizures.

7. Ethosuximide is the drug of choice for the control of uncomplicated absence seizures.

8. For carbamazepine, FDA-approved uses are for partial seizures, tonic–clonic seizures, and trigeminal neuralgia. However, it is often used for many other disorders, such as depression and bipolar disorder.

Apply Your Knowledge 17.3

CRITICAL THINKING

1. The major signs and symptoms of Parkinson's disease include tremors of the extremities and head, great difficulty in the coordination of fine muscle movement, and hypokinesia (an inability or slowness in initiating movements).

2. A central nervous system defect that leads to the illness exists in the basal ganglia portion of the midbrain known as the *substantia nigra*. This part of the brain is important in the initiation and control of muscular movement.

3. In the pathways of the substantia nigra, there is a balance between dopamine and acetylcholine in normal individuals. In patients with Parkinson's disease, a lack of dopaminergic activity leads to an imbalance between these neurotransmitters.

4. *Parkinsonism* is a term that refers to the symptoms produced by certain drugs, poisons, and traumatic lesions in the basal ganglia. When the cause is known, the disease is termed *secondary parkinsonism* as opposed to *primary parkinsonism*. Secondary parkinsonism is sometimes only temporary if the symptoms are caused by drugs.

5. Dopaminergic agents, such as levodopa, are metabolic precursors of dopamine, a catecholamine neurotransmitter. Unlike dopamine, levodopa readily crosses the blood–brain barrier. Its precise mechanism of action is unknown.

6. Dopaminergic agents should never be stopped abruptly because of a possible rebound of parkinsonism.

7. Anticholinergic agents work by inhibiting the muscarine receptors in the basal ganglia, lessening the imbalance between the extrapyramidal and pyramidal pathways by blocking the effect of acetylcholine.

8.
Generic name:	Trade name:
benztropine	Cogentin
Generic name: procyclidine	Trade name: Kemadrin
Generic name: levodopa	Trade names: Larodopa, L-Dopa
Generic name: amantadine	Trade name: Symmetrel
Generic name: bromocriptine	Trade name: Parlodel

Apply Your Knowledge 17.4

CRITICAL THINKING

1. Manifestations of schizophrenia include either positive or negative symptoms. Positive symptoms tend to be exaggerations of normal functioning. For example, a distortion of perceptions may manifest as hallucinations and as distortions of thought processes, which may manifest as delusions. Negative symptoms include terseness in speech, social withdrawal, anhedonia, and apathy.

2. The atypical antipsychotic agents are effective against the positive and the negative symptoms of schizophrenia.

3. The atypical agents are more expensive than the typical drugs but offer increased efficacy and higher rate of compliance with better outcomes. The atypical agents result in fewer hospital admissions and other emergency interventions.

4. Lithium is used in the control and prophylaxis of acute mania and the acute manic phase of mixed bipolar disorder.

5. Lithium should be avoided in pregnant women or patients with thyroid disorders.

6. Generic name: Trade name:
   haloperidol Haldol

   Generic name: Trade names:
   lithium Eskalith, Lithobid

   Generic name: Trade name:
   mesoridazine Serentil

   Generic name: Trade name:
   olanzapine Zyprexa

   Generic name: Trade name:
   clozapine Clozaril

Apply Your Knowledge 17.5

CRITICAL THINKING

1. Endogenous depression is caused by a chemical disorder in the brain. The majority of antidepressant medications are used chiefly in the management of endogenous depression.

2. Antidepressants are classified into several groups on the basis of their chemical structures and antidepressant action in the brain and include tricyclic antidepressants, monoamine oxidase inhibitors, and selective serotonin reuptake inhibitors.

3. The selective serotonin reuptake inhibitors (SSRIs) are relatively newer antidepressants—now considered the first-line drugs in the treatment of major depression.

4. The tricyclic antidepressants were the drugs of first choice before the development of SSRIs.

5. Generic name: Trade name:
   clomipramine Anafranil

   Generic name: Trade name:
   doxepin Sinequan

   Generic name: Trade name:
   phenelzine Nardil

   Generic name: Trade name:
   citalopram Celexa

   Generic name: Trade name:
   paroxetine Paxil

Apply Your Knowledge 18.1

CRITICAL THINKING

1. The two major systems controlling bodily functions are the nervous system and the endocrine system. They work closely with each other to control all of the body's functions.

2. The nervous system is divided into two main parts: the central nervous system, which comprises the brain and spinal cord, and the peripheral nervous system, which is the remainder of the nervous system.

3. The two primary neurotransmitters in the autonomic nervous system are acetylcholine and norepinephrine.

4. Neurons that release norepinephrine, epinephrine, or dopamine are termed *adrenergic*. Neurons that release acetylcholine are termed *cholinergic*.

5. Parasympathetic postganglionic neurons release acetylcholine. Sympathetic postganglionic neurons mostly release norepinephrine, although a few types release acetylcholine.

Apply Your Knowledge 18.2

CRITICAL THINKING

1. The fight-or-flight response is the reaction in the body when faced by a sudden threat or source of stress. It has been used to describe activation of the sympathetic nervous system during emergencies.

2. Norepinephrine and epinephrine are endogenous catecholamines, which are chemical compounds containing nitrogen that is derived from the amino acid tyrosine. The bind to adrenergic receptors and produce sympathetic effects.

3. The two main adrenergic receptors are alpha and beta. The alpha-adrenergic receptors are

divided into α_1 and α_2, and the beta-adrenergic receptors are divided into β_1 and β_2.

4. At times of "rest and digest," the parasympathetic nervous system dominates the sympathetic nervous system. Activation increases salivation, lacrimation, urination, digestion, and defecation.

5. The sympathetic nervous system causes the pupils to dilate, the heart rate and cardiac output to increase, and the dilation of the bronchial smooth muscle.

6. The effects of the parasympathetic nervous system include the contraction of the bladder wall, the erection of the penis, and bronchoconstriction. It has no effect on the uteruses of pregnant women.

7. Cholinergic receptors respond to cholinergic stimulation. Agents that bind to them also prevent acetylcholine from acting on them, which is known as *antagonism*.

8. The parasympathetic nervous system is also known as the *cholinergic nervous system*.

Apply Your Knowledge 18.3

CRITICAL THINKING

1. Alpha$_1$-receptor agonists cause vasoconstriction of blood vessels, dilation of pupils, decreased gastrointestinal motility, contraction of the external sphincter of the bladder, decreased bile secretion, and stimulation of sweat glands.

2. Beta$_1$-receptor agonists are used to treat circulatory shock, hypotension, and cardiac arrest.

3. Beta$_2$-receptor agonists are contraindicated in pediatric, pregnant, and lactating patients; in those sensitive to other sympathomimetic agents; and in patients with cardiac arrhythmias associated with tachycardia or digitalis intoxication, hyperthyroidism, preeclampsia, eclampsia, intrauterine infection, hypertension, diabetes mellitus, hypovolemia, thyrotoxicosis, asthma treated with beta-mimetics, hypersensitivity, coronary artery disease within 14 days of MAO inhibitor therapy, and angle-closure glaucoma.

4. Beta-receptor antagonists cause beta-blockade, resulting in vasodilation, decreased peripheral resistance, and orthostatic hypotension.

5.

Generic name:	Trade name:
propranolol	Inderal
Generic name: prazosin	Trade name: Minipress
Generic name: atenolol	Trade name: Tenormin
Generic name: metaproterenol	Trade name: Alupent
Generic name: dopamine	Trade name: Intropin

6. Cholinergic blockers inhibit the actions for acetylcholine by occupying the acetylcholine receptors.

7. The two types of cholinergic receptors are nicotinic and muscarinic. The nicotinic receptors affect skeletal muscles, and the muscarinic receptors innervate smooth muscle and slow the heart rate.

8.

Generic name:	Trade names:
bethanechol	Duvoid, Urabeth
Generic name: pilocarpine	Trade name: Pilocar
Generic name: nadolol	Trade name: Corgard
Generic name: metoprolol	Trade name: Lopressor
Generic name: terbutaline	Trade name: Brethine

Apply Your Knowledge 19.1

CRITICAL THINKING

1. General anesthetics are normally used to produce loss of consciousness before and during surgery. However, for certain minor procedures, an anesthetic may be given in small amounts to relieve anxiety or pain without causing unconsciousness. These are called *local anesthetics*. They numb small areas of tissue where a minor procedure is

to be done and are commonly used in dentistry and for minor surgery. Regional anesthesia affects a larger part of the body and is often used in obstetrics (labor and delivery). It does not make the person unconscious. Spinal and epidural anesthesia are examples of regional anesthesia.

2. The characteristics of anesthetic agents include rapid and pleasant induction and withdrawal from anesthesia, skeletal muscle relaxation, analgesia, high potency, a wide therapeutic index, nonflammability, and chemical inertness with regard to anesthetic delivery devices.

3. The four stages of anesthesia are analgesia, excitement (delirium), surgical anesthesia, and medullary paralysis. Two of the stages are dangerous. Sudden death can occur during stage 2, possibly because of vagal nerve inhibition. Stage 4 begins with respiratory failure and can lead to circulatory collapse. If it is reached, it is called an *anesthetic accident*.

4. Preanesthetics help to achieve sedation, reduced anxiety and amnesia, increased comfort, reduced gastric acidity and volume, increased gastric emptying, decreased nausea and vomiting, and reduced inspiration of aspiration by drying oral and respiratory secretions.

5. A combination of preoperative drugs may be ordered to achieve the desired outcomes with minimal side effects.

Apply Your Knowledge 19.2

CRITICAL THINKING

1. Balanced anesthesia is a technique of general anesthesia based on the concept that the administration of small amounts of several neuronal depressants increases the advantages but not the disadvantages of the individual components of the mixture.

2. Inhaled anesthetics include desflurane (Suprane), enflurane (Ethrane), halothane (Fluothane, Somnothane), isoflurane (Forane), methoxyflurane (Penthrane),

nitrous oxide (Entonox), and sevoflurane (Ultane).

3.
Generic name:	Trade name:
propofol	Diprivan
Generic name:	Trade name:
midazolam	Versed
Generic name:	Trade name:
ketamine	Ketalar
Generic name:	Trade name:
fentanyl	Sublimaze

4. A patient should stop taking herbal medications at least 2 to 3 weeks before surgery to decrease the risk of adverse effects.

5. Volatile liquids are those that are easily vaporized.

6. The anesthetic technique varies depending on the proposed type of diagnostic, therapeutic, or surgical intervention.

7. Desflurane (Suprane) and sevoflurane (Ultane) are the most widely used volatile anesthetics. They are often combined with nitrous oxide (Entonox).

8. Intravenous anesthetics are preferred because they are faster, less painful, and more reliable than intramuscular or subcutaneous injections.

Apply Your Knowledge 19.3

CRITICAL THINKING

1. The main groups of local anesthetics are the esters and amides.

2. The most common uses of local anesthetics include incision and drainage of abscesses, laceration repair, biopsy, wart treatment, vasectomy, neonatal circumcision, dental procedures, during labor and delivery, and for diagnostic procedures, such as gastrointestinal endoscopy.

3. It is important to keep track of the total amount of anesthetics being administered because they can lead to an abnormal heartbeat.

4. Ester-type local anesthetics have been in use longer than amides.

5. Generic name: Trade name:
procaine   Novocain

Generic name: Trade names:
tetracaine   Pontocaine, Dicaine

Generic name: Trade names:
bupivacaine   Marcaine, Sensorcaine

Generic name: Trade name:
lidocaine   Xylocaine

Generic name: Trade name:
ropivacaine   Naropin

Apply Your Knowledge 19.4

CRITICAL THINKING

1. Cryoanesthesia involves the reduction of nerve conduction by localized cooling. This may be accomplished with ice or by the use of a cryoanesthesia machine.

2. Field block anesthesia affects a single nerve, a deep plexus, or a network of nerves. It is a form of regional anesthesia.

3. During spinal anesthesia, an anesthetic agent is injected into the subarachnoid space through a spinal needle. It is most often used for gynecologic, obstetric, orthopedic, and genitourinary surgery.

4. Local infiltration anesthesia, which works by blocking nerves, is produced by the injection of a local anesthetic solution directly into an area that is painful or about to be operated upon. It is the simplest form of regional anesthesia.

5. Epidural anesthesia involves the injection of a local anesthetic into the epidural space via a catheter that allows repeated infusions. The anesthetic agent is very slowly absorbed into the cerebrospinal fluid. This is popular for labor and delivery.

Apply Your Knowledge 20.1

CRITICAL THINKING

1. The skin forms a barrier between our environment and ourselves. It is fundamental to the functioning of all other organs and vital in maintaining homeostasis. The skin helps to regulate body temperature, retards water loss from deeper tissues, houses sensory receptors, synthesizes various biochemicals, and excretes small quantities of wastes.

2. The outermost layer of the epidermis is the stratum corneum (horny layer). The deepest layer is the stratum basale or stratum germinativum.

3. The mainstay of treatment of acute or chronic inflammatory disorders is topical or oral corticosteroids.

4. Eczema is often considered synonymous with dermatitis (inflammation of the skin).

5. Generic name: Trade name:
amcinonide   Cyclocort

Generic name: Trade name:
fluocinonide   Lidex

Generic name: Trade name:
flurandrenolide   Cordran

Apply Your Knowledge 20.2

CRITICAL THINKING

1. Acne (vulgaris) is an inflammatory disorder of the sebaceous glands that commonly occurs during puberty. The incidence of acne tends to decline with age and is unusual in adults. It is defined as the overproduction of sebum, which blocks the ducts of glands, with bacteria becoming trapped beneath the sebum plug, forming a small abscess. Psoriasis is a chronic, relapsing inflammatory skin disorder that occurs at any age. It is marked by thickening of the dermis and epidermis, characterized by rounded plaques, covered by silvery white, scaly patches. The skin lesions are variably pruritic.

2. Actinic keratosis occurs on skin (especially fair skin) exposed to ultraviolet radiation. The lesion appears as a pigmented, scaly patch, which may develop into skin cancer.

3. Corns and calluses are localized hyperplastic areas of the stratum corneum layer of the epidermis.

4. Generic name: clindamycin	Trade name: Cleocin
Generic name: azelaic acid	Trade name: Azelex
Generic name: tretinoin	Trade name: Retin-A
Generic name: adapalene	Trade name: Differin

5. Generic name: masoprocol	Trade name: Actinex
Generic name: diclofenac sodium	Trade names: Solaraze
Generic name: salicylic acid with podophyllum	Trade names: Podocon-25, Podofin

6. Generic name: amphotericin B	Trade name: Fungizone
Generic name: haloprogin	Trade name: Halotex
Generic name: oxiconazole	Trade name: Oxistat
Generic name: nystatin	Trade names: Mycostatin, Nystex

Apply Your Knowledge 20.3

CRITICAL THINKING

1. The most common bacterial infections of the skin are caused by staphylococci and beta-hemolytic streptococci. They include impetigo, cellulitis, and folliculitis.

2. Impetigo is a common superficial bacterial infection of skin caused by either *Streptococcus spp.* or *Staphylococcus aureus*. The primary lesion is a superficial pustule that ruptures and forms a characteristic yellow-brown crust.

3. Candidiasis is a fungal infection caused by a related group of yeasts, mostly *Candida albicans*. This organism is a normal flora of the gastrointestinal tract, but it may overgrow and cause disease at a number of skin sites. Other predisposing factors include diabetes mellitus, oral contraceptive use, and cellular immune deficiency. It is a very common infection in HIV-infected individuals.

4. Pediculosis is a lice infestation, primarily affecting hairy areas of the body.

5. Scabicides are pharmacologic drugs that kill mites.

Apply Your Knowledge 21.1

CRITICAL THINKING

1. The cardiovascular system circulates blood throughout the body to provide it with oxygen and nutrients and to remove carbon dioxide and wastes. It also carries hormones from one part of the body to another. The blood is propelled by continuous rhythmic contractions of the heart. Blood circulates through three types of vessels: arteries, veins, and capillaries.

2. The layers of the heart are the endocardium (inside), myocardium (middle), and epicardium (outside).

3. The electrical conduction system of the heart consists of the sinoatrial (SA) node, which initiates the heart's rhythmic contractions; the atrioventricular (AV) node, which provides the only normal conduction pathway between the atrial and ventricular syncytial, with its fibers delaying impulse transmission; the bundle of His, which is bundle branches that allow electrical impulses to travel and cause the left and right ventricles to contract at the same time; and the Purkinje fibers, which branch off to become continuous with cardiac muscle fibers.

4. The four valves of the heart are the tricuspid, pulmonary, mitral, and aortic valves. The tricuspid valve is between the right atrium and right ventricle. The pulmonary valve is between the right ventricle and pulmonary artery. The mitral valve is between the left

atrium and left ventricle. The aortic valve is between the left ventricle and the aorta.

5. The pulmonary circulation carries oxygen-depleted blood away from the heart to the lungs. It also returns oxygenated blood back to the heart. The systemic circulation carries oxygenated blood away from the heart to the body and returns deoxygenated blood back to the heart.

Apply Your Knowledge 21.2

CRITICAL THINKING

1. The most common types of angina include classical (stable) angina, which often occurs during exertion, emotional stress, or indigestion; variant (vasospastic) angina, which usually occurs at rest; and unstable angina, which occurs at rest initially and often signifies a future myocardial infarction.

2. The three classes of antianginal drugs are organic nitrates, beta-adrenergic blockers (beta-blockers), and calcium channel blockers.

3. Nitroglycerin directly affects the vascular smooth muscle to dilate blood vessels.

4. The advantage of isosorbide mononitrate over isosorbide dinitrate is that there is no first-pass metabolism.

5. The organic nitrates used in the prophylaxis of angina pectoris include nitroglycerin, isosorbide mononitrate, erythrityl tetranitrate, and penterythritol tetranitrate.

6. The most common adverse effects of nitroglycerin include headache, hypotension, and tachycardia. The dizziness and lightheadedness of hypotension are better tolerated with time.

7. The trade names of nitroglycerin include Minitran, Nitrek, Nitro-Bid, Nitro-Dur, Nitro-Time, Nitroglycerin, Nitroglycerin in 5% Dextrose, Nitrolingual, and Nitrostat.

8. Unstable angina occurs at rest initially and then decreases in response to rest or nitroglycerin.

Apply Your Knowledge 21.3

CRITICAL THINKING

1. The insufficient supply of myocardium is the result of either a decreased flow of oxygen-rich blood to the heart muscle or an increased demand for oxygen by the myocardium that exceeds what the circulation can supply. Coronary artery disease, clot formation in the coronary artery or spasm of these arteries, stress, heavy exertion, and an abrupt increase in blood pressure are the main causes of acute myocardial infarction.

2. Acute myocardial infarction (AMI) is rare in childhood because for most patients, the disease is acquired from the lifelong deposition of atheroma and plaque, which causes coronary artery spasm and thrombosis.

3. The goal of treatment for AMI is to limit damage to the myocardium, thereby preserving enough myocardial function to sustain life.

4. In addition to intravenous fluids, pharmacotherapeutics are used as the first line of treatment for AMI. The mainstays of treatment include nitroglycerin, aspirin, thrombolytic drugs, morphine sulfate, beta-blockers, calcium channel blockers, and oxygen.

5. Bradycardia is defined as an abnormally slow heartbeat.

6. Potential side effects of morphine are the depression of respiration and the reduction of myocardial contractility. Hypotension and bradycardia secondary to morphine can usually be overcome by prompt elevation of the lower extremities.

Apply Your Knowledge 21.4

CRITICAL THINKING

1. Dysrhythmias can occur from heart disease or from chronic drug therapy. They can also be caused by drugs used to regulate dysrhythmia because they create an alteration of the heart's electrical impulse.

2. Antidysrhythmic drug therapy is the mainstay of management for most important dysrhythmias. There is no universally effective drug. Antidysrhythmic drugs include sodium channel blockers, beta-adrenergic blockers, potassium channel blockers, and calcium channel blockers.

3.

Generic name:	Trade names:
procainamide	Pronestyl, Procan-SR
Generic name:	Trade name:
phenytoin	Dilantin
Generic name:	Trade name:
moricizine	Ethmozine
Generic name:	Trade name:
esmolol	Brevibloc
Generic name:	Trade names:
amiodarone	Cordarone, Pacerone
Generic name:	Trade names:
diltiazem	Cardizem, Dilacor

4. Class I antidysrhythmic drugs bind to sodium channels. They are known as *sodium channel blockers.*

5. Examples of class Ia drugs are quinidine, procainamide, and disopyramide.

6. Class II antidysrhythmic drugs (beta-adrenergic blockers) may be the least toxic and most powerful drugs available. However, their antidysrhythmic effects are often overlooked.

7. Amiodarone is a powerful Class III antidysrhythmic.

8. The first calcium channel blocker approved by the FDA was verapamil.

LABELING

1. Generic name: morphine sulfate controlled-release

2. Drug class: analgesic; narcotic (opiate) agonist

3. Form of drug: tablet

4. Drug schedule: Schedule II

5. Adult dosage: controlled (sustained) release: 15 to 30 mg q812h

6. Typical use: symptomatic relief of severe acute and chronic pain after nonnarcotic analgesics have failed and as preanesthetic medication; also used to relieve dyspnea of acute left ventricular failure and pulmonary edema and pain of myocardial infarction

7. Body system that this drug targets: nervous system

8. Manufacturer: Purdue Pharma L.P.

9. Storage requirements: Store at 25°C (77°F); excursions permitted between 15° and 30°C (59°–86°F)

10. Pregnancy category: C (Pregnancy Category D in long-term use, high dose, or close to term

Apply Your Knowledge 22.1

CRITICAL THINKING

1. Prehypertension is classified as blood pressure of 120/80 mm Hg to 140/90 mm Hg; normal blood pressure is 119/79 mm Hg or less.

2. Uncontrolled hypertension can damage small blood vessels, causing the narrowing of the arteries, which can result in kidney failure, strokes, and cardiac arrest.

3. Lipoproteins are macromolecular complexes made up of the major plasma lipids (cholesterol and triglycerides) that are bound to proteins. These help to form the fatty material (plaque) that builds up in the lining of blood vessels and can cause angina, stroke, and myocardial infarction.

4. Lifestyle changes, such as the reduction of body weight; decreased intake of dietary total fat, cholesterol, saturated fatty acids, and salt; smoking cessation; increased exercise; and stress management can be effective for minor hypertension and hyperlipidemias. Pharmacologic methods combined with healthy lifestyle habits are usually necessary to treat chronic hypertension and serious hyperlipidemias.

5. The three main factors affecting blood pressure are cardiac output, peripheral resistance, and blood volume.

6. The walls of arteries contain three distinct layers: the tunica interna (innermost), tunica

media (middle), and tunia externa (outermost).

7. Hypertensive crisis is defined as severely elevated blood pressure, which may be fatal.

8. Primary (essential) hypertension accounts for 90% of the cases of hypertension in the United States.

Apply Your Knowledge 22.2

CRITICAL THINKING

1. Diuretics reduce circulating blood volume by blocking the reabsorption of sodium and chloride, which results in more water being retained in the kidney and the excretion of excess fluid.

2. Beta-adrenergic blockers competitively antagonize the responses to catecholamines that are mediated by beta-receptors. Alpha- and beta-blockers are indicated for severe hypertension. Their actions contribute to the blood pressure-lowering effect.

3. | Generic name: nadolol | Trade name: Corgard |
   |---|---|
   | Generic name: bisoprolol | Trade name: Zebeta |
   | Generic name: clonidine | Trade name: Catapres |
   | Generic name: methyldopa | Trade name: Aldomet |
   | Generic name: doxazosin | Trade name: Cardura |

4. The 10 most commonly prescribed angiotensin-converting enzyme (ACE) inhibitors for hypertension are benazepril, captopril, enalapril, fosinopril, lisinopril, moexipril, perindopril, quinapril, ramipril, and trandolapril.

5. Diuretics are classified as thiazide diuretics, thiazide-like diuretics, loop diuretics, and potassium-sparing diuretics.

6. Centrally acting adrenergic blockers are able to reduce the hyperactivity in the medulla oblongata of the brain. Sympathetic outflow from the medulla is diminished, and as a result, either systemic vascular resistance or cardiac output is decreased.

7. Peripherally acting adrenergic blockers are used for severe hypertension or as adjunctive therapy with other antihypertensive agents in the more severe form of hypertension.

8. Angiotensin-converting enzyme inhibitors may cause loss of taste, photosensitivity, severe hypotension, hyperkalemia, renal impairment, blood dyscrasias, dizziness, and angioedema.

9. Angiotensin II receptor blockers have beneficial effects on patients with congestive heart failure.

Apply Your Knowledge 22.3

CRITICAL THINKING

1. The term *congestive heart failure* (CHF) is used to describe the heart pumping at an insufficient rate, causing the kidneys to retain salt and water and fluid to accumulate in interstitial spaces.

2. CHF occurs when the heart pumps less blood than it receives, which results in blood accumulating in the heart chambers and the stretching of the heart walls. The underlying causes of CHF include arteriosclerotic heart disease, hypertensive heart disease, valvular heart disease, dilated cardiomyopathy, and congenital heart disease.

3. Inotropic drugs, such as cardiac glycosides, work by increasing the force and velocity of myocardial systolic contraction and decreasing conduction velocity through the atrioventricular node. They inhibit the enzyme ATPase, which is associated with the sodium pump, and the exchange between sodium and calcium is impaired.

4. Digoxin (Lanoxin) is the most commonly prescribed digitalis preparation for treating CHF.

5. Generic name: Trade name:
   inamrinone   Inocor

   Generic name: Trade name:
   milrinone   Primacor

   Generic name: Trade name:
   digoxin   Lanoxin

   Generic name: Trade name:
   digitoxin   Crystodigin

Apply Your Knowledge 22.4

CRITICAL THINKING

1. Bile acid sequestrants bind with bile salts in the intestinal tract to form an insoluble complex that is excreted in the feces, thus reducing circulating cholesterol and increasing serum low-density lipoprotein (LDL) removal rates.

2. The HmG-CoA reductase inhibitors (statins) are the most widely used drugs for lowering hyperlipidemia.

3. Generic name: Trade name:
   colestipol   Colestid

   Generic name: Trade name:
   clofibrate   Atromid-S

   Generic name: Trade name:
   dextrothyroxine   Choloxin

   Generic name: Trade name:
   gemfibrozil   Lopid

4. The seven generic and trade names of the HMG-CoA reductase inhibitors are:

   Generic name: Trade name:
   atorvastatin   Lipitor

   Generic name: Trade name:
   fluvastatin   Lescol

   Generic name: Trade names:
   lovastatin   Altoprev, Mevacor

   Generic name: Trade name:
   pravastatin   Pravachol

   Generic name: Trade name:
   rosuvastatin   Crestor

   Generic name: Trade name:
   simvastatin   Zocor

   Generic name: Trade name:
   simvastatin/ezetimibe Vytorin

5. Nicotinic acid (or niacin) appears to reduce the levels the very low-density lipoprotein (VLDL), LDL, and total cholesterol. It causes a decrease in liver triacylglycerol synthesis, which is required for VLDL production.

6. Gemfibrozil and clofibrate are derivatives of fibric acid that lower triglycerides and VLDL and increase high-density lipoprotein (HDL).

Apply Your Knowledge 23.1

CRITICAL THINKING

1. The three events of hemostasis are vascular spasms, formation of a platelet plug, and blood clotting.

2. Serotonin is a neurotransmitter released by platelets that causes the injured blood vessel to go into spasms, which decrease blood loss until clotting can occur.

3. A blood clot is formed by a series of chemical reactions that result in the formation of a netlike structure. The net is composed of protein fibers called *fibrin*, which seals off the opening in the injured blood vessel and stops the bleeding.

4. Most of the circulating clotting proteins are synthesized by the liver.

5. Clotting factors are plasma proteins involved in hemostasis.

6. There are 11 different clotting factors involved in hemostasis. They include the clotting factor prothrombin, which is converted to an enzyme called thrombin.

Apply Your Knowledge 23.2

CRITICAL THINKING

1. Three primary anticoagulants are standard (unfractionated) heparin, low-molecular-weight heparin (LMWH), and warfarin.

2. The major adverse effect resulting from heparin therapy is hemorrhage.

3. Protamine sulfate is the treatment for an overdosage of heparin.

4. Anticoagulants increase the length of clotting time and prevent thrombi from forming or growing larger. This action depends on the inhibition of thrombi and clot formation by blocking the conversion of prothrombin to thrombin and fibrinogen to fibrin.

5. Generic name: Trade name:
   dalteparin   Fragmin
   Generic name: Trade name:
   enoxaparin   Lovenox
   Generic name: Trade name:
   ardeparin   Normiflo
   Generic name: Trade name:
   danaparoid   Orgaran

6. Standard heparin is an animal extract (from pork). LMWH is derived from standard heparin. They are similar but not identical in their actions and pharmacokinetic characteristics. Standard heparin is produced by and can be released from mast cells throughout the body, especially in the liver, lung, and intestines. LMWHs offer greater bioavailability, longer-lasting effects, and dose-dependent clearance pharmacokinetics.

7. Warfarin is used when long-term anticoagulant therapy is indicated. Doses are adjusted to provide the desired outcomes.

8. Vitamin K is an antagonist of warfarin.

Apply Your Knowledge 23.3

CRITICAL THINKING

1. Platelet aggregation is the formation of blood clots caused by the binding together of platelets.

2. Aspirin in low doses inhibits platelet aggregation and prolongs bleeding time. It remains the first choice in antiplatelet therapy.

3. Ticlopidine and clopidogrel are structurally related drugs that irreversibly inhibit platelet activation, leading to the inhibition of platelet aggregation. Clopidogrel is preferred because of its better safety profile and lack of serious life-threatening side effects (leukopenia and thrombocytopenia) that can occur with ticlopidine. Clopidogrel is also more potent, better tolerated, and can be administered as a loading dose.

4. Percutaneous transluminal coronary angioplasty (PTCA) is commonly known as *stenting*.

5. Generic name: Trade name:
   abciximab   ReoPro
   Generic name: Trade name:
   dipyridamole   Persantine
   Generic name: Trade name:
   eptifibatide   Integrilin
   Generic name: Trade name:
   tirofiban   Aggrastat

Apply Your Knowledge 23.4

CRITICAL THINKING

1. *Idiopathic thrombocytopenic purpura* is another term for *platelet deficiency*.

2. Thrombolytics facilitate the conversion of plasminogen to plasmin, which subsequently hydrolyzes fibrin to dissolve blood clots (thrombi) that have already formed.

3. Thrombolytic drugs are indicated for the management of severe pulmonary embolism, deep vein thrombosis, and arterial thromboembolism. They are especially important for therapy after myocardial infarction and acute ischemic stroke.

4. The top five prescribed anticoagulants are heparin, warfarin, clopidogrel, enoxaparin, and fondaparinux.

5. Generic name: Trade name:
   anistreplase   Eminase
   Generic name: Trade name:
   urokinase   Abbokinase
   Generic name: Trade names:
   streptokinase   Streptase, Kabikinase
   Generic name: Trade name:
   tenecteplase recombinant   TNKase

Apply Your Knowledge 24.1

CRITICAL THINKING

1. Renin is a hormone that converts angiotensinogen to angiotensin I. Erythropoietin controls red blood cell production.

2. The formation of urine is achieved through the process of filtration, reabsorption, and secretion by the glomeruli and tubules within the kidneys.

3. Urea is the most abundant organic waste. Creatinine is a chemical waste molecule produced in skeletal muscle tissue by the breakdown of creatine phosphate, a high-energy compound that plays an important role in muscle contraction.

4. The nephrons reduce in number because of the aging process, different diseases, the use of various medications, and toxins.

5. The kidneys return filtered fluid to the internal environment through tubular reabsorption, selectively reclaiming just the right amounts of substances that the body requires, such as water, electrolytes, and glucose. Waste products and excess substances are processed out of the body.

6. The urine of infants and children is more dilute than that of adults because of pediatric higher blood flow and shorter loops of Henle.

7. Antidiuretic hormone (ADH) is also known as vasopressin.

8. The absence of ADH may cause diabetes insipidus.

Apply Your Knowledge 24.2

CRITICAL THINKING

1. Osmolality is the concentration of particles in plasma.

2. Water of metabolism makes up 10% of water intake and is a by-product of the oxidative metabolism of nutrients.

3. The electrolytes of greatest important to cellular function release sodium, potassium, calcium, magnesium, chloride, sulfate, phosphate, bicarbonate, and hydrogen ions.

4. Cations are positively charged ions. Sodium ions account for nearly 90% of all the cations in extracellular fluids. Anions are negatively charged ions. Chlorideions are the most abundant negatively charged ions in the extracellular fluids.

5. At birth, total body water represents about 75% to 80% of body weight.

Apply Your Knowledge 24.3

CRITICAL THINKING

1. The major classes of diuretics are osmotic diuretics, carbonic anhydrase inhibitors, thiazide diuretics, loop diuretics, and potassium-sparing diuretics.

2. Diuretics during pregnancy are not recommended because they may interfere with the normal expansion of fluid that occurs during pregnancy and disrupt the neurodevelopment of the fetus. Diuretic use increases the fetal risk of such conditions as schizophrenia, jaundice, blood problems, and potassium depletion.

3. Osmotic diuretics are highly effective treatments for cerebral edema and are used primarily for this purpose.

4. Examples of carbonic anhydrase inhibitors are acetazolamide, dichlorphenamide, and methazolamide.

5. The thiazide diuretics increase the urinary excretion of sodium and water by inhibiting sodium reabsorption on the distal convoluted tubules and collecting ducts. They also increase the excretion of chloride, potassium, and bicarbonate ions.

6. Examples of thiazide-like diuretics include chlorthalidone and indapamide.

7. Generic name: furosemide   Trade name: Lasix

   Generic name: acetazolamide   Trade name: Diamox (various)

   Generic name: mannitol   Trade name: Osmitro

   Generic name: chlorothiazide   Trade names: Diuril, Duragen

   Generic name: bumetanide   Trade name: Bumex

8. The potassium-sparing agents (diuretics) are used in the treatment of edema associated with congestive heart failure, hepatic cirrhosis with ascites, and the nephrotic syndrome.

9. The main adverse effects of potassium-sparing diuretics include hyperkalemia, acute renal failure, and kidney stones.

10. Loop diuretics are the drugs of choice in acute pulmonary edema, resulting in chronic heart failure.

Apply Your Knowledge 25.1

CRITICAL THINKING

1. The islets of Langerhans are small clusters of cells within the pancreas that have endocrine functions.

2. The anterior lobe of the pituitary secretes at least six separate hormones: growth hormone (GH, or somatotropin), adrenocorticotropic hormone (ACTH), thyroid-stimulating hormone (TSH), follicle-stimulating hormone (FSH), luteinizing hormone (LH), and prolactin (PRL).

3. GH insufficiency during childhood causes dwarfism (a condition in which the body is abnormally undersized).

4. Cushing's syndrome is caused by the hypersecretion of ACTH. It is a condition that affects the trunk of the body, in which a pad of fat develops between the shoulders, producing a "buffalo hump," and the face becomes round and moon shaped. Cushing's syndrome is called Cushing's disease when it is caused by a tumor in the pituitary gland.

5. The hypothalamic hormones control the secretion of specific trophic hormones; they in turn regulate other endocrine gland secretions and target tissues.

6. Excessive secretion of growth hormone before puberty—usually the result of a tumor of the anterior pituitary—causes gigantism. If excessive production of growth hormone occurs after puberty, it can result in acromegaly.

Apply Your Knowledge 25.2

CRITICAL THINKING

1. The two most common thyroid disorders are Graves's disease and Hashimoto's thyroiditis of the immune system, an autoimmune disease that attacks the thyroid gland, causing hypothyroidism. Graves's disease, an autoimmune disease in which antibodies overstimulate the thyroid gland, is characterized by hyperthyroidism—usually associated with an enlarged thyroid gland and exophthalmos. Graves's disease is also known as *thyrotoxicosis*.

2. Hypothyroidism during infancy causes congenital hypothyroidism, resulting in dwarfism and severe mental retardation. Myxedema is the most severe hypothyroidism developing in an older child or adult. It is characterized by swelling of the hands, feet, and face and can lead to coma and death.

3. Iodide is used alone for hyperthyroidism or in conjunction with antithyroid drugs and propranolol in treatment of thyrotoxic crisis. It is also prescribed for the treatment of persistent or recurring hyperthyroidism that occurs in patients with Graves's disease. It can be administered as a radiation protectant.

4. Parathyroid hormone (PTH) increases the reabsorption of calcium and the excretion of phosphate. It also increases the reabsorption of bone, with the release of calcium ions.

Another effect is the increased absorption of calcium and phosphate from the gastrointestinal tract. The gastrointestinal tract mediates calcitriol, a metabolite of vitamin D_3, which may be considered a hormone. PTH is a tropin for the renal synthesis of calcitriol.

5. Generic name: methimazole — Trade name: Tapazole

   Generic name: propylthiouracil — Trade name: PTU

   Generic name: levothyroxine — Trade name: Synthroid

   Generic name: potassium iodide — Trade names: Pima, SSKI

Apply Your Knowledge 25.3

CRITICAL THINKING

1. Diabetes mellitus exists in three forms: type 1, type 2, and gestational diabetes mellitus.

2. Some of the islets of Langerhans cells consist of alpha cells that secrete the hormone glucagon, which is secreted when blood glucose levels are low. Other clusters consist of beta cells that secrete the hormone insulin, which is essential for the maintenance of normal blood sugar.

3. Insulin is contraindicated during episodes of hypoglycemia or in patients sensitive to any ingredient in the formulation.

4. Examples of combination insulin products include insulin 70/30 (70% neutral protamine Hagedorn [NPH] and 30% regular), insulin 50/50 (50% NPH and 50% regular), and insulin 75/25 (75% Insulin Lispro Protamine [intermediate acting] and 25% Lispro).

5. Generic name: glipizide — Trade name: Glucotrol

   Generic name: rosiglitazone — Trade name: Avandia

   Generic name: tolbutamide — Trade names: Orinase

   Generic name: metformin — Trade names: Glucophage, Fortamet

Apply Your Knowledge 25.4

CRITICAL THINKING

1. The adrenal cortex secretes three types of steroid hormones: glucocorticoids (adrenocortical hormones), mineralocorticoids, and gonadal corticoids. As a group, these hormones are called *corticosteroids*. The glucocorticoids increase blood sugar levels, stimulate protein catabolism, mobilize fats, and decrease immunity and inflammatory responses.

2. Such glucocorticoids as cortisone and prednisone have diverse effects, including alterations in carbohydrate, protein, and lipid metabolism; the maintenance of fluid and electrolyte balance; and the preservation of normal function of the cardiovascular system, immune system, kidneys, skeletal muscle, endocrine system, and nervous system.

3. Mineralocorticoids are a group of hormones secreted from the adrenal cortex. The most important mineralocorticoid in humans is aldosterone.

4. Generic name: prednisolone — Trade names: Delta-Cortef, Key-Pred, Prelone

   Generic name: prednisone — Trade name: Deltasone

   Generic name: dexamethasone — Trade name: Decadron

5. Adrenocortical insufficiency is known as *Addison's disease*. It is accompanied by loss of sodium chloride and water, retention of potassium, lowering of blood glucose and liver glycogen levels, increased sensitivity to insulin, nitrogen retention, and lymphocytosis. The disturbances in electrolyte metabolism are the causes of morbidity and mortality in most cases of severe adrenal insufficiency.

Apply Your Knowledge 26.1

CRITICAL THINKING

1. The hormones that are essential for the development of secondary sex characteristics are testosterone (in males) and estrogen (in females).

2. The function of the prostate is to store and secrete a slightly alkaline fluid that is milky or white in appearance, which normally constitutes 25% to 30% of the volume of the semen. The seminal vesicles secrete a fluid that comprises about 60% of the volume of the semen. This fluid is slightly yellowish in color.

3. Testosterones are given to men and women for therapeutic purposes in various conditions. In men, they supplement low levels of testosterone to correct hypogonadism or cryptorchidism and to increase sperm production in cases of infertility. In women, they can be used in the palliative treatment of metastatic breast cancer or for the treatment of postpartum breast engorgement, endometriosis, and fibrocystic breast disorder.

4. Anabolic steroids include nandrolone, oxandrolone, oxymetholone, and stanozol.

5. Generic name: Trade name:
   oxandrolone   Oxandrin

   Generic name: Trade name:
   fluoxymesterone   Halotestin

   Generic name: Trade name:
   nandrolone   Durabolin

   Generic name: Trade name:
   stanozolol   Winstrol

6. Priapism is defined as a painful and prolonged erection.

Apply Your Knowledge 26.2

CRITICAL THINKING

1. A female's primary sex organs are the two ovaries, which produce the female sex cells and sex hormones.

2. Gonadotropin-releasing hormone (GnRH) is responsible for the release of follicle-stimulating hormone (FSH) and luteinizing hormone (LH) from the anterior pituitary.

3. FSH and LH play primary roles in controlling female sex cell maturation and in producing female sex hormones.

4. Estrogens stimulate the enlargement of accessory organs, including the vagina, uterus, uterine tubes, ovaries, and external reproductive structures. They also develop and maintain the female secondary sex characteristics. Estrogens bind to intracellular receptors that stimulate DNA and RNA to synthesize proteins responsible for the effects of these hormones.

5. The progestins are prescribed for secondary amenorrhea, functional uterine bleeding, endometriosis, and premenstrual syndrome. In combination with estrogens, they provide fertility control.

6. Salpingitis is the infection and inflammation of the fallopian tubes.

7. The contraceptive methods most commonly used in the United States include oral contraceptives, condoms, withdrawal, progestin injections, spermicides, diaphragms, progestin subdermal implants, and intrauterine devices.

8. Menorrhagia is defined as an abnormally heavy or prolonged menstruation. It is uterine bleeding that occurs independent of the normal menstrual period.

Apply Your Knowledge 26.3

CRITICAL THINKING

1. Examples of oxytocic drugs include ergonovine, methylergonovine, and oxytocin.

2. Oxytocic agents are used to initiate or improve uterine contraction at term only in carefully selected patients only after the cervix is dilated and after presentation of the fetus has occurred. They are also used to stimulate the letdown reflex in nursing mothers and to relieve pain from breast engorgement. They are prescribed for the management of an inevitable, incomplete, or missed abortion; the control of postpartum hemorrhage; and the promotion of postpartum uterine involution. They are also used to induce labor in cases of maternal diabetes and preeclampsia or eclampsia.

3. Two uterine relaxants are ritodrine and terbutaline.

4. Beta$_2$-adrenergic agonists are used to manage premature labor in selected patients.

5. Generic name: ritodrine — Trade name: Yutopar

Generic name: ergonovine — Trade name: Ergotrate

Generic name: terbutaline — Trade name: Brethaire

Apply Your Knowledge 27.1

CRITICAL THINKING

1. The three processes—digestion, absorption, and metabolism—begin in the mouth.

2. The small intestine receives secretions from the pancreas and liver.

3. Generic names of proton pump inhibitors include esomeprazole, lansoprazole, omeprazole, pantoprazole, and rabeprazole.

4. Trade names of H$_2$-receptor antagonists include Tagamet, Pepcid, Axid, and Zantac.

5. Prostaglandins produce a variety of actions on the body. The effects of these substances include inhibition of gastric acid and gastrin production, stimulation of mucus, and secretion of bicarbonate.

6. Generic name: ranitidine — Trade name: Zantac

Generic name: famotidine — Trade name: Pepcid

Generic name: pantoprazole — Trade name: Protonix

Generic name: omeprazole — Trade name: Prilosec

Generic name: esomeprazole — Trade name: Nexium

7. When gastric ulcers are caused by *Helicobacter pylori*, successful treatment usually includes a combination of such antibacterial agents as metronidazole, amoxicillin, or tetracyclines, along with such agents as colloidal bismuth or omeprazole.

8. The formation of hydrochloric acid depends on the production of hydrogen ions (protons) in the parietal cells, and proton pump inhibitors block this production.

Apply Your Knowledge 27.2

CRITICAL THINKING

1. Opioid antidiarrheals are the most effective drugs for controlling diarrhea.

2. The trade name of difenoxin hydrochloride with atropine sulfate is Motofen.

3. The generic name for Imodium is loperamide.

4. Opioid preparations are contraindicated in intestinal obstruction and should be avoided in children younger than 6 years old. In patients who have chronic diarrhea, treatment with opioids is not recommended.

5. The significant adverse effect of adsorbents is constipation, but it is usually mild and transient.

Apply Your Knowledge 27.3

CRITICAL THINKING

1. Laxatives are classified into several different categories depending on their mechanism of action: osmotic (saline) laxatives, stool softeners, stimulants, and bulk-forming laxatives.

2. Stool softeners may cause mild abdominal cramps, diarrhea, nausea, and a bitter taste.

3. Laxative stimulants include cascara sagrada and senna.

4. Bulk-forming laxatives absorb free water in the intestinal tract and oppose the dehydrating forces of the bowel by forming a gelatinous mass.

5. Osmotic laxatives work via osmosis, in which sodium and magnesium ions attract water into the bowel, causing a more liquid stool to be formed. The contents are

hypertonic, causing water to be retained, and if the osmotic pressure is great enough, it can pull water from the bowel's capillaries back into the bowel lumen. This results in a rise in pressure and volume in the colon and rectum, leading to the stimulation of the defecation reflex.

Apply Your Knowledge 27.4

CRITICAL THINKING

1. The vomiting center is in the medulla section of the brain.

2. Infectious diseases can directly irritate vomiting centers to inhibit impulses going to the stomach. Certain drugs, radiation, and chemotherapy may irritate the gastrointestinal tract or stimulate the chemoreceptor trigger zone and vomiting center. After surgery, particularly abdominal surgery, nausea and vomiting are common.

3. Ipecac syrup has central and peripheral emetic actions, but after oral administration, the peripheral action is predominant. Vomiting is triggered by intense irritation of the mucosal layer of the intestinal wall. The central action comprises stimulation of the vomiting center via the chemoreceptor trigger zone in the medulla.

4. Antiemetics are used for the prevention or treatment of nausea and vomiting, especially to treat motion sickness and radiation or postchemotherapy vomiting.

5. Ipecac syrup is contraindicated in comatose, semicomatose, and deeply sedated patients. It should not be used in patients who are in shock or having seizures or in patients with impaired cardiac function.

6. Generic name: chlorpromazine — Trade name: Thorazine
   Generic name: promethazine — Trade name: Phenergan
   Generic name: dimenhydrinate — Trade name: Dramamine

Apply Your Knowledge 28.1

CRITICAL THINKING

1. Obtaining oxygen and removing carbon dioxide are the primary functions of the respiratory system.

2. The lower respiratory tract consists of the larynx, trachea, bronchial tree, and lungs.

3. Asthma symptoms include breathlessness, cough, wheezing, and chest tightness. The airway becomes inflamed with edema (abnormal accumulation of fluid) and mucous plugs; hyperactivity of the bronchial tree adds to these symptoms.

4. Antiasthma drugs are classified as bronchodilators (beta$_2$-adrenergic agonists, xanthine derivatives, corticosteroids, leukotriene inhibitors, mast cell stabilizers, and combination drugs).

5. Generic name: cromolyn — Trade names: Intal, NasalCrom
   Generic name: montelukast — Trade name: Singulair
   Generic name: aminophylline — Trade names: Phyllocontin, Truphylline
   Generic name: terbutaline — Trade name: Brethine

Apply Your Knowledge 28.2

CRITICAL THINKING

1. Xanthine derivatives include aminophylline, dyphilline, oxtriphylline, and theophylline.

2. Leukotriene inhibitors include montelukast, zafirlukast, and zileuton

3. Bronchodilators include beta$_2$-adrenergic agonists, such as salmeterol, and xanthines, such as theophylline and aminophylline.

4. For asthma patients, the beta$_2$-adrenergic agonists produce bronchodilation by relaxing smooth muscles of the bronchial tree. This effect decreases airway resistance, facilitates mucus drainage, and increases vital capacity.

5. Xanthine derivatives are used for prophylaxis and the symptomatic relief of bronchial asthma as well as bronchospasm associated with chronic bronchitis and emphysema.

6. Mast cells are large cells found in connective tissue that contain a wide variety of biochemicals, including histamine. They are involved in inflammation secondary to injuries and infections, and they are sometimes implicated in allergic reactions. Their effects on the bronchial tree play a major part in asthma attacks.

7. Cromolyn (a mast cell stabilizer) is contraindicated in patients with coronary artery disease or a history of arrhythmias, dyspnea, acute asthma, or status asthmaticus. It should not be used during pregnancy or in children younger than 6 years old. It should be given cautiously to patients with renal or hepatic dysfunction.

8. Leukotriene inhibitors are used in the prophylaxis and treatment of chronic asthma or allergic rhinitis.

9. Xanthine derivatives must be used cautiously in older adults because their adverse effects include severe hypotension and cardiac arrest, which have higher fatality rates in this group of patients.

Apply Your Knowledge 28.3

CRITICAL THINKING

1. Antitussives are also called *cough suppressants.*

2. Antitussives are classified into two major groups: opioid and nonopioid.

3. Codeine and hydrocodone are generally not effective on the central cough center but are used because they elevate the cough threshold.

4. Generic name: Trade name:
   dornase alfa   Pulmozyme

   Generic name: Trade name:
   acetylcysteine   Mucomyst

5. Cystic fibrosis is a disorder marked by abnormal secretions of the exocrine glands, causing obstruction of bronchial pathways. Atelectasis is absence of gas from the lungs.

6. Decongestants may cause nervousness, insomnia, restlessness, dizziness, headaches, and irritability. They may also cause tachycardia, blurred vision, nausea, and vomiting.

7. Generic name: Trade name:
   pseudoephedrine   Sudafed

   Generic name: Trade name:
   fexofenadine-   Allegra D
   pseudoephedrine

   Generic name: Trade names:
   phenylephrine   Sinex,
                    Neo-Synephrine

8. Decongestants are vasoconstricting agents that shrink the swollen mucous membranes of the nasal airway passage of the upper respiratory tract.

Apply Your Knowledge 29.1

CRITICAL THINKING

1. Osteoporosis is a condition in which a reduction in bone mass is sufficient to compromise normal function. Reduction in bone mass begins between ages 30 and 40.

2. The five primary functions of the skeletal system are support, storage of minerals and lipids, blood cell production, protection, and leverage.

3. Parathyroid hormone and calcitonin coordinate the storage, absorption, and excretion of calcium ions.

4. Drugs used to treat or prevent osteoporosis include bisphosphonates, hormonal agents, calcitonin, and raloxifene hydrochloride.

5. The principal effects of calcitonin are to lower serum calcium and phosphate by action on the bones and kidneys. Calcitonin inhibits bone resorption and lowers serum calcium, increasing bone density and reducing the risk of vertebral fractures.

6. Raloxifene is used primarily to prevent and treat osteoporosis in postmenopausal women. It is also used to reduce the risk of breast cancer in postmenopausal women.

Apply Your Knowledge 29.2

CRITICAL THINKING

1. Rheumatoid arthritis (RA) is a systemic autoimmune disease that involves the inflammation of the membranes lining the joints and often affects internal organs. It can result in progressive joint destruction, deformity, and disability.

2. Antireumatic drugs include gold compounds, hydroxychloroquine, methotrexate, sulfasalazine, and, rarely, penicillamine.

3. Generic names of gold compounds include auranofin, aurothioglucose, and gold sodium thiomalate.

4. The adverse effects of gold compounds include hypersensitivity, syncope, bradycardia, thickening of the tongue, and a metallic taste in the mouth. Hematologic abnormalities are thrombocytopenia, leukopenia, and aplastic anemia.

5. Disease-modifying antirheumatic drugs (DMARDs) reduce or prevent joint damage and preserve joint function.

6. Methotrexate is a folic acid blocker and immunosuppressant that affects lymphocyte and macrophage function.

7. Sulfasalazine is effective in fighting RA and reduces the rate of appearance of new joint damage. It has been used in juvenile chronic arthritis and ankylosing spondylitis.

8. Gold compounds are contraindicated in patients with a gold allergy or a history of severe toxicity from previous therapy with gold or other heavy metals. Gold compounds should not be used in patients with uncontrolled diabetes mellitus, renal or hepatic insufficiency, or a history of hepatitis.

Apply Your Knowledge 29.3

CRITICAL THINKING

1. Gout is a metabolic disorder of sodium urate deposition, in which uric acid accumulates in the bloodstream or joint cavities, causing inflammation and pain. Gouty arthritis is caused by deposits of needle-like crystals of uric acid. It is one of the most painful rheumatic diseases.

2. Gout is classified as primary, secondary, or gouty arthritis. Primary gout has three manifestations: asymptomatic hyperuricemia, acute gouty arthritis, and chronic gouty arthritis.

3.

Generic name:	Trade name:
probenecid	Benemid
Generic name:	Trade names:
allopurinol	Aloprim, Zyloprim
Generic name:	Trade name:
sulfinpyrazone	Anturane

4. Colchicine is an anti-inflammatory agent specifically used for gout and is ineffective for any other disease. Its most common adverse effects are gastrointestinal disturbances, such as nausea, vomiting, diarrhea, and abdominal pain. It also may decrease the intestinal absorption of vitamin B_{12}.

5. Allopurinol reduces endogenous uric acid by selectively inhibiting the action for xanthine oxidase, the enzyme responsible for converting xanthine derivatives to uric acid.

6. Uricosuric agents include probenecid and sulfinpyrazone.

Apply Your Knowledge 29.4

CRITICAL THINKING

1. Neuromuscular junctions are spaces across which transmission of impulses from motor nerves to muscle cells occurs. They are sensitive to chemical changes in their immediate environment.

2. There are two types of muscle spasms: tonic and clonic spasms.

3. Nonpharmacologic treatments for muscle spasms include immobilization of the affected muscle, application of heat or cold, ultrasonography, hydrotherapy, and massage.

4. Baclofen is often a drug of first choice (of the centrally acting muscle relaxants) because of its wide safety margin.

5. Generic name: Trade name:
   lorazepam   Ativan

   Generic name: Trade name:
   baclofen   Lioresal

   Generic name: Trade name:
   methocarbamol   Robaxin

   Generic name: Trade name:
   dantrolene   Dantrium

Apply Your Knowledge 30.1

CRITICAL THINKING

1. The three layers of the eye are the outer layer (sclera), middle layer (choroid layer or "coat"), and inner layer (retina).

2. The ciliary body, which is the thickest part of the middle layer, extends forward from the choroid layer and forms an internal ring around the front of the eye, which constitutes the ciliary muscle.

3. The ability of the lens to adjust shape to facilitate focusing is called *accommodation*.

4. The iris is a thin diaphragm composed mostly of connective tissue and smooth muscle fibers. The pupil is a circular opening in the center of the iris.

5. The retina contains the visual receptor cells (photoreceptors).

6. Diabetic retinopathy is the degeneration of the blood vessels of the retina.

7. There are two types of glaucoma: acute angle-closure and chronic open-angle.

8. Risk factors for primary open-angle glaucoma include elevated intraocular pressure, older age, family history, black race, diabetes, hypertension, myopia, and the use of corticosteroids.

Apply Your Knowledge 30.2

CRITICAL THINKING

1. Generic name: Trade name:
   acetazolamide   Diamox

   Generic name: Trade name:
   methazolamide   Neptazane

   Generic name: Trade name:
   mannitol   Osmitrol

   Generic name: Trade name:
   cartelol   Ocupress

   Generic name: Trade name:
   apraclonidine   Lopidine

2. Beta-blocker agents are relatively safe, highly efficacious, act longer than the cholinergic agonists, and have no effects on pupil size or accommodation.

3. Osmotic diuretics are commonly used in patients needing eye surgery or for acute closed-angle glaucoma.

4. Examples of muscarinic agonists include carbachol, pilocarpine hydrochloride, and acetylcholine chloride.

5. Cholinesterase inhibitors produce severe miosis and muscle contractions. This causes a decreased resistance to aqueous outflow.

6. Sympathomimetics used in glaucoma include apraclonidine, brimonidine, dipivefrin, and phenylephrine.

7. Prostaglandin agonists are used in the treatment of open-angle glaucoma and intraocular hypertension to lower intraocular pressure. Travoprost can be used as first-line monotherapy or in combination with timolol.

8. Generic name: Trade name:
   bimatoprost   Lumigan

   Generic name: Trade names:
   pilocarpine   Isopto Carpine,
       Miocarpine

   Generic name: Trade name:
   phenylephrine   Neo-Synephrine

Apply Your Knowledge 31.1

CRITICAL THINKING

1. Major changes that occur during the impact process and impact health include gradual loss of the ability of the body to renew itself; slowing down of body functions; vital senses becoming less acute; changes in sensory processes; alteration of perception, motor skills, problem-solving ability, and emotions; changing roles and definitions of self; slower movements and less dexterity; cognitive changes; decreased income; increased health expenses; and unforeseen changes, such as death of a spouse.

2. Heart disease and cancer have been the two leading causes of death among people 65 and older for the past two decades.

3. The most important physiologic decline in elderly individuals appears to be in renal function.

4. Conditions that influence drug absorption in older adults include slower gastric emptying, altered nutritional habits, and greater use of over-the-counter medications.

5. Creatinine clearance is an indicator of the glomerular filtration rate.

6. Adverse effects of the following drugs are listed here:

   Morphine—shallow breathing, slow heartbeat, seizure (convulsions), cold and clammy skin, confusion, severe weakness or dizziness, lightheadedness, and fainting

   Thyroxine (which is known as levothyroxine in the United States)—headache, insomnia, nervousness or irritability, fever, hot flashes, sweating, changes in menstrual periods, appetite changes, and weight changes

   Warfarin—pain, swelling, hot or cold feelings, skin changes or discoloration; sudden and severe leg or foot pain, foot ulcers, purple toes or fingers; sudden headache, dizziness, or weakness; unusual bleeding; easy bruising; blood in the urine, stool, or vomitus; lightheadedness; tachycardia; dark urine; jaundice; abdominal or back pain; reduced urination; numbness or muscle weakness; illness with flu-like symptoms

   Aminoglycosides—allergic reaction; decreased hearing or ringing in the ears; reduced urination; dizziness.

7. Yohimbe is a natural supplement that is contraindicated in patients with hypertension, hepatic disease, renal disease, or peptic ulcer.

8. Polypharmacy is defined as the practice of prescribing multiple medicines to a single patient simultaneously. It increases the patient's costs for treatment as well as the changes for multiple adverse effects and drug interactions.

Apply Your Knowledge 31.2

CRITICAL THINKING

1. All elderly patients who receive antihypertensive drugs should be regularly monitored for orthostatic hypotension to avoid cerebral ischemia and falling.

2. Psychiatric depression is a leading cause of suicide in elderly adults and is often undertreated.

3. Cimetidine is not suggested for older adults because of its side effects and multiple potential drug interactions.

4. Elderly patients may be more or less sensitive to drug action because of age-related changes in the central nervous system (CNS), changes in the number of drug receptors, and changes in the affinity of receptors to drugs. If the patient is more sensitive to the drug's action, the dose may need to be lowered and vice versa. Changes in organ functions are important to consider in drug dosing.

5. People with Alzheimer's disease are often very sensitive to CNS toxicities of drugs that have antimuscarinic effects.

Apply Your Knowledge 32.1

CRITICAL THINKING

1. During the first few months of life, physiologic processes and their resulting pharmacokinetic variables change significantly. Factors such as blood flow at the site of administration and gastrointestinal function influence drug absorption. Physiologic conditions that can reduce the rate of blood flow to the site of administration include heart failure, cardiovascular shock, and vasoconstriction. Other factors include the percentage of body water, the rate of gastric emptying, amount of body fat, and the glomerular filtration rate (GFR).

2. A neonate is a newborn from birth to 28 days old. An infant is from 29 days old to walking age (typically 1 year). A toddler is a child from 1 to 3 years old.

3. Drugs given to a neonate with jaundice can displace bilirubin from albumin, and because of the greater permeability of a neonate's blood–brain barrier, large amounts of bilirubin may enter the brain and cause kernicterus, which is a serious form of jaundice in newborns.

4. Because of the lower metabolic activities in neonates, many drugs have slow clearance rates and longer half-life elimination times. Drug doses and dosing schedules must be altered appropriately. If not, the neonate may experience adverse effects from drugs that are metabolized in the liver.

5. The GFR rate is much lower in newborns than in older children. Based on body surface area, a neonate's GFR is only 30% to 40% that of an adult. Premature babies show an even lower rate. However, the rate improves greatly during the first week after birth. By the end of the third week, it is 50% to 60% that of an adult's. Drugs that require renal function for elimination are removed from the body very slowly during the first weeks of life.

Apply Your Knowledge 32.2

CRITICAL THINKING

1. Elixirs and suspensions are popular forms for pediatric administration.

2. Suspensions are dosage forms that contain undissolved drug particles and must be shaken to evenly distribute them. This is essential because if a suspension drug form is not adequately shaken, it will cause dangerous variations in dosages.

3. Major dosing errors may result from incorrect calculations because many pediatric doses are calculated by using body weight. A common but potentially fatal mistake is that 10 times the amount of medication is administered because a decimal point was placed incorrectly.

4. Heroin may be passed by a mother's breast milk, endangering the nursing infant. It can cause increased sleepiness and poor appetite in the infant, resulting in an undernourished baby. Other effects include an inadequate suckling reflex, tremors, restlessness, and vomiting.

5. It is not always safe to proportionally reduce adult doses to determine safe pediatric doses. The recommended pediatric dose—usually stated as milligrams per kilogram or milligrams per pound—should always be followed. The result of the difference in pharmacokinetics in children compared with those in adults may be greater drug effect or toxicity.

Apply Your Knowledge 33.1

CRITICAL THINKING

1. Drugs and other substances, including radiation, may be particularly harmful during the first trimester of pregnancy. Therefore, many medications are prohibited during this time.

2. During organogenesis, toxic agents may cause spontaneous abortion, birth defects, retarded development, functional disorders, such as autism, and transplacental carcinogenesis.

3. X-rays are a form of radiation, which can be particularly harmful during the first trimester of pregnancy. It may result in spontaneous abortion, low birth weight, stillbirth, birth defects, and chromosomal defects.

4. Fetal toxicity can be best prevented by avoiding use of all potentially harmful agents unless they are prescribed by a physician to ensure the health of the fetus.

5. When taken by pregnant women, the mild sedative thalidomide caused fetal limb deformities, many of which were extremely severe, in their children.

Apply Your Knowledge 33.2

CRITICAL THINKING

1. If hypertension exists before pregnancy, drug therapy should not be discontinued during pregnancy or lactation. It must be treated to maintain the health of the growing fetus.

2. Major physiological and anatomic changes occur in pregnant women. Some of these changes alter drug pharmacokinetics and pharmacodynamics. Changes in hormone levels as well as pressure exerted on the blood supply by the expanding uterus may affect the absorption of drugs.

3. Drug metabolism increases may cause higher doses of certain drugs to be used (primarily anticonvulsants). This is related to many other changes, including cardiac output, plasma volume, regional blood flow, lipid level alterations, and blood flow through the mother's kidneys.

4. The Food and Drug Administration (FDA) has created drug pregnancy categories because certain drugs may be teratogenic or have actions that are not yet understood. The

pregnancy categories are for the safety of the fetus and the mother.

5. Category X drugs are contraindicated in pregnant women. Examples include isotretinoin, misoprostol, and thalidomide.

Apply Your Knowledge 33.3

CRITICAL THINKING

1. During fetal development, common responses to toxic agents include restricted growth, structural malformations, functional impairment, fetal death, and transplacental carcinogenesis.

2. In general, drugs with shorter half-lives are preferable because those with longer half-lives (or active metabolites) can accumulate in the plasma of the infant. If possible, drugs with high-protein-binding abilities should be selected because they are not secreted into the milk as readily.

3. Drug toxicity may cause many structural malformations to occur during the period of organogenesis (between 20 and 70 days after the first day of last menstruation). They can also occur from 1 week before the missed menstruation until the woman is 44 days past due. Because organ and system maturation occurs beyond organogenesis and the prenatal period, responses may occur over a much longer period of time.

4. During pregnancy, gastrointestinal motility and the distribution to plasma proteins is decreased compared to other times during life. However, nearly all other resorptive, distributive, metabolic, and excretive processes are increased. Because total body water may be increased up to 81% during pregnancy, drugs can be distributed in a greatly increased volume.

5. During the last trimester, greatly increased renal plasma flow causes a more rapid elimination of drugs without being changed by the kidneys.

Apply Your Knowledge 33.4

CRITICAL THINKING

1. The placenta allows oral medications to pass between the maternal and fetal circulation. Drugs cross the placenta by passive diffusion.

2. By the third month of pregnancy, the liver of the fetus can activate or inactivate chemical substances by the process of oxidation.

3. Risks of toxicity concerning the embryo or fetus may be assessed via animal experimentation, epidemiological studies, case studies, and other methods.

4. Many analytical studies use the cohort approach, in which a specific adverse outcome is studied in women who were exposed to the same toxic agent.

5. Psychiatric illnesses in the mother may require long-term use of medications that have fetotoxic properties. Perinatal and postnatal effects may include premature birth, birth defects, stillbirth, neonatal death, toxicity, withdrawal symptoms, mental retardation, retarded development, metabolic and functional disorders, and such developmental disabilities as epilepsy or cerebral palsy.

Apply Your Knowledge 33.5

CRITICAL THINKING

1. The risk of each medication should be discussed between the pregnant woman and her physician before beginning use or before the patient even becomes pregnant. If the patient has already taken any medication and is pregnant, the physician should continue to communicate with her about potential outcomes. This communication should include whether diagnostic procedures may be required to assess any fetal harm and the consideration of termination of pregnancy if the harm is severe. It is not enough to rely on safety warnings printed on package inserts, reference books, and other sources to inform patients about the potential toxicities of medications.

2. Reproductive toxicology is the study of the effects of toxic agents during the entire reproductive process.

3. Teratogenicity is defined as a manifestation of developmental toxicity by induction or an increase of the frequency of structural disorders in embryos or fetuses.

4. Phenylketonuria is a genetic disorder characterized by an inability of the body to use phenylalanine. Symptoms are usually not present initially but eventually include mental retardation, seizures, hyperactivity, stunted growth, eczema, and microcephaly.

5. Dysmorphology is the study of birth defects.

Apply Your Knowledge 33.6

CRITICAL THINKING

1. Drugs that are highly fat-soluble (lipid-soluble) are most likely to enter the breast milk. Therefore, they can be passed more quickly to nursing infants.

2. Effects of cocaine on infants include hypertonia, tachycardia, excitation, and trembling.

3. Higher than normal amounts of caffeine usually cause infants to become irritable, jittery, not satisfied by breastfeeding, and unable to sleep normally and to have lower than normal amounts of iron.

4. If a mother consumes one serving of alcohol, she should wait 2 hours before breastfeeding.

5. Smoking tobacco products has been linked to poor milk supply, poor nursing, restlessness, and vomiting by the infant. Secondhand smoke causes a higher rate of infant respiratory illnesses. Secondhand smoke is dangerous for infants regardless of the manner of their feeding.

Index